Pathophysiology, Physical Assessment, & Pharmacology

Advanced Integrative Clinical Concepts

Pathophysiology, Physical Assessment, & Pharmacology

Advanced Integrative Clinical Concepts

Janie T. Best, DNP, RN, CNL
Associate Professor
Queens University of Charlotte
Presbyterian School of Nursing
Blair College of Health
Charlotte, North Carolina

Grace Buttriss, DNP, RN, FNP-BC, CNL
Associate Professor
Queens University of Charlotte
Blair College of Health
Charlotte, North Carolina

Annette Hines, RN, PhD, CNE
Professor
Queens University of Charlotte
Director, Presbyterian School of Nursing
Blair College of Health
Charlotte, North Carolina

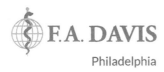
F.A. DAVIS

Philadelphia

F.A. Davis Company
1915 Arch Street
Philadelphia, PA 19103
www.fadavis.com

Printed in the United States of America

Last digit indicates print number: 10 9 8 7 6 5 4 3 2 1

Publisher, Nursing: Susan Rhyner
Manager, Content Development: William W. Welsh
Manager of Project and eProject Management: Catherine H. Carroll
Senior Content Project Manager: Julia L. Curcio
Digital Learning Project Manager: Sandra A. Glennie
Design and Illustration Manager: Carolyn O'Brien

As new scientific information becomes available through basic and clinical research, recommended treatments and drug therapies undergo changes. The author(s) and publisher have done everything possible to make this book accurate, up-to-date, and in accord with accepted standards at the time of publication. The author(s), editors, and publisher are not responsible for errors or omissions or for consequences from application of the book, and make no warranty, expressed or implied, in regard to the contents of the book. Any practice described in this book should be applied by the reader in accordance with professional standards of care used in regard to the unique circumstances that may apply in each situation. The reader is advised always to check product information (package inserts) for changes and new information regarding dose and contraindications before administering any drug. Caution is especially urged when using new or infrequently ordered drugs.

Library of Congress Cataloging-in-Publication Data

Names: Best, Janie T. author. | Buttriss, Grace, author. | Hines, Annette, author.
Title: Pathophysiology, physical assessment, and pharmacology : advanced
   integrative clinical concepts / Janie T. Best, Grace Buttriss, Annette Hines.
Description: Philadelphia : F.A. Davis Company, [2022] | Includes
   bibliographical references.
Identifiers: LCCN 2021023453 (print) | LCCN 2021023454 (ebook) |
   ISBN 9780803675674 (paperback) | ISBN 9780803675742 (ebook)
Subjects: MESH: Nursing Process | Nursing Care
Classification: LCC RT48 (print) | LCC RT48 (ebook) | NLM WY 100.1 |
   DDC 616.07/5—dc23
LC record available at https://lccn.loc.gov/2021023453
LC ebook record available at https://lccn.loc.gov/2021023454

This book is dedicated to:

My parents, Ray and Joyce Trogdon, for their encouragement as I pursued my childhood dream of becoming a nurse; my husband, Martin, my children, and their spouses (Steve & Brandy, Emily & Eric) for their unfailing love and support throughout my nursing career; and to my 5 grandchildren who are my source of joy and inspiration. To all the nurses, nursing students, doctors, and patients who have been an integral part of my nursing journey: Thank you!

Janie

My parents, Horace and Dorothy Baker, who met on a hospital ship caring for soldiers in WWII, and inspired me to become a nurse; my son, Joe, who has tolerated, advised, and unconditionally supported his working mom; and my husband, David, and many other family and friends (especially my Duke 'BSN 84 colleagues) who have cheered me on to write a textbook.

Annette

My parents, Ken and Eily O'Connor, who provided me with encouragement and hospital shadowing experiences to support my dream of becoming a Registered Nurse. Also, to my husband, Bert, and daughter, Darby, who just achieved her MSN, who believed in my abilities and have offered enduring love and support throughout this process and my lifelong learning journey. Thank you also to my colleagues, students, and patients who were the inspiration for this text.

Grace

Foreword

Nursing education is a curious field. We preach the need to deliver holistic patient care. However, we teach nursing care by dividing the elements of care categorically. We then expect the student, who is the least experienced member of the teaching/learning team, to integrate the information provided. We require students to intuitively identify the salient points and apply the knowledge they gain from the written word to a patient in the clinical setting.

This groundbreaking textbook, *Pathophysiology, Physical Assessment, and Pharmacology: Advanced Integrative Clinical Concepts,* facilitates knowledge in a way that enables student understanding for real world application. Integrating the concepts of physiology/pathophysiology, physical assessment, and pharmacology eliminates the silo approach to nursing education and guides the student to explore how each element impacts the other.

Drs. Best, Buttriss, and Hines collaborate to bring both clinical and academic experience to the forefront in *Pathophysiology, Physical Assessment, and Pharmacology.* Written with sound educational practices, this book will help students to reframe the way they provide patient care. Nursing faculty will appreciate the thoughtful integration of the "the 3Ps" in each chapter and exemplars that provide rich concepts for class design and implementation. *Pathophysiology, Physical Assessment, and Pharmacology* is the textbook that teaches like nursing students learn and practice.

TAMA L. MORRIS, RN, PhD, CNE
DEAN, BLAIR COLLEGE OF HEALTH & PRESBYTERIAN SCHOOL OF NURSING
QUEENS UNIVERSITY OF CHARLOTTE, CHARLOTTE, NORTH CAROLINA

Preface

As faculty at Queen's University of Charlotte, we decided to tackle a long-running curriculum issue: The "3 Ps" of Pathophysiology, Pharmacology, and Physical Assessment are the cornerstone of every nursing curriculum. Yet, students studying the "3 Ps" always struggle to relate and "connect" the content in one course to the content in the others. The traditional "separate course" approach was leaving both faculty and students frustrated; even our students requested a single 3 P course in order to keep up with the required content. We all know that studying each subject individually has its value, but the downside is that, in reality, nursing practice requires us to draw on our knowledge of Pathophysiology, Pharmacology, and Physical Assessment—simultaneously—every day with every patient encounter.

In nursing practice, nurses *have* to integrate them.

So, we asked ourselves: Why not try integrating them in a single nursing course?

And thus, the purpose and mission of a single "3 Ps course"—and this book—was born.

As instructors, we all know that students struggle to relate one course to the other, as they attempt to "pull" and apply information from the "3 Ps" simultaneously. In creating a single, integrated 3 Ps course and textbook, we saw that our students benefited from a different kind of pedagogical "scaffolding." It was easier to draw on their strengths in two "Ps" in order to advance their knowledge in the third "P" more smoothly. We were rewarded to see that students' mastery of the content deepened, and students demonstrated improved clinical thinking skills across the board.

After "road testing" our lectures, learning activities, and curricula with our students, we partnered with the publishing team at F.A. Davis to create this text, with the aim of providing a foundational, integrative course text to cover the 3 Ps of nursing. We believe this methodology promotes a deeper understanding of the concepts from these three essential—and challenging—content areas and guides students to recognize the importance of integration in the planning, delivery, and evaluation of nursing care. Equally important, we wanted to develop a text and graduate course based on the AACN guidelines and one that reflected our own commitment to application-based learning.

Table of Contents and Organization—Implementing a Life Span Approach

You'll notice that the table of contents for the text is organized in a life span approach. After an Introduction to the Foundations of Integrative Practice, the text is divided into six major sections, by population:

- Adult
- Maternity
- Newborn
- Pediatrics
- Geriatrics
- Mental Health Disorders Across the Life Span

Each population section covers key conditions and disorders that nurses—and especially advanced practice nurses—are likely to encounter within their scope of practice. We review the important pathophysiology, pharmacology, and physical examination and assessment information relative to each disorder. Finally, each section concludes with a case study that presents a new disorder relative to the population in that section, furthering our application-style approach.

Special Features

All chapters in the text follow a consistent organizational structure and feature set to facilitate the student's need to learn, apply, and retain this foundational knowledge. These features were designed to provide students with applicable clinical content across the life span for diverse care settings. Key features also highlight need-to-know information in a concise format to aid the pedagogical underpinnings of the text:

- Clinical and Assessment Pearls highlight information that is considered a priority when providing care across the life span in any clinical setting.
- Red Flag Alerts are featured within the pharmacology content to alert the student to potentially life-threatening situations.
- HIGH YIELD FACT FOR TESTING **High Yield Facts for Testing** highlight information commonly appearing on tests and examinations.
- **End-of-Chapter Review Questions** wrap up each chapter and help students review and test their knowledge of the essential content covered. These questions can also be assigned as a homework or course assignment.
- **Case studies** that focus on a supplementary disease process conclude each life span population and the mental health section. This book uses specific client scenarios to provide students with an interactive learning experience that is based on commonly encountered patient care diagnoses.

Who Is This Text Best Suited For?

Our partners at F.A. Davis collaborated with us to have the chapters for this text extensively reviewed by nursing faculty in high-level BSN and MSN programs, as well as DNP programs. We were grateful for all of the insightful and thoughtful reviews that we received every step of the way, which also helped us to understand how each segment of nursing found value in this text.

Faculty in MSN programs—especially APN areas such as clinical nurse leaders, clinical nurse educators, and clinical nurse managers—all appreciated the depth, breadth, and scope of the text, while noting the benefit of relying on a single text and course to bring "the 3Ps" together.

Faculty in DNP programs and NP tracks—all related that the text was a great "putting it all together" resource for their students, one that could be used across the curriculum to complement their major course texts as they continue to study each of the 3Ps in separate courses.

Faculty in BSN programs made similar observations about the "putting it all together" component of our text, plus noted that it served as great preparation for their students as they worked their way through clinicals, so especially challenging during the COVID-19 pandemic. Having access to case studies and a life span approach was reported as a great supplement to the guidance provided by clinical preceptors, to whom we all owe so much.

It is our sincere hope as fellow nursing educators that you and your students will find this textbook a valuable core resource as you partner together to maximize on all the touchpoints that connect pathophysiology, pharmacology, and physical examination and assessment. We hope your journey will be as enriching as ours has been.

Faculty Resources

In addition to the resources in this book, you will find a host of Instructor Resources available on FADavis.com.

The online Faculty Resources include:

- Instructor Test Bank: Hundreds of test questions that instructors can use to quickly create quizzes and exams.
- PowerPoint presentations: Provides a lecture overview for each chapter plus *case studies and follow-up questions* to use with students, in class or online.
- Active Classroom Instructor's Guide: Contains a multitude of ideas for student preparation; lecture points connected to the Power Point slides; pre-, post-, and in-class activities; and homework assignments.

Reviewers

Joseph Boney, MSN, RN, NEA-BC
Director of Adjunct Faculty Development
Nursing Lecturer
Second Degree BS in Nursing Program
Rutgers, The State University of New Jersey
Newark, New Jersey

Kathleen Bradbury-Golas, DNP, RN,
NP-C, ACNS-BC
Associate Clinical Professor
Drexel University
Philadelphia, Pennsylvania

Veronica J. Brady, PhD, FNP-BC,
BC-ADM, CDE
Assistant Professor
Cizik School of Nursing
University of Texas
Houston, Texas

Debra V. Craighead, PhD, RN, CNL
Associate Professor
CNL Track Leader
University of Louisiana Monroe
Monroe, Louisiana

Khoa (Joey) Dang, MSN, RN, FNP-C
Director of FNP Program
Assistant Professor
Western University of Health Sciences
Pomona, California

Janice Dunlap, DNP, APRN, AGPCNP-BC,
ACNS-BC
Contributing Faculty
University of St. Augustine Health Sciences
Hephzibah, Georgia

Mary P. Englert, DNP, NP-C, CNE
Associate Professor, MSN Program Chair
Rasmussen College
Bloomington, Minnesota

Ola Fox, DNS, CNL
Associate Professor Emerita
Spring Hill College
Mobile, Alabama

Catherine Frank, DNP, APRN, AGACNP-BC,
MSN, OHN
FNP Faculty
Xavier University
Cincinnati, Ohio

Masoud Ghaffari, PhD, RN, MT
Assistant Professor
Benedictine University
Lisle, Illinois

Cassandra Marie Godzik, MSN, PMHNP-BC
Adjunct Professor
Regis College
Weston, Massachusetts

Angie F. Hatley, DNP, MS, RN, NEA-BC, CNL
Chair, Graduate Studies in Nursing
Assistant Professor
Queens University of Charlotte
Charlotte, North Carolina

Nanette P. Leonardo, DNP, FNP-C
Assistant Professor
West Coast University
Los Angeles, California

Zhizhong Li, MSN, MA, RN, CNL
Assistant Professor
CNL Track Leader
Orvis School of Nursing
University of Nevada, Reno
Reno, Nevada

Paulette Melanson, DNP, RN, WHNP-BC
Assistant Professor
Framingham State University
Framingham, Massachusetts

Cyndi Moore, MSN, RN, CNL
Quality Improvement
UAB Hospital
Birmingham, Alabama

Richard Pembridge, ACNP, EDD
Lead Faculty at GCU for AGACNP program
Grand Canyon University
Phoenix, Arizona

Julie Poepoe, MSN, RN, FNP-BC
Associate Professor
Lead FNP Clinical Faculty
West Coast University
Los Angeles, California

Alicemarie Poyss, PhD, CNL, APRN-BC
CNL Track Director
College of Nursing and Health Professions
Philadelphia, Pennsylvania

Tina Ralyea, DNP, MS-NP, MBA, NE-BC, CNL, OCN, CCRN
Chief Nursing Officer
Prisma Health-Baptist and Baptist Parkridge
Adjunct Faculty
Queens University and Walden University
Columbia, South Carolina

Veronica Rankin, DNP, RN-BC, NP-C, CNL
Director of Professional Nursing Practice
Adjunct Graduate Nursing Faculty
Carolinas Medical Center-Central Division
Queens University of Charlotte
Charlotte, North Carolina

Kimberly P. Toole, DNP, APRN, CNP
Assistant Professor and Coordinator of
FNP Program
Xavier University
Cincinnati, Ohio

Missy Travelsted, DNP, APRN
Assistant Professor of Nursing
Western Kentucky University
Bowling Green, Kentucky

Eme Ukot, DNP, MBA, MS, MSN, FNP-BC, APRN
Professor
Rasmussen University
Houston, Texas

Rebecca Wilson, PhD, RN
Specialty Track Director
Nursing Education Master's and Certificate
Associate Professor
University of Utah College of Nursing
Salt Lake City, Utah

Contents

Foundations of Integrative Practice

LEARNING OBJECTIVES

LEARNING OBJECTIVES

Upon completion of this chapter the student will be able to:

- Describe integrative nursing practice using advanced knowledge of physiology, pathophysiology, assessment, and pharmacological management.
- Incorporate core competencies of graduate nursing education to achieve practice outcomes.
- Explain role of cultural competence across care settings.

Introduction

Masters-prepared nurses provide, supervise, coordinate, and evaluate care in increasingly complex care environments. In order to make decisions that promote quality outcomes, nurses must have advanced knowledge from many different areas, but particularly in the content domains of physiology/pathophysiology, physical assessment, and pharmacology. For advanced practice nurses in direct care roles (i.e., *certified registered nurse anesthetist* [CRNA], *certified nurse-midwife* [CNM], *clinical nurse specialist* [CNS], or *certified nurse practitioner* [CNP]), it is especially critical (and mandated by some accrediting bodies) that students are prepared by separate classes in each of these content areas (American Association of Colleges of Nursing [AACN], 2011). There are requirements for a clinical component for direct care roles, which can be met in traditional settings or through simulation (e.g., educators, *clinical nurse leader* [CNL]) (Halstead, 2007, 2018; National League for Nursing [NLN], 2012). In addition to the advanced knowledge, the nurse must integrate these concepts to function safely across inpatient and community-based health-care settings. For graduate students in tracks that lead to indirect care roles (e.g., administration, informatics), these concepts can be combined into one class (AACN, 2011; American Nurses Association [ANA], 2015).

Recommendations for graduate education are based in part on the Carnegie Foundation report (2009), *Educating Nurses: A Call for Radical Transformation*, which emphasizes the importance of advancing knowledge for masters-prepared nurses in clinical practice theory and experience for all direct care roles (Benner, Sutphen, Leonard, & Day, 2009). A scientific foundation for practice is formed from the three major areas (physiology/pathophysiology, physical assessment, and pharmacology) with opportunities to apply this knowledge in clinical settings, whether in traditional clinical or simulated settings. In this chapter, we provide an overview of how each of these subjects supports advanced practice in nursing and how their integration promotes patient and system outcomes.

Physiology/Pathophysiology

Nursing education includes physiology at the undergraduate level but often moves to a focus on pathophysiology for graduate students, with the expectation that students possess basic knowledge of physiology from nursing practice experience. It is also assumed that students and/or practicing nurses review physiology content as needed in order to better understand pathophysiology. Within a wide variety of health-care settings, nurses must be able to determine normal findings based on their understanding of physiology, and identify any deviations from normal findings, or pathophysiology. While nursing is based in science, there is also a human element that requires nurses to make judgments using both scientific knowledge of pathophysiology and understanding of best practices; therefore, as nurses progress in their educational preparation for advanced roles, an emphasis on scientific knowledge, along with clinical application of this information, is necessary (Rodgers, 2016).

Advanced Physical Assessment

While based on the sciences, nursing is described as both a science and an art; nowhere is this more evident than in the area of physical assessment. Learned as the first step in the nursing process, accurate assessment is crucial to all other components of care; students and practicing nurses cannot underestimate its importance. As the nurse develops knowledge in caring for patients, there are usually concomitant advances in clinical skills. Advanced assessment skills incorporate both physical assessment and clinical reasoning skills that support the nurse's ability to correlate assessment findings with possible diagnoses and treatment plans (Goolsby & Grubbs, 2019). The nurse's ability to assess a patient and their family is critical to making correct decisions regarding care. Expectations of masters-prepared nurses include expertise with advanced assessment skills; while there is a focus on the aspect of physical assessment, a holistic approach to assessment is the ultimate goal.

Pharmacology

Knowledge of medication and its safe use/administration is a priority in current health care. The landmark Institute of Medicine (IOM; now the National Academy of Medicine) report, *To Err Is Human* (1999), continues to guide clinical practice and motivate nurses to promote a safe clinical environment. Pharmacology has a vital role across the continuum of care; nurses must be able to manage its use in treating acute illness, managing chronic conditions, and preventing disease. It is the nurse's role to maximize the therapeutic effects of the pharmacological regimen, while minimizing the potential side effects and risk of complications. Nurses' advanced knowledge of pharmacology is key to their ability to practice in an advanced role and to be leaders in promoting quality care.

Integration of the Concepts

Students in graduate nursing programs have basic knowledge in each of these content areas and often have advanced understanding based on their clinical practice and continued education. The goal of this text is to present advanced information and highlight the relevant physiology/pathophysiology, advanced physical assessment, and pharmacology related to prevalent disease processes across the life span. This approach is designed to promote integration of these major concepts so they are understood at an advanced level and can be applied to current clinical practice.

Nurses are obligated to do much more than retrieve facts and apply knowledge; they must assimilate and then evaluate information from various sources (e.g., patient, family, health record) while planning and delivering care. While algorithms and standards of care are readily available electronically, the nurse must appraise the patient's situation and individual care through a process of problem-solving and decision making. Masters-prepared nurses are able to use integrated knowledge to promote outcomes at diverse levels (i.e., patient, unit, system) and through direct and indirect care roles with adequate preparation (Goolsby & Grubbs, 2019; Kenney, 2016).

Culturally Appropriate Care

Obtaining and maintaining cultural competence in nurses is an ongoing and intentional process (Jeffreys, 2016). For students in graduate nursing programs, there are many opportunities to engage in these valuable learning opportunities. First, the student assesses their own cultural knowledge and values in order to have realistic plans for cultural competency development, which is a necessary skill and growing challenge across health care. Cultural competence concepts must be addressed by students at an interpersonal level (i.e., with faculty and other students) in addition to being a comprehensive part of course work throughout the curriculum (Jeffreys, 2016).

While focusing on the traditional treatment, including pharmacological interventions, a masters-prepared nurse should be knowledgeable about nonpharmacological treatments and alternative strategies that may be used to promote health outcomes. Patients may adopt these practices as part of their cultural views of illness and health, or providers may offer information about them as an adjuvant or substitute for established regimens (Goolsby & Grubbs, 2019; Jeffreys, 2016). An integrated approach to holistic health considers the person's physical, mental, social, and spiritual circumstances as integral to planning preventive and medical care (Jeffrey, 2016; Shi & Singh, 2016). A review of current literature on the effect of providers' cultural competence concluded that patient satisfaction increases when providers are viewed as having this attribute (Govere & Govere, 2016). Further research is needed to examine the relationship between a provider's cultural competence and other outcomes, such as length of stay, infection rates, and readmission rates.

According to a recent study by Debiasi and Selleck (2017), nurses who have had education on cultural competence deliver improved care in this area. As a student, you may be asked to make a cultural self-assessment before engaging in educational modules and/or classes; research shows that students are more motivated to learn this content when they self-identify a lack of cultural competence. Even nurses who have practiced for years with a specific patient population may not be knowledgeable about how culture affects health for their patients. It is important for nurses to develop a practice that is culturally competent from the novice phase; graduate nursing education is an optimal time to reassess one's knowledge and improve proficiency in this area.

Any assessment should include what the patient believes about their individual health and what they do to promote health and/or prevent illness. There are benefits and drawbacks to performing a separate cultural assessment. First, this evaluation may be time consuming for the nurse who is already under a time constraint to gather and analyze data about the patient's current health condition. However, gathering this information may ultimately result in time saved, as the nurse is able to plan care that is more comprehensive and accurate. Also, the nurse may not feel comfortable asking questions about the person's culture for a number of reasons. The experienced nurse may think that they should have the knowledge related to the major cultures that they encounter and are therefore not presenting as a competent practitioner when they ask questions. However, the opposite is often true; patients appreciate the nurse's desire to understand their cultural beliefs regarding health. Next, if nurses use a framework to guide practice that promotes a physiological focus (i.e., Maslow's Hierarchy), they may not prioritize cultural aspects of care. While Maslow's Hierarchy is a very effective organizing framework, especially for novice nurses and in acute care settings, the advanced practice nurse should incorporate a holistic or integrated approach to each patient encounter if possible.

The nurse must present a nonjudgmental, accepting attitude for the patient to feel comfortable enough to share their beliefs. Effective communication is key to obtaining an accurate health history and performing an effective physical examination. The nurse takes into consideration all aspects of the patient's culture that affects communication, including language, nonverbal expressions, use of touch, and vocal characteristics. When planning care, additional cultural practices should be considered, such as herbal/nutritional supplements that may interact with prescribed medications and have potential side effects.

Theoretical Foundations for Nursing Practice

Many nurses base their clinical practice on basic knowledge and experiences that began with their initial nursing education, which may fail to incorporate evidence and holistic approaches to practice. Advanced nursing education introduces nurses to theoretical and evidence-based practice, which includes the patient's perspectives and wishes. Theory-based nursing practice incorporates the nursing process (assessment, diagnosis, implementation, evaluation) and provides the nurse with a framework that supports a consistent approach to holistic care planning (Kenney, 2016).

Whether in a direct or indirect care situation, a nurse in an advanced nursing role should integrate knowledge from various areas to make the best decisions at diverse levels. When subject content is learned across separate courses without intentional reflection and critical questioning, the graduate-prepared nurse may have only fragments of what is required for an advanced role. The authors have combined these major concepts in the in-depth study of common diseases across the life span in order to promote a deeper understanding to guide practice and decision making.

Key Points

- Advanced knowledge of physiology/pathophysiology is necessary for the masters-prepared nurse to plan care and anticipate potential outcomes, including complications.
- Advanced physical assessment skills are essential to understand the patient's individualized response to a disease.
- Pharmacology is part of most treatment plans and often monitored by nurses who must understand implications for planning and evaluating care.
- Masters-prepared nurses must be able to integrate the basic subject content that supports clinical care: physiology, pathophysiology, assessment, and pharmacological management.
- Cultural competence is a necessary component in all phases of nursing care and enables the nurse to provide holistic care that is consistent with the individual's preferences, values, and beliefs.

References

American Association of Colleges of Nursing. (2011). *The essentials of master's education in nursing*. Retrieved from http://www.aacn.nche.edu/education-resources/MastersEssentials11.pdf

American Nurses Association. (2015). *Nursing: Scope and standards of practice for nurse administrators* (3rd ed.). Silver Spring, MD: ANA Publishing.

Benner, P., Sutphen, M., Leonard, V., & Day, L. (2009). *Educating nurses: A call for radical transformation*. San Francisco, CA: Josey-Bass.

Debiasi, L. B., & Selleck, C. S. (2017). Cultural competence training for primary care nurse practitioners: An intervention to increase culturally competent care. *Journal of Cultural Diversity, 24*(2), 39–45.

Goolsby, M. J., & Grubbs, L. (2019). Assessment and clinical decision-making: An overview. In M. J. Goolsby & L. Grubbs (Eds.), *Advanced assessment: Interpreting findings and formulating differential diagnoses* (4th edition) (pp. 2–11). Philadelphia, PA: F.A. Davis.

Govere, L., & Govere, E. M. (2016). How effective is cultural competence training of healthcare providers on improving patient satisfaction of minority groups? A systematic review of literature. *Worldviews on Evidence-Based Nursing, 13*(6), 402–410. doi:10.1111/wvn.12176

Halstead, J. (2007). *Nurse educator competencies: Creating an evidence-based practice for nurse educators*. Washington, DC: National League for Nursing Publishing.

Halstead, J. (2018). *NLN core competencies for nurse educators: A decade of influence*. Washington, DC: National League for Nursing Publishing.

Institute of Medicine. (1999). *To err is human: Building a safer health system*. Retrieved from http://www.nationalacademies.org/hmd/~/media/Files/Report%20Files/1999/To-Err-is-Human/To%20Err%20is%20Human%201999%20%20report%20brief.pdf

Jeffreys, M. (2016). *Teaching cultural competence in nursing and health care* (93rd ed.). New York, NY: Springer.

Kenney, J. W. (2016). Theory-based advanced nursing practice. In S. M. DeNisco & A. M. Barker (Eds.), *Advanced practice nursing: Essential knowledge for the profession* (3rd ed., pp. 427–443). Burlington, MA: Jones & Bartlett Learning.

National League for Nursing. (2012). *The scope of practice for academic nurse educators*. Washington, DC: National League for Nursing Publishing.

Rodgers, B. L. (2016). The evolution of nursing science. In S. M. DeNisco & A. M. Barker (Eds.), *Advanced practice nursing: Essential knowledge for the profession* (3rd ed., pp. 401–426). Burlington, MA: Jones & Bartlett Learning.

Shi, L., & Singh, D. A. (2016). Beliefs, values, and health. In S. M. DeNisco & A. M. Barker (Eds.), *Advanced practice nursing: Essential knowledge for the profession* (3rd ed., pp. 179–209). Burlington, MA: Jones & Bartlett Learning.

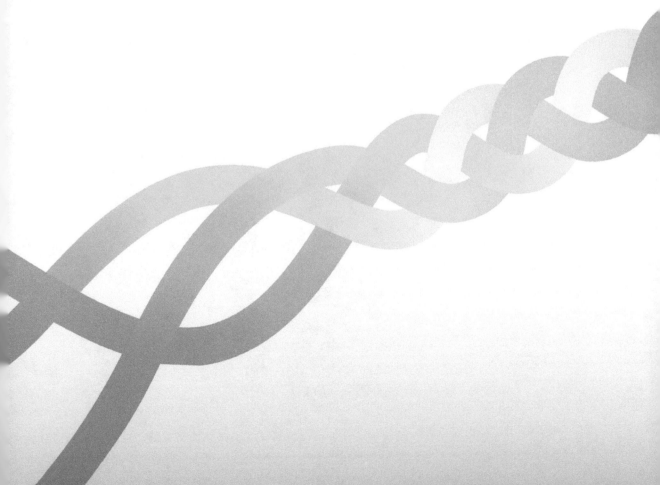

Section **1**

Adult

Chapter 1

Hypertension

Upon completion of this chapter the student will be able to:

- Integrate knowledge of the physiology, pathophysiology, assessment, and nonpharmacological and pharmacological management of hypertension into planning care.
- Appraise current standards of care for patients with hypertension.

Introduction

Elevated *blood pressure* (BP), or hypertension, is the most common chronic condition seen in primary care settings. It may lead to serious complications, such as cardiovascular disease, renal disease, and death if not identified early and treated appropriately (Cruickshank, 2013; Egan et al., 2013; James et al., 2014; Whelton et al., 2018). Hypertension affects approximately 26% of adults globally, with less than 20% controlled (Dagenais et al., 2020), and is expected to increase to 29% prevalence by 2025 (Alexander, 2019). Because nurses care for patients with hypertension in diverse settings, an in-depth understanding of this disease and its effect on an individual's health is crucial to the delivery of safe care. The nurse must understand the physiology of normal blood pressure, along with the pathophysiology associated with both primary and secondary hypertension.

According to *Healthy People 2020* objectives (at the writing of this text, *Healthy People 2030* is in proposal phase), the national goal is to increase the numbers of people who have had their blood pressure measured within the preceding two years and can report whether it is normal (*Healthy People 2020*). Accurate assessment is necessary in order to correctly identify high blood pressure and assess and/or prevent end-organ damage. Guidelines for pharmacological intervention for hypertension changed with the report from the *Eighth Joint National Committee* (JNC 8) (James et al., 2014); the evidence-based recommendations were amended in 2017 and are the new guide for the pharmacological treatment of hypertension (American College of Cardiology [ACC], 2017; Whelton et al., 2018).

Physiology

Blood pressure is the force exerted against arterial walls by the blood as it circulates through the body. The systolic component is the force during systole, or contraction of the heart; the diastolic component is the pressure in the arteries while the heart fills and does not contract. As one can deduct from the physiology of BP, systole is obtained at the highest pressure in the arteries, and diastole is achieved at the lowest, or resting, pressure. BP is affected by cardiac output (stroke volume × heart rate) and peripheral resistance (Bunker, 2014; Capriotti, 2020).

Blood pressure is dependent on several factors, including *cardiac output* (CO) and *peripheral vascular resistance* (PVR), as expressed in the following formula: CO = BP/PVR. The relationship of blood pressure and other hemodynamics is reflected in this calculation (Capriotti, 2020). First cardiac output is the amount of blood pumped by the heart and is approximately 5 liters/minute in a healthy adult; it is calculated by multiplying the stroke volume (amount of blood pumped by heart with each contraction) by the heartrate. Then the peripheral vascular resistance is dependent on arterial blood vessel size. As PVR increases, both BP and CO increase; a decrease in PVR also results in decreases in BP and CO (Capriotti, 2020).

Normal blood pressure is also dependent on normal functioning of other systems, especially the renal and endocrine systems. Specifically, the *renin-angiotensin-aldosterone system* (RAAS) functions to maintain normal blood pressure in response to a decrease in circulating blood volume or decreased blood pressure, but this mechanism may be blocked in order to lower blood pressure. Alterations in renal function that may affect the normal functioning of the RAAS and result in increased blood pressure include chronic kidney disease, polycystic kidney disease, and urinary tract obstruction. Normal endocrine function is necessary for normal blood pressure. In the endocrine system, the adrenal glands, located on each kidney, are responsible for secreting corticosteroids (both mineralocorticoids and glucocorticoids) that maintain normal blood pressure. Abnormalities of endocrine function that are causes of hypertension include acromegaly, adrenal hyperplasia, hyperaldosteronism, hyperthyroidism, hyperparathyroidism, and pheochromocytoma.

> **HIGH YIELD FACT FOR TESTING**
>
> Blood pressure is multifactorial and is dependent on normal functioning in multiple systems (cardiovascular, renal, musculoskeletal, and endocrine).

Pathophysiology

According to the 2017 American College of Cardiology/American Heart Association (ACC/AHA) guidelines and shown in Table 1-1, below-normal blood pressure must have both the systolic and diastolic readings below the recommended levels; if either is above the recommended level of 120/80, then the blood pressure is considered elevated and should be reassessed in a short period of time, usually 3 to 6 months (Whelton et al., 2018). At the time of BP measurement, the patient is also educated about lifestyle changes that will promote lower blood pressure (DASH diet, decreased sodium intake, limited alcohol intake, increased physical activity, smoking cessation); these nonpharmacological measures are part of the treatment plan for all subsequent stages of high blood pressure. In stage 1, a patient with concomitant heart disease and/or significant cardiac risk factors will start an antihypertensive medication, whereas patients without these risk factors will be reassessed in a few months without starting medication at that time. For patients with comorbidities, such as *chronic kidney disease* (CKD), heart failure, diabetes, and who are aged 18 or older, the BP should be less than 130/80 mm Hg; notably, there was insufficient evidence for the previously lower BP goals for this group (James et al., 2014).

Because the presence of hypertension causes negative effects in the cardiovascular system, it is important to identify it early and treat it appropriately. Damage to the linings of arteries and resistance against the left ventricle increase cardiac workload and lead to ventricular hypertrophy over time All body organs/systems are predisposed to injury when arteries and resulting blood flow are impaired from hypertension; especially vulnerable are the retinas, kidneys, brain, and lower extremities (Capriotti, 2020).

TABLE 1–1 Blood Pressure Categories from the American College of Cardiology/ American Heart Association

Category	Systolic		Diastolic	Plan
Normal	<120	and	<80	Reassess in 1 year.
Elevated	120–129	and	<80	Reassess in 3–6 months. Nonpharmacological management.
Stage 1	130–139	or	80–89	Nonpharmacological management and reassess in 3–6 months. If patient has heart disease or risk factors, start antihypertensive medication. Reassess in 1 month.
Stage 2	≥140	or	≥90	Start antihypertensive medication along with nonpharmacological management. Reassess in 1 month.
Hypertensive crisis	≥180	and/or	≥120	*Requires emergent intervention.*

(American College of Cardiology, 2017; Whelton et al., 2018)

Essential hypertension has no single identifiable cause but has been linked to several factors, including obesity, high dietary sodium intake, increased renin levels, genetics, age, insulin resistance, smoking, alcohol intake, and long-term stress. In comparison, secondary hypertension is associated with renal disease, adrenal gland malfunction, coarctation of the aorta, pregnancy, and/or medications (Capriotti, 2020; Whelton et al., 2018). Regardless of the cause of hypertension, the effects are the same. As a result of increased pressure in the heart and blood vessels, the cardiac muscle cells hypertrophy; this mechanism is considered a compensatory response to the higher pressures. In pathological cellular hypertrophy, however, there is no corresponding increased pressure in blood vessels to meet the needs of these hypertrophied cardiac cells. The increased pressure from hypertension creates a shearing force against endothelial arterial walls, which damages the cells and causes endothelial dysfunction. The weakened arterial walls may eventually lead to aneurysm formation (Capriotti, 2020).

As stated above, various factors, both genetic and environmental, are linked to the development of essential hypertension. Conversely, secondary hypertension is due to a clear cause, such as renal disease or Cushing syndrome. Some of these factors that are related to essential hypertension are described in more detail in what follows.

Aging

As people age, there are genetic alterations in the telomerase activity and shortening of the telomere DNA. These changes are related to increased stiffness in the arteries and a resulting increased pulse pressure (Cruickshank, 2013). With aging, arteries lose elasticity, and decreased renal function is responsible for diminished excretion of sodium. Blood pressure increases slightly with age, especially the systolic component; when arteries are damaged by additional factors, the aging person is at significant risk for developing hypertension (Capriotti, 2020).

Sodium Balance

Increased sodium reabsorption in the loop of Henle is associated with increased blood pressure (Cruickshank, 2013). An increased sensitivity to salt in the diet resulting in high blood pressure has a genetic component. Physiologically, increased sodium results in increased intravascular fluid volume and vascular dysfunction. Fluid volume greatly increases when increased sodium intake is coupled with impaired renal excretion of sodium, which often occurs in essential hypertension (Capriotti, 2020).

Altered Responses to Neurotransmitters

While the *sympathetic nervous system* (SNS) is vital to the maintenance of normal blood pressure, with overactivity in the SNS, the patient will experience an increased blood pressure. The role of *tyrosine hydroxylase* (TH) in catecholamine formation is a component of this hypertension-inducing process. A decreased response to beta$_2$-mediated vasodilation is also associated with increased blood pressure (Capriotti, 2020).

Diabetes Mellitus

Both types of diabetes mellitus (1 and 2) predispose a patient to the development of hypertension; because insulin is a vasodilator, and when there is a lack of insulin or resistance to its effect in the body, hypertension often results (Capriotti, 2020). With an increase in the prevalence of diabetes mellitus across the life span, patients are at higher risk for hypertension at a younger age.

Drug Use

Patients may not realize that many types of drugs have an impact on blood pressure. While street drugs, such as cocaine and methamphetamines, are associated with sometimes lethal increases in BP, over-the-counter NSAIDs can also cause an increase in BP. Nicotine, also considered a drug, is a potent vasoconstrictor that contributes to the development of hypertension (Capriotti, 2020).

Genetics

The role of family history, or genetics, is significant in the development of hypertension; despite following recommendations, the person with a family history of hypertension is likely to have high blood pressure at a relatively early age. This is a non-modifiable risk factor, but the patient can be counseled to monitor their blood pressure closely so hypertension can be diagnosed early. There is controversy over the efficacy of identifying hypertension in children, but a strong family history of hypertension may alert the nurse to the need for lifestyle modifications at an early age (Capriotti, 2020).

Environmental Factors

Workplace stresses, social conflicts, exposure to smoke or secondhand smoke, and physical inactivity have a significant impact on blood pressure (American Heart Association [AHA], 2018). Chronic stress activates the RAAS, leading to increased blood pressure (Capriotti, 2020).

Obesity

Obesity is the most important environmental risk factor for the development of hypertension, contributing about $254 billion to annual medical costs in the United States during 2011 (AHA, 2013). Overweight is defined as a *body mass index* (BMI) of 25.0 kg/m^2 or above, obesity is defined as a BMI of 30.0 kg/m^2 or above, and severe obesity is defined as a BMI of 40.0 kg/m^2 or above. Approximately 36.5% of adults in the United States were identified as obese in 2011 to 2014 (Centers for Disease Control and Prevention [CDC], 2017, August 31).

HIGH YIELD FACT FOR TESTING

Share the ACC/AHA categories of *hypertension* (HTN) with patients to improve their understanding of the impact of other health conditions on HTN and the importance of following the treatment plan.

Assessment

Auscultation of BP is one of the first skills learned as a nurse but is often replaced by automatic measurement and delegated to unlicensed personnel. When auscultating a BP, the cuff is inflated to restrict blood flow into the limb; when the blood flow returns, the first sound is the systolic reading. While this sound may change in pitch and clarity, the last sound heard is the diastolic, which indicates that blood flow is completely unrestricted. Automatic blood pressure cuffs work on the same principles, and usually also provide a *mean arterial pressure* (MAP). MAP is a calculated value that is defined as the average pressure in a patient's arteries during one cardiac cycle. Only invasive monitoring and complex calculations can determine true MAP; however, it can also be calculated using a formula of the *systolic blood pressure* (SBP) and the diastolic blood pressure (DBP).

$$MAP = SBP + 2 (DBP)/3.$$

Normal MAP is between 65 and 110 mm Hg (Capriotti, 2020).

Before taking the patient's BP, the nurse should palpate the radial and or brachial arterial pulse for strength and regularity. If any abnormality is noted in either of these characteristics, a manual BP should be assessed using a sphygmomanometer and stethoscope (see SENC Box 1-1). Because treatment decisions are based on accurate BP measurements, it is important to obtain a precise reading. Blood pressures are measured electronically in most settings, and this practice is considered the standard of care. There are certain situations that may require a manual reading, as shown in SENC Box 1-1.

When a patient has a slightly elevated BP reading (120/80 or higher but 140/90 or lower), it may be beneficial to conduct *ambulatory blood pressure monitoring* (ABPM). This assessment involves frequent measurement of BP throughout a 24-hour period during normal activities. Home BP monitoring may also be used to obtain an accurate representation of BP during a patient's day. These readings are especially useful if the patient tends to have elevated BP in the health-care setting (also known as "white coat syndrome"). An average of 14 readings taken at different times during a patient's waking hours may be used to determine a patient's BP and the need for pharmacological intervention (Bunker, 2014). There are differences between BP readings in arms, and a difference of 10 mm Hg or less is considered normal (Capriotti, 2020; Dillon, 2017).

Nonpharmacological Management

Based on the category of BP and presence of additional cardiac risk factors, nonpharmacological measures may be implemented before medication because changes in lifestyle can be very effective in lowering blood pressure (Bunker, 2014; James et al., 2014; Whelton et al., 2018). Often patients are motivated to make these modifications when they are able to forgo starting daily medication and when family members also adopt the changes and provide support (Whelton et al., 2018). However, patients should be

---

SENC BOX 1–1   Safe and Effective Nursing Care for Manual BP

Manual BP is indicated when:

1. Patient requires a cuff size not available with electronic measurement.
2. Clinician questions accuracy of electronic BP reading.
3. Calibration and confirmation of electronic measurement device for patient's home use is needed.

counseled that the need for medication does not represent a failure on their part, as blood pressure is dependent on many interrelated factors (Capriotti, 2020).

Healthy Lifestyle

First, weight loss is associated with decreases in both systolic and diastolic blood pressures, along with decreased stiffness of arteries in younger patients. As little as a 5- to 10-pound weight loss may lower BP (AHA, 2016). To safely lose weight, it is recommended that the patient decreases their calorie intake, based on an optimal weight and daily activity calculation and also increases their activity at the same time. Losing weight using medication is not recommended, as there are potential side effects (Whelton et al., 2018).

Exercise is effective in decreasing BP because the increased blood flow associated with BP causes a therapeutic stress to the endothelium and a resulting decrease in BP post-exercise. The American Heart Association (2016) recommends that healthy individuals should participate in at least 40 minutes a day for 3 to 4 days a week (120 to 160 minutes total each week) of physical activity that is of moderate intensity (e.g., brisk walking) for lowering BP and cholesterol (Whelton et al., 2018).

Healthy eating described in the *Dietary Approaches to Stop Hypertension* (DASH) diet is considered effective in lowering BP and is high in fruits and vegetables with reduced fat. For patients who are salt sensitive, their salt intake should be as low as possible, ideally less than 3.8 g/day. Increases in potassium consumption, when not contraindicated by a potassium-sparing diuretic or other medication, has been shown to promote normal BP (Whelton et al., 2018). Modifications in diet are usually more effective in lowering BP in hypertensive patients as compared to normotensive patients (Whelton et al., 2018).

If the patient smokes, education about cessation is an integral part of nonpharmacological management. Nicotine contained in tobacco is a powerful vasoconstrictor, which causes an immediate increase in blood pressure. The connection between smoking and hypertension is still under investigation, but there is evidence that smoking and exposure to secondhand smoke increases atherosclerosis, which is also accelerated by elevated blood pressure (AHA, 2018).

 RED FLAG ALERT

When an abnormal blood pressure reading is obtained, the first action is to wait 1 minute and retake to confirm the reading.

Drinking excessive alcohol can raise BP and contribute to the development of HTN. Recommended alcohol intake is specific to gender and is limited to 2 or fewer drinks per day for men and 1 drink per day (or none) for women (AHA, 2016). The caffeine in drinks like coffee, tea and sodas may cause elevations in BP and if patients are sensitive to caffeine, this may contribute to HTN (AHA, 2016). Last, stress may increase BP and over time will contribute to the causes of HTN (AHA, 2016).

ASSESSMENT PEARLS

Accurate evaluation of hypertension includes a complete history and physical examination.

Pharmacology

The JNC 8 presented recommendations for pharmacological intervention for HTN based on current evidence. Improved screening methods are necessary, and increased use of combination medications is required for optimal BP control. Medication should be initiated for BP of 130/80 or higher for patients with associated cardiovascular risk factors. The ACC clinical guidelines are based on randomized controlled trials and include broad options for initial therapy. Prescribers are recommended to initiate therapy and reassess BP in 1 month. If BP is not at goal when reassessed at 1 month, a second medication from a different class is added. A third medication may be added, at this time or later, as needed.

Choice of medications to manage HTN is based on cost, limitation of adverse effects, the patient's HTN classification, and presence of other risk factors or comorbidities (Robinson, 2020). Initial therapy may be from one of the following classifications of antihypertensive medications (James et al., 2014):

- Calcium channel blockers
- *Angiotensin-converting enzyme inhibitors* (ACE inhibitors)
- *Angiotensin-receptor blockers* (ARBs)

According to the JNC 8 recommendations, African American patients (including those with diabetes) should be prescribed a thiazide diuretic or calcium channel blocker as initial HTN therapy. If patients have CKD, then an angiotensin-converting enzyme inhibitor or angiotensin-receptor blocker should be used as initial therapy for hypertension because of its renoprotective properties. Evidence supports using a full assessment of the patient in order to individualize pharmacological treatment for hypertension (James et al., 2014). Table 1-2, located at the end of the Pharmacology section, provides a full list of medications used to treat hypertension.

It is important for the nurse to educate patients in certain general principles that they should follow when antihypertensive medication is initiated. First, they should take the medication at the same time each day. A single agent may be taken in either morning or evening, depending on patient preference. When a patient is on two antihypertensive medications, it may be more advantageous to take them at different times so there is more coverage across the 24-hour day. The patient's lifestyle, including work and sleeping schedules, affect the medication schedule. Patients need to achieve and maintain adequate fluid intake and change positions slowly to prevent orthostatic hypotension. No additional medications should be taken without consulting the prescriber. In addition, the nurse should caution the patient about safety considerations, including avoiding excessive alcohol intake and not exercising in hot weather (Robinson, 2020).

ACE Inhibitors (ACEI) and Angiotensin Receptor Blockers (ARBs)

Medications in these classifications work through their action on the *renin-angiotensin-aldosterone* (RAA) system to lower blood pressure. The ACEI medications decrease the production of both angiotensin II and aldosterone, which results in both decreased vasoconstriction and decreased fluid retention. The ARBs have similar actions by blocking the angiotensin II receptors in the adrenal cortex and smooth muscles of blood vessels with fewer reported side effects (Li, Heran, & Wright, 2014). Both are well absorbed via the oral route.

Most ACEIs are prodrugs that require conversion by the liver into active metabolites; however, lisinopril, unlike other ACEIs, is not a prodrug and is excreted unchanged in the urine. The most common side effects are headache, fatigue, orthostatic hypotension, and dry, hacking cough (cough is specific to ACEIs) (Woo & Wynne, 2020). While suspension of therapy for side effects occurs more often with ACEIs than with ARBs, there does not seem to be enough evidence to support use of an ARB instead of an ACEI in most hypertensive patients (Li et al., 2014). See SENC Box 1-2 for guidelines on caring for patients taking ACEI and ARB.

Beta Blockers

Medications in this classification are often used to decrease blood pressure because of their ability to decrease cardiac workload through negative chronotropic and

SENC BOX 1–2   Safe and Effective Nursing Care for Patients Taking ACEIs and ARBs

1. Monitor BP daily 1 hour after dose when the medication is initiated for a week and also daily for a week when the dose is changed.
2. Assess for any changes in voice or swelling of the tongue (signs of angioedema) with the first dose and report to the prescriber.
3. The prescriber will monitor lab values frequently (renal function for ACEIs and ARBs; liver function for ARBs).

SENC BOX 1–3   Safe and Effective Nursing Care for Patients Taking Beta Blockers

1. If you have diabetes, this medication may affect the signs and symptoms of hypoglycemia, so you need to check your blood glucose level if you suspect a problem.
2. Do not abruptly stop taking this medication; it will need to be weaned slowly by the prescriber.
3. Report wheezing or difficulty breathing immediately.
4. Food affects absorption, so take consistently, either with or without food.

inotropic effects but are not the first choice for initial pharmacological management. These medications also have an effect on the RAAS system but not as pronounced as the ACEIs and ARBs. Beta blockers are well absorbed orally (Robinson, 2020). Beta blockers are further classed based on their selectivity in blocking alpha and beta receptors. Nonselective adrenergic beta blockers block both alpha and beta receptors and may exacerbate asthma or bronchospasms because they cause the lungs to lose their bronchodilatation ability. Both nonselective alpha- and beta-adrenergic beta blockers may mask the patient's usual cues of hyperglycemia and hypoglycemia and should be used cautiously in these patients (Karch, 2017). The liver metabolizes most beta blockers, and some require dosage adjustment for patients with impaired renal function. The most common side effects are hypotension and bradycardia. Even though there are beta blockers that are beta$_1$ selective and do not cause bronchoconstriction, these medications are not considered safe for patients with respiratory illness (Woo & Wynne, 2020). See SENC Box 1-3 on caring for patients taking beta blockers.

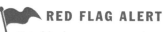 **RED FLAG ALERT**

Beta blockers are not used as primary agents for blood pressure control.

Calcium Channel Blockers (CCBs)

Calcium channel blockers (CCBs) work at the cellular level to block calcium influx, which results in vascular dilation. CCBs are absorbed orally and metabolized exclusively by the liver. Most CCBs are available in both short-acting and sustained-release forms. The most common side effects are due to vasodilation and include dizziness, hypotension, headache, syncope, fluid retention, constipation, and photosensitivity. Side effects are more pronounced with short-acting forms (Woo & Wynne, 2020). See SENC Box 1-4 on caring for patients taking calcium channel blockers.

Diuretics

Medications in this classification work to decrease blood pressure by decreasing *extracellular fluid* (ECF) volume. While there are several types of diuretics that exert physiological effects in different ways, the end result is decreased ECF. Thiazide-type

SENC BOX 1–4   Safe and Effective Nursing Care for Patients Taking Calcium Channel Blockers

1. Call your health-care provider if you experience chest pain.
2. This medication may interact with grapefruit juice, cold remedies, and alcohol.
3. Increase dietary fiber to prevent constipation.
4. Limit sun exposure and use sunscreen.

SENC BOX 1–5   Safe and Effective Nursing Care for Patients Taking Diuretics

1. Take this diuretic before 4 p.m. as it will cause you to urinate and interrupt your ability to sleep.
2. Weigh yourself weekly to monitor fluid balance.
3. You may need to change your diet to maintain normal electrolyte balance. Depending on the specific medication, you may need to increase potassium intake or limit it. You may also need to limit sodium intake so that the diuretic is more effective.
4. Taking this medication with food may decrease GI upset.

diuretics are considered to be the most effective in decreasing blood pressure. These drugs are mild diuretics that work in the loop of Henle to block chloride and sodium from being reabsorbed; they are also considered potassium-wasting drugs. Other types of diuretics include loop diuretics and potassium-sparing diuretics. Loop diuretics are also considered to be potassium-wasting diuretics. They also work in the loop of Henle similarly to thiazide diuretics and are useful with patients who have renal disease or acid–base/electrolyte imbalance (Karch, 2017).

Patients at risk of developing hypokalemia (cardiac arrhythmia or digitalis use) may benefit from a potassium-sparing diuretic. These drugs may be used along with a thiazide or loop diuretic to decrease risk of hypokalemia. Ultimately, the choice of diuretic should be based on the patient's renal function. The following side effects are common with all classes of diuretics: electrolyte imbalances, hypotension, blood glucose intolerance (which may be related to hypokalemia, which blocks glucose from entering cells) with prolonged use, and hyperlipidemia (Karch, 2017; Woo & Wynne, 2020). See SENC Box 1-5 on caring for patients taking diuretics. See Chapter 20, Table 20-4 for more information on loop diuretics.

 RED FLAG ALERT
Many drugs can cause lupus. Hydralazine, procainamide, and isoniazid are the three most common causes, with hydralazine use having the highest incidence. Generally, the symptoms are reversible after drug therapy is discontinued. Patients who are slow metabolizers are more likely to develop drug-induced lupus.

CLINICAL **PEARLS**
Ask patients if they have a scale in their home; it's a less judgmental approach as compared to asking, "Are you weighing yourself every day?"

Vasodilators

These medications work directly in the blood vessels, causing vasodilation with resultant drop in blood pressure. Their use is typically reserved for hypertensive crisis. Patients who have coronary heart disease, heart failure, tachyarrhythmia, or peripheral vascular disease should be given vasodilators with caution since a rapid drop in blood pressure may worsen their condition (Karch, 2017).

See Table 1-2 for an overview of medications affecting blood pressure.

TABLE 1–2 Medications Affecting Blood Pressure

Class	Example	Action	Dosage	SENC
Adrenergic agonists	Dopamine	Activates sympathomimetic response (alpha and beta). Treatment of shock that has not been responsive to fluid replacement.	Renal: IV: 0.5–3 mcg/kg/min Cardiac: IV: 2–10 mcg/kg/min	(SEs): Arrhythmias, hypotension, headache, mydriasis (high doses), vasoconstriction of peripheral circulation, extravasation. Close monitoring of cardiac rhythm, BP, urine output and IV site; administer in large veins to decrease risk of extravasation.
Alpha$_1$- and beta$_1$-(nonselective) adrenergic blocking agents Secondary agent	Labetalol	Vasodilation, decreased heart rate, and cardiac contractility.	Oral: 100 mg bid; max 2.4 g/day HTN crisis: IV: 20 mg slowly over 2 min	SEs: Fatigue, weakness, dizziness, bronchospasm, bradycardia, HF, pulmonary edema, orthostatic hypotension. Assess apical pulse prior to administration; assess for orthostatic hypotension, daily weights; assess for fluid overload.
	Amiodarone	Vasodilation; slows sinus rate; increases PR and QT. Hypertension; ventricular arrhythmias; SVT.	Oral: maintenance (ventricular) 400 mg/day IV: 150 mg over 10 min, then drip	SEs: Dizziness, malaise, fatigue, ARDS, CHF, bradycardia, hypotension, GI upset, photosensitivity, ataxia, and other CNS effects. Continuous ECG monitoring in IV therapy; assess lung sounds, has long half-life; monitor thyroid and liver function.
	Carvedilol	Decreases heart rate; improves cardiac output. Slows progression of heart failure.	Oral: 6.25 mg bid initial; max 25 mg bid ER: 29 mg daily; max 80 mg daily	SEs: Fatigue, weakness, dizziness, diarrhea, erectile dysfunction, hyperglycemia. Associated with hepatic failure. Assess apical pulse prior to administration. Assess BP, HR, I&O, and daily weights; teach patients not to abruptly stop drug; food slows absorption.
Nonselective beta-adrenergic blocking agents Secondary agent	Propranolol	Vascular tone is decreased by blocking of beta$_1$ receptors in heart.	Oral: 40 mg bid or 80 mg SR daily	SEs: Fatigue, weakness, bradycardia, arrhythmias, pulmonary edema, erectile dysfunction; masks hypo- and hyperglycemia. Assess HR and BP, blood glucose levels; take with meals or just after meals to enhance absorption.
Beta$_1$-selective adrenergic blocking agents Secondary agent	Atenolol	Reduce HR and BP by blocking beta$_1$ receptors in the heart.	Oral: 50 mg–100 mg daily	Fatigue, weakness, HF, bradycardia, pulmonary edema, erectile dysfunction. Masks hypo- and hyperglycemia. Pulse will not increase with exercise. Take pulse before giving, assess for HF. Caution: may lose selectivity in higher doses; caution with respiratory disease.

Drug Class	Drug	Action/Uses	Dosage	Side Effects/Nursing Considerations
Angiotensin-converting enzyme inhibitors (ACEIs) Primary agent	Lisinopril	Decrease BP by acting to block angiotensin I conversion to angiotensin II; prevents vasoconstriction and aldosterone release. Hypertension: first line in HF and with other drugs; helpful in diabetic neuropathy.	Oral: 10 mg daily; max 40 mg/day Can be compounded to suspension for those with dysphagia	SEs: Hypotension, dizziness, increased serum K+, decreased serum sodium; cough. Take on empty stomach 1 hour before a meal or 2 hours after a meal; decrease dose in renal failure; assess for angioedema. Caution use with NSAIDs. Change to another agent for persistent cough.
Angiotensin II receptor blockers (ARBs) Primary agent	Losartan	Decreases BP by binding with receptors of angiotensin II in vascular smooth muscle and adrenal glands. Use if ACE intolerant. May slow diabetic neuropathy and renal disease in diabetic patients.	Oral: 50 mg daily; may need to adjust does for patients with hepatic impairment.	SEs: Dizziness anxiety, fatigue, hypotension, angioedema. Assess for orthostatic hypotension, angioedema. Monitor daily weights and signs of fluid overload; liver function studies; many drug-drug interactions.
Calcium channel blockers Primary agent	Diltiazem	Inhibits calcium transport into the cells, resulting in vasodilation and decreased BP. Also treats angina pectoris, vasospastic angina, SVT; atrial flutter, atrial fibrillation with rapid ventricular rates.	Oral: 30–120 mg tid comes as SR, CD, or XR capsules Caution: dose no more than 240 mg daily when given with simvastatin (10 mg/day)	SEs: Hypotension, bradycardia, peripheral edema, abnormal dreams, confusion, dizziness, and other CNS effects; Stevens-Johnson syndrome. Interacts with grapefruit juice. Take pulse before administration; assess for HF, assess for rash intermittently during therapy; monitor serum K+. SR has fewer side effects.
Vasodilators Secondary agent	Hydralazine	Vasodilation by acting directly on peripheral arteries. Lowers BP and decreases afterload in HF.	Oral: maximum dose 300 mg/day IV: 5–40 mg may repeat as needed	SEs: Tachycardia, sodium retention, drug-induced lupus syndrome, dizziness, headache, drowsiness. Monitor BP and pulse carefully when starting therapy. Increased risk for toxicity in patients of Chinese, Alaska Native, and Japanese ethnicity.

(Adapted from Woo & Robinson, 2020)

SEs, side effects; BP, blood pressure; HF, heart failure; ARDS, acute respiratory distress syndrome; CHF, congestive heart failure; GI, gastrointestinal; CNS, central nervous system; ECG, electrocardiogram; HR, heart rate; I & O, intake and output; SVT, supraventricular tachycardia; SR, sustained release; CD, controlled delivery; XR, extended release

Complementary and Alternative Therapies (CAT)

Many *complementary and alternative therapies* (CAT) are implemented in the management of hypertension and considered lifestyle alterations. Patients may be educated in healthy lifestyle changes as part of safe and effective nursing care to lower blood pressure (see Table 1-3).

The nurse must have current knowledge of CAT in order to counsel patients regarding safety and efficacy of these therapies and educate the patient not to start any supplement without first consulting with their provider for potential interactions. Globally, there is increasing use of CAT among patients with hypertension but there is not supporting research of its efficacy. In a descriptive study of 127 patients with hypertension, 78.7% used CAT in the form of vitamins, herbs, and cognitive approaches (Akansel, Özdemir, Yıldız, Baran, & Dirik, 2017). The following box includes three current dietary supplements that are commonly used for lowering blood pressure, but research is not available to support their efficacy.

Caution should be used with any CAT, especially with patients who have significantly elevated blood pressure and comorbidities. In an integrated review of literature from 2011 through 2015, the most frequently used CAT for hypertension was phytotherapy (use of plant extracts), mainly in decoction (boiling and dissolving) and tea (de Fátima Mantovani, 2017). Similarly, Chen, Wang, Yang, Xu, and Liu (2015) conducted a meta-analysis and concluded Chinese medicine safely decreased blood pressure in hypertensive patients but also recommended more research before making a clinical recommendation. Patients should be asked in an accepting and nonjudgmental manner if they use CAT, and these therapies should be considered as a component of the patient history.

TABLE 1–3   Healthy Lifestyle for Lowering Blood Pressure

Dietary Changes	
Eat more: • Fruits, vegetables, and low-fat dairy foods • Whole grain products, fish, poultry, and nuts • Foods rich in magnesium, potassium, and calcium	Eat less: • Fatty foods (i.e., saturated fats, cholesterol) • Red meat • Sweets and simple sugars
Increase physical activity. 30–60 minutes 4–5 days/week is recommended.	
Stress Management	
• Deep breathing • Slow-movement activities (tai chi, yoga, qi gong)	

Dietary Supplements Used to Lower Blood Pressure

Amino acids:

• L-arginine
• L-taurine

Omega-3 fatty acids:

• EPA (eicosapentaenoic acid)
• DHA (docosahexaenoic acid)

Coenzyme Q10 (CoQ10)

Summary

While hypertension can usually be well controlled with a combination of lifestyle and pharmacological interventions, there are patients with treatment-resistant hypertension (those who take three or more BP medications and continue to have BP above the goal of 140/90). It is estimated that approximately 30% of patients with uncontrolled high BP while on medication have treatment-resistant hypertension and should be evaluated by a physician for optimal lifestyle and pharmacological intervention, and for consideration of innovative therapies, including complementary and alternative therapy options (Egan et al., 2013).

While the management of high BP should be directed by the JNC 8 guidelines, each patient's individual characteristics, lifestyle, and environment should be considered when initiating and monitoring the effectiveness of pharmacological and nonpharmacological interventions.

Key Points

- Current knowledge of hypertension is essential because it is the most common chronic illness in primary care settings.
- The Eighth Joint National Committee (JNC 8) has published current guidelines to manage hypertension.
- Definition of hypertension is dependent on age.
  - For patients younger than 60 years old: BP higher than 139/89.
  - For patients 60 and older: BP higher than 150/90.
- Most hypertension is considered essential and is multifactorial in nature.
- Factors that contribute to hypertension include age, sodium balance, sympathetic overstimulation, beta receptors, insulin resistance, drugs, obesity, and environmental factors.
- Reassess and confirm an abnormal blood pressure reading.
- Use nonpharmacological interventions first unless BP is emergently elevated.
- Incorporate both general and specific *Safe Effective Nursing Care* (SENC) interventions for patients taking antihypertensives that are both general and specific to the certain medication.

Review Questions

1. **The nurse anticipates that the patient will be placed on a diuretic to manage newly diagnosed hypertension. The specific medication has not been ordered, but the nurse teaches the patient and family the broad safety principles when taking any diuretic. Select all of the following that apply to taking a diuretic, no matter which category:**
   a. Take a diuretic on an empty stomach.
   b. Supplement your diet with potassium.
   c. Weigh yourself daily.
   d. Take medication at same time each day, preferably in the morning.
   e. Low blood pressure may be a side effect.

2. **The patient asks you, the nurse, if taking natural supplements is safe along with prescribed medications for elevated blood pressure. The nurse's best response is:**
   a. "Of course supplements are safe, as long as you take your medication as directed by the prescriber."
   b. "Bring in your supplements to your next visit and I'll look them up online for you."

c. "Let's involve a pharmacist in this discussion and confirm the safety of the combination of supplements and prescribed medications."

d. "You shouldn't take any supplements when you are on prescribed medications; it's not safe."

3. **The 63-year-old patient has had three monthly consecutive blood pressure readings that were above 144/86. The nurse anticipates that the following professionals/recommendations will be involved in the plan of care. Select all that apply.**

   a. Nutritionist will evaluate the patient's weight/diet and recommend DASH as appropriate.

   b. Social worker will determine whether medications will be covered by Medicare.

   c. Pharmacist will assess for drug-drug interactions.

   d. Physical therapist will evaluate for exercise program.

   e. Provider will determine whether prescribed medications are necessary.

4. **A 36-year-old obese woman has an elevated blood pressure reading of 160/98 at an annual gynecological and birth control planning appointment; she does not have a primary care provider. The appropriate follow-up care for her would include which of the following?**

   a. Refer her to the social worker to evaluate whether her insurance will pay for a primary care appointment.

   b. The gynecologist prescribes a diuretic for immediate blood pressure control.

   c. A test dose of an ACE inhibitor is administered in the office; the patient's blood pressure is monitored.

   d. The blood pressure is reassessed using a large cuff.

5. **The patient who is on an antihypertensive complains of headaches, dizziness, and ankle swelling. The nurse prioritizes which of the following assessments? Select all that apply.**

   a. Measuring blood pressure electronically.

   b. Comparing current weight to weight from last appointment.

   c. Assessing severity of ankle edema.

   d. Performing an ophthalmological exam.

   e. Obtaining accurate family medical history.

See the appendix for answers to review questions.

References

Akansel, N., Özdemir, A., Yıldız, H., Baran, A., & Dirik, M. (2017). The use of complementary and alternative medicine among hypertensive patients. *Rostrum of Asclepius/Vima Tou Asklipiou, 16*(3), 192–203. doi:10.5281/zenodo.821626

Alexander, M. (Ed.). (2019). What is the global prevalence of hypertension? Medscape RN. Retrieved from https://www.medscape.com/answers/241381-7614/what-is-the-global-prevalence-of-hypertension-high-blood-pressure

American College of Cardiology. (2017). New ACA/AHA blood pressure guidelines lower definition of hypertension. Retrieved from http://www.acc.org/latest-in-cardiology/articles/2017/11/08/11/47/mon-5pm-bp-guideline-aha-2017

American Heart Association. (2013). Statistical Fact Sheet 2014 Update. Retrieved from https://www.heart.org/idc/groups/heart-public/@wcm/@sop/@smd/documents/downloadable/ucm_462025.pdf

American Heart Association. (2016). Physical activity and blood pressure. Retrieved from http://professional.heart.org/professional/GuidelinesStatements/UCM_316885_Guidelines & Statements

American Heart Association. (2018). Get the facts about high blood pressure. Retrieved from http://www
.heart.org/HEARTORG/Conditions/HighBloodPressure/GettheFactsAboutHighBloodPressure/The
-Facts-About-High-Blood-Pressure_UCM_002050_Article.jsp#.Wzk2vNVKjHY

Bunker, J. (2014). Hypertension: Diagnosis, assessment and management. *Nursing Standard, 28*(42), 50–59.

Capriotti, T. (2020). *Pathophysiology: Introductory concepts and clinical perspectives* (2nd ed.). Philadelphia, PA:
F.A. Davis.

Centers for Disease Control and Prevention. (2017, August 31). *Adult obesity prevalence maps.* Retrieved from
https://www.cdc.gov/obesity/data/prevalence-maps.html

Chen, Z., Wang, L., Yang, G., Xu, H., & Liu, J. (2015). Chinese herbal medicine combined with conventional therapy for blood pressure variability in hypertension patients: A systematic review of randomized controlled trials. *Evidence-Based Complementary & Alternative Medicine, 2015,* 582751. doi:10.1155
/2015/582751

Cruickshank, J. M. (2013). *Essential hypertension.* Shelton, CT: People's Medical Publishing House.

de Fátima Mantovani, M. (2017). Complementary and alternative medicine in systemic arterial hypertension. *British Journal of Cardiac Nursing, 12*(4), 180–186. doi:10.12968/bjca.2017.12.4.180

Dagenais, G. R., Leong, D. P., Rangarajan, S., Lanas, F., Lopez-Jaramillo, P., Gupta, R., Diaz, R., Avezum, A.,
Oliveira, G., Wielgosz, A., Parambath, S. R., Mony, P., Alhabib, K. F., Temizhan, A., Ismail, N., Chifamba, J.,
Yeates, K., Khatib, R., Rahman, O., Zatonska, K., . . . Yusuf, S. (2020). Variations in common diseases,
hospital admissions, and deaths in middle-aged adults in 21 countries from five continents (PURE):
A prospective cohort study. *Lancet (London, England), 395*(10226), 785–794. https://doi.org/10.1016
/S0140-6736(19)32007-0

Dillon, P. (2017). *Nursing health assessment: A critical thinking, case studies approach.* (2nd ed.). Philadelphia,
PA: F.A. Davis Company.

Egan, B. M., Zhao, Y., Li, J., Brzezinski, W. A., Todoran, T. M., Brook, R. D., & Calhoun, D. A. (2013).
Prevalence of optimal treatment regimens in patients with apparent treatment-resistant hypertension
based on office blood pressure in a community-based practice network. *Hypertension, 62*(4), 691–697.

Healthy People 2020. (2016). Topics & objectives. Washington, DC: U.S. Department of Health and Human
Services, Office of Disease Prevention and Health Promotion. Retrieved from https://www.healthypeople
.gov/2020/topics-objectives

James, P. A., Oparil, S., Carter, B. L., Cushman, W. C., Denison-Himmelfarb, C., Handler, J., . . . Ortiz, E.
(2014). 2014 evidence-based guideline for the management of high blood pressure in adults: Report
from the panel members appointed to the Eighth Joint National Committee (JNC 8). *JAMA, 311*(5),
507–520. doi:10.1001/jama.2013.284427

Karch, A. M. (2017). *Focus on nursing pharmacology* (7th ed.). Philadelphia, PA: Wolters Kluwer.

Li, E. C. K., Heran, B. S., & Wright, J. M. (2014). Angiotensin converting enzyme (ACE) inhibitors versus
angiotensin receptor blockers for primary hypertension. *Cochrane Database of Systematic Reviews, 2014*(8),
CD009096. Retrieved from http://www.cochrane.org/CD009096/HTN_angiotensin-converting-enzyme
-ace-inhibitors-versus-angiotensin-receptor-blockers-for-primary-hypertension

Robinson, M. V. (2020). Hypertension. In T. M. Woo & M. V. Robinson (Eds.), *Pharmacotherapeutics for
advanced practice nurse prescribers* (5th ed., pp. 1195–1219). Philadelphia, PA: F.A. Davis.

Whelton, P., Carey, P., Aronow, W. S., Casey, D. E., Jr., Collins, K. J., Dennison Himmelfarb, C., . . .
Wright, J. T., Jr. (2018). 2017 ACC/AHA/AAPA/ABC/ACPM/AGS/APhA/ASH/ASPC/NMA/PCNA
2017 guideline for the prevention, detection, evaluation, and management of high blood pressure in
adults: A report of the American College of Cardiology/American Health Association Task Force on
Clinical Practice Guidelines. *Journal of the American College of Cardiology, 71,* e172–e248. Retrieved from
http://www.acc.org/latest-in-cardiology/ten-points-to-remember/2017/11/09/11/41/2017-guideline
-for-high-blood-pressure-in-adults

Woo, T., & Wynne, A. (2020). *Pharmacotherapeutics for nurse practitioner prescribers* (5th ed.). Philadelphia,
PA: F.A. Davis.

Chapter 2

Diabetes Mellitus

LEARNING OBJECTIVES

Upon completion of this section the student will be able to:

- Integrate knowledge of the physiology, pathophysiology, assessment, and nonpharmacological and pharmacological management for care of an adult patient with type 1 or type 2 diabetes mellitus.

- Appraise current standards of care for adult patients with diabetes mellitus.

Introduction

A chronic endocrine disorder, *diabetes mellitus* (DM) develops when glucose metabolism is impaired and blood glucose levels are consistently elevated above normal levels (Capriotti, 2020; Hendricks, 2018). There are four underlying causes of DM (Centers for Disease Control and Prevention [CDC], 2019, August 6; Hendricks, 2018):

- An autoimmune response—type 1
- Insulin resistance—type 2
- Glucose intolerance during pregnancy—gestational
- A variety of other conditions leading to elevated blood glucose levels

U.S. statistics from 2018 indicate that DM affects more than 34.1 million people, and it is estimated that more than 7.3 million of these individuals have not been diagnosed by a health-care provider. Additionally, approximately 88 million adults have *prediabetes* (above normal blood glucose levels but lower than required for a type 2 diabetes diagnosis). Of the total American diabetic population, only about 1.4 million children and adults have type 1 diabetes. Among causes of death, diabetes is listed as seventh, with approximately 80,000 deaths attributed to diabetes each year (American Diabetes Association [ADA], 2018, March 22; CDC, 2020).

During 2017, an estimated total $327 billion was spent on medical care for individuals with a diabetes diagnosis. This included approximately $237 billion in medical costs and $90 billion in lost productivity, disability, or premature death. Age-adjusted costs projected that those with diabetes spent approximately 2.3 times more in medical costs than individuals without diabetes, and about half of all outpatient visits made by diabetic patients was a direct result of diabetes (ADA, 2018a). Diabetes also contributes to several other chronic illnesses, including cardiovascular disease, cognitive impairment, kidney failure, amputations (particularly lower limb), and blindness, and is directly related to kidney failure in two-thirds of all American Indians and Alaska Natives who develop the condition (CDC, 2020; Lee & Halter, 2017).

For 2015, recommended preventive care for diabetic adults did not consistently meet the *Healthy People 2020* target goals. Reported figures that did not meet target goals included health-care professional foot examination (71.6%), diabetes self-management class attendance (54.4%), and daily blood glucose self-monitoring (63%). Only the rates for eye examination with dilation within the past year (61.6%) and hemoglobin A1c testing at least twice a year (71.4%) met the target (CDC, 2018). As the prevalence of diabetes and costs related to diabetes continue to rise, it is important to understand the disease process and the various preventive and treatment options available to the individual at risk for or who has developed diabetes.

Physiology

Normal cell function is dependent upon the availability of glucose, the primary energy source for cell metabolism, and insulin, the hormone that facilitates glucose transport into the cell. As shown in Figure 2-1, endocrine regulation of glucose occurs in the islets of Langerhans cells found in small numbers throughout the pancreas. Secretion of *glucagon* (by alpha cells) and secretion of *insulin* (by beta cells) counteract each other to regulate blood glucose levels. Insulin enters liver circulation in two ways: a *basal* or lower and consistent level of secretion (during fasting) and *prandial* (following food ingestion), which includes an initial release of insulin, followed by continued release over time until blood glucose levels fall back into normal range (Hendricks, 2018).

The role of insulin in normal metabolism is to maintain homeostasis of blood glucose and lipid levels. Insulin enables muscle cells of the heart and skeletal system to accept glucose where it is stored as glycogen (*glycogenesis*). It also inhibits the liver's processes of glycogen breakdown (*glycogenolysis*) and very low-density lipoprotein production. Insulin also supports protein conversion to glucose (*gluconeogenesis*) in muscle cells, and stimulates fat cells to store triglycerides (Hendricks, 2018). When insulin production or when ineffective insulin action within the cell membrane occurs, glucose is prevented from entering the cells, glucose levels in the blood rise, and metabolism is impaired (Renda, 2020).

The major source of glucose from foods is monosaccharides, formed by the breakdown of ingested carbohydrates (CHO) in the intestines. However, glucose is a large molecule, and flow of these large glucose molecules across the plasma membrane requires insulin and a process called *facilitated diffusion*. This process is triggered once glucose is absorbed into the bloodstream, glucose levels rise, and insulin is released by pancreatic beta cells. As insulin binds to insulin-specific receptors in the cell wall, cell wall permeability changes, allowing glucose to flow into the cells, where it is stored and used as an energy source for metabolism. Glucose and insulin levels are directly correlated, and the change in the rate at which glucose is absorbed, stored and used by the cell is dependent upon insulin secretion rates by the pancreas (Capriotti, 2020; Hendricks, 2018).

Glucose enters the cell where it is stored primarily in the liver and muscles as glycogen, a process called glycogenesis. Glycogen breakdown is triggered by low blood glucose levels, which occur when a person fasts or does not consume adequate CHO levels; it is facilitated by the release of epinephrine (adrenal gland) and glycogen (pancreas). In times of prolonged fasting, the process of gluconeogenesis can be used to convert amino acids and fats (fatty acids and glycerol) into glucose in the liver. While glycerol and amino acids are used to create glucose, the fatty acids are converted into *ketones* (or ketoacids)

HIGH YIELD FACT FOR TESTING

Glycogenesis, gluconeogenesis, and glycogenolysis are indirectly correlated to work in balance with each other. For example, while insulin promotes glycogenesis in the liver, it impedes glycogenolysis; and during gluconeogenesis, insulin inhibits ketogenesis (Capriotti, 2020; Hendricks, 2018).

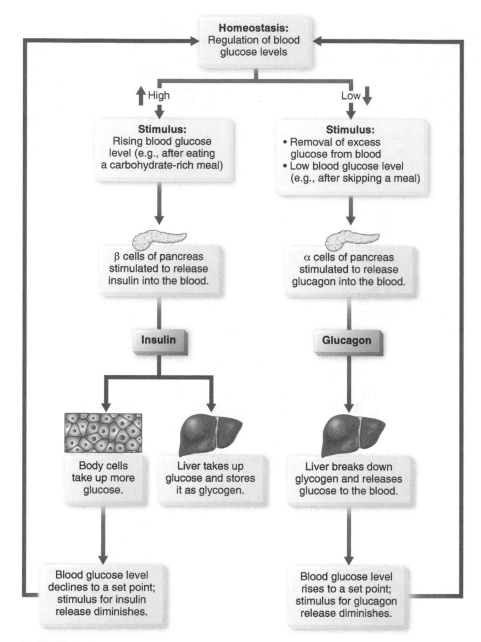

FIGURE 2–1 Glucose metabolism and insulin action *From Hoffman, J. J., & Sullivan, N. J. (Eds.). 2020. Davis's advantage for medical-surgical nursing, 2nd ed.*

and accumulate in the circulating blood supply. Cortisol, released from the adrenal gland, triggers the release of proteins from muscle tissues which are transformed into amino acids to make glucose during gluconeogenesis.

Pathophysiology

Diabetes develops when the regulation of blood glucose levels is impaired either by a failure to produce insulin, or by a reduction of insulin secretion or insulin activity with a corresponding rise in blood glucose levels to above normal levels (*hyperglycemia*).

Elevated blood glucose levels lead to disruption of normal metabolism and changes in the function of most body systems. In the blood, elevated glucose levels cause a fluid shift of water from the cells to the blood, depleting the cells of water, leading to increased feeling of thirst (*polydipsia*) and diluting blood sodium levels (*hyponatremia*). In the eye, changes in aqueous fluid osmolarity lead to changes in light refraction and blurring of vision. In the kidney, once the threshold of reabsorption of glucose is reached, glucose levels in the renal fluid increase. In diabetes, glucose absorption levels in the proximal tubule are exceeded at 300 to 500 mg/dL, causing an osmotic shift (high osmolality) that pulls water into the urine from the cells in the nephron tubules, leading to increases in the volume, frequency (*polyuria*), and glucose content (*glycosuria*) of urine (Capriotti, 2020; Hendricks, 2018).

In type 1 DM, an autoimmune response causes the destruction of islet of Langerhans beta cells, which prevents insulin production and results in hyperglycemia, as glucose is no longer able to move into cells for use as energy. The normal immune response fails because the body does not recognize pancreatic beta cells as belonging to the person, and antibodies attack the beta cells. The rate of beta cell destruction varies, so the onset of ketoacidosis may be delayed, explaining why some patients develop severe hyperglycemia as children, while others may not experience their first symptoms until they are adults (Capriotti, 2020; Hendricks, 2018). This abnormal immune response can also be triggered after a viral infection (Hendricks, 2018).

The patient with type 1 DM is typically diagnosed after they present with *ketoacidosis*. When the body is unable to produce insulin in amounts to maintain homeostasis following ingestion of glucose, excess glucose remains in the blood and blood glucose levels rise. As cells begin to starve without needed glucose, the individual experiences an increase in appetite but loses weight. The body compensates by triggering the liver to break down stored glycogen (gluconeogenesis) to meet cell needs for glucose, resulting in an elevation of blood glucose levels and an accumulation of ketones in the blood and other body fluids (saliva, sweat, urine). As ketone levels rise, the patient exhibits a fruity odor in the breath, body odor, and urine. Blood pH is altered to create a state of metabolic acidosis, or *diabetic ketoacidosis* (DKA). In DKA, the blood glucose level is typically greater than 250 mg/dL, arterial pH is less than 7.3, and serum bicarbonate is less than 15 mEq/L, and the patient has ketones in the blood and urine. Patients hyperventilate (*Kussmaul respiration*) to excrete excess acids as CO_2, thus lowering CO_2 blood levels, returning pH to a normal range. DKA is a medical emergency that, left untreated, can lead to coma and death (Capriotti, 2020; Hendricks, 2018).

Insulin resistance and insufficient insulin production to meet high glucose levels are the underlying causes of *type 2 DM*. In this form of DM, beta cell destruction does not occur, and ketoacidosis is a result of a stressor such as infection or other illness (Lee & Halter, 2017; Lew & Wick, 2015). Fat and muscle cells are more resistant to insulin, so glucose is prevented from entering these cells at a rate that would keep blood glucose levels within a normal range, and the pancreas is stimulated to produce more insulin to cover the rising blood glucose levels. The normal feedback mechanism is altered due to continuing elevated blood glucose levels that trigger the pancreas to produce more insulin. Eventually, the pancreas cannot produce enough insulin to meet the body's glycemic demands and pancreatic function is impaired. With an excessive number of fat cells, particularly in the abdominal area, the overweight or obese individual has higher insulin resistance and is more likely to develop type 2 DM. Other contributing factors to the development of type 2 DM include age, caloric intake that exceeds caloric expenditure, and sedentary lifestyle (Bostock-Cox, 2017; Hendricks,

2018; Kahn, Cooper, & Del Prato, 2014; Lee & Halter, 2017). The development of type 2 DM as one ages is influenced both by a reduction in beta cell function and the presence of risk factors for diabetes that lead to insulin resistance, which further impacts beta cell function (Lee & Halter, 2017).

While extremely elevated blood glucose levels and DKA in those with type 1 diabetes are directly related to the absence of insulin and breakdown of fats into ketones, in the type 2 diabetes patient, insulin resistance is the underlying cause of elevated blood glucose levels. Ketones are not present, and the elevated blood glucose levels are the result of osmolarity changes in the kidney (described above) that lead to glucosuria, and a condition called *hyperosmolar hyperglycemia syndrome* (HHS). The patient complains of thirst and increased need to void. As the condition evolves over time (up to several weeks), blood glucose levels rise to above 600 mg/dL and patients become confused and experience anorexia, tachycardia, weakness, and blurred vision. Underlying causes include infection or cardiovascular conditions including myocardial infarction, pulmonary embolus, or stroke (Capriotti, 2020).

Glucose intolerance during pregnancy is called *gestational diabetes mellitus* (GDM). While GDM occurs only during pregnancy and typically resolves following childbirth, the individual remains at increased risk for developing GDM during future pregnancies and for developing type 2 DM later in life (Hendricks, 2018; Pippitt, Li, & Gurgle, 2016). Currently, the underlying etiology of GDM is not clearly understood, but it is thought that the rise in estrogen levels and the weight gain that normally occur during pregnancy lead to insulin resistance and the pancreas's inability to produce enough insulin to cover the rise in blood glucose levels.

Hyperglycemia places both mother and fetus at risk as glucose crosses the placenta, creating hyperglycemia in the fetus, who stores the excess glucose in fat cells. The result is a larger-than-normal baby who may exhibit low blood sugars after delivery. Risk factors for GDM include hypertension, obesity, history of previous GDM, birth of a child weighing more than 9 pounds or with a birth deficit, or history of stillbirth (CDC, 2019, May 30; Hendricks, 2018). Current recommendations are for all nondiabetic patients to be screened for GDM at 24 to 28 weeks' gestation using a fasting (8 hours) oral glucose tolerance test (OGTT). Individuals who are diagnosed with GDM should be followed during the postpartum period and screened periodically for type 2 DM for the rest of their lives (Shaw & Robinson, 2016).

Other disease processes (endocrine disorders, pancreatitis, cystic fibrosis), and drug side effects that increase insulin resistance (e.g., corticosteroids) are among the secondary causes that lead to less than 5% of all DM cases (Hendricks, 2018). Regardless of the underlying cause, when insulin is not available to support the use of glucose for cell energy, the body breaks down stored fats and proteins as substitute energy sources. Hyperglycemia occurs as a response to lack of insulin and, if blood glucose levels remain elevated, over time creates a fluid and electrolyte imbalance that leads to the classic symptoms of DM: *polydipsia* (increased thirst), *polyphagia* (increased appetite), and *polyuria* (increased urination) (Hendricks, 2018).

Patients with DM may experience *hypoglycemia* (blood glucose less than 70 mg/dL) as a response to overmedication with antidiabetic drugs, extreme physical activity, illness, infection, inadequate nutritional intake, or stressful situations (including surgery). Alcohol abuse is another underlying factor in development of hypoglycemia, particularly for individuals who require insulin to manage their diabetes. The carbohydrates contained in alcohol cause a rise in blood glucose levels, which may lead to hypoglycemia as the alcohol metabolizes. Additionally, alcohol consumption prevents the liver from adequately responding to the presence of insulin by converting a sufficient amount glycogen to glucose to maintain normal blood glucose levels. Alcohol consumption at night may lead to dangerously low blood glucose levels during the night for all diabetics, with the risk of delayed hypoglycemic events being further increased if the individual uses insulin to control their diabetes (Diabetes Digital Media Ltd., 2018; Hendricks, 2018). Signs and symptoms are reflective of the underlying compensatory mechanisms that low glucose levels trigger and include neurological symptoms (confusion, disorientation, dizziness, headache, inability to concentrate, seizures, tremors, loss of consciousness), along with heart palpitations, hunger, and sweating. Hypoglycemia unawareness may develop over time as autonomic neuropathy develops and the sympathetic compensatory responses no longer warn the patient of their rapidly falling blood glucose levels (Capriotti, 2020).

Common long-term complications include peripheral neuropathy and autonomic neuropathy, along with changes to the microvasculature, leading to cardiovascular disease and lower extremity amputation. Diabetic retinopathy and diabetic nephropathy are the result of changes to the microvasculature of the eyes and kidneys and are leading causes of blindness and end-stage renal disease. Other common complications of diabetes include immunosuppression, skin conditions (ulcerations, delayed wound healing, acanthosis nigricans, and candida infections), anxiety, and depression or eating disorders (Capriotti, 2020).

CLINICAL PEARLS
Each year about 2% to 10% of all pregnant individuals develop GDM related to the normal changes of pregnancy (CDC, 2019, May 30).

Assessment

Classification of DM is based on the underlying cause (Capriotti, 2020; Hendricks, 2018; Pippitt et al., 2016). Prior to developing diabetes, an individual may be at risk based on specific criteria. *Prediabetes*, a precursor to diabetes, is described as an impaired glucose tolerance that increases an individual's risk for developing cardiovascular disease and diabetes. Fasting blood glucose levels in prediabetes are above normal limits but are not high enough to be considered at diabetic levels (ADA, 2018b; Capriotti, 2020). The CDC (2020, March 31) estimates that 88 million adults meet prediabetic criteria. Another condition that is often a precursor to development of type 2 DM, *metabolic syndrome* affects about 23% of Americans and is closely related to insulin resistance. Diagnosis is based on the presence of at least three of the following conditions:

- *Central obesity* (abdominal girth greater than 40 inches in men or greater than 35 inches in women)
- Elevated fasting blood glucose (above 100 mg/dL)
- *Hypertension* (130/85 mm Hg or higher)
- *Elevated triglycerides* (150 mg/dL or higher)
- *Low levels of high-density lipoprotein* (HDL) *cholesterol* (less than 40 mg/dL in men or less than 50 mg/dL in women)
- Antidiabetic medication

Individuals diagnosed with metabolic syndrome are at high risk for cardiovascular disease, stroke, and DM (American Heart Association [AHA], 2016, August; Hendricks, 2018).

Screening for DM is important even if the individual does not exhibit classic symptoms. Patients are not typically screened for type 1 DM since it usually presents as an acute episode of ketoacidosis and there are no interventions to prevent the disease from developing. In general, screening for type 2 DM should start at 45 years (ADA, 2018b). However, a risk-based screening assessment and early interventions for type 2 DM is recommended for adults and for children older than 10 years or for those who have reached puberty and who are at risk due to body mass index (BMI) or other risk factors. Early diagnosis is important to delay disease development and progression (ADA, 2018b; Pippitt et al., 2016).

A comprehensive assessment of all patients with DM should include both the physical examination and a laboratory evaluation. Additionally, all diabetic patients should have a psychosocial screening with appropriate referrals for emotional, financial, or social support. The individual's ability to comply with blood glucose testing and with drug, diet, and activity regimens is dependent on their socioeconomic status and must be included to ensure their ability to self-manage and comply with any treatment plan (ADA, 2018b; Funnell & Piatt, 2017). Table 2-1 outlines current risk-based screening recommendations for asymptomatic adolescents, children, and adults who meet the risk weight criteria.

Because red blood cells have a limited life span (about 120 days) and red blood cells are continuously being replaced, hemoglobin saturation with glucose is difficult to accurately measure. To accurately measure the average blood glucose levels over time, the hemoglobin A1c (HA1c) test was developed to provide a weighted average of blood glucose levels over a 2- to 3-month period (Corbett & Banks, 2013). Notably, false readings may occur in acute blood loss or hemolytic anemia (false low), or in aplastic anemias or following splenectomy (false high). HA1c is used in the initial assessment for diabetes to evaluate the severity of disease and is used in conjunction with fasting blood glucose, glucose tolerance tests, and postprandial blood glucose levels to diagnose diabetes (Pippitt et al., 2016). HA1c goals for the diabetic patient include maintaining levels below 7% but can be adjusted upward to a higher level of less than 8% if the patient has a history of severe hypoglycemic events (ADA, 2018b). Blood glucose screening includes oral glucose tolerance tests (OGTTs), glycated hemoglobin A1c, and fasting and random blood glucose levels. Criteria for a prediabetes or

TABLE 2–1   Screening Recommendations for Diabetes

Risk Factor	Adults	Children and Adolescents
Weight	BMI ≥25 kg/m²	BMI ≥85th percentile Weight >120% of ideal weight
Ethnicity/Race	African American, Asian American, Native American, Latino, Pacific Islander	African American, Asian American, Native American, Latino, Pacific Islander

History	Parent or sibling with diabetes
	    Polycystic ovary syndrome (women)
	    Sedentary lifestyle
		Mother had GDM during pregnancy of this child.
		    Family history extends to 2nd degree relatives who have been diagnosed with DM.

Physical/Laboratory Findings	Evidence of insulin resistance
	    Blood pressure ≥140/90 mm Hg
	(or being treated for HTN)
	    Low HDL cholesterol (<35 mg/dL
	    Elevated triglycerides >250 mg/dL
		Evidence of insulin resistance

(ADA, 2018b)

BMI, body mass index; GDM, gestational diabetes mellitus; HDL, high-density lipoprotein; HTN, hypertension

TABLE 2–2 Diagnostic Criteria for Diabetes Mellitus

Laboratory Test	Value*	Interpretation
Fasting blood glucose OR	Greater than or equal to 126 mg/dL 100–125 mg/dL	DM Prediabetes
2-hr postprandial OR	Greater than or equal to 200 mg/dL 140–199 mg/dL	DM Prediabetes
Hemoglobin A1c OR	Greater than or equal to 6.5% 5.7%–6.4%	DM Prediabetes
Random blood glucose level	Greater than or equal to 200 mg/dL	DM if accompanied by classic signs/symptoms of hyperglycemia

From Hoffman, J. J., & Sullivan, N. J. (Eds.). 2020. *Davis's advantage for medical-surgical nursing*, 2nd ed. Philadelphia, PA: F.A. Davis.
*In the absence of unequivocal signs of hyperglycemia, criteria 1 to 3 should be confirmed by repeated testing on a different day.
DM, diabetes mellitus

diabetes diagnosis based on blood glucose testing are found in Table 2-2 (ADA, 2018b; Capriotti, 2020).

Assessment of the diabetic patient also includes screening for conditions that arise from the chronic, long-term pathological processes of diabetes, such as neuropathy, retinopathy, nephropathy, immunosuppression, and skin conditions. Current guidelines recommend an eye examination be conducted within the first 5 years after diabetes diagnosis to establish a baseline for comparison (ADA, 2018b).

Psychosocial assessment includes an assessment for *diabetes distress*, a common negative reaction to the challenges of self-management of a chronic disease. Patients with diabetes distress are overwhelmed by the challenges of managing the disease. They experience anger, fear, frustration, guilt, or shame as they struggle to live with diabetes and are often unable to meet target self-management goals including hemoglobin A1c. These patients may also be experiencing some of the complications of diabetes. Approximately 48% of diabetic adults experience diabetes distress, but only about 24% report this stress to their health-care providers (ADA, 2018b).

ASSESSMENT PEARLS

Attention to patient symptoms is another important key to accurate diagnosis of DM. Patients with diabetes complain of increased thirst, increased appetite, and the need to frequently urinate. Other symptoms include complaints of blurred vision, difficulty concentrating, fatigue, and unexplained weight loss (Capriotti, 2020; Pippitt et al., 2016).

Nonpharmacological Management

Creation of a comprehensive treatment plan that includes referrals (diabetes educator, nutritionist), glucose monitoring, antidiabetic medications, and lifestyle management is central to nonpharmacological management of DM.

Diabetes self-management education (DSME) is the cornerstone of enabling the diabetic to own and self-manage their condition. Engaging patients by providing information about the disease and possible complications, then helping them decide on behavioral changes that are key to promoting a healthy lifestyle is essential (ADA, 2017; Burden, 2017; Renda, 2020). Evidence-based care for the patient with diabetes includes consideration of the patient's understanding of the disease and their personal preferences and values. It begins with assessing the patient's current lifestyle activities (particularly diet and exercise). Lifestyle modifications (nutrition, exercise, weight loss) are essential components of the treatment plan for a patient diagnosed with prediabetes or diabetes. Compliance with these changes may be encouraged by a positive emphasis on the benefits of exercise and healthy eating rather than introducing nutritional changes as a "diet" and suggesting exercises that are not appealing or not within the patient's ability to undertake. Decreasing intake of saturated fats and cholesterol, increasing fiber and omega-3 fatty acids, along with increasing physical activity work together to correct abnormal lipid levels and blood glucose levels. Increasing physical exercise to 150 minutes of moderate-level aerobic exercise a week in addition to dietary changes is known to improve glycemic goals (ADA, 2017, 2018b; Shaw & Robinson, 2016).

Blood Glucose Monitoring

Accurate and regular blood glucose monitoring is an important teaching point for all diabetics. Since one of the most common errors in technique is obtaining a blood sample that is too small, periodic observation of the patient's technique is important to ensuring that their results accurately reflect blood glucose levels. They should be taught how to use their individual monitoring device and how to clean the skin prior to obtaining the sample. Teach the importance of documenting the blood glucose result, any medications, exercise, and when they consumed a meal or snack to provide a complete picture of their glucose control. While the number of times a day that a diabetic should monitor blood glucose levels is individualized, it is suggested that insulin-dependent diabetics monitor their blood glucose levels before meals and at bedtime. Blood glucose levels should be checked more frequently than usual anytime the dose of medication is changed, during illness, following a hypoglycemic event, or when the patient is taking a drug that masks normal hypoglycemic symptoms. An additional time that monitoring may be increased is when the HbA1c results are not consistent with the individual's fasting or postprandial levels (Renda, 2020).

Nutrition

Nutritional goals include a plant-based diet (e.g., the Mediterranean diet) and limiting caloric intake if weight loss is a part of the treatment plan. Weight loss has been shown to be beneficial in preventing prediabetes progression to type 2 DM and facilitates the type 1 and type 2 diabetic to achieve glycemic goals (ADA, 2017, 2018). Having a consistent mealtime and including small snacks during the day and restricting carbohydrate intake to 45 to 60 grams per meal are important in controlling glucose levels. Carbohydrates should come from healthy dairy, fruit, legumes, and vegetables, rather than carbohydrate foods that are high in fat, sodium, or sugars. Non-nutritive sweeteners may have some benefit; however, in some studies they have been associated with weight gain. Fat intake should be limited to approximately 7% of all calories per day. Alcohol consumption should be limited to decrease the risk for hypoglycemic episodes, particularly for the patient who requires insulin therapy (ADA, 2017, 2018b; Shaw & Robinson, 2016). Patients and their caregivers need to be taught to shop for foods that are nutritious and cost effective and to understand that "diabetic" foods are not required to follow a heart-healthy and limited carbohydrate diet.

Portion control for both carbohydrates and proteins is an important part of nutrition education (Burden, 2017).

Exercise

Physical exercise should be incorporated into the patient's daily routine, preferably combining moderate to intense aerobic exercise three times a week with resistance training twice a week (for a total of 150 minutes). Some patients may be reluctant to start an exercise program for fear of developing hypoglycemia, especially during the night, so it is important to teach the patient appropriate self-monitoring to avoid hypoglycemic episodes. Caution patients to monitor their blood glucose levels prior to and after exercise, to keep a diary of their blood glucose levels along with the type and duration of the exercise, and to eat a snack with a carbohydrate content of 10 to 30 grams if their blood glucose falls to 100 mg/dL or lower (ADA, 2018b; Greener, 2017; Shaw & Robinson, 2016). In addition, prolonged sitting should be avoided by changing positions and ambulating every 30 minutes, as a general increase in activity has been shown to benefit blood glucose levels. Both aerobic and muscle-strengthening exercises should be included in the weekly exercise program. To reduce fall risks, older patients should incorporate some type of balance training like tai chi or yoga into their weekly exercise routines (ADA, 2017, 2018b).

Dealing With Sick Days

Planning for sick days is an important part of diabetes self-management. Blood glucose levels are difficult to regulate when the patient is sick, and an established sick day plan may decrease challenges associated with the sick experience. In addition to the patient, at least one or two close contacts (family or friends) should also be trained to use the glucometer and follow the sick day protocol. On sick days, drinking 4 to 6 ounces of water every 30 minutes will help prevent dehydration. If the patient is unable to eat a meal, every 4 hours they should plan to consume about 50 grams of a carbohydrate either as food or sugar-containing liquids. Also, the patient should monitor their temperature at least twice a day, access their blood glucose levels every 4 hours, monitor urine ketone levels, and weigh every day to monitor for unexpected weight loss, which is a sign of elevated blood glucose levels (CDC, 2020). Additional guidelines for sick days, including when to contact the health-care provider during an illness, should be provided as part of the initial education and reviewed with each visit. The CDC Web site provides the following information on when to seek emergent care:

- Blood glucose less than 60 mg/dL
- Diarrhea/vomiting that lasts more than 6 hours
- Drowsiness and inability to think clearly
- Dyspnea
- Elevated urine ketone
- Fever above 101°F for longer than 24 hours
- Unable to keep fluids down for longer than 4 hours or solids down for longer than 24 hours

CLINICAL **PEARLS**
  Advise patients to have a "Sick Box" prepared ahead of time with all the supplies that will be needed to manage a sick day. Over-the-counter medications for fever, pain, and gastrointestinal (GI) symptoms, along with a thermometer, sports drinks, water, crackers, and other nonperishable foods, should be included in the box.

Psychosocial Concerns

Addressing psychosocial issues is another component of the comprehensive care plan for the diabetic patient. Setting achievable goals that enable the patient to have an acceptable quality of life is a key to successful self-management of this chronic disease. Periodic evaluation of the patient's mood and perception of self-care management success, as well as their financial needs, is important. Additionally, the older adult with diabetes should be assessed for cognitive decline and depression (ADA, 2018b; Funnell & Piatt, 2017). Prevention of distress is an important part of the initial patient education, as the feelings patients experience are common and sharing those feelings with their provider is important to gaining self-confidence in managing the various aspects of their disease. Once diabetes distress is identified, the patient needs to be provided education and achievable options for management of those areas of self-care that are proving to be stressful and difficult to manage (ADA, 2018b; Funnell & Piatt, 2017).

Pharmacology

Individuals with type 1 DM and GDM require insulin therapy to control hyperglycemia, while drug therapy for type 2 diabetes is most frequently oral and may or may not include insulin therapy. Patients must understand that to adequately control blood glucose levels, a comprehensive treatment plan that includes appropriate use of antidiabetic drugs, lifestyle changes (diet that limits alcohol and sugar), exercise, and avoiding smoking will be needed (Capriotti, 2020). This section discusses pharmacological interventions used to treat diabetes.

Type 1 diabetics do not produce insulin, so insulin replacement is required to control blood glucose levels. The type of insulin chosen is dependent on the onset, peak, and duration of action required by the patient to control blood glucose levels. Currently, most insulins are synthetically manufactured, which has eliminated the sensitivity issues that occur with animal-based insulins. Insulins are thus categorized based on their peak, onset, and duration of action. Insulin analogs have been designed to estimate the body's normal pattern of insulin secretion and include rapid acting (lispro and aspart), short duration, short acting (regular), longer duration, intermediate acting (NPH), and long acting (glargine and detemir). Insulin can be delivered subcutaneously as an injection, through an injector or insulin pen, or through an external insulin pump. Rapid-acting insulin can also be administered intravenously, but because of the careful monitoring required, IV insulin administration is often reserved for the critical care setting (Capriotti, 2020; Freeland, 2016; Karch & Tucker, 2020). Intermediate and long-acting insulins are used to mimic how the body normally makes insulin, while shorter-acting insulins are used to mimic the insulin needs after carbohydrate ingestion (Freeland, 2016).

It is important to individualize insulin type and dose and to provide patients with appropriate education regarding administration, rotation of injection sites, blood glucose monitoring, and what to do for hypoglycemia, hyperglycemia, and how to adjust insulin during times of illness (Capriotti, 2020; Karch & Tucker, 2020). In the hospital setting, timing insulin administration according to the patient's home schedule can help avoid inadequate glucose management (Freeland, 2016). Table 2-3 shows common insulin types and actions.

For patients with type 2 DM, oral drugs are most often the first line of drug therapy. These drugs work in the pancreas (increase insulin release), kidney (enhance glucose excretion), liver (enhance insulin sensitivity and inhibit glucose production), brain (promote satiety), GI tract (inhibit carbohydrate absorption and delay gastric emptying), and in fat and muscles (enhance insulin sensitivity), all with a common effect of reducing elevated blood glucose levels (Lew & Wick, 2015).

TABLE 2–3   Insulin Types and Their Action

Brand Name/Generic	Onset	Peak	Duration	Purpose
RAPID ACTING*				Prandial insulin used within 0–15 minutes prior to eating or used as correction insulin for blood glucose elevations; used in combination with long-acting insulin.
Humalog/lispro	15–30 min	30–90 min	3–5 hr	Also available in U-200 concentrated form for people requiring larger dosages.
NovoLog/aspart	10–20 min	40–50 min	3–5 hr	
Apidra/glulisine	20–30 min	30–60 min	1–2.5 hr	
SHORT ACTING				Prandial insulin used for meals eaten within 30 to 60 min after administration; used in combination with long-acting insulin.
Regular Humulin/NPH	30–60 min	2–5 hr	5–8 hr	
INTERMEDIATE ACTING				Covers insulin needs for approximately half the day or overnight; used in combination with rapid-acting or short-acting insulin.
NPH	1–2 hr	4–12 hr	18–24 hr	
LONG ACTING				Basal insulin; used in combination with rapid-acting or short-acting insulin.
Lantus, Toujeo, and Basaglar/glargine	1–1.5 hr	No peaks or valleys	20–24 hr	Glargine as Toujeo is U-300, three times the concentration for patients on large dosages.
Levemir/detemir	1–2 hr	No peaks or valleys	24 hr	
Tresiba/degludec	1 hr	Steady state achieved at 8 days	24–42 hr	The very long half-life helps maintain glycemic control if dosage is late. Also available in U-200 for people who require large dosages.

From Hoffman, J. J., & Sullivan, N. J. (Eds.). 2020. *Davis's advantage for medical-surgical nursing*, 2nd ed. Philadelphia, PA: F.A. Davis.
   *Prandial insulin of choice for both multiple injections and the insulin pump.

Like insulin, it is important to individualize pharmacological therapy to consider the efficacy of the drug and its impact on the patient's risk for hypoglycemic events, weight, kidney function, and side effects, and to consider the patient's cardiovascular history. The most commonly ordered oral drug for the treatment of type 2 DM is metformin (ADA, 2018b; Lew & Wick, 2015). Caution the diabetic patient who is also taking a beta-adrenergic blocker to be consistent with their diet, exercise, and blood glucose monitoring, since these drugs are known to mask the symptoms of hypoglycemia (Capriotti, 2020). Table 2-4 describes some of the most commonly prescribed oral antidiabetic agents.

🚩 **RED FLAG ALERT**

Incretin mimetics carry risk for C-cell tumors of the thyroid and for GI side effects in renal impairment.

TABLE 2–4   Oral Drugs Used to Treat Type 2 Diabetes Mellitus

Class	Example	Action	Dosage	SENC
Biguanides	metformin	Increases liver sensitivity to insulin and inhibits glucose production.	500 mg daily titrated to 500 mg to bid; max dose 2,500 mg/day (adults) Max dose 2,000 mg/day (children)	The only oral drug approved for use by children (≥10 years). Titration helps relieve GI side effects. Vitamin B_{12} deficiency is possible. Must produce some insulin for metformin to be effective. Contraindicated in renal disease (lactic acidosis risk).
Sulfonylureas 1st generation	chlorpropamide tolbutamide	Bind to beta cell receptors stimulating insulin secretion.	100–250 mg/day	Adjunctive therapy for type 2 DM. Beta cell function is required for these drugs to be effective. Hypoglycemia and weight gain.
2nd generation	glipizide		5 mg/day; titrate to max of 15 mg/day	
Dipeptidyl peptidase-4 inhibitors	sitagliptin	Prolong insulin secretion in the pancreas; slow gastric emptying to moderate blood glucose levels.	100 mg daily	Monotherapy or combination therapy. May be adjusted for use in renal impairment.
Glucagon-like peptide-1 receptor agonists (GLP-1)	Liraglutide	Stimulates insulin secretion; inhibits glucagon secretion; slows gastric emptying.	0.6 mg subq daily for 1 week; titrate to max of 1.8 mg/daily	Given as adjunct with insulin; increases hypoglycemia risks. GI side effects.
Incretin mimetics	Liraglutide	Stimulates incretin factors in GI tract to enhance insulin secretion in the pancreas; slows gastric emptying to moderate blood glucose levels.	0.6 mg daily subq injection; initial titrated to max of 1.8 mg/day	Do not need to correlate injection with meals. Risk for C-cell tumors of the thyroid and for GI side effects in renal impairment.
Thiazolidinediones	Pioglitazone	Increase glucose metabolism in adipose tissues and skeletal muscle.	15–30 mg/day; may titrate to max of 45 mg/day	Side effects: weight gain, fluid retention. Caution in cardiovascular disease–heart failure.

(ADA, 2018; Karch & Tucker, 2020; Shaw & Robinson, 2016; Vallerand & Sanoski, 2020)
   DM, diabetes mellitus; GI, gastrointestinal; subq, subcutaneous.

Summary

Diabetes is a serious chronic disease that affects individuals across the life span. The effects of the disease and its complications have a major impact on the patient's physical and emotional health, quality of life, and financial resources. Understanding the disease process and the assessment, education, and follow-up required to manage the disease is important for all health-care providers. Evidence-based management of diabetes includes assessment, diagnosis, and creation of a comprehensive patient-centered treatment plan that considers the patient's psychological, physical, and socioeconomic needs.

Key Points

- Diabetes is classified by the underlying cause of glucose metabolism dysfunction and includes type 1 (no insulin secretion) and type 2, gestational, and other disease processes where limited pancreatic beta cell activity results in inadequate glucose metabolism.

- A complete health history including identification of risk factors, laboratory tests, and patient signs and symptoms aids in accurate assessment of diabetes.

- A comprehensive, patient-centered treatment plan must consider the patient's cultural values, physical condition, and financial ability to purchase equipment and medications.

- Self-management of diabetes is dependent on appropriate resource allocation and patient education about their disease process and lifestyle changes that support glycemic control.

Review Questions

1. **One role of insulin is to inhibit the liver from breaking down glycogen. This process is called:**

   a. Gluconeogenesis
   b. Glycolysis
   c. Glycogenesis
   d. Glycogenolysis

2. **The best response by the nurse when the newly diagnosed type 1 diabetic patient states, "I thought only children are diagnosed with type 1 diabetes" is:**

   a. "Type 1 diabetes is a common diagnosis in the adult population."
   b. "The rate of beta cell destruction determines when the disease is diagnosed."
   c. "This is true; you have type 2 diabetes."
   d. "The pancreas can still produce insulin in type 1 diabetes."

3. **The patient with type 2 diabetes asks the nurse how to prevent hypoglycemia when exercising. The nurse's best response is:**

   a. "Check your blood glucose level before each meal."
   b. "Eat a high-protein snack before you exercise."
   c. "Eat a snack if your blood glucose is low after exercising."
   d. "Exercise at the same time every day to avoid low glucose levels."

4. **Which of the following would indicate to the nurse that the female patient may be diagnosed with metabolic syndrome? Select all that apply.**

   a. Abdominal girth of 38 inches
   b. Blood pressure of 138/88
   c. HDL cholesterol of 35 mg/dL
   d. Triglyceride level of 140 mg/dL

5. **The nurse is caring for a diabetic patient who has experienced several hypoglycemic events this week. Which of the following statements best explains the new hemoglobin A1c (HA1c) goals?**

   a. "Adjust your insulin and diet so that your HA1c levels are still below 7% in 2 months."
   b. "A higher HA1c level of less than 8% may help prevent future hypoglycemic events."
   c. "Fasting blood glucose is a better indicator of your risk for hypoglycemia."
   d. "The HA1c level does not reflect your blood glucose over time and is not adjusted."

See the appendix for answers to review questions.

References

American Diabetes Association. (2017). Lifestyle management. *Diabetes Care, 40*(Suppl. 1), S33–S43. doi:10.2337/dc17-S007

American Diabetes Association. (2018, March 22). *Statistics about diabetes.* Retrieved from www.diabetes.org /diabetes-basics/statistics/?loc=db-slabnav

American Diabetes Association. (2018a). Economic costs of diabetes in the U.S. in 2017. *Diabetes Care, 41*(5), 917–928. Retrieved from https://doi.org/10.2337/dci18-0007

American Diabetes Association. (2018b). Standards of medical care in diabetes—2018 abridged for primary care providers. *Clinical Diabetes Journal, 36*(1), 14–37. Retrieved from https://doi.org/10.2337 /cd17-0119

American Heart Association. (2016, August). *Why metabolic syndrome matters.* Retrieved from http://www .heart.org/HEARTORG/Conditions/More/MetabolicSyndrome/Why-Metabolic-Syndrome-Matters _UCM_301922_Article.jsp#.WvrxAoAvzIU

Bostock-Cox, B. (2017). Understanding the link between obesity and diabetes. *Nursing Standard, 31*(44), 52–62.

Burden, M. (2017). Supporting patients to self-manage their diabetes in the community. *British Journal of Community Nursing, 22*(3), 120–122.

Capriotti, T. (2020) *Pathophysiology: Introductory concepts and clinical perspectives* (2nd ed.). Philadelphia, PA: F.A. Davis.

Centers for Disease Control and Prevention. (2018). *Diabetes report card 2020.* Retrieved from https://www .cdc.gov/diabetes/pdfs/data/statistics/national-diabetes-statistics-report.pdf

Centers for Disease Control and Prevention. (2019, May 30). *Gestational diabetes.* Retrieved from https://www.cdc.gov/diabetes/basics/gestational.html

Centers for Disease Control and Prevention. (2019, August 6). *Diabetes quick facts.* Retrieved from https://www.cdc.gov/diabetes/basics/quick-facts.html

Centers for Disease Control and Prevention. (2020, March 31). *Managing sick days.* Retrieved from https://www.cdc.gov/diabetes/managing/flu-sick-days.html

Corbett, J. V., & Banks, A. D. (2013). *Laboratory tests and diagnostic procedures with nursing diagnoses* (8th ed.). Upper Saddle River, NJ: Pearson Education.

Diabetes Digital Media Ltd. (2018). Alcohol and hypoglycemia. Retrieved from https://www.diabetes.co.uk /alcohol-and-hypoglycemia.html

Freeland, B. (2016). Hyperglycemia in the hospital setting. *MEDSURG Nursing, 25*(6), 393–396.

Funnell, M. M., & Piatt, G. A. (2017). Incorporating diabetes self-management education into your practice: When, what, and how. *The Journal for Nurse Practitioners, 13*(7), 468–474.

Greener, M. (2017). Exercise and type 1 diabetes: Overcoming the barriers. *Practical Diabetes, 34*(8), 277–279.

Hendricks, S. (2018). Care of patients with diabetes mellitus. In D. D. Ignatavicius, L. Workman, & C. R. Rebar (Eds.), *Medical-surgical nursing: Concepts for interprofessional collaborative care* (9th ed.). St. Louis, MO: Elsevier.

Hoffman, J. J., & Sullivan, N. J. (Eds.). 2020. *Davis's advantage for medical-surgical nursing,* 2nd ed. Philadelphia, PA: F.A. Davis.

Kahn, S. E., Cooper, M. E., & Del Prato, S. (2014). Pathophysiology and treatment of type 2 diabetes: Perspectives on the past, present, and future. *Lancet, 383,* 1068–1083. Retrieved from http://dx.doi.org /10.1016/S0140-6736(13)62154-6

Karch, A. M., & Tucker, R. G. (2020). *Focus on nursing pharmacology* (8th ed.). Philadelphia, PA: Wolters Kluwer.

Lee, P. G., & Halter, J. B. (2017). The pathophysiology of hyperglycemia in older adults: Clinical considerations. *Diabetes Care, 40,* 444–452. doi:10.2337/dc16-1732

Lew, K. N., & Wick, A. (2015). Pharmacotherapy of type 2 diabetes mellitus: Navigating current and new therapies. *MEDSURG Nursing, 24*(6), 413–419, 438.

Pippitt, K., Li, M., & Gurgle, H. E. (2016). Diabetes mellitus: Screening and diagnosis. *American Family Physician, 93*(2), 103–109.

Renda, S. (2020). Coordinating care for patients with diabetes mellitus. In J. J. Hoffman & N. J. Sullivan (Eds.), *Medical-surgical nursing: Making connections to practice* (2nd ed.). Philadelphia, PA: F.A. Davis.

Shaw, K., & Robinson, M. (2016). Diabetes mellitus. In T. M. Woo & M. V. Robinson (Eds.), *Pharmacotherapeutics for advanced practice nurse prescribers* (4th ed.). Philadelphia, PA: F.A. Davis.

Vallerand, A. H., & Sanoski, C. A. (Eds.). (2020). *Davis's drug guide for nurses* (17th ed.). Philadelphia, PA: F.A. Davis.

Obesity

Introduction

An individual is diagnosed as overweight or obese when their weight exceeds the range that is considered healthy for their height. The calculation of the ratio of height to weight is made using the *body mass index* (BMI) calculator, with obesity defined as a BMI ≥30 kg/m^2 and overweight as a BMI ≥25 kg/m^2 (Centers for Disease Control and Prevention [CDC], 2016a; World Health Organization [WHO], 2018). Several risk factors have been linked to the development of obesity including age, gender, excessive caloric intake, sedentary lifestyle, genetic predisposition, endocrine disorders, and smoking cessation (Capriotti, 2020; CDC, 2017; Fruth, 2017; WHO, 2018).

Global obesity rates have rapidly increased since 1975, with approximately 13% of all adults and 18% of all children currently classified as either overweight or obese. In fact, in all areas of the world except Asia and sub-Saharan Africa, more individuals die of conditions related to obesity than die from being underweight (WHO, 2018). In the United States, more than 36.5% of the adult population is currently identified as being *obese* (CDC, 2017). While geographically a global health problem, in the United States obesity impacts individuals in all 50 states. Obesity increases risk for several chronic illnesses including diabetes mellitus, cancer, cardiovascular disease, and obstructive sleep apnea, creating far-reaching impacts on health and health-care costs (CDC, 2017).

The financial impact of treating obesity in the United States is almost $210 billion each year (Trust for America's Health and Robert Wood Johnson Foundation, 2018), with a nationwide estimated annual cost of $3.38 billion to $6.38 billion attributed to lost productivity (CDC, 2017). The 2014 health-care costs of treating conditions directly related to obesity was estimated at $427.8 billion. Additionally, pharmaceutical costs are increased as the moderately obese individual is prescribed medications to treat co-morbidities more than twice as often as those who are not obese (Milken Institute, 2016). From a financial perspective, addressing risk factors for obesity, maintaining a healthy weight and decreasing comorbidities associated with obesity are one key to controlling health-care costs.

While the focus on obesity often centers on the exogenous factors (excessive intake of high-calorie, high-fat, or high-sodium foods) that lead to increased BMI, the condition is complex, and often impaired metabolic function contributes to development of the disease. Disturbances of hypothalamus functioning related to the appetite regulation may lead to obesity, and endocrine or metabolic (endogenous) conditions are often underlying causes of obesity (O'Brien, Hinder, Callaghan, & Feldman, 2017). Additionally, medications used to treat many chronic conditions may contribute to the development of obesity, including corticosteroids, NSAIDs, antidepressants, antiepileptics, antihypertensives, estrogens, and some oral agents used to treat type 2 diabetes mellitus (Willis & Rebar, 2018).

Physiology

The body's ability to regulate weight is a complex balance between the *central nervous system* (CNS), *gastrointestinal* (GI) organs, and adipose tissues. In response to consumption of nutrients, hormones are released from the hypothalamus and adipose tissues, energy is used, and excess energy is stored in adipose tissues. Because of this complex process, weight fluctuates in response to signals from adipose tissues to the CNS. If a balance between energy intake and expenditure exists, weight is maintained (Chaptini & Peikin, 2016; Willis & Rebar, 2018).

As shown in Figure 3-1, the hypothalamus lies deep within the brain and is divided into anterior, intermediate, and posterior regions, with each region having a distinct and critical role in homeostasis, regulating functions of the autonomic and endocrine systems and exercising some control over behavior. Among its other functions, the hypothalamus balances energy use by receiving and integrating signals from the gut hormone leptin and from ghrelin, which is secreted from an empty stomach, about hunger and satiety (feeling full). Together, leptin and ghrelin work to stimulate and suppress the appetite; thus, they influence body weight through a complex process of homeostasis. Nuclei in the intermediate region of the brain function to impact leptin's effects on energy balance and to signal satiety. Posterior hypothalamic nuclei control hunger and the desire to eat and also influence reward-seeking behaviors that can lead to eating as a response to stress (Braine, 2009; Perry & Wang, 2012).

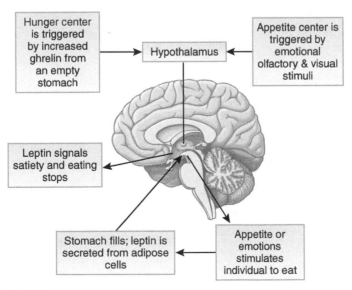

FIGURE 3–1 Anatomy of appetite

The healthy gut has a balance of microbiota that survive on ingested food and consequently play a role in metabolism. Two main types of microbes are prevalent in the gut: those of the phyla Bacteroidetes and Firmicutes. The composition of gut microbiota fluctuates in response to age, diet, and medication use (antibiotics are well known to interrupt normal gut flora). Individuals with lower numbers of bifidobacteria in the gut are often overweight or obese. However, the ratio of Firmicutes is similar among overweight, obese, and normal weight individuals. Although the relationship is not clearly understood, how the imbalance in normal gut microbiota results in fat storage and a corresponding weight gain and how diet and the use of prebiotics and probiotics impacts weight will continue to be the focus of obesity research (Burton-Shepherd, 2015; Tseng & Wu, 2019).

Adipose tissue plays an important role in protecting organs, insulating the body, and storing and releasing energy (O'Brien et al., 2017). Found with adipose tissues, adipocytes (fat-storing endocrine cells) produce several adipokines, including adiponectin, leptin, and resistin, which directly impact metabolic processes related to obesity. As the number of adipocytes increases and these cells hypertrophy, more fat can be stored and more adipokines are secreted, changing insulin sensitivity and glucose production in the liver. These changes impact fat breakdown, fat storage, and lipid levels. As the amount of adipose tissue increases, the impact of adipokines on metabolism increases (Capriotti, 2020).

Adiponectin protects against arteriosclerosis by increasing insulin sensitivity at the cellular level. As the amount of adipose tissue increases, the production of adiponectin decreases, resulting in elevated blood glucose levels, triglycerides, and lower levels of *high-density lipoproteins* (HDL). *Leptin* has roles in regulation of inflammation, metabolism, sympathetic nerve function, and energy regulation. Leptin levels rise as food is consumed, triggering a negative feedback loop in the brain that signals satiety. Leptin also influences both insulin sensitivity and triglyceride levels and functions to decrease the accumulation of body fat. The role of *resistin*, an adipokine identified in the blood of obese individuals, is not clearly understood. Resistin has an opposite effect of the other adipokines, so an increase in resistin levels causes elevated triglyceride and glucose levels and lowered HDL levels and increases the individual's risk of arteriosclerosis (Capriotti, 2020; Chaptini & Peikin, 2016; Imayama & Prasad, 2017; Perry & Wang, 2012).

Other adipokines also have an impact on an individual's risk for developing diseases associated with obesity. An increased number of adipocytes results in several changes that impact cardiovascular disease. First, an increase in *angiotensinogen* levels raises blood pressure and increases risk of development of hypertension and arteriosclerosis. Second, an excess release of *tissue plasminogen activator* (tPA) blocks *fibrinolysis*, increasing clot formation and stroke risks. Finally, *lipolysis* (increased free fatty acids) results from an increase in the production of the adipokines interleukin-6 and tumor necrosis factor alpha. Elevated free fatty acids cause tissue damage in the pancreas, liver, and heart muscle, and lead to glucose intolerance as the pancreas decreases the production of insulin (Capriotti, 2020).

In summary, as the underlying hormonal imbalance continues, adipocyte cells hypertrophy and cause a low-grade inflammatory response in adipose tissues. As overstimulation of receptors occurs and the negative feedback loop that triggers a feeling of satiety is blocked; thus, individuals who are obese become resistant to the feeling of satiety (Perry & Wang, 2012). This triggers the individual's desire to eat more food than is required in order to maintain an energy balance. Insulin resistance develops, which further contributes to the amounts of free fatty acids in circulation (Braine, 2009; Campbell, 2018; Capriotti, 2020; O'Brien et al., 2017).

HIGH YIELD FACT FOR TESTING

The complex mechanism by which appetite is controlled is influenced by signals to the brain that are based on cognitive and sensory triggers that result in the desire to eat when hungry and to stop eating when the stomach is distended to the point of feeling full. Emotional responses to these signals, social circumstance, and the way food or drink is prepared are among the external influences that trigger eating (Benelam, 2009; O'Brien et al., 2017).

CLINICAL PEARLS
As BMI increases and obesity develops, the number of adipocytes available to produce adipokines increases. Thus, obesity itself increases the influence on metabolism, glucose production, insulin resistance, hunger, and satiety.

Pathophysiology

Understanding the physiological aspects of obesity is the first step in assessing and treating this challenging condition. A metabolic disorder, obesity occurs when there is an imbalance between energy intake and expenditure. When more calories are absorbed than are used during metabolism and physical activity, excess fat is stored and weight gain results. However, adipocyte (fat cell) hypertrophy and genetics also impact an individual's predisposition to becoming overweight or obese (Braine, 2009; Capriotti, 2020; Venes, 2017). Box 3-1 describes the five main types of obesity.

Dyslipidemia, a result of increased adipose tissue storage, is distinguished by an increase in low-density lipoproteins and triglycerides and a decrease in high-density proteins; these along with chronic inflammation form the basis of changes in the endothelial tissues of the vascular system that increase risk of cardiovascular disease (Capriotti, 2020; DeMarco, Aroor, & Sowers, 2014; Fruth, 2017). As lipids accumulate in the liposomes of liver cells, they enlarge (steatosis), leading to the development of cirrhosis or nonalcoholic fatty liver disease (Heymsfield & Wadden, 2017).

The function of major organs is affected by excess lipid accumulation and contribute to a variety of conditions that impact overall health. An increased volume of adipose tissue around the kidneys constricts kidney function and results in increased blood pressure, contributing to the development of hypertension (Heymsfield & Wadden, 2017). The presence of visceral fat (abdominal obesity) increases intra-abdominal pressure, elevating risk for *gastroesophageal reflux disease* (GERD) and esophageal disorders including Barrett's esophagus. Excess visceral fat is also a major contributor to the development of type 2 diabetes mellitus. As fat cells become enlarged and fatty acid levels increase, there is a decreased need for glucose to meet the body's energy requirements. This imbalance results in hyperglycemia and the development of insulin resistance. In the musculoskeletal system, as weight increases so does the mechanical load for weight-bearing joints, leading to the development of osteoarthritis (Bostock-Cox, 2017; Chaptini & Peikin, 2016; Heymsfield & Wadden, 2017).

Finally, as the individual's BMI increases, the accompanying increase in neck size and volume of soft tissues in the pharynx contributes to the development of obstructive sleep apnea as the airway collapses from the extra weight when the individual reclines. Periods of snoring and apnea often lead to significant levels of hypoxemia. Oxygenation

---

BOX 3-1   Types of Obesity

- Abdominal (android) – fat deposits are concentrated in the abdomen and waist and the person has an apple-shaped appearance.
- Endogenous – endocrine or metabolic condition is an underlying cause of obesity.
- Exogenous – excessive intake of high-calorie, high-fat, or high-sodium foods is the cause of obesity.
- Hypothalamic – appetite-regulating disturbance of the hypothalamus is caused by excess secretion of adipokines.
- Adult-onset and juvenile obesity are defined by the age of obesity onset. Individuals with juvenile diabetes are at increased risk to remain or become obese in adulthood.

is further impaired because of visceral fat deposits that limit lung expansion, leading to decreased lung volume and oxygen availability (Eckert & Malhotra, 2008; Fruth, 2017; Heymsfield & Wadden, 2017).

Many chronic conditions are directly associated with obesity. Where the individual stores fat impacts their risk for development of these conditions, which include cardiovascular disease, dyslipidemia, gastroesophageal reflux, hypertension, nonalcoholic fatty liver disease, polycystic ovary syndrome, osteoarthritis, type 2 diabetes mellitus, and obstructive sleep apnea (Capriotti, 2020; CDC, 2017; Fruth, 2017; Milken Institute, 2016). In addition to the physical comorbidities of obesity, the disorder has been associated with difficulty sleeping, low self-esteem, and depression and other mental health conditions (Fruth, 2017).

A diagnosis of overweight or obesity is based on an individual's percentage of lean body mass. One method of obtaining this percentage is to use skinfold calipers to measure three separate body areas on three separate occasions and input this information into a mathematical calculation (weight × percentage of body fat). Areas measured for women include the suprailiac, triceps, and thigh areas; for men, abdomen, chest, and thigh measurements are used. Lean body mass equal to or exceeding 32% for women and 26% for men is considered obese (Capriotti, 2020).

More common in use and easier to estimate is the BMI formula, where a weight-to-height ratio is compared to a standard. Height and weight are entered into a calculation tool to determine the BMI (see Box 3-2). The BMI calculator uses standardized weights and heights of men and women as the standard, and while it is not as accurate as calculations using caliphers, it is an easy population-level way to estimate lean body mass (Capriotti, 2020; WHO, 2018). An additional measurement of waist -to-hip ratios serves as an adjunct measurement of the amount of fat in the abdominal area and helps identify risk for diseases related to obesity (O'Brien et al., 2017). See Box 3-2 on calculating BMI.

Many risk factors predispose an individual to become overweight or obese. Unmodifiable risk factors include age, gender, and some genetic predispositions and diseases (e.g., Cushing's and hypothyroidism). Modifiable risk factors include lifestyle choices, such as a sedentary instead of an active lifestyle and amount/types of food consumed. An individual's socioeconomic status and their location (rural vs. urban) may impact their access and means to purchase healthy foods; also, adults who are committed to smoking cessation are at increased risk of substituting eating for smoking (Bryant, Hess, & Bowen, 2015; Capriotti, 2020; WHO, 2018). The WHO identifies urbanization, agricultural, and food-processing changes, along with an increase in sedentary working conditions and the tendency to choose fast-food options as societal impacts that increase in worldwide obesity rates (WHO, 2018). When assessing risk and discussing weight management strategies, it is important for the nurse to use a nonjudgmental approach

---

BOX 3–2   Calculating BMI

- Underweight <18.5
- Normal weight 18.5–24.9
- Overweight 25–29.9
- Obesity ≥30
- Morbid obesity ≥40

(Capriotti, 2020)

that focuses on the personal benefits to health and quality of life that accompany weight loss (Fruth, 2017).

Physically, individuals tend to store fat differently, and the location of fat stores affects risk factors for certain health problems. In central obesity, fat is stored in the abdominal area (creating an apple-shaped body). Central obesity, combined with an increase in insulin resistance, elevated blood pressure, and dyslipidemia (metabolic syndrome), places the individual at increased risk for diabetes, cardiovascular disease, and stroke (Capriotti, 2020; Chugh & Sharma, 2012).

HIGH YIELD FACT FOR TESTING

Obesity is a multifactorial condition impacted by genetics and environmental factors, including eating habits, physical activity, medications used to treat chronic conditions, and socioeconomic status.

CLINICAL PEARLS

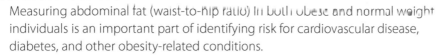

Measuring abdominal fat (waist-to-hip ratio) in both obese and normal weight individuals is an important part of identifying risk for cardiovascular disease, diabetes, and other obesity-related conditions.

Nonpharmacological Management

One of the most important outcomes of weight loss for obese or overweight individuals is a reduction in obesity-related comorbidities and mortality. It is estimated that even a small weight loss is beneficial in decreasing risk of cardiovascular disease and stroke (Fruth, 2017; Novosel, Grant, Dormin, & Coleman, 2017). One must decrease daily caloric intake by 500–1,000 calories or burn off at least 500–1,000 calories each day to achieve a weight loss of 1–2 pounds a week (CDC, 2016b, 2018).

Understanding the individual's motivators and barriers to behavioral changes is one of the first steps to successful weight loss. Lifestyle changes (diet and exercise) form the foundation of weight-loss interventions and successful weight management. Individuals who set realistic and measurable goals for healthy eating, physical activity, and the amount of weight loss to be expected (between 5% and 15% of current body weight) are most successful in achieving and sustaining weight loss (Fruth, 2017; Novosel et al., 2017). Combining realistic goals for weight loss with dietary and activity diaries and scheduled follow-up appointments is important to an individual's motivation to continue working on lifestyle changes that result in adherence to the program (Fruth, 2017).

Healthy eating is a core component of dietary changes that support weight loss and maintenance. Integral to supporting the patient's eating choices is an understanding of their culture/ethnicity, socioeconomic status, and ability to access and purchase health foods (Bryant et al., 2015; Trust for America's Health and Robert Wood Johnson, Foundation, 2014). A healthy diet includes a balance of fruits, vegetables, milk products (low fat or fat free), and lean meats and other protein-rich foods; a healthy diet is also low in added sugars, fats, and sodium (CDC, 2016c). Helping the individual understand their motivation to eat and learn ways to control eating decisions is a key to healthy eating (Fruth, 2017).

Along with dietary changes, increasing physical activity is an important part of a weight-loss plan. Brisk walking is considered a safe activity for most adults and is one of the best aerobic activities that an individual can add to their daily routine. Previously sedentary individuals and those with chronic conditions should consult with their provider before starting a new exercise program and should start slowly and progress over time to a moderate intensity of activity to decrease risk for cardiac events or injury (CDC, 2018). Recommendations for physical activity include approximately 50 minutes of moderate-intensive activities like brisk walking each week, along with muscle-strengthening exercises twice a week (CDC, 2016b).

> **SENC BOX 3–1   Safe and Effective Nursing Care: The 5-A Framework for Behavioral Modifications in Obesity**
>
> 1. **Assess** behavioral risk and motivations.
> 2. **Advise** based on a discussion of the individual's health risks and benefits.
> 3. **Agree** mutually on a care plan.
> 4. **Assist** the individual to change behavior.
> 5. **Arrange** follow-up support that includes making adjustments to the plan as needed.

(Novosel et al., 2017)

Motivation to make dietary and exercise changes and then assimilation of the changes into daily routines is essential to successful weight management (Fruth, 2017). The Centers for Medicare and Medicaid Services (CMS) suggests a 5-A framework for addressing behavioral modifications in obesity, as shown in SENC Box 3-1.

The CDC provides links to pencil-and-paper and Web-based food and physical activity diaries to assist individuals with achieving a healthy balance in eating and exercise (CDC, 2016b). In addition to the CDC resources, other resources that may be useful in weight management include the Obesity Action Coalition, the Stop Obesity Alliance, and the UConn Rudd Center's resources for providers who want to learn more about their role in obesity management (Fruth, 2017). Helping patients with weight management requires ongoing discussion and guidance to set personal goals that are realistic and include activities that are sustainable over time. Part of this discussion includes setting goals for weight loss. Using the SMART acronym, patients are encouraged to set *specific* goals, decide how to *measure* their progress in meeting the goals, decide if the goals are *achievable*, and *relevant* to their overall weight loss plan, and finally to identify a short-term *time* to reach their goals. By using the SMART guide for goal development, nurses can help patients identify specific behaviors related to eating and activity that are measurable, achievable, and relevant to their overall weight-loss plan and set a time limit on reaching these goals (Rethink Obesity®, 2019).

Pharmacology

While management of obesity is often directed at lifestyle changes (diet and exercise) with a goal of weight loss and prevention of weight gain, pharmacological interventions may be required as adjuncts to other weight-loss interventions (Chugh & Sharma, 2012; Lee & Dixon, 2017). Pharmacological therapy is generally reserved for individuals whose "BMI ≥30 kg/m², or ≥27–28 mg/m²" (Jones & Bloom, 2015, p. 941) if the individual has a comorbid condition associated with obesity.

Some drugs used to treat obesity target the hypothalamus, particularly the appetite pathways that signal dopaminergic or serotoninergic receptors. Other drugs target satiety-signaling pathways, acting to increase the expenditure of the body's energy supplies, to reduce appetite and reduce the amount of food an individual consumes by creating a sensation of satiety from a smaller meal that lasts for a longer period. Weight-loss drugs must be considered with respect to the risk and benefits of their use and in conjunction with the patient's commitment to lifestyle changes. Consideration of costs of adjunct drug therapy is also important because not all insurance companies include weight-loss drugs in their formulary (Jones & Bloom, 2015; Lee & Dixon, 2017; National Institute of Diabetes and Digestive and Kidney Diseases [NIDDK], 2016).

As the understanding of how energy balance is regulated has increased, drugs have been developed that influence these pathways and control appetite with fewer adverse side effects. The oldest drug currently on the market is orlistat, a lipase inhibitor that works in the intestine to reduce fat absorption. Lorcaserin, approved for use in 2012, is a 5-HT serotonin stimulator whose major adverse effect is an increased risk for cardiovascular valve disease. In addition to its action to release insulin in the presence of elevated glucose levels, liraglutide delays gastric emptying and suppresses appetite and has been approved for treating obesity. There are combination drugs approved for use. All these drugs have major contraindications for use (Jones & Bloom, 2015; Lee & Dixon, 2017; Vallerand & Sanaski, 2020). Table 3-1 describes the most common obesity drugs on the market today.

TABLE 3–1   Common Drugs to Treat Obesity

Class	Example	Action	Dosage	SENC
Glucagon-like-peptide (GLP-1)	Liraglutide (Saxenda)	Controls hyperglycemia.	Subcutaneous injection 0.6 mg daily, does not have to be given with a meal. Usually titrated over a 5-week period.	Side effects include GI upset, constipation. Symptomatic gallstone, pancreatitis may also develop. Contraindicated in severe hepatic or renal insufficiency, pancreatitis, pregnancy, or history of psychiatric disorders including major depression.
Lipase inhibitor	Orlistat (Xenical)	Decreases fat absorption (30%) by inhibiting excretion of gastric and pancreatic lipase.	Oral, 120 mg tid taken with (just before, during, or just after) meals.	Side effects are related to decreased fat absorption and high-fat diet and include steatorrhea, flatulence, fecal incontinence, deficiencies of fat-soluble vitamins, and renal calculi (calcium oxalate). Contraindicated during pregnancy. Caution: multivitamin supplement should be taken 2 hours before or after orlistat.
Combination therapies				
Dopamine & norepinephrine-reuptake inhibitor, μ-opioid antagonist	Naltrexone-bupropion (Contrave)	Bupropion inhibits reuptake of dopamine and norepinephrine, and naltrexone, an opioid antagonist.	Oral, 16 mg/ 180 mg bid. Usually titrated over a 4-week period to a maintenance dose.	Side effects are usually mild and include GI upset (constipation or diarrhea, nausea), dry mouth, headache, insomnia. Contraindicated with use of MAOIs or in patients with bipolar disease, seizures, anorexia nervosa, withdrawal (alcohol or opiates), end-stage renal disease.

Continued

TABLE 3–1   Common Drugs to Treat Obesity—cont'd

Class	Example	Action	Dosage	SENC
Combination therapies				
Anorectic sympathomimetic amine and an antiepileptic drug	Phentermine/ topiramate (Qsymia)	Phentermine, a sympathomimetic that suppresses appetite, and topiramate, typically used for migraine or seizure treatment. that causes satiety sooner.	Oral, slow-release (15, 30, or 40 mg) pill. Once daily in the morning. Usually titrated to reach the mainte-nance dose.	Side effects include agitation, constipation, dry mouth, insomnia or tachycardia. Contraindicated in patients with a history of anxiety, cardiovascular dis-ease, hyperthyroidism, sub-stance abuse, MAOI drugs, pregnancy, and lactation. Monitor blood pressure closely. Caution: for short-term (maximum of 12 weeks) use only, as the drug has poten-tial for addiction.

(Jones & Bloom, 2015; Lee, 2017; Vallerand & Sanoski, 2015)
    MAOI, monoamine oxidase inhibitor.

 CLINICAL PEARLS
    Because the obese individual has a larger mass for distribution of medications, loading doses may need to be larger; however, maintenance doses do not need to be larger because medications are still metabolized in the body at the same rate.

Surgical Management of Obesity

Surgical intervention is another adjunct therapy for some indi-viduals who need to achieve significant weight loss to decrease complications from obesity-related comorbidities (Colquitt, Pickett, Loveman, & Frampton, 2014; Novosel et al., 2017). Individuals qualify for a bariatric procedure if they have not responded to lifestyle changes or pharmacotherapies, and are classified as morbidly obese, or are obese with significant obesity-related risk factors (Willis & Rebar, 2018).

The laparoscopic (or open) Roux-en-Y gastric bypass, lapa-roscopic (or open) adjustable gastric banding, and laparoscopic sleeve gastrectomy are frequently performed procedures for individuals who are classified as morbidly obese and who need to achieve significant weight loss in a short amount of time to improve health. In a Cochrane review, findings indicate that surgery does improve outcomes for weight loss and obesity-related comor-bidities in general and particularly for those who are morbidly obese, but that evidence is lacking for surgical interventions for those who are classed as overweight and do not meet the criteria for bariatric surgical intervention (Colquitt et al., 2014; Willis & Rebar, 2018). Table 3-2 describes the most common bariatric surgical procedures.

 CLINICAL PEARLS
    Bariatric surgery for older adults is covered by Medicare only for individuals with comorbid conditions and who have not been successful with nonsurgical weight-loss treatment; however, the long-term effectiveness of surgery in this population has not been determined.

TABLE 3-2 Common Weight-Loss Surgical Procedures

Surgical Procedure	Action on GI track	Considerations
Roux-en-Y gastric bypass (RYGB, or gastric bypass)	Creates approximately a 1-ounce-capacity stomach pouch by dividing stomach and reconnecting a section of divided small intestine, changing capacity and gut hormones to suppress hunger, increase satiety, and control of blood glucose.	• Significant weight loss can be maintained over time. • Procedure decreases absorptive area and decreased vitamin and mineral absorption. • Requires commitment to following diet, vitamin/mineral supplements, and follow-up care. • Requires the longest hospital stay.
Sleeve gastrectomy	Removes about 80% of stomach, leaving a tubular pouch that holds less volume, changes gut hormones, increases satiety, suppresses hunger, and controls blood glucose.	• Compares with Roux-en-Y gastric bypass in terms of weight loss over time. • Does not re-route flow of food through the GI track. • Decreases absorptive area and results in decreased vitamin and mineral absorption. • Has a higher complication rate in the early postoperative period than an adjustable gastric band procedure.
Biliopancreatic diversion with duodenal switch gastric bypass (BPD/DS)	Small stomach pouch created by removing part of the stomach, bypassing the proximal duodenum, connecting the stomach pouch to the distal duodenum, and reconnecting the proximal duodenum to the terminal small intestine.	• Creates malabsorption while allowing consumption of larger amounts of food than other procedures. • Reduces appetite and increases satiety, and is most effective in controlling blood glucose. • Higher rates of complications and mortality. • Longer length of stay post-procedure. • Numerous vitamin/mineral deficiencies and risk for protein deficiency because most of absorption area of small intestine is bypassed.
Adjustable gastric band	Creates smaller stomach capacity by inflating a band around the upper stomach, which divides upper and lower stomach and reduces the amount of food that can be ingested at one time, reducing hunger.	• Does not re-route flow of food through the GI track. • Band can be adjusted or removed. • Lowest early complication rate of all the weight-loss procedures. • Complications include band slippage, band erosion, or esophageal dilation if overeating. • Diet and follow-up visits must be strictly followed.

(American Society of Metabolic and Bariatric Surgery, 2018)

Summary

As society becomes increasingly more automated, socioeconomic status continues to impact access to and affordability of healthy food. Participation in sedentary activities is more common than aerobic physical exercise, so the obesity epidemic remains a chronic disease that impacts morbidity and mortality and has economic impacts for all persons around the world (Chugh & Sharma, 2012; Heymsfield & Wadden, 2017).

Nurses have a key role in helping patients to understand obesity and to create effective weight management plans. Understanding the relationships of the hypothalamus, endocrine function, and individual patient choices in the development of obesity is

HIGH YIELD FACT FOR TESTING

Treatment of obesity at any age should include a comprehensive assessment and focused interventions that address behavioral, dietary, and activity changes as central components of effective weight management. All surgical procedures, except the adjustable gastric banding procedure, increase risk of vitamin/mineral deficiencies and require supplementation.

an important first step to creating effective weight management plans. While behavioral changes in diet and exercise form the foundation of these plans, some individuals may also need to incorporate weight-loss medications or surgical interventions to obtain a faster weight loss if comorbidities put them at high risk for death. Taking time to listen actively and engage the patient in a positive dialogue about their weight, thus raising awareness of and encouraging individuals to develop healthy lifestyles, eating, and physical activity "habits," is an important responsibility for nurses and health-care providers.

Key Points

- Active engagement of the patient in developing and implementing individualized strategies that address nutrition, exercise and other behavior changes are key to successful weight management.
- Obese individuals are at significant risk for developing significant comorbidities, including cancer, cardiovascular disease, diabetes, and obstructive sleep apnea.
- Weight-loss drugs should be used cautiously after assessing for contradictions for use and with ongoing monitoring for adverse effects.

Review Questions

1. **The nurse is discussing a healthy eating plan for an adult client who has been diagnosed with obesity. What is the nurse's best response when the client asks, "Why can't I just take a pill to lose weight"?**

   a. "Following a healthy diet and increasing your exercise will be more effective to losing and keeping weight off than taking a pill."
   b. "If you don't think you can follow a Mediterranean diet, you should ask your provider to order you a diet pill."
   c. "You should ask the provider to write you a prescription for a weight-loss pill."
   d. "Weight-loss drugs are only ordered when the BMI is over 25 kg/m^2."

2. **A 75-year-old widow has been diagnosed with type 2 diabetes as a result of obesity. Which of the following interventions for this client would be most effective in helping with weight-loss program?**

   a. Describe the reasons why the client should change their eating habits.
   b. Engage with the client in finding a support system for their exercise goals.
   c. Explore reasons why the client is not walking as a part of their daily routine.
   d. Sign the collaborative behavior change agreement as a witness.

3. **The nurse is providing patient education to a client who has been pre-scribed orlistat, a lipase inhibitor. Which of the following should be included in the education?**

   a. "Have someone monitor your blood pressure daily while on the medication."
   b. "Side effects of the drug include dry mouth, headache, or fatigue."
   c. "Take this drug three times a day with meals."
   d. "You will need to learn to give yourself the injection once a day with breakfast."

4. **Which of the following statements made by the nurse best describes the role of leptin in hunger and satiety?**

   a. Circulating leptin triggers a negative feedback loop in the hypothalamus.
   b. Leptin levels increase and body weight decreases.
   c. Secretion of leptin by the pancreas results in elevated blood glucose levels.

5. **The hypothalamus secretes leptin as a response to increased gut hormones. The nurse is providing education to an adult client who has been diagnosed with obesity. Which of the following interventions would be appropriate to include in the initial instructions? (Select all that apply.)**

   a. "Eat a well-balanced diet and cut your caloric intake by 500–1,000 calories a day."
   b. "Increase the amount of fruit, legumes and vegetables you eat every day."
   c. "Limit the amount of fatty foods and processed sugars in your diet."
   d. "Start running at least a mile a day so that you don't have to decrease your calories."

See the appendix for answers to review questions.

References

American Society of Metabolic and Bariatric Surgery. (2018). *Bariatric surgical procedures.* https://asmbs.org/patients/bariatric-surgery-procedures

Benelam, B. (2009). Satiation, satiety and their effects on eating behaviour. *Nutrition Bulletin, 34*(2), 126–173.

Bostock-Cox, B. (2017). Understanding the link between obesity and diabetes. *Nursing Standard, 31*(44), 52–61. doi:10.7748/ns.2017e10106

Braine, M. (2009). The role of the hypothalamus, part 1: The regulation of temperature and hunger. *British Journal of Neuroscience Nursing, 5*(2), 66–72. http://onlinelibrary.wiley.com/doi/10.1002/14651858.CD012114/epdf

Bryant, P. H., Hess, A., & Bowen, P. G. (2015). Social determinants of health related to obesity. *The Journal for Nurse Practitioners, 11*(20), 220–225.

Burton-Shepherd, A. (2015). Prebiotics and probiotics as novel therapeutic agents for obesity. *Nurse Prescribing, 13*(3), 136–139.

Campbell, A. W. (2018). The epidemic of obesity. *Alternative Therapies, 24*(1), 9–10.

Capriotti, T. (2020). *Pathophysiology: Introductory concepts and clinical perspectives* (2nd ed.). Philadelphia, PA: F.A. Davis.

Centers for Disease Control and Prevention. (2016a). *Defining adult overweight and obesity.* https://www.cdc.gov/obesity/adult/defining.html

Centers for Disease Control and Prevention. (2016b). *Finding a balance.* https://www.cdc.gov/healthyweight/calories/index.html

Centers for Disease Control and Prevention. (2016c). *Healthy eating for a healthy weight.* https://www.cdc.gov/healthyweight/healthy_eating/index.html

Centers for Disease Control and Prevention. (2017, Aug. 31). *Adult obesity prevalence maps.* https://www.cdc.gov/obesity/data/prevalence-maps.html

Centers for Disease Control and Prevention. (2018, Feb. 3). *Physical activity and health.* https://www.cdc.gov/physicalactivity/basics/pa-health/index.htm

Chaptini, L., & Peikin, S. (2016). Physiology of weight regulation. In N. J. Talley, K. R. DeVault, M. B. Wallace, B. A. Aqel, & K. D. Lindor (Eds.), *Practical gastroenterology and hepatology board review toolkit* (2nd ed.). New York: John Wiley & Sons. http://www.practicalgastrohep.com/pdf/c102.pdf

Chugh, P. K., & Sharma, S. (2012). Recent advances in the pathophysiology and pharmacological treatment of obesity. *Journal of Clinical Pharmacy and Therapeutics, 37*, 525–535. doi:10.1111/j.1365-2710.2012.01347.x

Colquitt, J. L., Pickett, K., Loveman, E., & Frampton, G. K. (2014). Surgery for weight loss in adults [Review]. *Cochrane Database of Systematic Reviews, 2014*(8):CD003641. http://onlinelibrary.wiley.com/doi/10.1002/14651858.CD003641.pub4/epdf/abstract

DeMarco, V. G., Aroor, A. R., & Sowers, J. R. (2014). The pathophysiology of hypertension in patients with obesity. *Nature Reviews Endocrinology, 10*(6), 364–376. http://doi.org/10.1038/nrendo.2014.44

Eckert, D. J., & Malhotra, A. (2008). Pathophysiology of adult obstructive sleep apnea. *Proceedings of the American Thoracic Society, 5*(2), 144–153. http://doi.org/10.1513/pats.200707-114MG

Fruth, S. M. (2017). Obesity: Risk factors, complications, and strategies for sustainable long-term weight management. *Journal of the American Association of Nurse Practitioners, 29*, 53–514.

Heymsfield, S. B., & Wadden, T. A. (2017). Mechanisms, pathophysiology, and management of obesity. *The New England Journal of Medicine, 376*(3). doi:10.1056/NEJMra1514009

Imayama, I., & Prasad, B. (2017). Role of leptin in obstructive sleep apnea. *Annals of the American Thoracic Society, 14*(11), 1607–1621. doi:10.1513/AnnalsATS.201702-181FR

Jones, B. J., & Bloom, S. R. (2015). The new era of drug therapy for obesity: The evidence and the expectations. *Drugs, 75*, 935–935. doi:10.1007/s40265-015-0410-1

Lee, P. C., & Dixon, J. (2017). Pharmacotherapy for obesity. *Australian Family Physician, 46*(7), 472–477.

Milken Institute. (2016, Nov. 30). *Americans' obesity weighs down U.S. economy by $1.4 trillion.* http://www.milkeninstitute.org/newsroom/press-releases/view/316

National Institute of Diabetes and Digestive and Kidney Diseases. (2016, July). Prescription medications to treat overweight and obesity. https://www.niddk.nih.gov/health-information/weight-management /prescription-medications-treat-overweight-obesity

Novosel, L. M., Grant, C. A., Dormin, L. M., & Coleman, T. M. (2017). Obesity and disability in older adults. *The Nurse Practitioner, 42*(4), 40–47.

O'Brien, P. D., Hinder, L. M., Callaghan, B. C., & Feldman, E. L. (2017). Neurological consequences of obesity. *The Lancet Neurology, 16*(6), 465–477. http://dx.doi.org/10.1016/S1474-4422(17)30084-4

Perry, B., & Wang, Y. (2012). Appetite regulation and weight control: The role of gut hormones. *Nutrition and Diabetes, 2*(1), e26. doi:10.1038/nutd.2011.21

Rethink Obesity®. (2019). Setting SMART goals. https://www.rethinkobesity.com/talking-with-patients /setting-smart-weight-loss-goals.html

Trust for America's Health and Robert Wood Johnson Foundation. (2014). *Special Report: Racial and ethnic disparities in obesity.* https://stateofobesity.org/disparities/

Trust for America's Health and Robert Wood Johnson Foundation. (2018). *The healthcare costs of obesity.* https://stateofobesity.org/healthcare-costs-obesity/

Tseng, C. H., & Wu, C. Y. (2019). The gut microbiome in obesity. *Journal of the Formosan Medical Association, 118*, 53–59.

Vallerand, A., & Sanaski, C. (2020). *Davis's drug guide for nurses* (17th ed.). Philadelphia, PA: F.A. Davis.

Venes, D. (Ed.). (2017). *Taber's cyclopedic medical dictionary.* Philadelphia, PA: F.A. Davis.

Willis, L. M., & Rebar, C. (2018). Care of patients with malnutrition: Undernutrition and obesity. In D. D. Ignatavicius, M. L. Workman, & C. R. Rebar (Eds.), *Medical-surgical nursing: Concepts for interprofessional collaborative care* (9th ed.). St. Louis, MO: Elsevier.

World Health Organization. (2018). *Obesity and overweight* [Fact sheet]. http://www.who.int/mediacentre /factsheets/fs311/en/

Chapter 4

Irritable Bowel Syndrome and Inflammatory Bowel Disease

LEARNING OBJECTIVES

Upon completion of this section the student will be able to:

• Integrate knowledge of the physiology of intestinal mobility and digestion; the pathophysiology of irritable bowel syndrome (IBS) and inflammatory bowel disease (IBD); along with the assessment and nonpharmacological and pharmacological management for care of an adult patient with these conditions.

• Appraise current standards of care for adult individuals with IBS and IBD.

Introduction

Irritable bowel syndrome (IBS), a dysfunction of intestinal motility, is a commonly diagnosed condition afflicting an estimated 20% of American adults (Cromar, 2018a; Office on Women's Health [OWH], 2019). IBS symptoms are reported by 20% to 40% of all individuals who visit a gastroenterologist (International Foundation for Functional Gastrointestinal Disorders [IFFGD], 2016a). The condition is characterized by chronic impaired mobility and bowel habit alterations that include abdominal pain, diarrhea, and/or constipation without the presence of a structural cause of the symptoms (Buono, Carson, & Flores, 2017; Schub & Karakashian, 2018). Diagnosis is typically made following the exclusion of other conditions such as celiac disease, gluten intolerance, or food allergies (Williams, 2018). More women (60%–65%) than men (35%–40%) report IBS symptoms, with the onset of symptoms typically between ages 30–50 years (IFFGD, 2016a; OWH, 2019; World Gastroenterology Organization [WGO], 2015). The severity of symptoms varies, with mild symptoms being reported by 40% of IBS patients, while 35% report moderate symptoms and (25%) report more severe symptoms (IFFGD, 2016b).

The cost of IBS is difficult to estimate, because many adults do not seek medical help for their symptoms. However, the yearly number of visits to a health-care provider for IBS symptoms is estimated to be 2.4 to 3.5 million, with 12% of all primary care visits attributed to IBS symptoms. Additionally, GI specialists report that IBS is the most commonly diagnosed disorder in their practice (IFFGD, 2016b; Weinberg,

Smalley, Heidelbaugh, & Sultan, 2014). Taking both the costs of medical care for diagnosis, treatment, and follow-up of IBS symptoms and the indirect costs related to lost productivity and absenteeism in the workplace, IBS annual costs are estimated to be around $21 billion. Additionally, more women report IBS symptoms, and women with IBS symptoms are 47% to 55% more likely to undergo gynecological (hysterectomy or ovarian) surgery than their counterparts without IBS (IFFGD, 2016b). Women frequently report an increase in their IBS symptoms during menstruation, suggesting a hormonal component to the condition (Crohn's & Colitis Foundation of America [CCFA], 2014). IBS diagnosis is frequently delayed, as the diagnosis is determined by eliminating more serious conditions as a source of the patient's symptoms (Luthy, Larimer, & Freeborn, 2017; Williams, 2018). The psychosocial burdens on individuals, family, or caregivers while awaiting a diagnosis and of the ongoing and often activity-limiting symptoms experienced by the patient significantly impacts quality of life, and these intangible costs cannot be quantified in dollars (Buono et al., 2017).

Inflammatory bowel disease (IBD) occurs when the bowel walls become chronically inflamed and the *gastrointestinal* (GI) tract becomes damaged. The inflammatory process is progressive, with intermittent times of exacerbations of symptoms with subsequent periods of remission (Mehta, 2016). *Crohn's disease* (CD) presents as inflamed patches of intestinal wall that are adjacent to healthy intestinal walls. These patches can be found anywhere in the GI tract but are more commonly found in the small intestine. *Ulcerative colitis* (UC) presents as continuous inflammation that originates in the rectum and spreads upward throughout the colon. An estimated 3.1 million adults were diagnosed with IBD in 2015 (Centers for Disease Control and Prevention [CDC], 2019, March 21; Dahlhamer, Zammitti, Ward, Wheaton, & Croft, 2016). Statistics for that year revealed that IBD was more common in adults 45 years or older, in people who do not have a high school diploma or the equivalent, and in people who are unemployed and who live below the poverty level and are suburban dwellers. Ethnic groups most commonly diagnosed with IBD include those of Hispanic origin and European origin. Rates of IBD did not significantly differ based on the categories of sex, marital status, or region of the country, or by type of health-care insurance (Dahlhamer et al., 2016). Onset of Crohn's typically begins between the ages of 20 and 30, while onset of ulcerative colitis is most common between the ages of 30 and 40 (Mehta, 2016).

Although IBD was the eighth-leading cause of primary care visits in 2009, it was determined to be first in direct costs of treatment, particularly the costs of diagnosis, pharmacological interventions (both over the counter and prescription), and outpatient and hospital care, which were predicted to reach between $11 and $28 billion for the year 2014 (Mehta, 2016). More recent cost estimates suggest the yearly direct costs of CD are around $15.5 billion, while UC costs are similar and approach $14.9 billion (Click, Binion, & Anderson, 2017). Indirect costs are attributed to loss of productivity and time away from work and from leisure activities. As with IBS, those with an IBD diagnosis have psychosocial concerns related to impacts of delays in diagnosis, direct and indirect costs, and the impact on their family, friends, and caregivers. Lack of adequate coping strategies may lead to increased anxiety or depression, inability to adhere to the treatment regimen, increased costs related to complications, and, eventually, poor outcomes (Click et al., 2017; Cromar, 2018b). Accurate diagnosis and effective management of symptoms have been suggested to be the best way to decrease the costs of living with IBD (Mehta, 2016).

Thus, to provide patient-centered care based on best practice and outcomes, it is important to understand the physiology and pathophysiology of GI motility to accurately assess, diagnose and manage these common GI conditions.

Physiology

The function of the GI tract is to ingest and process food, absorb needed nutrients, and eliminate solid waste. The walls of the GI tract consist of five layers, as shown in Figure 4-1. The *inner* layer has two distinct types of cells that absorb electrolytes and fluids (columnar epithelial cells) and lubricate and protect the intestines by producing mucus (goblet cells). These cells live only a few days, at which time they shed and are digested as endogenous protein (Capriotti, 2020; Huether, 2012). The *submucosal*

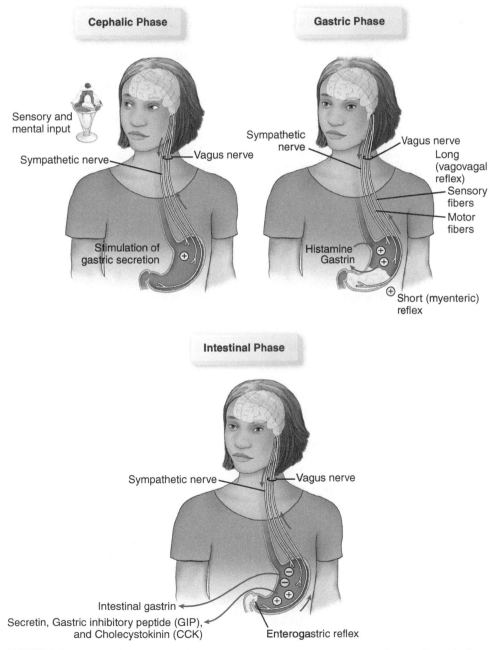

FIGURE 4–1 Anatomy of the GI tract *(From Hoffman, J. J., & Sullivan, N. J. (2020). Davis advantage for medical-surgical nursing (2nd ed.). Philadelphia, PA: F.A. Davis.*

(middle) layer consists of blood vessels, connective tissue, nerves, and structures that secrete digestive enzymes. The submucosal connective tissue (lamina propria) is responsible for production of immunoglobulins by its plasma cells and lymphocytes (Huether, 2012). *Peristalsis* is facilitated by the muscle layers (*circular* and *longitudinal*), while the outer layer (*peritoneum*) functions to loosely attach and cover the entire intestine (Capriotti, 2020).

The communication pathways between the autonomic, central, and enteric nervous systems and the hypothalamic-pituitary-adrenal axis is called the *brain-gut axis*. The coordination of these systems is key to effective facilitation of the digestive process. Disturbances in nerve innervation and impulse responsiveness or the amounts of amines, peptides, and peripheral hormones disrupt the normal function of these systems and may contribute to the underlying cause of infective gut motility (Weaver, Melkus, & Henderson, 2017). In the initial phase of gastric secretion (cephalic phase), the vagal nerve responds to both mental and sensory stimulation to initiate gastric secretion. In the second phase (gastric), the presence of food in the stomach triggers release of digestive enzymes. In the final (intestinal) phase, the duodenum responds to the production of chyme (partially digested food and digestive enzymes) by stimulating the release of gastrin in the intestine. As gastric acid and chyme enter the small intestine, signals from the duodenum initiate the inhibition of gastric secretion (Goodwin, 2017).

GI motility, the process of moving food and liquids through the digestive system, is controlled by hormonal influences along with innervation from the autonomic (parasympathetic and sympathetic) nervous system. Additionally, the *enteric nerve innervation* within the GI tract controls motility in two ways: the *myenteric plexus* controls motility of entire gut, while the *submucous plexus* controls motility in each segment of the colon, independent of other sections. The myenteric plexus has an additional role in secretion while the submucous plexus has a role in both absorption and secretion. Motility is stimulated by parasympathetic activity and inhibited by sympathetic activity. Parasympathetic activity also controls pain sensation, intestinal relaxation, and secretion in the intestinal tract (Capriotti, 2020; Huether, 2012).

Chyme is moved through the intestine in a coordinated kneading and mixing process. The autonomic nervous system triggers the circular smooth muscles of the intestinal wall to contract and relax in a coordinated way (*haustrations*) that allows for bacteria accumulation and electrolytes and water to be absorbed. The mucosal folds formed by the smooth muscles slow progress of intestinal contents and are covered with villi and microvilli, which secrete enzymes that enhance absorption of nutrients. The villi move as short sections of smooth muscles contract (*peristalsis*), further enhancing the digestive process. While the stomach and colon absorb some water, the majority of all water (85%–90%) is absorbed in the small intestine, which is also responsible for absorption of carbohydrates, fats, minerals, proteins, and vitamins (Capriotti, 2020; Huether, 2012).

Bulk movement of intestinal contents is typically initiated after eating as the contraction of a large portion of the intestine propels contents forward (*propulsion*). These contractions occur periodically throughout the day and last about 10 to 30 minutes to move fecal contents along to the sigmoid colon and then into the rectum, where the feces are expelled from the body. The gastrocolic reflex, which controls the awareness of one's need to defecate, is accelerated by parasympathetic stimulation and the enzymes cholecystokinin and gastrin (relaxes the internal anal sphincter) and inhibited by sympathetic stimulation with epinephrine (contracts the internal anal sphincter). Sympathetic innervation is responsible for large intestine feelings of pain and fullness (Capriotti, 2020; Huether, 2012).

Microorganisms of the intestines play an important role in the digestive process. The large intestine has no flora at birth, and it takes about 3 to 4 weeks for a normal distribution of intestinal bacteria to develop. Acids keep the stomach relatively bacteria free; in the duodenum, production of antibodies, secretion of bile acids, and intestinal motility work together to inhibit bacterial growth (Huether, 2012). The largest proportion of bacteria is found in the large intestine where bacteria are responsible for breaking down unabsorbed proteins (amino acids) into ammonia, which is transported to the liver to be changed to urea. Colon bacteria also change unabsorbed carbohydrates into organic acids that can be absorbed by the body, and they absorb bile and help in the metabolism of some hormones (androgens and estrogens) and lipids. Approximately one-third of the feces bulk is bacteria and 95% of colon bacteria are anaerobic, with the most common types being anaerobic lactobacilli, *Bacteroides*, *Clostridia*, and *Escherichia coli* (Capriotti, 2020; Huether, 2012).

Bacterial fermentation generates gas in the intestinal tract and this, along with the gas ingested by swallowing, which can be as much as 500 mL during a meal, creates bowel sounds (borborygmic). Gas is eliminated through burping (eructation) or by passing from the rectum as flatus (Capriotti, 2020). Dysfunction of any of the steps of digestion can result in signs and symptoms that range from mild to severe and can be attributed to a variety of GI conditions including IBS or IBD.

Pathophysiology

The differentiation between GI conditions is often difficult to make because of the similarity in symptoms, and accurate diagnosis requires a systematic assessment to successfully identify the source of GI symptoms. IBS symptoms are often similar to those of *lactose intolerance* (LI) and are characterized by psychological and physiological variables. The symptoms are related to changes in peristaltic activity involved in digestion. In contrast, symptoms of Crohn's disease and ulcerative colitis, both IBD, are more severe and are the result of pathological changes in the immune system that lead to inflammation in the intestines (Crohn's & Colitis Foundation, 2019a; Weaver et al., 2017; Wehkamp, Götz, Herrlinger, Steurer, & Stange, 2016). Table 4-1 provides a comparison of the pathological findings in IBS and IBD.

Irritable Bowel Syndrome (IBS)

While the underlying pathology of IBS is not clearly understood, there are several different mechanisms that are thought to contribute to the symptoms that are the result of changes in bowel patterns with chronic abdominal pain. Symptoms may occur as constipation (IBS-C), diarrhea (IBS-D), or fluctuation between both. A heightened

TABLE 4–1   Comparison of Pathological Findings in IBS and IBD

Irritable Bowel Syndrome (IBS)	Crohn's Disease	Ulcerative Colitis

No pathological findings	Lesions found anywhere in GI tract
	    Skip lesions
	    Cobblestoning
	    Transmural (entire wall thickness involved)
	    Anal fistulas and fissure
	    No increased risk for colorectal cancer
		Lesions in large intestine progressing from rectum upward
		    Pseudopolyps
		    Mucosa and submucosal involvement
		    No anal fistulas or fissures
		    Increased risk for colorectal cancer

(Capriotti, 2020; CCFA, 2019a; CCFA, 2019b; OWH, 2018; Weaver et al., 2017)

visceral sensitivity may be attributed to dysfunction of the brain-gut axis, which changes how nociceptive information is processed and leads to changes in intestinal motility (diarrhea, constipation, or both). It is thought that brain-gut axis changes could be related to genetics, intestinal infection, or stress (Drossman, 2013; Weaver et al., 2017). There is some correlation between anxiety, depression, and stress and brain-gut axis dysfunction associated with IBS (Anastasi, 2013; Capriotti, 2020; Cromar, 2018a; Dudley-Brown & Huether, 2012).

IBS is diagnosed in some individuals who have recently experienced a bout of infectious gastroenteritis, linking inflammation and alteration of mucosal immune function to IBS symptoms. It is also thought that gut microflora alterations lead to an overgrowth of small intestine bacteria and excessive fermentation of intestinal contents, which then leads to the bloating and constipation symptoms of IBS (Anastasi, 2013). Another suggested association with IBS is the presence of a food allergy or intolerance of certain foods such as those containing gluten, beverages that contain carbonation or caffeine, and dairy products (Anastasi, 2013; Capriotti, 2020; Cromar, 2018a; Dudley-Brown & Huether, 2012). Celiac disease is an autoimmune disease that develops because the small intestine does not tolerate gluten and may present with IBS symptoms. Removal of gluten from the diet may significantly reduce symptoms (Luthy et al., 2017). An inadequate amount of the enzyme lactase in the presence of foods that contain lactose also leads to GI symptoms of boating, gas, abdominal discomfort, and diarrhea. LI symptoms are most commonly experienced after eating foods and liquids containing lactose. While LI generally begins in childhood, the presence of lactase declines as one ages, leading to the development of these symptoms in adults. In contrast, irritable bowel symptoms are typically worse in the morning and after meals and may not be connected to the presence of inadequate lactose enzyme secretion (Luthy et al., 2017).

Inflammatory Bowel Disease (IBD)

Crohn's disease is a slowly progressive inflammatory disease of exacerbations and remissions. While the inflammatory changes of CD (or regional enteritis) can occur anywhere in the GI tract, they are most commonly found in the ascending right colon and the terminal ileum. Inflammation of the bowel wall mucosa extends throughout the submucosal layers. Crohn's lesions are segmental, reddish-purple, and edematous patches of inflamed tissue that are interspersed between healthy areas of tissue (*skip lesions*) (Capriotti, 2020; Crohn's & Colitis Foundation, 2019a; Cromar, 2018b; Davis, Robinson, Vess, & Lebel, 2018). As the lesions become more inflamed, fissures form and fistulas and abscesses develop. Chronic inflammation causes enlargement in the adjacent lymph nodes, granulomas (*inflammatory cobblestoning*) develop, the bowel tissues become fibrotic and scarred, and thickened bowel walls create a narrowed lumen and shorten the colon, impairing digestion and absorption of nutrients (Capriotti, 2020). Presence of lesions in the small intestine severely impact absorption of nutrients, leading to malnourishment and debilitation (Cromar, 2018b).

UC is also an inflammatory bowel disease of exacerbation and remissions that is caused by abnormal immune system response that identifies intestinal bacteria and food as foreign material. However, in contrast to the sporadic lesions of Crohn's, the lesions of UC are widespread, beginning in the rectum and extending upward through the colon as the disease progresses. Inflammation of the colon's lining causes the intestinal goblet cells to secrete mucus, although as the disease progresses, the number of goblet cells diminishes, and affected tissues become edematous, reddened, and hyperemic (Capriotti, 2020; Crohn's & Colitis Foundation, 2019b; Cromar, 2018b; Davis et al., 2018).

Excessive blood flow to inflamed areas leads to erosions, ulceration of the mucosa, and bleeding. A cycle of ulceration, granulation tissue formation, and inflammation of granulation tissue develops, leading to continuous areas of inflammation and overgrowth of tissue (*pseudopolyps*), which are characteristic of UC. Necrotic tissue develops as ulcerated areas abscess (*crypt abscess*), intestinal walls thicken, and the intestinal lumen narrows (Cromar, 2018b).

Toxic megacolon is an emergency complication of IBD. As IBD progresses, intestinal nerves are damaged, motility is impaired, and the colon can become paralyzed (*ileus*). Next, the colon dilates, obstructs the flow of bowel contents, inhibits absorption of nutrients, and may lead to bowel perforation and peritonitis.

CLINICAL PEARLS

Another complication of IBD is the risk for colorectal cancer, as bowel changes cause the development of precancerous lesions in the intestinal wall (Capriotti, 2020; Cromar, 2018b).

Risk Factors

Risk factors for IBS include age (typical onset between 30 and 50 years), gender (women at greater risk than men), family history, personal history of gastroenteritis, symptoms in the presence of dietary triggers (dairy, fructose, sorbitol, wheat), and psychological issues, including anxiety, depression, and childhood adversity (CCFA, 2014). While IBD is typically diagnosed in early adulthood, gender is not a significant risk factor. Ethnicity, education level, family history, and socioeconomic factors (poverty or suburban living) are the most prevalent risk factors for developing IBD. Additionally, CD is associated with a history of smoking (CDC, 2019; CCFA, 2014).

Assessment

The nurse must understand the complex presentations of the signs and symptoms of gastrointestinal diseases and the difficulty many patients have in accurately describing how their daily lives are affected. Abdominal symptoms may be mild to severe and may be caused by conditions other than GI disease, making the comprehensive assessment an important foundation of accurate diagnosis and treatment. The assessment for all individuals with GI symptoms begins with a comprehensive health history including general history, past medical history, family history, nutritional history, current symptoms, and self-management interventions. This is followed by a physical examination (Goolsby & Grubbs, 2015), as described in SENC Box 4-1 (Capriotti, 2020). The order of the abdominal examination is important for an accurate assessment.

SENC BOX 4-1   Safe and Effective Nursing Care for the Order of Steps for Abdominal Examination

1. Conduct a general inspection of the abdomen for signs of distension, asking patient to identify any painful areas.
2. Auscultate for bowel sounds proceeding from pain-free areas to painful or tender areas.
3. Percuss for abnormal tones (dullness indicates air has been replaced with fluid or solid tissue).
4. Palpate for any guarding, rigidity, or tenderness, proceeding from pain-free areas to painful or tender areas.

Finally, a digital rectal examination helps identify the presence of fissures or hemorrhoids, and the presence of occult blood in any feces that may be in the rectum (Goolsby & Grubbs, 2015).

Additional laboratory or diagnostic tests may be ordered based on assessment findings. Classification of diarrhea symptoms is an important component of the assessment for IBS and IBD and is based on the severity of diarrhea, absence or presence of blood in the stool, and presence and severity of other symptoms (Cromar, 2018b; Davis et al., 2018).

Individuals with IBS present with abdominal bloating, fullness, discomfort/pain, and/or flatulence, and they describe an alteration in their bowel habits (constipation, diarrhea, or alternating constipation and diarrhea) for at least 3 months. Typically, symptoms of pain are relieved once the patient has had a bowel movement (Goolsby & Grubbs, 2015; OWH, 2019). Women may experience an increase in their IBS symptoms during menstruation (OWH, 2019).

Because IBS is a functional, not pathological condition, diagnostic evaluation has a primary goal of ruling out pathological conditions. Diagnostic testing includes endoscopic evaluation of the GI tract, abdominal *computed tomography* (CT) or ultrasound, and a hydrogen breath test to exclude fructose or lactose intolerance as contributors to IBS symptoms (Capriotti, 2020). The Rome IV criteria is used, along with diagnostic tests, to confirm IBS based on symptoms. IBS symptoms must be present for at least 6 months and also present within the last three months and occur at least once a week. Abdominal pain must be related to defecation and associated with changes in frequency and form, which is categorized using the Bristol Stool Form Scale. IBS subtypes are based on the type of stool—*IBS-C* (constipation), *IBS-D* (diarrhea), or *IBS-M* (mixed)—and treatment is based on the particular subtype diagnosed (Goolsby & Grubbs, 2015; Weaver et al., 2017).

Symptoms of IBD vary according to the severity of the onset. In UC, continuous abdominal cramping and pain accompany severe, frequent, and often bloody diarrhea. The bleeding and fluid loss of persistent diarrhea, along with chronic inflammation, lead to anemia, dehydration, fever, and weight loss (CCFA, 2014; Dudley-Brown & Huether, 2012). In contrast, symptoms of CD may not appear early in the disease process and will vary according to the location of bowel inflammation. However, as in UC, abdominal pain and weight loss are common in CD. Diarrhea is the most frequent symptom of UC and CD, and rectal bleeding accompanies involvement of the colon. Deficiencies of vitamin D and folic acid and resultant anemia accompany disease in the ileum. Both types of IBD have periods of exacerbations and remissions and, over time, lead to comorbidities including liver dysfunction, altered coagulation, and polyarthritis (Dudley-Brown & Huether, 2012). Symptoms of CD and UC are highlighted in Table 4-2.

TABLE 4–2   Comparison of Symptoms in IBS and IBD

Irritable Bowel Syndrome (IBS)	Crohn's Disease	Ulcerative Colitis
• Abdominal cramps/pain relieved with bowel movements • Diarrhea/constipation or a mixture often occurring after eating • Sensations of inability to completely evacuate the bowel	• Abdominal cramps/pain • Persistent diarrhea • Sensations of urgency and inability to completely evacuate the bowel • Rectal bleeding	• Abdominal cramps/pain • Urgent, persistent diarrhea with progressively looser stools • Bloody stools • Loss of appetite • Weight loss

(Anastasi et al., 2013; Crohn's & Colitis Foundation, 2019a,b; Luthy et al., 2017)

Laboratory testing for IBD includes a *complete blood count* (CBC), renal and hepatic function panels, and tests for inflammation. Stool analysis is performed to rule out infectious disease, particularly that caused by *Clostridium difficile* (Wehkamp et al., 2016). The gold standard test for a differential diagnosis of IBD is endoscopic evaluation with intestinal wall biopsies and laboratory tests in addition to a comprehensive health history and physical examination. For those with suspected CD, the colonoscopy includes examination of the terminal ileum, along with a capsule endoscopy or small bowel series, because CD may begin anywhere in the GI tract (Davis et al., 2018; Dudley-Brown & Huether, 2012; Wehkamp et al., 2016).

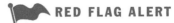 **RED FLAG ALERT**

Some symptoms suggest serious disease, including iron deficiency anemia, rectal bleeding, nocturnal diarrhea, weight loss, and family history of celiac disease, colorectal cancer, or IBD. Individuals with these symptoms are typically referred to a gastroenterologist for colonoscopy (OWH, 2019).

ASSESSMENT PEARLS
Patients with IBS or IBD often report other symptoms including anxiety, depression, and fatigue. Patients with IBD may also report fever, loss of appetite, night sweats, and weight loss.

Nonpharmacological Management

Dietary modifications are often prescribed to treat IBS and IBD because some symptoms are associated with particular foods. Avoiding the foods that trigger symptoms is an important part of self-management of these chronic conditions. Individuals are encouraged to avoid caffeine, carbonated drinks, alcohol, spicy foods, or foods known to contribute to bloating and gas such as beans, broccoli, or cabbage (CCFA, 2014). IBS symptoms are often relieved by making dietary changes. Health-care providers may prescribe a diet low in glutens, lactose, and fermentable sugars (disaccharides, monosaccharides, oligosaccharides, and polyols), commonly referred to as FODMAPs. Avoidance of foods high in sugar content has been shown to decrease fermentation and osmosis within the gut, thus decreasing bloating, diarrhea, and abdominal pain (Weaver et al., 2017; Williams, 2018).

Pharmacology

Pharmacological management of IBS is based on the severity of abdominal pain and the type of bowel symptoms (constipation or diarrhea). Pain is treated using antispasmodics, selective serotonin reuptake inhibitors, tricyclic antidepressants or peppermint oil. The focus of *IBS-C* treatment is on decreasing constipation and includes the use of chloride channel activators, guanylate cyclase-C agonists, polyethylene glycol, or psyllium. The focus of *IBS-D* treatment is on controlling diarrhea and may include use of antibiotics, bile acid sequestrants, mixed opioid receptor modulators, opioid agonists, probiotics, or serotonin-3 agonists (Weaver, 2016). One of the most commonly prescribed medications used to treat IBS-D is dicyclomine hydrochloride (Buono et al., 2017).

The antibiotic rifaximin is approved by the U.S. Food and Drug Administration (FDA) for use in IBS, as it has been shown to be helpful in reducing IBS symptoms in some patients (Drossman, 2013). Examples of drugs used to treat IBS are found in Table 4-3. Pharmacological interventions for IBD are chosen to control inflammation, diarrhea, pain, and anemia that may result from GI bleeding. Drugs to treat UC and CD are similar and include a combination of antidiarrheals, aminosalicylates, glucocorticoids, and immunomodulators (Cromar, 2018b). Examples from each drug class are found in Table 4-4.

TABLE 4–3   Drugs Used to Treat IBS

Class	Example	Action	Dosage	SENC
Serotonin 5 HT$_3$ antagonist	Alosetron hydrochloride	Blocks serotonin receptors to decrease pain perception in the GI tract, decreased GI motility, and increases transit time of colon contents	Initial: 0.5 mg bid to 1 mg bid Maintenance: 0.5 mg to 1 mg daily	Used for IBS-D: women only. Black box warning: discontinue with symptoms of constipation or ischemic colitis.
Chloride channel activator	Lubiprostone	Increase chloride in intestinal secretions with changing chloride/potassium balance; softens stool, increases GI motility.	8 mcg bid	Used for IBS-C in adults. Take with food to decrease nausea. Report diarrhea.
Anticholinergic/antispasmodic	Hyoscyamine	Decreases GI spasms.	0.125 mg 30–60 min before meals; max dose 1.5 mg/24 hr.	Antacids decrease drug absorption; take them at least 1 hr after taking hyoscyamine.
	Dicyclomine hydrochloride	Decreases GI motility and smooth muscle tone.	10–20 mg tid to qid, max dose of 160 mg/day.	Assess for urinary retention and constipation. Take 30 min–1 hr before meals.
Antidepressant	Amitriptyline	Antidepressant and anticholinergic effects	Up to 75 mg/day in divided doses	May be helpful for some patients with IBS. Take 30–40 min before meals.
Antibiotics	Rifaximin	Decreases bloating and distention of IBS; decreases diarrhea severity.	550 mg tid for 14 days.	Off label use for IBS-D; at risk for *C. difficile* up to several weeks after use.
Antidiarrheals	Loperamide	Inhibits peristalsis, decreases volume and increases viscosity of feces; decreases fluid and electrolyte loss associated with diarrhea.	4 mg initial dose; 2 mg following each loose stool up to 8 mg/day (OTC) and 16 mg/day if prescribed.	IBS-D; may cause dry mouth; take only as directed and instruct not to exceed recommended dose.
Fiber supplements	Psyllium	Increase bulk of stool.	1 tsp or 1 packet in cold water 1–3 times a day.	Used for IBS-C. Indicated for short-term use.

(Crohn's and Colitis Foundation, 2019a,b; Karch, 2013; Vallerand & Sanoski, 2017; Woo, 2020)
   OTC, over the counter

Surgical Management

Conservative treatment of IBD may eventually fail, leading to surgical removal of inflamed and necrotic portions of the colon. Colostomy or ileostomy is performed based on the location of damage (Capriotti, 2020; Wehkamp et al., 2016). Currently, these procedures may be minimally invasive, which decreases recovery time and minimizes postoperative pain (Wehkamp et al., 2016). Preoperative education and planning

TABLE 4–4   Drugs Used to Treat Inflammatory Bowel Disease

Class	Example	Action	Dosage	SENC
Aminosalicylates	Sulfasalazine	In the colon produces local anti-inflammatory effects; reduces symptoms.	Initial 500 mg every 6–12 hr; up to 1 g every 6–12 hr. Maintenance: 500 mg every 6 hr.	Used for UC. Assess for sulfonamide and salicylate allergy. Monitor for blood dyscrasias (CBC with differential and liver function tests).
Glucocorticoids	Prednisolone	Inhibit the inflammatory response by decreasing leukotriene and prostaglandin production.	5–60 mg /day.	Caution: may suppress signs/symptoms of infection.
Immunomodulators	Azathioprine	Suppresses immunity and antibody formation by inhibiting synthesis of DNA and RNA.	50 mg daily, may increase by 25 mg/day over 1–2 weeks with a max dose of 2–3 mg/kg/day.	Used in CD and UC. Caution: teratogenic properties; avoid exposure to live viruses or infectious diseases.
Biological response modulators	Infliximab Adalimumab	Anti-inflammatory response by inhibiting tumor necrosis factor-alpha (TNF-alpha), used to help heal fistulas of CD.	IV: initial dose 5 mg/kg; repeat at 2 and 6 weeks; maintenance 5 mg/kg every 8 weeks.	Used for CD when other drugs fail to control symptoms. Monitor for signs/symptoms of infection.
Antibiotics	metronidazole	Inhibits protein synthesis; used with anaerobic bacterial caused infections.	250–500 mg tid to qid for 10–14 days.	Treatment of diarrhea caused by *C. difficile*. Caution: increases risk of Stevens-Johnson syndrome.

(Crohn's & Colitis Foundation, 2019a,b; Vallerand & Sanoski, 2017; Woo, 2020)
    CBC, complete blood count; TNF, tumor necrosis factor

are essential components of the plan of care for the IBD patient who must undergo ostomy procedures. A consultation with the *certified wound ostomy care nurse* (CWOCN) is an essential adjunct to learning self-management techniques following surgery.

Complementary and Alternative Therapies (CAT)

Some studies indicate that the presence of *bifidobacteria* in the intestinal tract decreases bloating and gas, and that addition of probiotics containing these helpful bacteria to the diet may be effective in relieving abdominal distension in some cases of IBS (Drossman, 2013; Weaver et al., 2017). Another dietary supplement that may help IBS symptoms is peppermint oil, which acts to block calcium channels and may act as an antispasmodic to relieve abdominal

HIGH YIELD FACT FOR TESTING

Planning for the perception of an altered body image and how to care for the ostomy, understanding dietary constraints, and knowing how to obtain supplies are all part of the preoperative planning (Cromar, 2018b).

pain. It is best consumed as an enteric-coated peppermint oil capsule, as the oil causes heartburn and the enteric coating delays absorption (Anastasi, 2013).

Moderate physical exercise has been shown to improve IBS symptoms, and individuals with IBS who practice yoga have decreased severity of symptoms, decreased anxiety, and improved quality of life. Individuals with IBS or IBD are encouraged to incorporate at least 30 minutes of physical exercise into their daily routine at least 5 times a week (CCFA, 2014).

Use of other complementary therapies such as acupuncture or moxibustion (heat application) has demonstrated mixed results. Individuals who participate in educational sessions to learn self-management strategies (diet, relaxation, and cognitive-behavior modifications) are more successful in managing symptoms, have fewer symptoms over time, and report an improved quality of life (Anastasi, 2013; Weaver et al., 2016).

Summary

Abdominal pain and altered intestinal motility impact the individual through direct care costs and indirect costs and are life-altering conditions. Because the symptoms of IBS and IBD may be similar in the early stages of disease, a delay in diagnosis causes increased stress both to the individual and to those around them. Understanding the underlying causes and risk factors for these common GI conditions is a key to early diagnosis and initiation of appropriate interventions. IBS and IBD are chronic diseases requiring a partnership between the health-care provider and patient that includes acknowledgment by providers of the role of stress on symptoms, along with open communication and agreement on a treatment plan for effective management of symptoms (Best, 2015). Ongoing assessment of the individual's understanding of their disease process and their ability to self-manage a chronic condition are important components of the diagnostic and follow-up care of both IBS and IBD (Davis et al., 2018).

Key Points

- Irritable bowel syndrome is a noninflammatory, functional disorder of gastrointestinal motility presenting with abdominal pain and diarrhea, constipation, or a mixture of the two extremes of bowel function without pathological changes in the GI mucosa.
- Inflammatory bowel disease presents with abdominal pain and diarrhea with either continuous inflammation starting in the rectum and progressing upward (ulcerative colitis) or as inflamed patches of intestinal wall at any point in the intestines (Crohn's).
- While assessment and diagnostic testing are similar for IBS and IBD, accurate diagnosis relies on intestinal wall biopsies collected during endoscopic procedures.
- Treatment of IBS and IBD takes a comprehensive approach to managing symptoms, including pharmacological and complementary therapies.

Review Questions

1. **The patient who is newly diagnosed with Crohn's disease asks the nurse why they need to take a vitamin D supplement. Which of the following statements is the nurse's best response?**

    a. "Crohn's disease does not impair absorption of vitamins, so supplements are not needed."

    b. "Chronic irritation causes scarring of the abdominal wall, which impairs absorption of nutrients."

c. "You only need to take a vitamin supplement if your disease progresses upward from the rectum."

d. "You will not need a vitamin supplement if you can control your diarrhea with other medications."

2. **When conducting a physical assessment of the abdomen, which of the following is correct?**

a. Auscultating bowel sounds after percussion and palpation ensures an accurate assessment.

b. Beginning with inspection, proceed to auscultation moving from pain-free to painful areas.

c. Palpation of unpainful areas should proceed auscultation in order to have an accurate assessment.

d. Percussion of the abdomen from right upper quadrant to left lower quadrant before auscultation.

3. **The primary goal of diagnostic assessment of irritable bowel syndrome is to:**

a. Choose the appropriate immunomodulator to treat diarrhea.

b. Determine which portion of the colon has developed ulcerations.

c. Identify the cause of the patient's vitamin deficiency.

d. Rule out underlying pathological causes of symptoms.

4. **When discussing dietary alterations for the patient with IBS or IBD, which of the following foods should be avoided? (Select all that apply.)**

a. Alcohol

b. Broccoli

c. Carbonated sodas

d. Cabbage

e. Low-fat dairy foods

5. **The patient with IBS tells the nurse that someone has suggested the use of peppermint oil to help with their abdominal pain. Which of the following statements does the nurse include in her response?**

a. "Acupuncture would be a better option for relieving abdominal cramps associated with IBS."

b. "Peppermint oil taken as an enteric-coated capsule may be useful in relieving abdominal cramping."

c. "There are no known dietary supplements that have been shown to help with IBS symptoms."

d. "Use of any type of peppermint oil is not recommended for IBS symptoms."

See the appendix for answers to review questions.

References

Anastasi, J. K. (2013). Managing irritable bowel syndrome. *American Journal of Nursing, 113*(7), 42–52.

Best, C. (2015). Examining the extent to which stress contributes to disease in the gastrointestinal tract: A literature review. *Gastrointestinal Nursing, 13*(2), 16–21.

Buono, J. L., Carson, R. T., & Flores, N. M. (2017). Health-related quality of life, work productivity, and indirect costs among individuals with irritable bowel syndrome with diarrhea. *Health and Quality of Life Outcomes, 15*(35). doi:10.1186/s12955-017-0611-2

Capriotti, T. (2020). *Pathophysiology: Introductory concepts and clinical perspectives* (2nd ed.). Philadelphia, PA: F.A. Davis.

Centers for Disease Control and Prevention. (2019, March 21). *Inflammatory bowel disease (IBD)*. https://www.cdc.gov/ibd/data-statistics.htm

Click, B., Binion, D. G., & Anderson, A. M. (2017). Predicting costs of care for individuals with inflammatory bowel diseases. *Clinical Gastroenterology and Hepatology, 15*(3), 393–395.

Crohn's & Colitis Foundation of America. (2014). Inflammatory bowel disease and irritable bowel syndrome: Similarities and differences. http://www.crohnscolitisfoundation.org/assets/pdfs/ibd-and-irritable-bowel.pdf

Crohn's & Colitis Foundation. (2019a). What is Crohn's disease? www.crohnscolitisfoundation.org/what-are-crohns-and-colitis/what-is-crohns-disease/

Crohn's & Colitis Foundation. (2019b). What is ulcerative colitis? http://www.crohnscolitisfoundation.org/what-are-crohns-and-colitis/what-is-ulcerative-colitis/

Cromar, K. (2018a). Care of patients with non-inflammatory intestinal disorders. In D. D. Ignatavicius, L. Workman, & C. R. Rebar (Eds.), *Medical-surgical nursing: Concepts for interprofessional collaborative care* (9th ed.). St. Louis, MO: Elsevier.

Cromar, K. (2018b). Care of patients with inflammatory intestinal disorders. In D. D. Ignatavicius, L. Workman, & C. R. Rebar (Eds.), *Medical-surgical nursing: Concepts for interprofessional collaborative care* (9th ed.). St. Louis, MO: Elsevier.

Dahlhamer, J. M., Zammitti, E. P., Ward, B. W., Wheaton, A. G., & Croft, J. B. (2016, Oct. 28). Prevalence of inflammatory bowel disease among adults aged ≥ 18 years—United States, 2015. *Morbidity and Mortality Weekly Report, 65*(42), 1166–1169. https://www.cdc.gov/mmwr/volumes/65/wr/mm6542a3.htm

Davis, S. C., Robinson, B. L., Vess, J., & Lebel, J. S. (2018). Primary care management of ulcerative colitis. *The Nurse Practitioner, 43*(1), 19.

Drossman, D. (2013). Irritable bowel syndrome (IBS). *International Foundation for Functional Gastrointestinal Disorders* [IFFGD].

Dudley-Brown, S., & Huether, S. E. (2012). Alterations of digestive function. In S. E. Huether & K. L. McCance (Eds.), *Understanding pathophysiology* (5th ed.). St. Louis, MO: Elsevier Mosby.

Goodwin, J. (2017). Assessment of gastrointestinal function. In J. J. Hoffman & N. J. Sullivan (Eds.), *Medical-surgical nursing: Making connections to practice* (pp. 1195–1216). Philadelphia, PA: F.A. Davis.

Goolsby, M. J., & Grubbs, L. (2015). *Advanced assessment: Interpreting findings and formulating differential diagnoses* (3rd ed.). Philadelphia, PA: FA Davis.

Hoffman, J. J., & Sullivan, N. J. (2020). *Davis advantage for medical-surgical nursing* (2nd ed.). Philadelphia, PA: F.A. Davis.

Huether, S. E. (2012). Structure and function of the digestive system. In S. E. Huether & K. L. McCance (Eds.), *Understanding pathophysiology* (5th ed.). St. Louis, MO: Elsevier Mosby.

International Foundation for Functional Gastrointestinal Disorders. (2016a). *Facts about IBS.* https://www.aboutibs.org/what-is-ibs/facts-about-ibs-2.html

International Foundation for Functional Gastrointestinal Disorders. (2016b). *Facts about IBS: Statistics.* https://www.aboutibs.org/facts-about-ibs/statistics.html

Karch, A. M. (2013). *Focus on nursing pharmacology* (6th ed.). Philadelphia, PA: Wolters Kluwer/Lippincott Williams & Wilkins.

Luthy, K. E., Larimer, S. G., & Freeborn, D. S. (2017). Differentiating between lactose intolerance, celiac disease, and irritable bowel syndrome-diarrhea. *The Journal for Nurse Practitioners, 13*(5), 348–353.

Mehta, F. (2016). Economic implications of inflammatory bowel disease and its management. *The American Journal of Managed Care, 22*(3), S51–S60.

Office on Women's Health. (2019, April 1). Irritable bowel syndrome. https://www.womenshealth.gov/a-z-topics/irritable-bowel-syndrome

Schub, T., & Karakashian, A. L. (2018, April 20). Irritable bowel syndrome. *CINAHL nursing guide.* EBSCO Publishing, Ipswich, Massachusetts.

Vallerand, A. H., & Sanoski, C. A. (Eds.). (2020). *Davis's drug guide for nurses* (17th ed.). Philadelphia, PA: F.A. Davis.

Weaver, K. R., Melkus, G. D., & Henderson, W. A. (2017). Irritable bowel syndrome. *American Journal of Nursing, 117*(6), 48–55.

Wehkamp, J., Götz, M., Herrlinger, K., Steurer, W., & Stange, E. F. (2016). Inflammatory bowel disease: Chrohn's disease and ulcerative colitis. *Deutsches Ärzteblatt International, 113*, 72–82. doi:10.3238/arztebl.2016.0072

Weinberg, D. S., Smalley, W., Heidelbaugh, J. J., & Sultan, S. (2014). American Gastroenterological Association Institute guideline on the pharmacological management of irritable bowel syndrome. *Gastroenterology, 147*, 146–148. http://dx.doi.org/10.1053/j.gastro.2014.09.001

Williams, M. (2018). Irritable bowel syndrome: The latest thinking. *Journal of Community Nursing, 32*(1), 28–33.

World Gastroenterology Organization. (2015). *Irritable bowel syndrome: A global perspective.* http://www.worldgastroenterology.org/UserFiles/file/guidelines/irritable-bowel-syndrome-english-2015.pdf

Woo, T.M. (2020). Drugs affecting the gastrointestinal system. In T. M. Woo & M. V. Robinson, *Pharmacotherapeutics for advanced practice nurse prescribers* (5th ed.). Philadelphia, PA: F.A. Davis.

Myocardial Infarction

LEARNING OBJECTIVES

Upon completion of this section the student will be able to:

- Integrate knowledge of the physiology, pathophysiology, assessment, and nonpharmacological and pharmacological management of myocardial infarction into planning care.
- Appraise current standards of care for patients with a myocardial infarction.

Introduction

Myocardial infarction (MI) is defined as the "loss of living heart muscle as a result of coronary artery occlusion" (Venes, 2021, p. 1239). The annual U.S. incidence of MI is approximately 1.5 million and continues to increase; while the age-adjusted mortality rate is decreasing, the number of MI deaths in the United States has not decreased, and it is fatal in more than one-third of cases. With more than 8 million survivors of MI living in the United States, nurses must understand the complex care of this disease in the acute and rehabilitative phases (Campion, Anderson, & Morrow, 2017; Davies, 2016; Hoffman & Sullivan, 2020; Norton, 2017). While the initial injury is to the heart muscle, multiple systems are often impacted by this event (cardiovascular, renal, and respiratory) (Capriotti, 2020; Hoffman & Sullivan, 2020).

Atherosclerotic cardiovascular disease (ASCVD), caused by plaque buildup in arterial walls (especially the coronary arteries), often leads to the following conditions: *coronary heart disease* (CHD), MI, angina, and coronary artery stenosis (American College of Cardiology [ACC], 2017; American Heart Association [AHA], 2017; Capriotti, 2020). ASCVD remains the leading cause of mortality and major morbidity in the United States. Its incidence increases with each decade of life after 45 years of age, independent of other factors such as sex and racial/ethnic groups. According to the AHA, *coronary artery disease* (CAD) prevalence is higher in European American men than in African American and Hispanic American men (7.7%, 7.1%, and 5.9%, respectively). Among women, Hispanic American women have the highest prevalence rate, followed by African American and European American women (6.1%, 5.7%, and 5.3%, respectively). Across men and women, the prevalence of CAD in Native Americans and Alaskan Natives is estimated to be highest of all groups at 9.3% (AHA, 2017; Hoffman & Sullivan, 2020).

As nurses plan care with patients, they often encounter older adults who have modifiable risk factors, including elevated blood pressure, dyslipidemia, smoking, and diabetes (Hoffman & Sullivan, 2020). By using tools and guidelines, such as the Million Hearts Initiative, which has the goal of preventing 1 million MIs and strokes, the nurse implements preventive therapies, including prophylactic aspirin, antihypertensive medications, statins, and/or smoking cessation (Lloyd-Jones et al., 2017).

First, it is necessary to focus on the pathophysiology of MI so the nurse can accurately assess the risk factors and intervene, based on an individualized evaluation. The term *myocardial infarction* refers to the destruction of heart muscle that results from ischemia (lack of oxygenated blood supply) to the myocardium (heart muscle). While an MI can occur from a variety of conditions and/or events that results in myocardial ischemia, the most common cause of MI is obstruction of the coronary arteries due to atherosclerosis (Capriotti, 2020; Hoffman & Sullivan, 2020). Atherosclerosis is the gradual buildup of plaque along arterial walls; a rupture of this plaque results in thrombus formation and resulting obstruction of coronary artery flow. With impaired oxygenation to the myocardium, there is ischemia and death of heart muscle. Pharmacological management of the patient with an MI follows specific guidelines developed by the ACC and AHA but must be individualized to address specific risk factors, both modifiable and nonmodifiable (ACC, 2017; AHA, 2017). Nonpharmacological strategies may also be effective in promoting both acute recovery and sustainability of a return to or adoption of an active lifestyle (ACC, 2017; Stone et al., 2014; Thygesen et al., 2012).

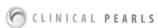 CLINICAL PEARLS
Nurses encounter many cardiovascular disorders in adult patients, including MI.

Physiology

Coronary arteries provide the only blood supply for the myocardial muscle (Figure 5-1); the adequacy of heart muscle perfusion is directly dependent on unimpeded blood flow through these arteries. Normal blood flow through arteries is dependent on several factors, including blood volume, hypoxemia, blood viscosity, lumen size that is affected by atherosclerotic plaques, and presence of thrombi (Capriotti, 2020). If blood volume is insufficient and/or the blood isn't fully oxygenated, these deficits will affect the adequacy of nutrient and oxygen transport to the myocardial cells (Davies, 2016; Hoffman & Sullivan, 2020; Norton, 2017).

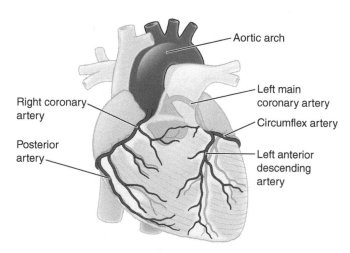

FIGURE 5–1 Structure of the heart and coronary arteries *(From Capriotti, T. (2020). Pathophysiology: Introductory concepts and clinical perspectives (2nd ed.). Philadelphia, PA: F.A. Davis.)*

The process of ASCVD begins in the arteries. Cholesterol is one of three major classes of lipids, which all animal cells use to construct their membranes and which is thus manufactured by all animal cells. Cholesterol is also the precursor of the steroid hormones and bile acids. Because cholesterol is insoluble in water, it is transported in the blood plasma within protein particles (lipoproteins). Lipoproteins are classified by their density (Stone et al., 2014; Venes, 2021):

- *Very low-density lipoprotein* (VLDL-C)
- *Low-density lipoprotein* (LDL-C)
- *Intermediate-density lipoprotein* (IDL)
- *High-density lipoprotein* (HDL-C)

The lumen of a coronary artery becomes smaller as atherosclerotic plaques, composed of cholesterol, form along the intima and impede blood flow. Thrombi often form along the intima walls as an inflammatory response to the plaques; when plaques rupture into the vessel lumen, clot formation can occur (AHA, 2017; Capriotti, 2020).

While blood viscosity and lumen size are risk factors for impaired blood flow in the coronary arteries, they do not usually affect the heart sounds. The normal closing(s) of the heart valves between the chambers are responsible for heart sounds. When there is turbulent blood flow due to valvular dysfunction, the provider may hear a murmur. The atrioventricular (mitral and tricuspid) valves' closing results in the *first heart sound* (S1); semilunar (aortic and pulmonic) valves' closing causes the *second heart sound* (S2). Any change in the blood flow through the valves or their mechanical functioning may affect the resultant sounds. A *third heart sound* (S3) may be normal, or physiological, in certain populations (children, young adults, and pregnant women) due to early ventricular filling. A *fourth heart sound* (S4) is due to resistance during ventricular filling and is usually considered pathological (Dillon, 2017; Goolsby & Grubbs, 2019).

> **HIGH YIELD FACT FOR TESTING**
>
> An MI occurs when the normal functioning of the coronary arteries is affected by impaired blood flow.

Pathophysiology

Acute coronary syndrome (ACS) can take one of two forms: *unstable angina* (UA) or *acute MI* (AMI). Acute MI is categorized as either *ST-elevation myocardial infarction* (STEMI) or non-ST-*elevation myocardial infarction* (NSTEMI) (Capriotti, 2020; Hoffman & Sullivan, 2020; Norton, 2017; Reed, Rossi, & Cannon, 2017; Thygesen et al., 2017). The differences between these categories of MI is shown in Figure 5-2. In most cases, an MI is due to an atherosclerotic plaque breaking away from the arterial wall, causing erosion of the coronary artery endothelium. Stenoses within the coronary artery are unlikely to cause a STEMI because they are less likely to rupture and have

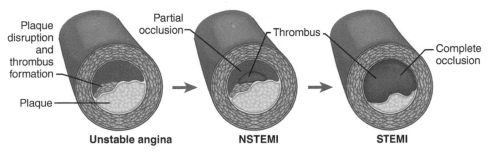

FIGURE 5–2 Extent of Occlusion in UA, NSTEMI, and STEMI. *(From Hoffman, J., & Sullivan, N. (2020). Medical-surgical nursing: Making connections to practice (2nd ed.). Philadelphia, PA: F.A. Davis.*

compensatory collateral circulation. In contrast, atherosclerotic plaques are at high risk to rupture; this releases thrombogenic components, causes platelet activation, initiates the coagulation cascade, and leads to further formation of atherosclerotic debris. These processes result in myocardial cell (myocyte) necrosis, detectable by elevation of cardiac biomarkers in the peripheral blood. Severity of ischemia and/or necrosis is due to the following (Campion et al., 2017; Capriotti, 2020; Reed, Rossi, & Cannon, 2017):

• Occlusion percentage
• Duration of impaired blood supply
• Area of myocardium supplied by the coronary artery
• Presence of collateral circulation
• Reperfusion

When there is an interruption to blood flow in a coronary artery, the muscle distal, or *downstream*, does not receive necessary oxygen and nutrients and metabolic wastes build up. If the lack of blood supply is prolonged, the myocardial muscle infarcts, or dies. At the cellular level, there is a decrease in aerobic respiration due to a lack of oxygen, which causes decreased energy production, ischemia to the cells, and, ultimately, cellular death. This cellular injury, or infarction, affects the pumping ability of the myocardial cells and their ability to supply blood to both the heart muscle and entire body. When a there is a blockage in a coronary artery, the damage will be manifested in a specific area of the heart (Reed et al., 2017; Venes, 2021). (See Figure 5-1.) While the focal damage to the myocardial muscle can be correlated directly to the involved coronary artery, the systemic effects of the myocardial damage are not as predictable.

When atherosclerosis is present in a coronary artery, there is a buildup of plaque, platelets, fibrin, and cellular debris, which eventually occludes the lumen and resulting blood flow; angiotensin II acts as a growth catalyst for this mass of cells. With exercise there is an increased demand for blood supply to the myocardium. When blood flow through the coronary arteries is compromised due to the atherosclerotic changes, the increased demand for oxygenated blood cannot be met by an increase in heart rate alone (Norton, 2017; Thygesen et al., 2012). A coronary occlusion may be due to a thrombus that forms after an atherosclerotic plaque ruptures from the vessel wall, causing bleeding and thrombus, or clot, formation. When the thrombus lodges in the vessel, it occludes blood flow through it (Capriotti, 2020; Norton, 2017).

An MI is usually initiated by the rupture or erosion of an atherosclerotic plaque that exposes the circulating coronary artery blood to thrombogenic materials present in the plaque. A thrombus that causes total occlusion of an artery usually leads to a STEMI (Campion et al., 2017; Norton, 2017). As noted earlier, the term *ST-elevation myocardial infarction* refers to an MI that presents with an ST segment elevation; with this condition, the patient is at higher risk for serious complications, including arrhythmias, cardiogenic shock, and cardiac arrest (O'Gara et al., 2013). When placed in a hypoxic state, the myocardium converts to anaerobic metabolism, and lactic acid, a byproduct of this type of metabolism, accumulates. The nerves of the myocardium are irritated by lactic acid and subsequently transmit pain to the cardiac nerves and upper thoracic posterior nerve roots, which causes chest pain of ischemia. Necrosis of myocardial cells occurs after an average of 2 to 4 hours of ischemia and is dependent on the following factors: collateral circulation, completeness of coronary arterial occlusion, myocyte sensitively to ischemia, and individualized oxygen demand. Healing after an MI usually takes at least 5 to 6 weeks and is also dependent on the above factors (Thygesen et al., 2012).

TABLE 5–1   CAD Risk Factors

Nonmodifiable Risk Factors	Modifiable Risk Factors
Increased age: >45 for men, >55 for women Male sex Postmenopausal women Family history 　　Race (highest rates in Native Americans and Alaskan Natives)	Dyslipidemia (high total cholesterol, high LDL, low HDL, high triglycerides) Sedentary lifestyle Cigarette smoking Hypertension Diabetes Increased C-reactive protein levels Stress Excessive alcohol consumption Obesity, especially central

(ACC, 2017; AHA, 2017; Capriotti, 2020; Hoffman & Sullivan, 2020)

Coronary Artery Disease (CAD)

As the leading cause of death in industrialized countries, CAD is responsible for approximately 600,000 deaths in the United States annually. The disease is due to narrowing of the coronary arteries, usually the result of atherosclerosis. Several major causative factors for CAD are reviewed in Table 5-1.

Based on these factors, a person's individualized risk for developing CAD can be estimated (O'Gara et al., 2013; Thygesen et al., 2012). A related condition, *coronary microvascular disease* (CMD), may be responsible for reducing blood flow to the myocardium. Because the changes in the coronary arteries are not visible on angiography, the condition can lead to an MI if left untreated. A coronary spasm, or closure of the opening due to a contraction of muscles, may also lead to occlusion of an artery and resulting MI (Norton, 2017; O'Gara et al., 2013).

Dyslipidemia

Dyslipidemias include any disorder of lipid metabolism. All the lipoproteins carry cholesterol, but elevated levels of the lipoproteins other than HDL-C (termed non-HDL-C cholesterol), particularly LDL-C-cholesterol, are associated with an increased risk of atherosclerosis and coronary heart disease. In contrast, higher levels of HDL-C cholesterol are protective (Stone et al., 2014). Specifically, hypercholesterolemia is elevated cholesterol in the blood and triglycerides are fats that are carried in the blood. Elevated triglycerides and LDL-C are risk factors for cardiovascular disease and may result from diet, obesity, and genetics (such as LDL-C receptor mutations in familial hypercholesterolemia).

CLINICAL PEARLS
　An MI is necrosis of the myocardial tissue due to ischemia, regardless of the pathobiology (Thygesen et al., 2012).

Assessment

Subjective assessment data are critical to accurate identification of an MI. Through focused interviewing, the nurse guides the patient to convey pertinent symptoms, leading to an accurate diagnosis. Patients often deny and/or misinterpret symptoms related to an MI. Typically, persons with an MI will experience chest pain; however, there may be great variance among patients in the pain characteristics (Norton, 2017).

While the pain may be crushing, burning, and/or suffocating, it is often accompanied by shortness of breath and increases with physical exertion. Cardiac-origin pain often radiates to the jaw, arm, and shoulders, making it difficult to correlate to its cardiac source.

Women, older adults, and people with diabetes may not have typical symptoms and when having an MI may experience fatigue, indigestion, and/or upper-back and jaw pain (Davies, 2016; Thygesen et al., 2012). Rarely, a patient has an MI without experiencing any symptoms, which is known as a *silent MI*. These asymptomatic patients have *electrocardiography* (EKG) changes, usually a new pathological Q wave, which should be evaluated further with cardiac imaging. A silent MI occurs in 9% to 37% of all non-fatal MI events and is associated with a significantly increased mortality risk. Because improper lead placement may be responsible for Q waves, a repeat EKG is the first action when this abnormality is identified.

On inspection, the patient having an MI will often appear anxious with pale, diaphoretic skin. Otherwise, there may not be any outward manifestations of this life-threatening event. Jugular venous distension may be present if there is concomitant fluid volume overload due to decreased myocardial function. Palpation during an MI may reveal that the patient has compromised peripheral circulation resulting in decreased pulses. Otherwise, there are usually not any useful palpable physical findings; nor is percussion an effective assessment tool for the patient with an MI. Cardiac percussion is generally used for assessment of pericardial effusion when x-ray isn't available and is not applicable to assessment of an MI patient (Dillon, 2017; Goolsby & Grubbs, 2019).

Auscultation during an MI may reveal some significant findings. First, the patient's blood pressure may be elevated due to multiple factors, including compensatory adrenergic mechanisms to maintain circulation, reaction to pain, and anxiety. If myocardial ischemia is substantial, cardiac output will decrease and hypotension occurs. Accurate and frequent auscultation of blood pressure is necessary to identify these changes. Heart sounds are often affected by the physiological changes that occur to blood flow when there is myocardial ischemia and damage. Additional heart sounds, S3 (ventricular gallop) and S4 (atrial gallop), are often present in an MI. An S3 may be one of the first assessment findings that results from myocardial damage and often portends a poor prognosis. An S4 almost always occurs with an MI and is not necessarily an ominous finding (Dillon, 2017; Goolsby & Grubbs, 2019).

In order to auscultate the heart accurately, the nurse must use the stethoscope bell correctly and listen at the precise precordial area. For an S3, listen at the *left lower sternal border* (LLSB), also known as tricuspid area at the fourth to fifth intercostal space, with the patient supine or in a left recumbent position. It is a soft sound, difficult to hear, and best identified using the bell. An S4 is also best heard at the LLSB or apex with the bell. The timing of the sound in the cardiac cycle may be what distinguishes these two sounds. An S3 occurs in early diastole, creating a galloping sound, whereas the S4 is in late diastole, just before the S1, and is described as an atrial gallop. Other abnormalities may be auscultated during an MI due to resistance to blood flow through the heart, but murmurs are not necessarily diagnostic of an MI and occur as sequelae of the initial event. A rub may develop if pericarditis is a complication of an MI. Arrhythmias and conduction abnormalities may also be responsible for murmurs after an MI (Dillon, 2017; Goolsby & Grubbs, 2019). Other tools may also be used to assess patients' risk for a major cardiac event (mortality, MI, or coronary revascularization). One tool, the HEART Score, is used in the emergency department to place patients with chest pain in a risk group (low, moderate, and high). HEART is an acronym of History, EKG, Age, Risk factors, and Troponin; each component is scored with 0, 1, or 2 points, with

BOX 5-1   Myocardial Infarction (MI) Diagnostic Criteria

- Abnormal cardiac biomarker (cardiac troponin is the most predictive)
- Subjective reports of ischemia
- New changes in ST-segment–T wave (ST–T) or new left bundle branch block (LBBB)
- New Q waves
- Myocardium damage or abnormal wall motion
- Intracoronary thrombus (diagnosed by angiography or autopsy)

the resulting categories: low = 1–3; moderate = 5–6; high is more than 6 (Backus, 2017; Dubin et al., 2017).

According to the ACC/AHA guidelines (Norton, 2017; O'Gara et al., 2013; Thygesen et al., 2012), one of the criteria listed in Box 5-1 must be met for the diagnosis of MI.

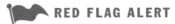 **RED FLAG ALERT**

An S4 is almost always present in a patient with expected myocardial ischemia.

ASSESSMENT PEARLS
Abnormal heart sounds during an MI are early signs of potential complications.

Diagnostic Tests

Changes in the cardiac system during a STEMI may be initially diagnosed and/or confirmed by diagnostic tests. After an accurate assessment of the patient's symptoms and risk factors, the appropriate test will be scheduled and analyzed in order to provide data related to the patient's cardiac status and severity of myocardial damage. Timing of these tests is crucial to their correct interpretation.

A 12-lead EKG is used to diagnose an MI by evaluation of ST elevation and/or depression, arrhythmias, and/or conduction abnormalities. An example of such an EKG is shown in Figure 5-3, where A = normal EKG; B = ST depression with ischemia; C = ST elevation with AMI; D = Q waves after AMI; and E = EKG waveform changed after AMI. According to current ACC guidelines, patients with suspected MI should have an EKG within 10 minutes of clinical presentation. Because the initial EKG is often nondiagnostic and the EKG may change during an ischemic event, serial or continuous 12-lead EKGs may be required to identify an evolving MI (Goolsby & Grubbs, 2019; Norton, 2017). If the patient experiences any symptoms during each EKG, use these EKGs as a comparison with asymptomatic EKGs.

Any acute or evolving changes in the ST-T waveforms and Q waves provide the nurse the following data: timing of the cardiac event, identification of causative artery, amount of myocardial damage, and anticipated medical interventions (Norton, 2017). Significant ST-segment changes (1 mm change from baseline in at least two contiguous precordial or two adjacent limb leads) or T-wave inversion in multiple leads is associated with large regions of myocardial damage (Campion et al., 2017; Davies, 2016). In an acute MI, there may also be the following findings on EKG: arrhythmias, conduction delays (*bundle branch blocks* [BBB]), and decreased R-wave amplitude (Hoffman & Sullivan, 2020).

Cardiac biomarkers are also used to diagnose an MI. Abnormal values indicate damage to myocardial cells regardless of the causative mechanism. Two laboratory values are used to diagnose an MI: *cardiac troponin* (cTn) and the MB fraction of *creatine kinase* (CK-MB) (Campion et al., 2017; Thygesen et al., 2012). The timing of these abnormalities is key to correct identification of cardiac injury. Because of their high sensitivity and specificity, if biomarkers are evaluated at appropriate times and are normal, an MI is excluded and no further diagnostic measures are indicated. Specifically, the

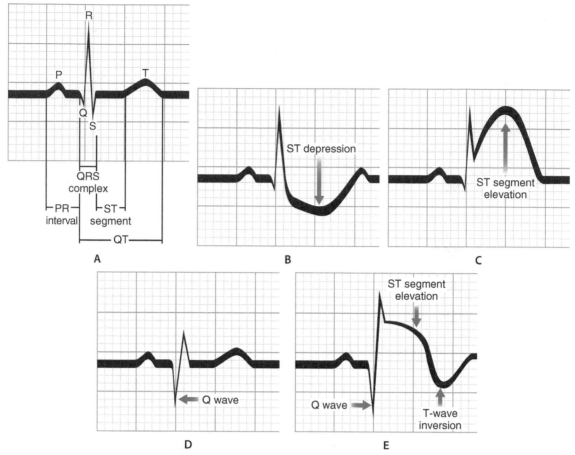

FIGURE 5–3 EKG Waveforms in an MI. **A.** Normal EKG waveform; **B.** EKG Waveform with ST depression indicating ischemia; **C.** ST elevation in acute myocardial infarction (AMI); **D.** Q waves after AMI; **E.** EKG waveform illustrating changes that occur with AMI

troponin level is the more sensitive indicator, rising at 4 hours after injury and staying elevated for 7 to 10 days. The cTn value must exceed the 99th percentile of the reference value, which is determined for each specific assay and provided with the results for accurate interpretation (Campion et al., 2017; Capriotti, 2020; Hoffman & Sullivan, 2020).

While the CK-MB level may rise earlier during an MI, it generally returns to normal in 72 hours and is affected by other factors related to muscular damage that is not necessarily cardiac in origin. Because normal cardiac function is rarely present in an acute MI, accurate imaging is useful for early identification of MI. Additional diagnostic tests may be indicated as providers seek to confirm a diagnosis of an MI based on the above criteria. These include *guided exercise test* (GXT) or *treadmill stress test* (TST), EKG, *magnetic resonance imaging* (MRI), and cardiac catheterization (Hoffman & Sullivan, 2020).

HIGH YIELD FACT FOR TESTING

Accurate diagnosis of a STEMI is based primarily on EKG but must also include cardiac biomarkers measured at accurate intervals.

 CLINICAL PEARLS

When the nurse provides a calm, supportive environment, the patient will be better able to share pertinent information and accurately convey their symptoms.

Nonpharmacological Management

During the acute phase, the use of nonpharmacological interventions is not necessarily a priority but may provide substantial physiological and psychological benefits. While patients may expect that they will have to take medications after an MI, they are often surprised that their recovery can be positively impacted by lifestyle changes. The combination of these changes with medication has a synergistic effect. Involving the family in these interventions will also help to embed them into daily routines and for them to become habits more quickly and (possibly) easily. While lifestyle changes that focus on modifiable risk factors are important for all patients, a systematic review and meta-analysis by Zhang et al. (2017) revealed that these changes are particularly impactful with patients who have diabetes, as their risk of developing cardiovascular disease is high. In this study, lifestyle interventions resulted in significant improvement in the following measurements: systolic blood pressure, diastolic blood pressure, total cholesterol (increased HDL-C and decreased LDL-C), and triglycerides (Norton, 2017; Zhang et al., 2017).

Stress Reduction

This modifiable cardiac risk factor may be the most difficult to correctly identify and treat. According to a meta-analysis by Roest, Martens, de Jonge, and Denollet (2010), anxiety was an independent risk factor for the development of coronary heart disease and cardiac mortality. Also, Burke, Lam, Stussman, and Yang (2017 conducted a secondary analysis on 2012 National Health Interview Survey data (n = 34,525) to investigate factors related to use of meditation as a stress management strategy. The 12-month prevalence for meditation practice was 6.6% of the sample, broken down as shown here:

Spiritual meditation (3.1%)—approximately 7.0 million adults
Mindfulness meditation (1.9%)—approximately 4.3 million adults
Mantra meditation (1.6%)—approximately 3.6 million adults

People who used conventional health-care services were also more likely to use one of these forms of meditation, which would include patients after a STEMI who are in traditional cardiac rehabilitation. In this study, the majority of subjects (74%) were motivated by seeking wellness and prevention, but almost a third of the sample (30%) used meditation to treat a specific disease. These numbers support the belief that patients after a STEMI may use meditation both to promote general wellness and to prevent further progressions of CHD. Some patients are able to independently make lifestyle changes that dramatically decrease their stress level. Other patients may require professional intervention to attain and sustain the necessary changes to decrease this risk. The AHA (2017) recommends substituting healthy behaviors for the stressful ones, such as physical activity, talking with others, and getting adequate sleep.

Diet Changes

There are multiple recommendations for the best diet to follow after an MI. Patients with hyperlipidemia will be instructed in a low-fat diet to address this issue. A Mediterranean diet may be indicated, as it limits saturated and hydrogenated oils (trans fats) and replaces them with monounsaturated fats that have antioxidant properties. Specifically, linolenic acid (contained in monounsaturated fats) lowers triglycerides, decreases blood clotting, and is associated with decreased risk of an MI. Even for patients with normal lipid profiles, a Mediterranean diet is considered appropriate to decrease the risk of another cardiac event. This type of diet often leads to weight loss, which is associated with improved cardiac performance by lowering blood pressure and promoting arterial compliance (ACC, 2017; AHA, 2017).

Exercise

After an acute MI, patients may either begin or resume an exercise plan; however, this must be medically supervised so the patient is not at risk for increased cardiac workload and resulting ischemia. With an appropriate plan, patients can reach the exercise goal for healthy individuals of moderate intensity physical activity for at least 30 minutes a day for 5 days a week (150 minutes total each week) (O'Gara et al., 2013).

Pharmacology

The nurse can expect medications administered during an MI will be aimed at increasing coronary blood flow, decreasing blood coagulability, and decreasing cardiac workload. First, if an MI is expected, an aspirin should be chewed and swallowed for its antiplatelet activity. Oxygen is considered a drug and is administered in order to decrease ischemia. Nitroglycerin is dose titrated to achieve vasodilation and improved cardiac output. Nitroglycerin is available for delivery via various routes: oral, sublingual, transdermal, and IV (Hoffman & Sullivan, 2020; Woo & Robinson, 2020).

Aspirin

Acetylsalicylic acid (ASA), or aspirin, is used in both the acute treatment and secondary prevention of MI (Woo & Robinson, 2020). It inhibits platelet production and aggregation by inhibiting the synthesis of thromboxane A2, which decreases the destructive effect of an extant thrombus as the causative factor and prevent other thrombi formation while the patient is in a hypercoagulable state. If an MI is suspected, the patient is to chew and swallow a 325 mg ASA for best absorbability. After the acute event, a daily dose of 81 to 100 mg may be administered in enteric form to decrease potential gastric irritation (Woo & Robinson, 2020). Care for patients on an aspirin regimen is shown in SENC Box 5-1.

Oxygen

While oxygen continues to be used as standard treatment during an MI, the evidence is not conclusive that its use decreases myocardial damage. According to Nehme et al. (2016), supplemental oxygen in the first 12 hours after STEMI has been associated with increases in cardiac troponin and CK levels. In a meta-analysis by Khan et al. (2019), meta-regression revealed that evidence on the safety and efficacy of oxygen was weak and inconsistent. Similarly, Hofmann et al. (2017) found that 1-year mortality was not improved with use of supplemental oxygen in patients with suspected MI.

SENC BOX 5–1   Safe and Effective Nursing Care for Patients on Aspirin During and/or After an MI

1. Assess for aspirin allergy.
2. Assess for increased bleeding risk from recent surgery or trauma, such as a fall or motor vehicle crash.
3. Monitor for toxicity, often manifested as tinnitus or decreased hearing.
4. The dose with a suspected MI must be chewed to increase its absorption.

> **SENC BOX 5-2** Safe and Effective Nursing Care for Patients on Oxygen During and/or After an MI
>
> 1. Administer and titrate the lowest dose to maintain oxygen saturation above 90%.
> 2. Assess oxygenation in the patient's overall condition, cardiac and respiratory systems, and peripheral circulation.
> 3. When available, partner with the interprofessional team, especially respiratory therapists, to manage oxygen therapy.
> 4. Treat oxygen as a medication that should be dosed at the lowest effective rate for the shortest period of time.

At the cellular level, high oxygen levels decrease the diameter of arterioles, which also decreases oxygen transport to muscle. When this occurs in coronary arteries, it results in decreased oxygen to the myocardial muscle at a time when it is needed most (Siela & Kidd, 2017). According to the ACC, no data support or refute the use of supplemental oxygen to treat patients with acute STEMI (O'Gara et al., 2013). A Cochrane analysis indicated that MI patients treated with oxygen had a three times higher risk for death as compared to patients receiving room air (Siela & Kidd, 2017). Therefore, it is recommended that patients be evaluated for hypoxia/hypoxemia and treated based on an individualized assessment, as indicated in SENC Box 5-2.

Nitroglycerin

Nitroglycerin remains a first-line treatment for acute MI. Nitroglycerin converts to nitric oxide, which causes vasodilation and increases blood flow to the myocardium. At low doses, nitroglycerin causes venous dilation, which decreases venous return; this positively affects the transmyocardial gradient and allows for more transport of oxygen between the coronary arteries and the myocardium. At higher doses, nitroglycerin causes arterial dilation, which decreases systemic vascular resistance (afterload). While nitroglycerin may dilate the coronary arteries directly, its effect is minimal when arteries are atherosclerotic (ACC, 2017; Woo & Robinson, 2020).

Patients may develop tolerance during continuous delivery of nitroglycerin due to inactivation of *aldehyde dehydrogenase 2* (ALDH2), an enzyme that is responsible for the conversion. Like aspirin, this drug may be effective in both an acute MI and in the prevention of further cardiac events; the sublingual, transdermal, or IV route is preferred for rapid absorption. If a transdermal patch is already on the patient having chest pain, it is recommended that the patch be removed when the IV infusion is started in order to achieve accurate titration based on pain relief and hemodynamic improvement (Campion et al., 2017; Hoffman & Sullivan, 2020; Woo & Robinson, 2020). SENC Box 5-3 provides care information for patients on nitroglycerin.

Beta Blockers

Also known as beta-adrenergic antagonists, these medications preferentially block the beta1 receptors, located in myocardial muscle. At higher doses, there is a concomitant blockade on the $beta_2$ receptors in the bronchioles and vascular muscles (Goldberger et al., 2015). Both $beta_1$-selective and nonselective agents decrease the myocardial contractility, heart rate, and conduction velocity. Their effect on decreasing systemic vascular resistance and blood pressure also decreases afterload. These medications are effective in decreasing mortality by 30% to 40% post-MI by limiting the infarct size, preventing arrhythmias, and preventing subsequent cardiac events due to coronary

SENC BOX 5–3   Safe and Effective Nursing Care for Patients on Nitroglycerin During and/or After an MI

1. Because of the risk for hypotension, patients should be instructed to sit down when they self-administer nitroglycerin.
2. Patients may take prophylactic acetaminophen to prevent post-administration headache.
3. Nitroglycerin tablets must be stored in their original container in a cool place.
4. Sublingual tablet should "fizz" and slightly burn when placed under tongue.
5. Expiration date should be followed; expired medication should be discarded and replaced.
6. Patients may be on a prophylactic daily dose of nitroglycerin and also need to understand how to administer sublingual doses for acute chest pain.

occlusion. Decreased heart rate results in decreased cardiac output and workload; however, because a decreased cardiac output may lead to cardiogenic shock, they are contraindicated when there is widespread ischemia or existing signs/symptoms of shock (Woo & Robinson, 2020).

While current evidence supports the use of beta blocker therapy after acute MI to improve survival, there isn't agreement about its dosing. For example, in a multisite study of 7,057 patients with acute MI, at 2-year follow-up there was lower mortality among patients on a beta blocker ($p < 0.0002$) as compared to patients who were not on a beta blocker; however, higher doses of a beta blocker were not associated with better outcome (Goldberger et al., 2015).

Statins

Statins are the most frequently used lipid-lowering medications for patients after a STEMI. They are also known as HMG-CoA reductase inhibitors because they block that particular enzyme necessary for the formation of cholesterol in the liver. Statins are used effectively in both primary and secondary prevention of cardiovascular disease. Side effects of statins may include the following: muscle pain, increased risk of developing diabetes mellitus, and liver and/or muscle/tendon damage (Kheloussi, 2018). These medications may be used when diet and lifestyle changes are not effective in achieving normal cholesterol levels. Based on evidence, these medications are responsible for a decrease of LDL-C cholesterol by 1.8 mmol/L (70 mg/dL), which is associated with a 60% decrease in the risk of a cardiac event, including myocardial infarction (ACC, 2017; Norton, 2017; Stone et al., 2014; Woo & Robinson, 2020).

While statin medications to lower cholesterol were once considered necessary for all patients who had a history of MI, the current guidelines are to use statins for the following four situations:

• Documented atherosclerotic cardiovascular disease (ASCVD) (e.g., ACS, MI, angina, stroke)
• No documented ASCVD but with LDL-C greater than 190 mg/dL
• Diabetics, aged 40 to 75, with LDL-C 70 to 189 mg/dL but without clinical ASCVD
• Patients aged 40 to 75 (without diabetes or ASCVD) but with LDL-C 70 to 189 mg/dL (Kheloussi, 2018).

Statins are also deemed less effective in reducing LDL-C in familial hypercholesterolemia. However, statins are used primarily to decrease LDL-C and its atherosclerotic plaques in coronary arteries (ACC, 2017; Hoffman & Sullivan, 2020; Kheloussi,

SENC BOX 5–4   Safe and Effective Nursing Care for Patients on Statins During and/or After an MI

1. Patients must understand the importance of reporting all myalgias, as this may be a precursor to tendon rupture.
2. Patients should have labs measured after 6–8 weeks of medication and then are reevaluated at 8- to 12-week intervals for the first year of therapy.
3. Lifestyle changes (increased activity, healthy eating, and smoking cessation) should also be incorporated to the therapeutic regiment.
4. Evaluate for drug and food interactions.

TABLE 5–2   Non-Statin Medications for Dyslipidemia

Medication	Usage Before and During MI with SENC
Nicotinic acid (niacin)	• Decreases production of VLDLs • Increases clearance of triglycerides from blood • Increases HDL-C. • Often difficult to tolerate side effects of flushing and nausea.
Bile acid–binding resins	• May be first line pharmacological therapy and used as monotherapy. • May be combined with a statin to decrease LDL-C. • Primarily GI side effects: constipation, abdominal pain, bloating, vomiting, diarrhea, heartburn, weight loss, and gallstones.
Fibric acid derivatives/fibrates	• Most effective at decreasing triglycerides. • Should not be used when patient is on statin due to increased risk of rhabdomyolysis (muscle symptoms) • Often used for patients with diabetes and/or familial dysbetalipoproteinemia.

(Hoffman & Sullivan, 2020; Woo & Robinson, 2020)

2018; Norton, 2017; Stone et al., 2014). Care for patients on statins is shown in SENC Box 5-4.

Non-Statins

These medications may be used as an adjuvant to a statin if outcomes are not obtained with the statin alone and/or there are contraindications to the patient taking a statin for dyslipidemia (Woo & Robinson, 2020). The most commonly used non-statins are presented in Table 5-2 with their SENC.

Anti-hypertensive Agents in Post-STEMI Care

Angiotensin-converting enzyme (ACE) *inhibitors* block the formation of angiotensin II and are effective post-MI by decreasing peripheral vascular resistance and cardiac workload. They are also effective in preventing further thickening of coronary arteries and ventricular muscular walls. (See additional information about ACE inhibitors in Chapter 1.) Direct renin inhibitors have the same effects as the ACE inhibitors and do so by blocking renin; they may be used because they cause less risk of cough and angioedema. *Calcium channel blockers* (CCB) decrease the flow of calcium into cells, which results in peripheral vasodilation; non-dihydropyridine

TABLE 5–3   Medications During and After a STEMI

Class	Example	Action	Indication	Adverse Effects	SENC
Antiplatelet	Aspirin (ASA) 80–325 mg/day	Inhibits platelet aggregation	Acute MI and secondary prophylaxis	Gastric irritation, gastric bleeding, tinnitus	Use with caution in impaired liver function. Monitor for bleeding.
Nitroglycerin	Nitrostat 0.3–0.6 mg sublingual up to 3 tabs	Dose- related venous and arterial Dilation	Chest pain Unstable angina	Hypotension, headache, tachycardia	Only take when sitting or lying down to decrease hypotension.
Statins	Atorvastatin 10–40 mg/day up to 80 mg/day	Inhibits HMG-CoA Increases LDL-C uptake and catabolism	Hyperlipidemia Decreases LDL-C and triglycerides	Muscle pain, tendon rupture, liver failure	Minimize alcohol intake. Lipid and liver laboratory tests will be monitored.

(AHA, 2017; Woo & Robinson, 2020)

CCBs also decrease heart rate and myocardial contractility, which decrease myocardial oxygen demand (Campion et al., 2017; Woo & Robinson, 2020). (Also see CCB in Chapter 1.)

RED FLAG ALERT

Adverse effects of statins are most common in the first 12 months and in patients with the following: diabetes, hyperuricemia, and a history of tendon disorders. Patents who participate in strenuous sports may also experience adverse effects.

HIGH YIELD FACT FOR TESTING

Patients using medications such as sildenafil citrate (i.e., Viagra) should be educated on the increased risk of hypotension when taking nitroglycerin.

Additional Medications

Ranolazine is an anti-anginal that does not affect heart rate or blood pressure, but decreases late inward sodium current, which normalizes the intracellular ion homeostasis and related oxygen requirements, so angina is avoided. Additional anticoagulants may also be indicated post-MI, such as P2Y12 inhibitors, heparin, and/or glycoprotein inhibitors, used based on individual risk factors and treatments. After a STEMI in the anterior wall, it is necessary for the patient to be anticoagulated with warfarin to maintain an *international normalized ratio* (INR) target of 2.0 to 3.0 to prevent a left ventricular thrombus. Usually after 9 months on warfarin, the patient may be changed to dual anticoagulant with ticagrelor (P2Y12 inhibitor) and low-dose ASA. Other medications administered post-STEMI are shown in Table 5-3. Glycoprotein IIb/IIIa inhibitors are used to treat certain types of MI and are given in combination with heparin or aspirin to prevent clotting before and during invasive heart procedures, such as *percutaneous coronary intervention* (PCI).

Interventional Cardiology

Patients with a STEMI often benefit from reperfusion that limits the size of an infarct with a primary PCI. Abrupt disruption of the atherosclerotic plaque that occurs in a STEMI leads to intense coagulation and formation of a thrombus that evolves into an occlusive fibrin-rich thrombus built around the initial platelet plug. It is crucial to restore blood supply to the myocardium and prevent a worsening hemodynamic state

(Davies, 2016; Norton, 2017). Based on a review of more than 25 clinical studies and numerous meta-analyses, Brener (2017) determined that PCI is more effective than fibrinolytics and has less risk. Additionally, PCI restores normal antegrade blood flow in approximately 90% of patients, as compared to 40% to 60% of patients treated with fibrinolytics. The salvage index (myocardium recovering function as proportion of myocardium at risk at beginning of STEMI) is much higher with PCI (50%–60%) as compared to fibrinolytics (Brener, 2017). The *Door-to-Balloon* (D2B) Initiative established by the ACC in 2006 set the goal of 90 minutes for patients with a STEMI to receive primary PCI. This 90-minute time frame is divided into the following 30-minute intervals: *emergency medical services* (EMS), emergency department care, and the cardiac catheterization laboratory (ACC, 2017).

> **HIGH YIELD FACT FOR TESTING**
>
> Caring for the STEMI patient who requires a cardiac intervention is based on a strict timeline of assigned tasks and transition of care from one area to another.

Complementary and Alternative Therapies (CAT)

Increasingly, patients are requesting that *complementary and alternative therapies* (CAT) are part of their care, and this may mean including them during the acute and rehabilitative care for a STEMI. Kramlich (2016) summarizes that reasons for CAT-inclusive care for critically ill patients include improved quality of life, management of unrelieved symptoms, collaborative decision making, holistic care, concerns related to invasive procedures, and cultural influences (Chandrababu et al., 2017). Also according to Kramlich in an earlier article (2014), CAT may decrease stress and anxiety that patients and families experience during an acute illness. If the patient and their families have established CAT practices, it is usually safe to continue these. Notably, CAT such as music, guided imagery, and massage may contribute to the healing environment without the potential for side effects. Positive physiological effects of these therapies may include improved sleep; decreased anxiety and pain; lowered heart rate, respiratory rate, and blood pressure; decreased stress hormones; improved immune system functioning; and normalized intestinal motility. With these positive changes, patients often require less pharmacological analgesia and sedation. In a related issue, however, patients are not always forthcoming about their use of CAT, and herbal remedies may have significant cardiac side effects. Specifically, hypertensive crisis and cardiac arrhythmias have been associated with the herbals ginseng, yohimbe, and ephedra, and these should be avoided in patients with coronary heart disease (Kramlich, 2014).

While CAT may not be included in the standard clinical pathway for the STEMI patient, post-STEMI may be an optimal time to educate patients and their families about CAT as part of a healthy lifestyle. Post-STEMI patients may be particularly motivated to learn about CAT during and after resolution of the acute event (see Box 5-2, Healthy Lifestyle After an MI). In a literature review, Chandrababu et al. (2017) examined the prevalence and predictors of CAT use in patients with CHD and those at risk for CHD. Included in this review was a study by Kristoffersen et al. (2017), using *Protection Motivation Theory* (PMT) to frame a large study (n = 11,103) that compared subjects without CHD but with a family risk factor (35.8%), to people with CHD (30.2%), and people with no CHD or family risk factor (32.1%) and their use of CAT; the four predictors of CAT in the people with no CHD but a family history were: self-rated health, expectations for future health, preventive health beliefs, and score on the health behavior index. Specific outcomes of CAT use were not measured by Kristoffersen. Based on an analysis of 28 studies, Chandrababu et al. (2017) found strong but inconsistent evidence supporting CAT

BOX 5–2   Healthy Lifestyle After an MI

SMOKING CESSATION
- Plan for a non-smoking life.
- Use medication if necessary.
- Involve family and friends in the plan.

TREAT OBESITY AS A DISEASE
- Eat more fruits, vegetables, and whole grains.
- Achieve and/or maintain a normal body mass index (BMI): 18.5–25 kg/m^2.
- Set realistic goals to achieve a normal BMI.

ADD PHYSICAL ACTIVITY TO DIETARY MODIFICATIONS
- AHA exercise recommendations for lowering blood pressure and/or cholesterol: 40 minutes of moderate- to vigorous-intensity aerobic activity 3 or 4 times per week.

MANAGE STRESS
- Practice meditation.
- Engage in regular physical activity.
- Get adequate sleep.
- Develop healthy relationships.

(ACC, 2017; AHA, 2017; Hoffman & Sullivan, 2020)

---

for CHD patients; twenty-five of the studies reported improved outcomes with use of CAT, but evidence is still inconclusive.

According to the AHA (2017), approximately 20% of patients over age 45 who survive an MI will have another MI within 5 years; therefore, adherence to both pharmacological and nonpharmacological measures is critical to promoting a healthy heart. When patients are faced with complex medication regimens, they may become overwhelmed and have difficulty incorporating all recommended changes into their lives. Technology, such as activity trackers and mobile applications (e.g., My Cardia Coach™ by AHA), may support the patient's success with lifestyle changes.

Summary

The nurse must have current knowledge of pathophysiology, assessment, and pharmacological and nonpharmacological management of MI in order to care for patients during and after a STEMI. The complete occlusion of a coronary artery by an atherosclerotic plaque that has ruptured from the arterial wall results in interrupted blood flow to the myocardium. Then myocardial ischemia begins; the longer the blood supply is occluded, the greater the amount of heart muscle that is lost. In order to have a proactive approach to care management of the patient with after a STEMI, an accurate assessment of ASCVD risk factors must be performed, including information about diabetes mellitus, chronic renal disease, hypertension, and dyslipidemia. The cardiovascular assessment history should include both present and past history; family members and medical records may be useful secondary sources of data. The pharmacological management of STEMI follows a protocol based on the individual patient profile and concomitant disease processes but generally is aimed at improving delivery of oxygenated blood to the myocardium, lowering cardiac workload by maintaining a normal blood pressure, and addressing the specific aspects of dyslipidemia (i.e., elevated triglycerides, elevated LDL-C).

Patients are experiencing a life-changing event that may result in opportunities for positive lifestyle changes if approached in this manner by nurses who manage their care. This potentially life-threatening condition may have constructive outcomes for the patient and their family.

Key Points

- Current knowledge of myocardial infarction is essential because mortality has decreased, and nurses are likely to encounter these patients in primary care settings.
- The ACC/AHA guidelines are used to plan care in both the acute and rehabilitative phases of a STEMI.
- A STEMI can result in life-changing disabilities but can also be an opportunity to implement healthy lifestyle behaviors.
- Factors that contribute to risk of CAD and a resulting STEMI include age, sex, family history, hypertension, diabetes, obesity, sedentary lifestyle, and smoking.
- Use diagnostic tests to guide diagnosis and treatment plan.
- Use nonpharmacological interventions as adjuvants to medical interventions in all stages of STEMI care.
- Incorporate both general and specific Safe and Effective Nursing Care (SENC).
- Interventions for patients who are on medications after a STEMI.

Review Questions

1. **A 64-year-old female patient presents with fatigue and intermittent chest heaviness for several days. The nurse anticipates she will have which of the following assessments/interventions. Select all of the following that apply to this clinical situation.**

   a. Initial and serial troponin, Ck-MB levels

   b. EKG

   c. Fasting lipid panel

   d. Gallbladder ultrasound

   e. Chew 325 mg aspirin

2. **When caring for the patient with an acute STEMI, the patient's family asks the nurse, "What changes will we need to make in our lifestyle with this diagnosis?" The nurse's best response is:**

   a. "Supplements are safe; as long as you take them without food."

   b. "These changes must be initiated by the patient in order for them to be effective"

   c. "We have a support group for cardiac patients that will contact you about classes."

   d. "Let's talk about your current eating and exercise habits so we can make some small changes first."

3. **The 63-year-old patient post-STEMI is being discharged on nitroglycerin sl prn. The nurse anticipates that the following patient education will be part of the plan of care. (Select all that apply.)**

   a. "If you have any chest pain, you should call 911 before you take any medication."

   b. "If you are wearing a nitro patch, remove it to take additional nitroglycerin."

   c. "Contact the MD even when pain is relieved by nitroglycerin; we may need to adjust the dose."

   d. "Take a nitroglycerin before strenuous activity."

   e. "This medication should burn as it dissolves under your tongue."

4. **A 66-year-old obese diabetic woman has had a STEMI and is being discharged to home. What medications do you expect will be used to manage her dyslipidemia? Choose all that apply.**

   a. Statin
   b. Nicotinic acid
   c. Bile acid–binding resins
   d. Nonpharmacological interventions only
   e. Fibrate/fibric acid derivatives

5. **A STEMI is most likely to occur in which of the following situations?**

   a. Stenosis of a coronary artery
   b. Rupture of an atherosclerotic plaque from a coronary artery
   c. Hypercoagulable state after a stroke
   d. Coronary artery spasm

See the appendix for answers to review questions.

References

American College of Cardiology. (2017). Guidelines and clinical documents. http://www.acc.org/guidelines

American Heart Association. (2017). Acute myocardial infarction toolkit. https://www.heart.org/HEARTORG/Conditions/HeartAttack/Acute-Myocardial-Infarction-Toolkit_UCM_487847_SubHomePage.jsp

Backus, B. (2017). HEART score for major cardiac events. https://www.mdcalc.com/heart-score-major-cardiac-events

Brener, S. (2017). PCI for STEMI. *The Cardiology Advisor.* http://www.thecardiologyadvisor.com/cardiology/pci-for-stemi/article/583820/

Burke, A., Lam, C. N., Stussman, B., & Yang, H. (2017). Prevalence and patterns of use of mantra, mindfulness and spiritual meditation among adults in the United States. *BMC Complementary and Alternative Medicine, 17*(1), 316. doi:10.1186/s12906-017-1827-8

Campion, E. W., Anderson, J. L., & Morrow, D. A. (2017). Acute myocardial infarction. *New England Journal of Medicine, 376*(21), 2053–2064. https://ezproxy.queens.edu:2048/login?url=https://search.proquest.com/docview/1902164191?accountid=38688

Capriotti, T. (2020). *Pathophysiology: Introductory concepts and clinical perspectives* (2nd ed.). Philadelphia, PA: F.A. Davis.

Chandrababu, R., Nayak, B. S., Baburaya, V., Patil, N. T., George, A., George, L. S., & Sanatombi Devi, E. (2017). Effect of complementary therapies in patients following cardiac surgery: A narrative review. *Holistic Nursing Practice, 31*(5), 315–324. doi:10.1097/HNP.0000000000000226

Davies, N. (2016). Treating ST-elevation myocardial infarction. *Emergency Nurse, 24*(3), 20. doi:10.7748/en.24.3.20.s26

Dillon, P. (2017). *Nursing health assessment: A critical thinking, case studies approach* (2nd ed.). Philadelphia, PA: F.A. Davis.

Dubin, J., Kiechle, E., Wilson, M., Timbol, C., Bhat, R., & Milzman, D. (2017). Mean HEART scores for hospitalized chest pain patients are higher in more experienced providers. *The American Journal of Emergency Medicine, 35*(1), 122–125. doi:10.1016/j.ajem.2016.10.037

Goldberger, J. J., Bonow, R. O., Cuffe, M., Liu, L., Rosenberg, Y., Shah, P. K., . . . Smith, S. J. (2015). Effect of beta-blocker dose on survival after acute myocardial infarction. *Journal of the American College of Cardiology (JACC), 66*(13), 1431–1441. doi:10.1016/j.jacc.2015.07.047

Goolsby, M., & Grubbs, L. (2019). *Advanced assessment: Interpreting findings and formulating differential diagnoses* (4th ed.). Philadelphia, PA: F.A. Davis.

Hoffman, J., & Sullivan, N. (2020). *Medical-surgical nursing: Making connections to practice* (2nd ed.). Philadelphia, PA: F.A. Davis.

Hofmann, R., James, S. K., Jernberg, T., Lindahl, B., Erlinge, D., Witt, N., . . . Pernow, J. (2017). Oxygen therapy in suspected acute myocardial infarction. *New England Journal of Medicine, 377*(13), 1240–1249. doi:10.1056/NEJMoa1706222

Khan, A. R., Abdulhak, A. B., Luni, F. K., Farid, T. A., Riaz, H., Ruzieh, M., . . . Bolli, R. (2019). Oxygen administration does not influence the prognosis of acute myocardial infarction: A meta-analysis. *American Journal of Therapeutics, 26*(1), e151–e160. doi:10.1097/MJT.0000000000000475

Kheloussi, S. (2018). Considerations in the approach to appropriate statin selection. *U.S. Pharmacist, 43*(7), 22–26.

Kramlich, D. (2014). Introduction to complementary, alternative, and traditional therapies. *Critical Care Nurse, 34*(6), 50–56. doi:10.4037/ccn2014807

Kramlich, D. (2016). Strategies for acute and critical care nurses implementing complementary therapies requested by patients and their families. *Critical Care Nurse, 36*(6), 52–58. doi:10.4037/ccn2016974

Kristoffersen, A. E., Sirois, F. M., Stub, T., & Hansen, A. H. (2017). Prevalence and predictors of complementary and alternative medicine use among people with coronary heart disease or at risk for this in the sixth Tromsø study: A comparative analysis using protection motivation theory. *BMC Complementary and Alternative Medicine, 17*(1), 324. doi:10.1186/s12906-017-1817-x

Lloyd-Jones, D., Huffman, M. D., Karmali, K. N., Sanghavi, D. M., Wright, J. S., Pelser, C., . . . Goff, D. C. (2017). Estimating longitudinal risks and benefits from cardiovascular preventive therapies among Medicare patients. *Journal of the American College of Cardiology, 69*(12), 1617–1636. doi:10.1016/j.jacc.2016.10.018

Nehme, Z., Stub, D., Bernard, S., Stephenson, M., Bray, J. E., Cameron, P., . . . for the AVOID Investigators. (2016). Effect of supplemental oxygen exposure on myocardial injury in ST-elevation myocardial infarction, *Heart, 102*(6), 444–451.

Norton, C. (2017). Acute coronary syndrome: Assessment and management. *Nursing Standard, 31*(29), 61–71. doi:10.7748/ns.2017.e10754

O'Gara, P. T., Kushner, F. G., Ascheim, D. D., Casey, D. E. Jr., Chung, M. K., de Lemos, J. A., . . . Zhao, D. K. (2013). 2013 ACCF/AHA Guideline for the management of ST-elevation myocardial infarction. *Journal of the American College of Cardiology, 61*(4), e78–e140. doi:10.1016/j.jacc.2012.11.019

Reed, G. W., Rossi, J. E., & Cannon, C. P. (2017). Acute myocardial infarction, *The Lancet, 389*(10065), 197–210. doi:10.1016/S0140-6736(16)30677-8

Roest, A. M., Martens, E. J., de Jonge, P., & Denollet, J. (2010). Anxiety and risk of incident coronary heart disease. *Journal of the American College of Cardiology, 56*(1), 38–46. doi:10.1016/j.jacc.2010.03.034

Siela, D., & Kidd, M. (2017). Oxygen requirements for acutely and critically ill patients. *Critical Care Nurse, 37*(4), 58–70. doi:10.4037/ccn2017627

Stone, N. J., Robinson, J. G., Lichtenstein, A. H., Bairey Merz, C. N., Blum, C. B., Eckel, H. H., . . . American College of Cardiology/American Heart Association Task Force on Practice Guidelines. (2014). 2013 ACC/AHA guideline on the treatment of blood cholesterol to reduce atherosclerotic cardiovascular risk in adults: A report of the American College of Cardiology/American Heart Association Task Force on Practice Guidelines. *Circulation, 129*(25 Suppl. 2), S1–45. http://circ.ahajournals.org/lookup/suppl/doi:10.1161/01.cir.0000437738.63853.7a/-/DC1

Thygesen, K., Alpert, J. S., Jaffe, A. S., Simoons, M. L., Chaitman, B. R., & White, H. D. (2012). Third universal definition of myocardial infarction. *Journal of the American College of Cardiology, 60*(16), 1581–1598. doi:10.1016/j.jacc.2012.08.001

Venes, D. (Ed.). (2021). *Taber's cyclopedia medical dictionary.* (24th ed.). Philadelphia, PA: F.A. Davis.

Woo, T., & Robinson, M. (2020). *Pharmacotherapeutics for advanced practice nurse prescribers* (5th ed.). Philadelphia, PA: FA Davis.

Zhang, X., Devlin, H. M., Smith, B., Imperatore, G., Thomas, W., Lobelo, F., . . . Geiss, L. S. (2017). Effect of lifestyle interventions on cardiovascular risk factors among adults without impaired glucose tolerance or diabetes: A systematic review and meta-analysis. *PLoS One, 12*(5). doi:doi.org/10.1371/journal.pone.0176436

Case Study 1 (Adult): Glaucoma

LEARNING OBJECTIVES

Upon completion of this case study the student will be able to integrate knowledge of the pathophysiology, assessment, and pharmacological and nonpharmacological care options for care of an adult patient with glaucoma.

Introduction to Glaucoma

Glaucoma is a disease of *elevated intraocular eye pressure* (IOP) above normal for a period of time that leads to long-term damage of the optic nerve, visual impairment, and blindness. An individual is considered visually impaired when their vision is determined to be at best 20/40 even with glasses, while legal blindness is diagnosed when visual acuity is 20/200 or worse with limitation of the visual field to <20 degrees diameter (American Academy of Ophthalmology [AAO], 2018). Glaucoma is a "silent" disease with only about 50% of all people having an awareness of their condition. At least 3 million Americans have been diagnosed with a form of glaucoma, and about 120,000 of these Americans are designated as blind (Centers for Disease Control and Prevention [CDC], 2017; Glaucoma Research Foundation [GRF], 2017b). *Primary open-angle glaucoma* (POAG) is the most common form of the disease. The 2050 projected incidence of POAG in the United States is estimated to be 7.32 million, with the highest prevalence expected to be among the 70-to-79-year-old age-group (32%). While currently the disease is most prevalent in non-Hispanic European American women, by 2050 the highest prevalence is expected to shift to Hispanic American men (AAO, 2018). Around the world, only cataracts cause more blindness than glaucoma. The economic burden of glaucoma to the U.S. government ($1.5 billion each year) is extensive in terms of health expenditures, use of Social Security benefits, and lost revenue as individuals are unable to work (GRF, 2017b). Based on the prevalence of glaucoma, the impacts of the disease on quality of life, productivity, and overall health-care costs, *Healthy People 2020* selected improvement of visual health with a goal of decreasing blindness as one of its objectives (AAO, 2018).

Meet Mrs. SM

Mrs. SM is a 62-year-old African American woman who has come to her health-care provider with complaints of headaches and blurred vision that have become worse over the past few weeks. When taking the health history, Nurse NN learns that Mrs. SM is employed as an administrative assistant to a local bank manager. She has a history of hypertension controlled with lisinopril, and her blood pressure at this visit is 128/60 mm Hg taken with a manual cuff. Today she reports a headache with a pain level of 5 on a 0 to 10 scale and says that she takes ibuprofen for headaches. She reports using a 5-day prednisone dose pack for a sinus infection last year and admits to smoking two packs of cigarettes a week.

Physiology and Pathophysiology

The anterior chamber of the eye is composed of the aqueous and vitreous chambers. (See Figure CS1–1.) The *vitreous humor* is a gel-like substance whose primary responsibility is to form the eye's shape and form. Ciliary bodies, found between the iris and the lens, secrete approximately 5 mL of *aqueous humor* each day (about 1 mL of fluid circulating at any given time), and provides nutritional support to the cornea and lens. The fluid is reabsorbed via the canal of Schlemm and the trabecular meshwork. (See Figure CS1–2.) Contraction of the ciliary muscle, which is attached to the trabecular meshwork, facilitates aqueous fluid drainage, while muscle relaxation obstructs the canal. Innervated by both sympathetic (relaxation) and parasympathetic (contraction) pathways, changes in stimulation can change IOP (Capriotti, 2020).

The balance in the volume of fluid being formed, circulated, and reabsorbed establishes eye pressure, with normal pressure being between 12 and 22 mm Hg. Buildup

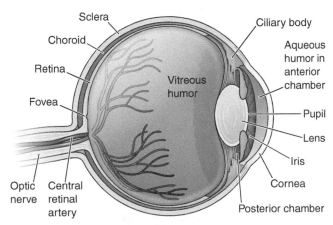

FIGURE CS1–1 Cross section of the eye *(From Capriotti, T. (2020). Pathophysiology: Introductory concepts and clinical perspectives (2nd ed). Philadelphia, PA: F.A. Davis.)*

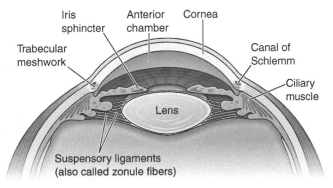

FIGURE CS1–2 Close-up view *(From Capriotti, T. (2020). Pathophysiology: Introductory concepts and clinical perspectives (2nd ed). Philadelphia, PA: F.A. Davis.)*

of fluid either by an imbalance in the amount of fluid or a blockage in the flow of aqueous fluid being created raises the IOP to a level that compresses blood vessels, photoreceptors, and nerve fibers of the optic nerve and results in ischemia and cell death. This destruction of the visual tissues typically begins in the peripheral areas of the retina and progresses to the central visual fields. Left untreated, elevated IOP can cause significant visual impairment and blindness (Belden, DeFriez, & Huether, 2012; Borchers & Borchers, 2018b; GRF, 2017c; Tsai, 2017; Weinreb, Aung, & Medeiros, 2014).

In POAG, the most common form of the disease, elevated eye pressure occurs as a result of inadequate drainage of aqueous fluid via the canal of Schlemm and trabecular meshwork systems, even though the space for the fluid to drain is "open." Fluid continues to be made at the normal rate, and as the volume of circulating fluid increases, the IOP increases. Damage is slowly progressive as neural pathways from the retina to the brain are destroyed and is often unnoticed until neural damage of peripheral vision is advanced (Belden et al., 2012; Borchers & Borchers, 2018b; Weinreb et al., 2014).

Acute angle-closure glaucoma (AACG) is less common but is responsible for more severe visual impairment and blindness than POAG (Weinreb et al., 2014). In this acute emergency condition, the iris is pushed forward against the cornea as the ciliary muscle relaxes, the trabecular meshwork is obstructed, and the canal of Schlemm is closed, preventing aqueous fluid from flowing out of the anterior chamber to be reabsorbed (Borchers & Borchers, 2018a; Capriotti, 2020). Relaxation of the ciliary muscle can be the response to anticholinergic medications or sympathetic activity (Capriotti, 2020). AACG is typically an acute condition that abruptly raises IOP and causes pain and acute visual impairments (Belden et al., 2012). Prevalence of AACG is most common in older adults in their 60s and 70s, especially women whose eye anatomy has a shallow anterior chamber (Capriotti, 2020).

A third, less common type of glaucoma is *congenital closure*. In this rare type of glaucoma, elevated IOP is the result of either a genetic abnormality or congenital malformation (Borchers & Borchers, 2018b). Regardless of the origin of elevated IOP, screening, early detection and appropriate treatment, and ongoing follow-up are essential to decreasing compression of visual pathways, minimizing visual acuity loss, and improving quality of life of patients with glaucoma (Boyd, 2018; Khanna, Leske, & Holmes, 2018; Sharts-Hopko & Glynn-Milley, 2009). Risk factors for glaucoma are highlighted in Table CS1–1.

TABLE CS1–1   Risk Factors for Glaucoma

Open Angle	Acute Closed
• Age >60 years or African American and age >40 years • Family history • Race • Hypertension • Diabetes mellitus • Hypothyroidism • Long-term corticosteroid use • Smoker • Eye pathology (myopia or thin cornea)	• Age >60 (or >40 and African American) • Family history • Race (ethnic Chinese) • Sex (female) • Eye pathology (iris, lens abnormalities; hyperopia)

(International Council of Ophthalmology, 2015; Sharts-Hopko & Glynn-Milley, 2009; Weinreb et al., 2014)

Gathering Information

Nurse NN assesses Mrs. SM's medical and social history. When questioned further about her symptoms and history, Mrs. SM states that she has not seen an eye doctor in several years, and that her brother has been diagnosed with glaucoma and uses eye drops. Additionally, her mother was diagnosed with glaucoma when she was 42 years old and used eye drops until she passed away last year. Mrs. SM reports that while she is employed, she does not have medical insurance, stating, "It is just too expensive, and I have to pay my bills."

Assessment and Diagnosis

Diagnosis of glaucoma is based on a review of the patient's history to identify risk factors; patient's reported symptoms; and a comprehensive eye examination with administration of dilating and numbing drops. During the examination, visual field limitations are identified and eye pressure is measured using tonometry; IOP measurements higher than 22 mm Hg indicate probable glaucoma, particularly if the individual is experiencing other symptoms (Tsai, 2017). A gonioscopy exam is conducted to directly visualize the interior of the eye and to observe drainage angles of aqueous humor (Boyd, 2019). During the direct ophthalmic visualization, the optic nerve's shape and color are observed, and, using a pachymetry test, the thickness of the cornea is determined (GRF, 2017a; International Council of Ophthalmology [CIO], 2015).

Diagnosis

During Mrs. SM's examination, her primary care provider notices that her pupils are equal but are slow to accommodate to light and her peripheral vision is slightly reduced. Mrs. SM is referred to an ophthalmologist for further testing. Nurse NN reinforces the importance of keeping the appointment with the ophthalmologist.

At the ophthalmologist's office, the technician (Miss AJ) conducts preliminary visual testing, and the ophthalmologist performs a dilated examination. Snellen visual acuity tests results indicate that Mrs. SM has 20/40 visual acuity in both eyes. Tonometry testing indicates that her IOP is elevated in both eyes at 26 mm Hg (normal range is 12 to 22 mm Hg). Additional examination results include minimal atrophy and cupping of the optic disk, and a minimal loss of peripheral vision in the right eye. Gonioscopic examination indicates that the iris/cornea angle is normal width and open to flow of fluid. Mrs. SM is diagnosed with primary open-angle glaucoma.

Treatment Options

Treatment options are aimed at lowering the IOP to about 20% to 50% lower than the IOP at time of diagnosis (Sharts-Hopko & Glynn-Milley, 2009). Pharmacological treatment with prostaglandin analogs (the first line drugs of choice), topical beta-adrenergic antagonists, alpha$_2$-adrenergic agonists, carbonic anhydrase inhibitors, or cholinergic agonists are prescribed. Treatment goals include utilization of the fewest medications possible to reduce IOP and with minimal adverse effects (Weinreb et al., 2014). Frequently used topical eye drops for glaucoma are highlighted in Table CS1–2.

These drugs, though prescribed as eye drops, often have systemic side effects, and often patients are noncompliant due to "forgetting" or to the lack of adequate resources for purchase of the prescribed medication (Sharts-Hopko & Glynn-Milley, 2009).

TABLE CS1–2   Drugs Commonly Used to Treat Glaucoma

Class	Example	Action	Dosage	SENC
Prostaglandin analogs	Latanoprost	Selective prostaglandin agonist; increases aqueous humor outflow rate.	*1–2 drops in the affected eye bid to qid.	Must space out 5–10 min between administration of latanoprost and thimerosal to avoid precipitation of latanoprost; iris may darken over time and eyelashes will grow longer.
Topical beta-adrenergic antagonists	Timolol maleate	Decrease aqueous humor production.	Extended release: 1 drop in the affected eye daily in the morning.	Has additive effects systemically; may interact with oral beta blockers and other cardiac drugs.
Alpha 2-adrenergic agonists	Iopidine*	Decrease aqueous humor production and increase outflow of aqueous humor.	*1–2 drops in the affected eye bid to qid.	Avoid with monoamine oxidase inhibitors (MAOIs). Because pupils dilate with these meds, patient should wear sunglasses outdoors; monitor for vasovagal response.
Cholinergic agonists (miotics)	Pilocarpine	Indirect-acting cholinesterase inhibitor; decreases resistance to aqueous outflow.	1–2 drops in the affected eye up to 6 times a day to get effect.	No significant drug–drug interactions. Systemic side effects include headache, flushing, sweating, and increased salivation.
Carbonic anhydrase inhibitors	Brinzolamide	Slows bicarbonate ion production, which slows sodium/fluid transport and decreases aqueous humor production.	1 drop in the affected eye tid; wait 10 min before administering another type of eye drop.	Rarely used due to adverse effects (aplastic anemia); many serious drug–drug interactions that decrease effectiveness or result in toxic levels of those drugs.

(Borchers & Borchers, 2018b; Vallerand & Sanoski, 2017; Woo, 2020)

*The range for most eye drops is 1 to 2 drops in the affected eye bid to qid. Specifically identified doses are listed.

Patient education regarding proper eye drop administration is important to successful treatment and is found in SENC Box CS1–1.

Surgical interventions may be indicated when glaucoma has been nonresponsive to pharmacological interventions, when there is progression of visual field impairment, or for those patients who have been noncompliant with their eye drops. *Trabeculoplasty* (argon or selective) laser surgery is performed as an office procedure. Small holes are burned into the trabecular meshwork to improve aqueous humor drainage. If the first eye responds well and the patient tolerates the procedure, it is repeated for the other eye. The advantage of selective laser surgery is the option to repeat the procedure if indicated. Patients should be taught to expect some localized soreness and inflammation following the procedure. *Selective laser trabeculoplasty* (SLT), may be effective for individuals whose eye pressure has not been adequately reduced by medications. When applied to the drainage area of the eye, the resulting tissue changes can improve fluid drainage, which reduces IOP. Results are typically seen within 1 to 3 months, but the procedure is determined to be ineffective if the pressure does not remain lower after 12 months. While the procedure may be repeated in select patient

SENC BOX CS1-1   Safe and Effective Nursing Care for Eye Drop Administration Education

1. Wash hands with soap and water prior to and following eye drop or eye ointment administration.
2. Avoid touching the dropper with fingers and do not touch the eye with the dropper.
3. Hold eye drop container in the dominant hand.
4. Tilt the head back and use the nondominant hand pointer finger to gently pull the lower eyelid down to create a pocket.
5. Place the drop onto the lower eyelid pocket and release the eyelid.
6. Close eye and look down. For 3 to 5 minutes, gently apply pressure to the inside corner of the eye to help avoid systemic absorption of the eye drop solution.
7. Wait 5 minutes before instilling another type of eye medication.
0. Do not rub the eyes after administration of eye drops.

Teach patients the following:

- Check the eye drops for name and expiration date, and check the color and clarity of the solution.
- The importance of not touching the dropper.
- That all eye drops may cause some burning or stinging, but prolonged burning / stinging and severe pain should be promptly reported.
- Never to stop their antiglaucoma medications abruptly.
- Remove contact lens prior to administration of eye drops and do not replace them for at least 10 to 15 minutes after medication is instilled (depending on the medication) to avoid discoloration of the contact lens.
- If drops are to be instilled only in one eye, avoid use of the drops in the other eye.

(Borchers & Borchers, 2018a, 2018b; Karch, 2020; Woo, 2020)

populations, a repeated trabeculoplasty is not usually as effective as the first procedure (Francis, 2019).

Trabeculectomy may be considered if medication or SLT have not been effective in lowering IOP. In this procedure, tissue is removed from the drainage canal in an effort to form a new pathway for fluid to flow from the eye. The procedure is effective for about 70% of patients; however, if not effective, while a repeat procedure can be performed, the results are typically less successful (Bedinghaus, 2020).

Treatment and Follow-Up

Following her diagnosis of primary open-angle glaucoma, Mrs. SM is prescribed a prostaglandin analog to reduce IOP, is given directions on how to use eye drops, told where she can fill the prescription for an affordable price, and given written information on her condition. Mrs. SM is scheduled for a follow-up visit in 4 months.

At the follow-up visit, Mrs. SM's IOP remains high at 25 mm Hg and she reports that the drops "sting" and blur her vision, and she does not use them every day because she often forgets. Due to her noncompliance with the eye drops, Mrs. SM is scheduled for laser trabeculoplasty as an alternative treatment. The procedures are scheduled (each eye at a separate time) and another follow-up appointment is scheduled 6 weeks after the last procedure. At this appointment, Mrs. SM reports no headaches, IOP is now 20 in each eye, and there has been no progression of peripheral visual loss since her initial visit. Mrs. SM will be followed at 4- to 6-month intervals and is taught the importance of reporting a return of headaches or visual impairment, and of keeping her scheduled visits.

Summary

Glaucoma is a "silent" disease that, left undiagnosed and untreated, robs the affected individual of sight and changes quality of life. Nurses have an integral role in patient education as they help patients to understand the disease process and the importance of identifying risk factors, and they encourage individuals to seek regular eye examinations. A key component of this education includes working with patients to identify methods to help them adhere to treatment plans. Engaging the patient in self-management of the disease and encouraging independence in their activities are key to improving quality of life for this patient population (Borchers & Borchers, 2018b).

Key Points

- The first signs of glaucoma are often nonreversible visual impairments, particularly of peripheral visual fields.
- Acute angle-closure glaucoma is a medical emergency requiring prompt treatment to minimize visual impairment.
- Treatment of the patient with glaucoma includes identification of barriers to obtaining and properly administering eye drops.
- Surgical treatment may be indicated if pharmacological treatment is not effective or is not followed by the patient. Some surgical treatment may provide only short-term improvement.

Review Questions

1. **The nurse is reviewing the health history of a 62-year-old African American female. The nurse understands that which of the following increases the patient's risk for glaucoma? (Select all that apply.)**

   a. Age
   b. History of hypertension
   c. Observed lens abnormality in the left eye
   d. Smokes two packs of cigarettes a week

2. **When explaining a trabeculoplasty procedure to a patient, which of the following statements made by the nurse is correct?**

   a. "A laser is used to make a little hole in the meshwork of the eye to allow fluid to flow."
   b. "A small incision is made in the eye canal while you are under anesthesia in the operating room."
   c. "Any inflammation should be reported immediately, as you should have no aftereffects from the procedure."
   d. "This procedure is only used because you refused to take your eye drops every week."

3. **Which of the following statements made by the patient indicates accurate understanding of a nurse's instructions on the proper administration of eye drops?**

   a. "Eye drops are topical, and I do not need to worry about any systemic effects."
   b. "I can put the drops in and immediately afterward put in my contact lens."

c. "I will place light pressure on the inside corner of the eye for 3 to 5 minutes after I put the drops in."

d. "I will clean the dropper with a clean cloth after putting my eye drops in."

4. **The nurse is providing education about newly prescribed eye drops to the patient newly diagnosed with primary open-angle glaucoma. Which of the following statements made by the patient indicates a need for further education?**

a. "I need to inform my cardiologist that I am taking timolol drops for glaucoma."

b. "I should not stop my eye drops unless I've talked to the eye doctor and have permission."

c. "My doctor only ordered drops for one eye but using them in both will help my eye pressures."

d. "The eye drops may sting and burn for a few minutes after I put them in, but that is normal."

5. **The nurse understands that a frequent cause of progression of glaucoma is which of the following? (Select all that apply.)**

a. Not seeking treatment for severe eye pain

b. Failure to use eye drops daily as directed

c. Lack of resources to purchase eye drops

d. Use of the Internet to find out more about glaucoma symptoms

See the appendix for answers to review questions.

References

American Academy of Ophthalmology. (2018). U.S. eye disease statistics. Retrieved from https://www.aao.org/eye-disease-statistics

Bedinghaus, T. (2020, March 28). Trabeculectomy for glaucoma. Retrieved from https://www.verywellhealth.com/trabeculectomy-3421700

Belden, J., DeFriez, C., & Huether, S. E. (2012). Pain, temperature, sleep, and sensory function. In S. E. Huether & K. L. McCance (Eds.), *Understanding pathophysiology* (5th ed.). St. Louis, MO: Elsevier Mosby.

Borchers, S. A., & Borchers, A. A. (2018a). Assessment of the eye and vision. In D. D. Ignatavicius, M. L. Workman, & C. R. Rebar (Eds.), *Medical-surgical nursing: Concepts for interprofessional collaborative care* (9th ed.). St. Louis, MO: Elsevier.

Borchers, S. A., & Borchers, A. A. (2018b). Care of patients with eye and vision problems. In D. D. Ignatavicius, M. L. Workman, & C. R. Rebar (Eds.), *Medical-surgical nursing: Concepts for interprofessional collaborative care* (9th ed.). St. Louis, MO: Elsevier.

Boyd, K. (2018). What is glaucoma? Retrieved from https://www.aao.org/eye-health/diseases/what-is-glaucoma

Boyd, K. (2019). What is gonioscopy? Retrieved from https://www.aao.org/eye-health/treatments/what-is-gonioscopy

Capriotti, T. (2020). *Pathophysiology: Introductory concepts and clinical perspectives* (2nd ed). Philadelphia, PA: F.A. Davis.

Centers for Disease Control and Prevention. (2017). *Don't let glaucoma steal your sight!* Retrieved from https://www.cdc.gov/features/glaucoma-awareness/index.html

Francis, B. A. (2019). *Selective laser trabeculoplasty: 10 commonly asked questions*. Retrieved from https://www.glaucoma.org/treatment/selective-laser-trabeculoplasty-10-commonly-asked-questions.php

Glaucoma Research Foundation. (2017a). Five common glaucoma tests. Retrieved from https://www.glaucoma.org/glaucoma/diagnostic-tests.php

Glaucoma Research Foundation. (2017b). Glaucoma facts and stats. Retrieved from https://www.glaucoma.org/glaucoma/glaucoma-facts-and-stats.php

Glaucoma Research Foundation. (2017c). High eye pressure and glaucoma. Retrieved from https://www.glaucoma.org/gleams/high-eye-pressure-and-glaucoma.php

International Council of Ophthalmology. (2015). ICO guidelines for glaucoma eye care. Retrieved from http://www.icoph.org/downloads/ICOGlaucomaGuidelines.pdf

Karch, A. M. (2020). *Focus on nursing pharmacology* (8th ed.). Philadelphia, PA: Wolters Kluwer / Lippincott Williams & Wilkins.

Khanna, C. L., Leske, D. A., & Holmes, J. M. (2018). Factors associated with health-related quality of life in medically and surgically treated patients with glaucoma. *JAMA Ophthalmology, 136*(4), 348–355. doi:10.1001/jamaophthalmol.2018.0012

Sharts-Hopko, N. C., & Glynn-Milley, C. (2009). Primary open-angle glaucoma. Catching and treating the "sneak thief of sight." *American Journal of Nursing, 109*(2), 40–47.

Tsai, J. C. (2017, Oct. 29). High pressure and glaucoma. *Glaucoma Research Foundation.* Retrieved from https://www.glaucoma.org/gleams/high-eye-pressure-and-glaucoma.php

Weinreb, R. N., Aung, T., & Medeiros, F. A. (2014). The pathophysiology and treatment of glaucoma: A review. *JAMA, 311*(18), 1901–1911.

Woo, T. M. (2020). Drugs used in treating eye and ear disorders. In T. M. Woo & M. V. Robinson (Eds.), *Pharmacotherapeutics for advanced practice nurse prescribers* (5th ed.). Philadelphia, PA: F.A. Davis.

Vallerand, A. H., & Sanoski, C. A. (Eds.). (2017). *Davis's drug guide for nurses* (15th ed.). Philadelphia, PA: F.A. Davis.

Maternity

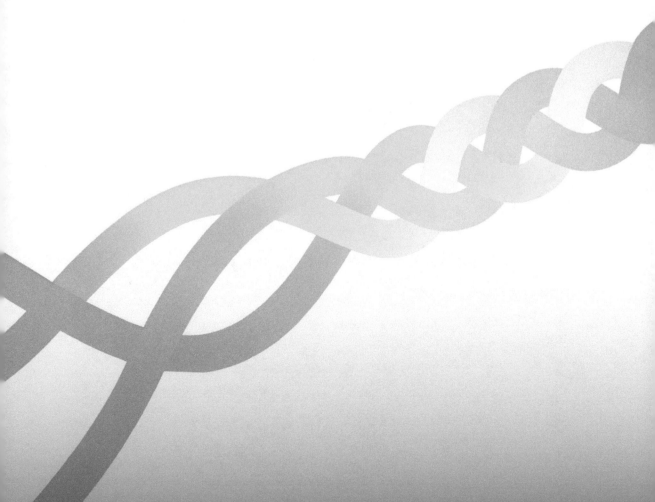

Hypertensive Disorders of Pregnancy

Introduction

The diagnosis of hypertensive disorder during pregnancy is a common manifestation secondary to the diagnosis of pregnancy and the second-leading cause of pregnancy complications. Hypertensive disorders complicate up to 5% to 10% of all pregnancies worldwide and are a major contributor to maternal mortality. A diagnosis of embolic disorders in pregnancy is the most common complication of pregnancy. These complications can be caused by a blood clot leading to a thrombus, a fat particle causing a fat embolism, a bubble of air, or a foreign body or material (Ward & Hisley, 2016).

Hypertensive disorders are also a major contributor to neonatal morbidity and mortality and can lead to significant maternal- and neonatal-related complications. Maternal complications may include aspiration pneumonia, placenta abruption, adult respiratory distress syndrome, cerebral hemorrhage, liver and renal failure, pulmonary edema, and *disseminated intravascular coagulation* (DIC) (American College of Obstetricians and Gynecologists [ACOG] in Ward & Hisley, 2016). Neonatal complications can include premature rupture of membranes, premature labor and delivery, and all the complications associated with early gestation, intrauterine growth restriction, and admission into the neonatal intensive care unit.

According to the ACOG 2018 guidelines, the term *gestational hypertension*, or high blood pressure that has developed during a pregnancy, is used to diagnose any pregnant patient who experiences an increase in blood pressure after 20 weeks of pregnancy. A pregnant patient who experiences hypertension prior to 20 weeks of pregnancy is diagnosed with *chronic hypertension*, based on the consideration that the elevation in blood pressure likely "predated" the pregnancy (Ward & Hisley, 2016).

The differentiation between gestational hypertension (or benign hypertension secondary to pregnancy) and the diagnosis of pre-eclampsia must also be considered.

Pre-eclampsia is a significantly more serious diagnosis in pregnancy and must be appropriately treated to prevent severe maternal and neonatal complications (Ward & Hisley, 2016). Unfortunately, the diagnosis of pre-eclampsia has increased by 25% during the past 20 years worldwide and is a leading cause of both maternal and neonatal complications to include premature birth and death.

Physiology

The physiological changes that occur in pregnancy are widespread and significant. The systems and processes with the most significant alterations include the cardiovascular, hematological, and coagulation areas. The blood volume increases in pregnancy as much as 50% over a woman's pre-pregnancy state for a pregnancy with one fetus. This increase in maternal blood volume results from a combination of plasma and erythrocytes. Additional erythrocytes are necessary to compensate for the additional oxygen requirements needed in pregnancy for placental tissue and the increasing maternal supply of oxygen needed for the growing fetus.

There are many hormones responsible for the preservation of pregnancy, and each one has a certain function related to the embryo and developing fetus. Progesterone and estrogen are the primary hormones produced by the placenta in pregnancy, with progesterone being responsible for pregnancy maintenance and estrogen being responsible for fetal growth. Estrogen is also responsible for hyperplasia related to a woman's uterus and breasts and prepares for the contractility necessary for the delivery process. Progesterone relaxes the smooth muscles within the body and increases vasodilation with an increase of blood flow to the entire body.

In response to the maternal increase in blood volume, the *cardiac output* (CO) increases by 30% to 50% of pre-pregnancy levels with secondary vasodilation. This reaction is responsible for relaxing the vascular smooth muscle and decreasing the maternal blood pressure during pregnancy. Due to the decrease in blood pressure, the heart rate normally increases to circulate the level of increased blood volume. In addition, the *systemic vascular resistance* (SVR) also decreases in response to the increased levels of circulating progesterone. This SVR response can begin as early as the 5th week of pregnancy and normally maintains a minimal reduction in blood pressure readings (Ward & Hisley, 2016).

Pathophysiology

The hormonal influences of pregnancy can cause complications associated with hypertension. Alterations in the woman's clotting mechanisms can begin as early as 11th week of pregnancy and continue into the postpartum period for up to 4 weeks post-delivery. This alteration increases the body's ability to form abnormal blood clots, decreases the body's capacity to break down any clots that form, and inhibits the woman's ability to break down clots throughout the body. These changes, in addition to the stressors of pregnancy, contribute to the potential for excessive clot formation in patients with pre-existing cardiovascular disease. These cumulative changes, in addition to a diagnosis of hypertension in pregnancy, can compound the risk of cerebrovascular complications in pregnancy. This combination can lead to cerebrovascular problems that can include a *cerebrovascular accident* (CVA), or stroke (Davis & Sanders, 2019).

According to Capriotti (2020), "hypertension (HTN) has two major effects on the cardiovascular system (p. 339)." The influence of hypertension on the body can damage the lining of the arteries and create resistance against the functioning of the left ventricle of the heart. This resistance can eventually create a larger-than-normal ventricle due to the excessive workload required of the ventricular muscle. The new size of the ventricle will eventually require additional blood flow and oxygen levels to compensate for the larger muscle. The body's respiratory and cardiac systems are often unable to deliver the needed supplies, and further damage and long-term complications can develop secondary to the uncontrolled HTN.

The long-term effects of hypertension that has not been detected or controlled can be significant to all body systems. The systems most often affected include the brain, kidneys, lower extremities, and the retina of the eye. The effect of hypertension on these systems can cause substantial acute complications with secondary chronic problems, such as renal failure, limb amputation, embolic and hemorrhagic stroke, and limited vision or even complete blindness (Capriotti, 2020).

Pregnancy-induced hypertension (PIH) has been previously classified as a secondary hypertension, one that is caused secondarily to the pregnancy diagnosis, and this diagnosis is the source of elevation in maternal blood pressure. Secondary hypertension is also considered an effect of a systemic disorder or diagnosis. The main pathophysiological feature found in PIH is vasospasm with concurrent endothelial damage (Ward & Hisley 2016). A patient may also be predisposed to the development of hypertension based on other diagnoses present that can influence and elevate the patient's potential for a diagnosis of both primary and secondary hypertension during pregnancy (Capriotti, 2020).

The new ACOG guidelines (2019) suggest using the diagnosis of gestational hypertension and pre-eclampsia to replace a diagnosis of PIH. The ACOG Task Force on Hypertension has recommended that the following classifications be assigned to patients who experience hypertension during pregnancy (Ward & Hisley, 2016):

- Chronic hypertension
- Gestational hypertension
- Transient hypertension
- Pre-eclampsia/eclampsia
- Pre-eclampsia superimposed on chronic hypertension

Chronic hypertension is defined as hypertension that is present before a woman becomes pregnant or hypertension diagnosed in a pregnant patient before the 20th week of pregnancy. *Gestational hypertension* is defined as a "blood pressure of 140 mm Hg systolic or a diastolic of 90 mm Hg or higher, or the increase in both systolic and diastolic readings with two separate readings 4 hours apart" if able based on symptoms (ACOG, 2019, p. 2). If the patient is not critical, another BP reading is taken after 4 hours. If the patient is critical, the first reading is used and the patient is treated. The diagnosis is made after 20 weeks of gestation in a pregnant patient with prior normal blood pressure readings without protein in the urine (ACOG, 2019). *Transient hypertension* is used only to describe women in the postpartum period who experience an elevation in blood pressure that returns to a normal level within 3 months after delivery. There is an increased risk for ongoing hypertension and associated complications if left untreated. If the blood pressure remains elevated after a 3-month time frame, the diagnosis converts to chronic hypertension (Ward & Hisley, 2016).

Pre-eclampsia/Eclampsia

Pre-eclampsia is a pregnancy complication that is usually diagnosed after the 20th week and up to the end of the pregnancy, or 40 weeks. A new onset of increase in maternal blood pressure is the main indicator of this condition. Pre-eclampsia occurs only in pregnancy, and its effects are systemwide in nature. Proteinuria may or may not be present in conjunction with the increase in blood pressure, and proteinuria and edema are no longer considered factors when making the diagnosis (Davis & Sanders, 2019).

Eclampsia occurs with a new onset of seizures in conjunction with pre-eclampsia and no previous history of seizure activity. The seizures can manifest as tonic-clonic, focal, or multifocal without other causes or a record of seizures. The seizure activity can cause both maternal and fetal hypoxia and trauma or aspiration of gastric contents, which may lead to aspiration pneumonia.

According to ACOG (2019), there are multiple theories related to the onset of pre-eclampsia and eclampsia in pregnancy. These theories include a decreased blood flow to the placenta and uterus; blood vessel imbalances; and a decreased or increased immune system response to the pregnancy. A combination of these factors has also been proposed but not clinically proven to be the etiology for this diagnosis. It is known that the placenta has a major role in the development of pre-eclampsia, and, because of this connection, the diagnosis can only be made during a molar or actual pregnancy.

Patients with pre-eclampsia often have less blood volume than normal pregnant women and are found to have blood that is significantly more concentrated than normal. Blood vessel vasospasms are common due to the interface of vasoactive agents, which include prostacyclin (a prostaglandin and potent vasodilator that decreases blood pressure and platelet adhesions) and thromboxane (a vasoconstrictor synthesized in platelets from prostaglandins that increase blood pressure and promotes platelet adhesions). These vasospasms may also increase sodium and water retention and lead to a reduced urinary and uric acid output with secondary proteinuria present (ACOG, 2019; Ward & Hisley, 2016).

The decreased blood flow to the uterus and placenta often leads to *intrauterine growth restriction* (IUGR), low amniotic fluid volume (oligohydramnios), and the potential for a placental abruption. When a pregnant patient with pre-eclampsia is placed on an external fetal monitor, it often reveals a fetal monitoring pattern that is not reassuring for the continuation of the pregnancy. Early or premature labor often ensues due to the decrease in placental blood flow, causing premature rupture of membranes and delivery of an infant before 37 weeks of gestation (ACOG, 2019). Figure 6-1 illustrates the pathophysiological changes in pre-eclampsia.

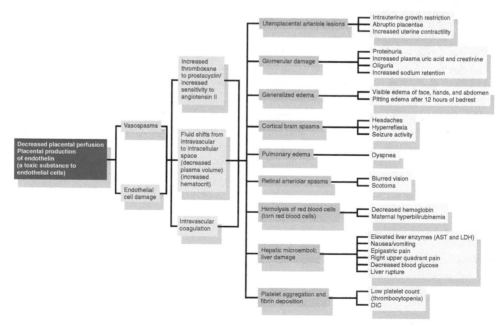

FIGURE 6–1 Pathophysiological changes in pre-eclampsia *(Ward, S. L., & Hisley, S. M. (2016).* Maternal-child nursing care. *Philadelphia, PA: F.A. Davis.)*

Pre-eclampsia or eclampsia in pregnancy can also increase a patient's risk of hypertension and stroke later in life. The American Heart Association (AHA) and the American Stroke Association (ASA) determined in 2014 that pre-eclampsia should be added to the gender-specific risk factors for a future stroke and have added the diagnosis to their prevention guidelines. A woman's risk for stroke should be considered across her life span because several of the risk factors can compound during her childbearing years (Davis & Sanders, 2019).

Risk Factors for Pre-eclampsia/Eclampsia

The following are risk factors for pre-eclampsia in pregnancy (ACOG, 2019):

- Pregnant for the first time (nulliparity)
- Multifetal gestations
- Pre-eclampsia in a previous pregnancy or a family history thereof
- Chronic hypertension
- Pre-gestational diabetes
- Gestational diabetes
- Thrombophilia
- Systemic lupus erythematosus
- Pre-pregnancy body mass index greater than 30
- Antiphospholipid antibody syndrome
- Maternal age 35 years or older
- Kidney disease
- Assisted reproductive technology
- Obstructive sleep apnea
- Obesity
- Diabetes
- Lupus

These risk factors can increase the potential for a diagnosis of pre-eclampsia in pregnancy, but the majority of newly diagnosed patients with pre-eclampsia are healthy, nulliparous (never given birth) women with no discernable risk factors for the diagnosis. The roles of environmental and genetic factors are emerging as potential components for an increased risk of developing pre-eclampsia. Although a clear connection has not been determined between these factors, these areas remain under review as potential maternal and neonatal risk factors (ACOG, 2019).

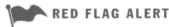 **RED FLAG ALERT**
Any patient diagnosed with pre-eclampsia during pregnancy should be screened for hypertension annually.

HIGH YIELD FACT FOR TESTING

The stabilization and reduction of hypertension in a patient diagnosed with pre-eclampsia may decrease the potential for a premature delivery.

Assessment

Hypertensive disorders in pregnancy are defined and classified according to specific criteria and symptoms experienced by the pregnant woman. The blood pressure measurements for chronic hypertension can include a systolic blood pressure greater than or equal to 140 mm Hg or a diastolic reading greater than or equal to 90 mm Hg. The guidelines for elevations in blood pressure leading to a diagnosis of chronic hypertension include the following (Ward & Hisley, 2016):

- Elevated Blood Pressure: Systolic between 120 and 129 and diastolic less than 80 mm Hg
- Stage 1 Hypertension: Systolic between 130 and 139 or diastolic between 80 and 89 mm Hg
- Stage 2 Hypertension: Systolic at least 140 or diastolic at least 90 mm Hg

Diagnostic Criteria for Pre-eclampsia

BLOOD PRESSURE ASSESSMENT

- Systolic blood pressure of 140 mm Hg or more or diastolic blood pressure of 90 mm Hg or more on two occasions at least 4 hours apart after 20 weeks of gestation in a woman with a previously normal blood pressure.
- Systolic blood pressure of 160 mm Hg or more or diastolic blood pressure of 110 mm Hg or more. (Considered to be severe hypertension and should be diagnosed quickly to initiate treatment.)

PROTEIN IN URINE

- 300 mg or more per 24-hour urine collection, or
- Protein/creatinine ratio of 0.3 mg/dL or more, or
- Urine dipstick reading of 2+.
- In the absence of protein in the urine, new-onset hypertension with the new onset of any of the following:
  - Thrombocytopenia: Platelet count less than 100,000.
  - Renal insufficiency: Serum creatinine levels greater than 1.1 mg/dL or a doubling of the serum creatinine concentration in the absence of renal disease.
  - Impaired liver function: Elevated blood concentrations of liver transaminases to twice normal concentration.
    - Pulmonary edema.
    - New-onset headache unresponsive to medication and not caused by other diagnoses or visual symptoms.

SEVERE DIAGNOSTIC CRITERIA

- Systolic blood pressure of 160 mm Hg or more, or diastolic blood pressure of 110 mm Hg or more, on two occasions at least 4 hours apart.
- Thrombocytopenia (platelet count less than 100,000).
- Impaired liver function as indicated by abnormally elevated blood concentrations of liver enzymes.
- Severe persistent right upper quadrant or epigastric pain unresponsive to medication and not related to other diagnoses.
- Renal insufficiency.
- Pulmonary edema.
- New-onset headache unresponsive to medication and not related to other diagnoses.
- Visual disturbances.

The diagnosis of pre-eclampsia must be considered in any pregnant patient who has any known risk factors or who experiences symptoms that fall under the diagnostic criteria for this diagnosis. See the box Diagnostic Criteria for Pre-eclampsia (ACOG, 2019).

Trace edema is present in the majority of pregnant patients and often resolves after rest and elevation of the lower extremities. A new onset of rapidly progressing or substantial maternal edema on a 0 to 4+ scale, edema that does not respond to rest and leg elevation, generalized edema or a weight gain of over 2 pounds per week always warrant a closer assessment. This brisk increase in maternal edema may indicate deteriorating symptoms associated with a hypertensive disorder and should raise a high index of suspicion for the progression of pre-eclampsia or eclampsia by a healthcare provider (Ward & Hisley, 2016). Figure 6-2 provides an assessment scale for edema (Dillon, 2016).

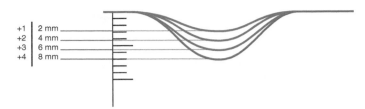

FIGURE 6–2 Edema Assessment Scale *(From Dillon, P. M. (2016).* Nursing health assessment. *Philadelphia, PA: F.A. Davis.)*

To assess for edema, press the index finger over the bony prominence of the tibia or medial malleolus. Orthostatic (pitting) edema results in a depression that does not rapidly refill and resume its original contour. It is not usually accompanied by thickening or pigmentation of the overlying skin. The severity of edema can be graded on a scale of +1 to +4, as shown in the following (Dillon, 2016):

+1 Slight pitting with about 2 mm depression that disappears rapidly. No visible distortion of extremity.

+2 Deeper pitting with about 4 mm depression that disappears in 10 to 15 seconds. No visible distortion of extremity.

+3 Depression of about 6 mm that lasts more than a minute. Dependent extremity looks swollen.

+4 Very deep pitting with about 8 mm depression that lasts 2 to 3 minutes. Dependent extremity is grossly distorted.

A more severe diagnosis of pre-eclampsia is the HELLP syndrome. This syndrome presents with the symptoms of **H**emolysis of red blood cells, **E**levated **L**iver enzymes and a **L**ow blood **P**latelet count, and correlates with a significant increase in morbidity and mortality. The laboratory values include a *lactate dehydrogenase* (LDH) level of 600 IU/L or higher, *aspartate aminotransferase* (AST) and *alanine aminotransferase* (ALT) elevated over twice the upper normal limit, and platelet counts of less than 100,000. HELLP syndrome may manifest in the third trimester of pregnancy or after delivery in the postpartum period. The symptoms are often vague and may only include hypertension, proteinuria, right upper quadrant pain, fatigue, nausea, and vomiting (ACOG, 2019).

With eclampsia, the pregnant patient can experience symptoms prior to seizure activity onset, including hyperreflexia of the deep tendon reflexes, headache, blurred vision, photophobia, or a change in level of consciousness. The seizure activity can begin during pregnancy, in labor, or post-delivery. The seizure may also occur without any warning or symptoms during pregnancy or post-delivery (ACOG, 2019).

A diagnosis of pre-eclampsia can also be made in combination with a diagnosis of chronic hypertension. This diagnosis is labeled *superimposed pre-eclampsia.* The criteria for this diagnosis are specific and include the following:

• High blood pressure and no protein in the urine before 20 weeks, with a new onset of protein in the urine.

• An increase in protein in the urine without evidence of a urinary tract infection.

• An increase in blood pressure readings after a period of controlled blood pressure.

• Evidence of thrombocytopenia (platelets less than 100,000).

• A surge in the liver enzymes ALT and AST.

The diagnosis of superimposed hypertension is very serious due to the potential for a significant increase in complications for both the mother and fetus. The elevated blood pressure must be controlled quickly to avoid ominous problems from arising (Ward & Hisley, 2016).

"Fifty percent of pregnant patients diagnosed with gestational hypertension will eventually develop protein in their urine and a form of organ dysfunction that is often associated with a diagnosis of pre-eclampsia (ACOG, 2019, p. 1)." This conversion to pre-eclampsia often occurs when a diagnosis of gestational hypertension is made before 32 weeks of pregnancy. In the event that systolic readings increase to over 160 mm Hg or diastolic readings over 110 mm Hg, the maternal diagnosis will convert to pre-eclampsia. This is based on the severe symptoms and will be associated with an increased risk for both maternal and neonatal complications. This can occur during the pregnancy, in the post-partum period, and long term with the potential for chronic hypertension (ACOG, 2019).

Assessment Techniques

Blood pressure measurements should be carried out using the gold standard measurement devices. The traditional sphygmomanometer is considered by many to be the optimal measurement tool for obtaining accurate blood pressure readings. The appropriate cuff size for the patient's arm or leg is also important to precisely obtain a true interpretation of a patient's blood pressure. The measurement should ideally occur with a patient seated or lying, and the blood pressure cuff should be positioned at the level of a patient's heart. The use of automated blood pressure recording systems in health care has often been found to provide inaccurate readings. Blood pressures obtained with the use of these devices are often found to be lower than the patient's actual reading, and treatment is then inaccurately based on the charted readings that are erroneous (Ward & Hisley, 2016).

It is helpful to use the SPASMS method of assessing a patient with symptoms of pre-eclampsia. This method follows the first letter of the mnemonic and highlights symptoms of pre-eclampsia progression:

- S—Significant blood pressure changes that may occur without warning.
- P—Proteinuria is a sign of renal involvement.
- A—Arterioles are affected by vasospasms that cause endothelial damage and leak intravascular fluid into tissues.
- S—Significant diagnostic changes that denote progression (liver function tests and platelet counts).
- M—Multiple system involvement (cardiac, renal, hepatic, hematology, central nervous system).
- S—Symptoms begin after 20 weeks of pregnancy (Ward & Hisley, 2016).

All patients experiencing a hypertensive disorder of pregnancy should be fully assessed using a head-to-toe method that should include a measurement of vital signs, fundal height, edema, fetal heart rate, and *deep tendon reflexes* (DTRs). The assessment of reflexes may provide information related to central nervous system involvement and irritability. The level of irritability provides information about the potential for the onset of maternal seizure activity. Reflexes are graded on a scale of 0 to 4+ as shown in the following (Thompson, 2018):

0 Absent
1+ A slight response but diminished
2+ Normal response with average strength
3+ Very brisk or exaggerated response; may or may not be normal
4+ A tap elicits a repeating abnormal reflex (clonus); always abnormal

Assessment of deep tendon reflexes involves both tendons and muscles to elicit a comparison reflex on both the left and right sides of the patient's body. To provide an accurate reflex assessment, the patient should be relaxed during assessment, through distraction provided by talking to the patient. An assessment of the patellar tendon reflex involves having the patient dangle their legs freely if possible and tapping the patellar tendon below the right and left patella. An assessment is made of the reaction of the legs to the tapping and is graded according to the reflex grading scale. Any increase in reflexes may indicate neurological complications and decreased reflexes may be due to medications or an altered level of alertness (Thompson, 2018).

Auscultation of heart, lung, breath, and bowel sounds should also be performed. Daily weights should be recorded, with an assessment of skin turgor and capillary refill noted. The patient should be provided with the management plan to include pharmacological agents, their effects and any potential side effects (Ward & Hisley, 2016).

Nonpharmacological Management

A pregnant patient diagnosed with a hypertensive disorder of pregnancy will be monitored closely for worsening symptoms or further complications to both mother and fetus. The optimal care provided should include a plan for delivery as needed. The stability of maternal symptoms may provide for a term delivery of the newborn with a reduced risk of acute and chronic complications and optimal neonatal benefit. It is essential to take into consideration the gestational age of the neonate versus the maternal stability of symptoms and progression of symptoms. Ongoing maternal surveillance should include serial ultrasounds for assessment of fetal growth, placental positioning in the uterus, and placental functioning with amniotic fluid measurements (ACOG, 2019).

Numerous studies have been initiated to review the causes and possible prevention of pre-eclampsia with progression to eclampsia in pregnancy. To date, there have been no equivocal data supporting any single intervention to prevent the onset of this diagnosis. Optimal nutrition, bedrest, sodium restriction, prenatal vitamins, fish oil, aspirin, metformin therapy, and garlic supplementation are a few of the areas researched with the prospect of discovering prevention strategies. Ongoing surveillance, monitoring, and serial ultrasounds as needed to assess fetal growth and amniotic fluid levels have been found to reduce the potential for current and future complications associated with hypertensive disorders of pregnancy.

Blood pressure monitoring, laboratory analysis for proteinuria, and complete blood counts including platelet counts and liver enzymes should be assessed as necessary. If severe symptoms begin to manifest in the pregnant patient, delivery rather than expectant assessments may be warranted to reduce further complications associated with a continuation of the pregnancy. A plan should also be in place and agreed on by both the provider and family to provide for a transfer to a health-care facility that has the ability and designation to ensure the best possible outcome for both the mother and her baby or babies if a preterm delivery is anticipated. A consultation with the neonatal intensive care unit team should also be provided in preparation for a preterm delivery if warranted (ACOG, 2019).

Home Care Management

If reasonable and possible, a pregnant patient may choose to be treated at home instead of in the hospital for a diagnosis of mild hypertensive disorder of pregnancy and or clotting issues. This decision will be made in combination with and supported by her health-care provider. If home care is a choice, frequent maternal and fetal assessments will be required and documented. This can be achieved through visiting home nurses or remote fetal and maternal monitoring or a combination of the two approaches. In the event the maternal blood pressure increases and is associated with further symptoms, it will be necessary to admit the mother for blood pressure management and possible early delivery (ACOG, 2019).

Pharmacology

The management of a pregnant woman experiencing a diagnosis of hypertension of pregnancy requires specific pharmacological precautions and monitoring. Evidence supports using a full assessment of the patient in order to individualize pharmacological treatment for hypertension. The provider should prescribe the safest medication at the lowest appropriate dosage initially and monitor the patient for any new complications associated with the medication before any alterations are made to the dosage. The effectiveness of all medications prescribed for hypertension should be closely supervised to determine whether additional or supplementary medications need to be included. SENC Box 6-1 gives general SENC practices that should be shared with patients.

The antihypertensive medications for adults discussed in Chapter 1 can be referenced for information related to their administration during pregnancy. The majority have been shown to have a good safety profile in pregnancy. The specific classes of antihypertensive medications to be avoided from Table 1-2 include *angiotensin-converting enzyme* (ACE) inhibitors, angiotensin II receptor blockers, and renin inhibitors. It has been established that these medications have been found to have an increased risk of maternal side effects and adverse neonatal outcomes. Table 6-1 lists the most common medications administered to pregnant women and provides information about normal dosages and specific SENC practices for each.

Summary

The risk factors and symptoms associated with pre-eclampsia and eclampsia may be indicators of underlying pre-existing factors or a precursor to future cardiovascular events. Women with a history of pre-eclampsia and eclampsia have a higher-than-normal risk for the development of *cardiovascular disease* (CVD) for a minimum of 10 years post-delivery. They are more likely to have elevations in blood pressure, meet the criteria for a diagnosis of hypertension, and require antihypertensive medications than women without a diagnosis of pre-eclampsia/eclampsia in pregnancy. There is also a risk for the development of metabolic syndrome, an elevation in serum lipid levels, insulin resistance, and a high waist-to-hip ratio with a previous diagnosis of pre-eclampsia/eclampsia during a single pregnancy or multiple pregnancies (Davis & Sanders, 2019).

SENC BOX 6-1 Safe and Effective Nursing Care for Patients on Antihypertensive Medications

1. Take the medication at the same time each day.
2. Maintain fluid intake and change positions slowly.
3. Do not take any other medications without consulting the prescriber.
4. Avoid excessive exercise in hot weather.

TABLE 6–1   Medications Used to Treat Hypertensive Disorders of Pregnancy

Class	Example	Action	Dosage	SENC
Beta blocker	Labetalol	Relaxes blood vessels and decreases heart rate to increase blood flow and decrease blood pressure. Blocks epinephrine.	200 mg PO q 12 hr, increasing to 800 mg PO q 8–12 hr prn, max of 2,400 mg/day.	May decrease blood flow to extremities, which is exacerbated with smoking. Light-headedness, fatigue, weight gain, instability in blood glucose levels, dizziness.
Calcium channel blocker	Nifedipine	Relaxes blood vessels by affecting the movement of calcium into the cells of the heart and blood vessels. Blocks the flow of calcium into the muscle cells around the heart. Increases the blood supply and oxygen to the heart while decreasing the workload.	30–60 mg/day with a maximum dose of 90 mg/day.	May cause headache, dizziness, flushing, edema, nausea, constipation, muscle cramps, wheezing, gum hyperplasia, hypotension.
Central alpha-adrenergic inhibitor	Alpha-methyldopa	Centrally active sympatholytic agent. Reduces concentration of epinephrine, norepinephrine, dopamine, and serotonin to dilate blood vessels.	0.5–3.0 g PO/day in 2–3 divided doses.	Safe in breastfeeding. May cause maternal edema and anemia.
Loop diuretic	Furosemide	Inhibits the luminal 1Na/1K/2Cl co-transporter in the ascending loop of Henle	12.5–50 mg PO/day	May induce neonatal thrombocytopenia when breastfeeding on medication. Assess for dizziness, drowsiness, hypotension, and electrolyte disorders.
Anticonvulsant	Magnesium sulfate	Causes a resolution of eclampsia by decreasing muscular excitability and neurotransmission.	40 g in 1,000 cc of lactated Ringer's solution, run at ordered rate IV. Loading dose 4–6 g over 15–30 min, maintenance dose 1–3 g/hr.	Do not use with hypermagnesemia, hypocalcemia, anuria, or heart block. The therapeutic range for magnesium is 4.8–9.6 mg/dL. Can decrease respirations and cause drowsiness and hypotension. Magnesium levels should be monitored. Calcium gluconate should be available as an antidote for hypermagnesemia.

Continued

TABLE 6-1   Medications Used to Treat Hypertensive Disorders of Pregnancy—cont'd

Class	Example	Action	Dosage	SENC
Peripheral arteriolar vasodilator	Hydralazine	Lowers blood pressure by exerting a peripheral vasodilating effect by relaxing vascular smooth muscle.	50–300 mg PO/day in 2–4 divided doses.	Use with labetalol to prevent reflex tachycardia. May cause tachycardia, dizziness, anorexia, and headache.
Vasodilator	Sodium nitroprusside	Relaxes vascular smooth muscle and dilates peripheral arteries.	0.25 mcg/kg/min (increase by 25 mcg/kg/min every 5 min to a maximum of 5 mcg/kg/min).	Reserve for extreme emergencies due to the potential for cyanide toxicity. Monitor for maternal cerebral edema.
NSAIDs	Aspirin	Reduces inflammation, has analgesic and antiplatelet properties.	60–100 mg PO/day.	Monitor for congenital defects and pregnancy loss with higher doses.

(Ward & Hisley, 2016)

Prenatal care is essential for the early diagnosis and treatment of all complications including hypertensive disorders of pregnancy. The ability for a pregnant woman to have access to early, consistent maternity care is fundamental to ensuring a reduction in risk for both the mother and fetus. Continued maternal/fetal management is contingent on the results of consistent assessments and gestational age. The decision to move forward to delivery whether term or preterm must always be a balance between the maternal and fetal risks and the potential for additional complications related to prematurity in the newborn.

All women diagnosed with hypertensive disorders of pregnancy should be educated about their future risk for cardiovascular disease, chronic hypertension, and stroke. These risks should be assessed at every annual visit to their health-care provider in conjunction with a close review of blood pressure readings and risk factors. National guidelines related to screening should be created to ensure consistency with follow-up. In addition, recommendations for review and treatment of both modifiable and non-modifiable risk factors and the potential for future complications related to a history of pre-eclampsia should be generated.

Key Points

- Patients with a diagnosis of pre-eclampsia in pregnancy are at future risk for developing chronic hypertension.
- All health-care personnel providing care for pregnant patients must be educated in the signs and symptoms of hypertensive disorders of pregnancy.
- Early, consistent prenatal care is essential in reducing the potential for pregnancy-related complications.
- The level of irritability in the assessment of reflexes provides critical information about the potential for maternal seizure activity and a diagnosis of eclampsia.
- The definition of elevated blood pressure in pregnancy is defined as a systolic blood pressure between 120 and 129 and diastolic less than 80 mm Hg.

Review Questions

1. **The pathophysiology of hypertensive disorders of pregnancy includes which of the following?**

   a. Relaxation of smooth muscles
   b. Vasospasm of blood vessels
   c. Increased urinary output
   d. Onset of respiratory depression

2. **Which of the following can be symptoms of pre-eclampsia? (Select all that apply.)**

   a. Nausea and vomiting
   b. Hyporeflexia
   c. Headache
   d. Restlessness

3. **Which of the following converts a diagnosis of pre-eclampsia to eclampsia? (Select all that apply.)**

   a. An increase in systolic blood pressure
   b. A seizure
   c. Proteinuria
   d. Elevated liver enzymes

4. **Which of the following must be present to diagnose a pregnant patient with pre-eclampsia?**

   a. Hypertension and proteinuria
   b. Elevated liver enzymes
   c. 4+ in the lower extremities
   d. HELLP syndrome

5. **Which of the following is the most common complication of pregnancy?**

   a. Hypertensive disorders
   b. Embolic disorders
   c. Preterm delivery
   d. Anemia

See the appendix for answers to review questions.

References

American College of Obstetricians and Gynecology. (2019). ACOG Practice Bulletin No. 202: Gestational hypertension and preeclampsia. *Obstetrics and Gynecology, 133*(1), 1. doi:10.1097/AOG.0000000000003018

Capriotti, T. (2020). *Pathophysiology: Introductory concepts and clinical perspectives* (2nd ed.). Philadelphia, PA: F.A. Davis.

Davis, M., & Sanders, B. (2019). Preeclampsia and future stroke risk in women: What NP's need to know. *The Nurse Practitioner, 44*, 50–54. doi:10.1097/01.NPR0000554088.97825.ad

Dillon, P. M. (2016). *Nursing health assessment*. Philadelphia, PA: F.A. Davis.

Gilbert, E. S., & Harmon, J. S. (2003). *Manual of high-risk pregnancy and delivery* (3rd ed.). St. Louis, MO: Mosby.

Thompson, J. M. (2018). *Essential health assessment*. Philadelphia, PA: F.A. Davis Company.

Ward, S. L., & Hisley, S. M. (2016). *Maternal-child nursing care*. Philadelphia, PA: F.A. Davis.

Gestational Diabetes

Introduction

A pregnant patient may begin a pregnancy with either a diagnosed or undiagnosed complication. One of the complications that can adversely affect a pregnancy is diabetes mellitus. This condition, if left undiagnosed and untreated, can lead to further, major complications for both the mother and fetus. It is imperative for pregnant patients to receive early and consistent prenatal care to determine whether this (or any other) complication or problem exists or develops that can complicate the pregnancy and put both patients in a high-risk situation.

Patients at risk for diabetes in pregnancy can conceivably prevent a diagnosis of diabetes by preemptively losing weight, actively exercising, and altering their nutritional habits prior to becoming pregnant. These preventive measures can significantly reduce the potential for diabetes-related complications for both mother and fetus during a pregnancy. The diagnosis of diabetes mellitus in pregnancy is broad and includes a host of potential problems. According to the Centers for Disease Control and Prevention (CDC, 2019), up to 10% to 14% of all pregnancies can be affected by a type of diabetes mellitus during the pregnancy.

A patient can be diagnosed with *pregestational diabetes* prior to becoming pregnant. This diagnosis is a chronic state of hyperglycemia due to a decrease in or an absent production of insulin in the pancreas or a blend of the two processes.

Type 2 diabetes mellitus is the most common form of diabetes and is a combined etiology of decreased insulin production with an evident level of insulin resistance. Type 2 diabetes may also be diagnosed in a patient either before or during the pregnancy. The signs and symptoms of diabetes mellitus type 2 may be recognized for the first-time during pregnancy and may remain post-pregnancy as a diagnosis of diabetes (ACOG, 2019b).

Type 1 diabetes mellitus can also affect pregnancy and accounts for approximately 5% to 10% of all diagnoses of diabetes. Type 1 diabetes mellitus is caused by an autoimmune response in the body that destroys the actions of the beta cells in the pancreas, with a resultant complete insulin deficiency (Ward & Hisley, 2016).

Gestational diabetes is the final category of diabetes and the one with which this chapter is primarily concerned. In it, an elevated level of glucose remains in the bloodstream instead of being utilized to supply the body with energy. This diagnosis is associated with pregnancy and occurs secondary to the normal physiological changes of pregnancy or due to an underlying level of insulin resistance of pregestational diabetes.

Any diagnosis of diabetes in pregnancy is a serious one that can affect both maternal and fetal outcomes. Each of these diagnoses must have an interdisciplinary team approach to providing pregnancy care and to reducing the potential for diabetes-associated problems. The most important purposes of pregnancy-related diabetes care are to prevent complications and encourage normoglycemia throughout the pregnancy. Patient education is key and should provide information related to optimal diabetes management from the preconception to postpartum phases. All patients who are of childbearing age should be educated regarding the importance of maintaining normal blood glucose levels before, during, and after pregnancy. Education related to the prospective of complications arising with inadequate glucose control should be provided expectantly to decrease the advent of pregnancy-related complications that can affect the mother and fetus. The control of maternal blood glucose levels is also an essential element of future fetal outcomes secondary to a diabetes diagnosis. Ongoing future care is essential for a pregnant patient diagnosed with gestational diabetes due to the increased potential for a diagnosis of diabetes type 2 post-pregnancy (Ward & Hisley, 2016).

Physiology

The body requires a continuous source of energy for normal processes to occur. Adequate glucose levels primarily supply this energy, which enters the cells to sustain normal metabolism. When glucose enters the cells, the pancreas is stimulated to produce insulin in response to the intake of glucose into the body.

The body naturally produces several hormones to control the normal functioning processes within the human body. One of these key hormones is insulin, which is responsible for controlling the blood glucose levels within the bloodstream. Insulin is produced in the beta cells of the islets of Langerhans within the pancreas (see Figure 2-1 in Chapter 2). Insulin acts as a glucose transporter into the cells to provide the body with energy. This process synchronizes the levels of glucose, glucose entry into cells, insulin secretion, and utilization of insulin, which is critical to the body's normal processes (Ward & Hisley, 2016).

The significant physiological changes that occur in pregnancy are systemwide and are intensified by the changes that occur in fat, protein, and carbohydrate metabolism. The normal action in a non-pregnant state is to move glucose into cells for energy and then provide energy use through the action of insulin produced within the body. An imbalance occurs when the decreased action of insulin on movement of glucose into the cells no longer provides adequate energy and support to physiological functioning.

Pregnancy growth and development are dependent on many hormones for pregnancy maintenance. The primary hormones are estrogen and progesterone, but cortisol, growth hormones, and *human placental lactogen* (HPL) are also responsible for pregnancy maintenance, fetal growth, and progression. During the third trimester of pregnancy, the levels of estrogen, progesterone, cortisol, insulinase, growth hormones, and HPL block the effects of normally occurring maternal insulin. This blockade of insulin's action is referred to as a state of *insulin resistance*. This process decreases the amount of insulin entering the body's cells, causing the glucose levels to increase within the maternal blood and a state of maternal hyperglycemia to occur.

In addition, the amount of weight gain experienced during pregnancy contributes to the state of insulin resistance and the ability of the body to use both insulin and glucose effectively.

The first 20 weeks of pregnancy is considered to be a state of anabolism, with the body storing protein and fat in addition to the increased production of estrogen and progesterone. These processes cause maternal hyper insulin levels and hyperplasia with a resultant uptake of glycogen and fat stores in the liver and tissues. The second 20 weeks of pregnancy is viewed as a state of catabolism, with a breakdown of protein and fat stores. Insulin resistance is elevated due to increasing hormone levels with a potential for distorted metabolism of carbohydrates and subsequent further increasing of glucose levels (Ward & Hisley, 2016).

 CLINICAL PEARLS

Normal weight gain during pregnancy is 25 to 35 total pounds. Any additional weight gained by the mother significantly increases the potential for additional insulin resistance and leads to a diagnosis of gestational diabetes.

Pathophysiology

During pregnancy, the mother's pancreas is in overdrive to produce adequate insulin to compensate for the increasing hormonal effects. A woman's body is unable to generate an adequate supply of insulin to counteract the antagonistic effects of pregnancy. As noted earlier, this condition is also identified as a state of insulin resistance, which increases the body's need for effective insulin to reduce blood glucose levels. This additional insulin attempts to lower maternal glucose levels but cannot lower the fetal levels. The ability of insulin to pass through the placenta and lower the effects of hyperglycemia levels that reach the fetus is inadequate to decrease the elevated blood glucose levels. The result may be a form of maternal diabetes.

Gestational Diabetes

Gestational diabetes causes a decrease in the ability of the body to metabolize carbohydrates. This diagnosis is made during a pregnancy and may occur in patients with previously undiagnosed type 1 or 2 diabetes mellitus. This type of diabetes mellitus is often characterized by the following:

- An increased risk for diabetes mellitus type 2 in the future with a 70% chance of developing it.
- Diagnosed after 24 weeks of pregnancy secondary to increasing hormone levels.
- Can be associated with 10% to 14% of all pregnancies.
- Increasing prevalence secondary to the increasing rates of obesity in adults.
- Symptoms minor and nonemergent when diagnosed.
- Initial treatment including alterations in nutrition and exercise levels.
- Ongoing treatment including the addition of oral medications and or insulin based on the glucose-level response to diet and exercise (Ward & Hisley, 2016).

Gestational diabetes often will not have associated signs and symptoms, but will be suspected based on maternal risk factors and will be confirmed with testing, which is normally completed between 24 and 28 weeks of pregnancy. If a patient is considered high risk for diabetes, testing may occur earlier in the pregnancy to avoid potential complications. Earlier testing can reveal a new diagnosis of type 1 or 2 diabetes that was previously undiagnosed and untreated, leading to treatment that decreases potential maternal and fetal complications related to the diagnosis.

Type 1 Diabetes

Type 1 diabetes is characterized by abrupt onset of symptoms, which requires an acute medical intervention in conjunction with the new diagnosis. An acute onset of symptoms includes the 3 Ps—polyuria, polydipsia, polyphagia—with a substantial acute onset of weight loss. The diagnosis typically occurs in patients under 30 years of age. It requires the administration of insulin to decrease blood glucose levels, because insulin levels are minimal to nonexistent (Ward & Hisley, 2016).

Type 2 Diabetes

Diabetes mellitus type 2 is not a type of diabetes that characteristically results in *diabetic ketoacidosis* (DKA). Classically diagnosed in adults over 30 years of age, it is now often diagnosed in pediatric patients due to mounting obesity rates within this population. Onset is usually slow without overt symptoms, with gradual development of symptoms and complications. It can be treated with diet, exercise, and oral agents if the patient is compliant; insulin may be prescribed but is not always required (Ward & Hisley, 2016).

Effects on Fetal Development

Increased maternal glucose levels easily cross the placenta to the fetus but without insulin, which is unable to cross effectively. The growing fetus responds by increasing the fetal production of insulin, which has the capability of acting as a growth hormone while also decreasing the surfactant production. The effects of increased fetal growth hormone contribute to a diagnosis of *macrosomia* in the fetus with associated potential pulmonary complications. These diagnoses increase the risks for further fetal and maternal complications and a preterm birth of a larger-than-normal newborn with pulmonary complications.

Based on the late onset of insulin resistance and gestational diabetes during pregnancy, the fetus's organ development is not normally affected. However, fetal growth and birth weight can be accelerated based on higher-than-normal levels of glucose in the mother's body that cross the placenta for use by the fetus. Macrosomia is diagnosed in a newborn whose weight, length, and head circumference are assessed above the 90th percentile for gestational age. This is also known as a *large for gestational age* (LGA) newborn and occurs with approximately 25% of all patients diagnosed with diabetes or beginning a pregnancy with a diagnosis of diabetes. Depending on the size of the fetus in relationship to the mother's pelvis, a baby diagnosed with macrosomia and/or the mother may experience or require the following:

- Delivery through a cesarean section
- Shoulder dystocia
- Birth trauma
- Permanent newborn injuries
- Difficult labor process
- Excessive vaginal bleeding in the postpartum period
- Vaginal tears
- First through fourth degree lacerations (ACOG, 2019a)

Risk Factors

Several risk factors have been associated with the diagnosis of gestational diabetes. These include the following:

- Physical inactivity
- Age over 25 years

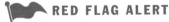

HIGH YIELD FACT FOR TESTING

Maternal hyperglycemia is a teratogen to a developing fetus.

RED FLAG ALERT

Fetal growth to include weight and size can be accelerated with a diagnosis of gestational diabetes.

- History of insulin resistance
- Overweight or obese
- History of a stillbirth, miscarriage, or congenital anomalies
- Diagnosis of gestational diabetes in a prior pregnancy
- Diagnosis of macrosomia in a prior pregnancy (9 pounds or more)
- History of hypertension or cardiac disease
- History of *polycystic ovarian syndrome* (PCOS)
- Ethnic background of Pacific Islander, Hispanic, African American, Native American, or Asian (ACOG, 2019b)

The regulation of maternal glucose levels and the amount of glucose entering cells in pregnancy is critical to the normal development of a fetus in utero and the progression of a pregnancy to term. It is essential to maintain normoglycemia to reduce the potential for perinatal and neonatal mortality and morbidity. In addition, the level of glucose can have a negative effect on the incidence of congenital abnormalities and the rate of normal fetal growth and development.

Assessment

All patients experiencing insulin resistance or gestational diabetes during pregnancy should have frequent prenatal assessments and fetal monitoring due to the potential for complications for both the mother and fetus. Blood glucose self-assessments will be necessary to determine optimal treatment, medication dosages, and risk reduction throughout the pregnancy. A glucose meter should be provided to the patient to self-test blood glucose levels, and a record should be kept to determine whether any changes in the treatment plan are indicated and required. If a pregnant patient's fasting blood glucose levels are over 105 mg/dL, insulin treatment will be necessary to maintain normal glucose levels and reduce the potential for complications.

The control of maternal blood glucose levels is essential to reducing potential problems. A *hemoglobin A1c level* (HbA1c), or glycosylated hemoglobin, is used to measure the blood glucose levels over a period of time. This diagnostic test examines the average level over the previous 3 months and is the primary test used to assess diabetes treatment and management. Elevated blood glucose levels will cause an increase in the attachment of glucose to hemoglobin within red blood cells and is reported as a percentage. A level less than 5.7% is considered normal (National Institute of Diabetes and Digestive and Kidney Diseases, 2018). Table 7-1 provides the HbA1c interpretations.

The glucose challenge test or the *oral glucose tolerance test* (OGTT) is used to assess for diabetes in pregnancy between 24 and 28 weeks' gestation. The initial blood test is nonfasting and 1 hour after the ingestion of 50 g of oral glucose. If the level is over 140 mg/dL, a 3-hour fasting test is ordered with the ingestion of 100 g of glucose and an assessment of blood at 1-hour intervals. A diagnosis of gestational diabetes is made if two of the four blood levels are abnormal. Table 7-2 provides the 3-hour test plasma values used to diagnose gestational diabetes.

TABLE 7-1 Hemoglobin A1c Result Interpretations

Normal	Below 5.7%
Prediabetes	5.7–6.4%
Diabetes	6.5% or above

(National Institute of Diabetes and Digestive and Kidney Diseases, 2018)

TABLE 7–2   Three-Hour Glucose Tolerance Testing Plasma Values for Diagnosing Gestational Diabetes

Fasting blood sugar	<105 mg/dL
1-hour	<190 mg/dL
2-hour	<165 mg/dL
3- hour	<145 mg/dL

(Ward & Hisley, 2016)

A head-to-toe assessment with auscultation of heart, lung, breath, and bowel sounds should be performed. Maternal weights should be monitored to determine weight gain throughout pregnancy, as excessive weight gain is associated with additional complications and a higher risk for gestational diabetes in pregnancy.

Hypoglycemia and hyperglycemia are both complications that must be assessed for during pregnancy. Hypoglycemia is more common in pregnancy and occurs when a blood glucose level falls below 60 mg/dL. Patients must be educated about the symptoms, management, and resultant problems related to fluctuating blood glucose levels. Education should include the following.

- Symptoms, including light-headedness, sweating, hot flashes, shaking, nervous feelings, chills, clamminess, tachycardia, hunger, nausea, pallor, sleepiness, weakness, blurry vision, impaired vision, and seizures.
- Management, including instructions to:
  - Drink milk instead of juice for glucose maintenance.
  - Have glucagon available for decreased level of consciousness or severe symptoms (American Diabetes Association, 2019).
- Family education related to disease and symptoms.
- Increased incidence in pregnancy (Ward & Hisley, 2016).

In addition, multiple problems can occur to both the mother and fetus with a diagnosis of gestational diabetes. These can include:

- Pre-eclampsia
- Eclampsia
- Spontaneous miscarriage
- Increased infection rates
- Polyhydramnios
- Postpartum hemorrhage
- Cesarean delivery
- Diagnosis of diabetes later in life
- Increased risk for congenital anomalies (Ward & Hisley, 2016)

HIGH YIELD FACT FOR TESTING

Hypertension and pre-eclampsia are four times more common in women diagnosed with gestational diabetes during pregnancy. Any patient diagnosed with pre-eclampsia during pregnancy should be screened for hypertension annually.

It is important to have an understanding of the patient's diagnosis; their management plan; the potential for complications associated with disease progression and possible mismanagement; and pharmacological agents ordered and their effects and potential side effects. Women diagnosed during pregnancy should also be reevaluated after delivery to determine whether type 2 diabetes is present and diagnosed (Ward & Hisley, 2016).

ASSESSMENT PEARLS
Multiple risk factors can predispose a pregnant patient to a diagnosis of gestational diabetes.

Nonpharmacological Management

Many nonpharmacological measures can be taken to manage diabetes mellitus. It is essential for patients to receive adequate education regarding the diagnosis, appropriate care, and treatment throughout pregnancy and beyond, and to have the support of interdisciplinary team members available for referrals as needed. These team members may include maternal–fetal medicine provider, endocrinologist, diabetic educator, neonatologist, and nutritionist.

When a pregnant patient is diagnosed with insulin resistance or gestational diabetes, the first step is to provide education regarding the new diagnosis. This education should include nutrition and meal choice counseling with an exercise plan to initiate during the pregnancy. Food choices can potentially exacerbate altered blood glucose levels and increase the probability for complications. Regular meals with smaller snacks in between should be implemented, ideally to include three healthy meals and two or three snacks per day. This regimen will assist in maintaining normoglycemia without harmful exaggerated increases and decreases in blood glucose levels. Nutritional planning will also be useful to guide normal weight gain during pregnancy and reduce the potential for excessive weight gain or weight that is gained too quickly. It is widely thought that following a Mediterranean diet can decrease the potential for diagnoses of prediabetes, gestational diabetes, and diabetes mellitus type 2.

According to Ward and Hisley (2016), a pregnant patient with a normal pre-pregnancy weight should ingest 30 kcal/kg/day and an obese patient should ingest 25 kcal/kg/day. Fifty percent of daily calories should be from complex, high-fiber carbohydrates, with 20% protein and 30% unsaturated fats ingested. A small nutritional snack before sleep is advisable to reduce the potential for unrecognized hypoglycemia during sleep with deleterious effects.

Regular exercise is optimal for all pregnant patients and is especially important to include in patients diagnosed with gestational diabetes. Moderate exercise is recommended 5 days per week for a minimum of 150 minutes per week. Walking is an accepted form of weekly exercise during pregnancy and can also be effective throughout the day following nutrition intake to support the control of blood glucose levels with a reduction in insulin resistance and an increase in insulin sensitivity.

Ongoing diagnostic testing should be ordered to monitor the health of the pregnancy and fetus. These tests will also guide the treatment plan and management and provide accurate information related to potential or definite complications. The testing may include the following:

- A *biophysical profile* (BPP), which monitors the fetal heart rate and includes an ultrasound examination to determine the amniotic fluid levels. Fetal muscle tone, movement, and breathing are also assessed.
- A nonstress test, which assesses the fetal heart rate alterations with fetal movement. There is no stress placed on the pregnancy or fetus during this test.
- Fetal movement counts or (kick counts), which assesses how often a mother feels the fetus move during a period of time. A healthy fetus will move in a similar pattern each day throughout the pregnancy. The health-care provider should be notified if alterations occur (ACOG, 2019a).

Pregnant women may be unaware they have diabetes or have undiagnosed diabetes prior to pregnancy. These patients will continue to experience the signs and symptoms of diabetes mellitus type 2 post-delivery and will convert to a diagnosis of diabetes mellitus type 2. This diagnosis may require lifestyle modifications to include nutritional alterations and increased exercise. It may also require prescription of medications to increase the functioning of naturally occurring insulin, increase the patient's exogenous insulin, or a combination of the two treatments.

Gestational diabetes can affect future pregnancies and can affect blood glucose levels, leading to a diagnosis of type 2 diabetes mellitus in the future that is not associated with a pregnancy. The combination of gestational diabetes, hypertension, and pre-eclampsia can have a substantial impact on future maternal health if not controlled. This combination of diagnoses can lead to maternal heart disease and stroke at a higher-than-normal rate.

The offspring of mothers with gestational diabetes are also at a higher risk for becoming overweight or obese and, in conjunction with weight gain, can develop type 2 diabetes mellitus. The maternal history is an important component of a child's ongoing follow-up with a health-care provider to monitor their growth and weight gain, and to work importantly to prevent a diagnosis of diabetes and associated complications (ACOG, 2019b).

CLINICAL PEARLS

Current research is ongoing to determine whether pre-pregnancy bariatric surgery can reduce the potential for gestational diabetes in pregnancy. Unfortunately, this procedure has also been found to increase the potential for *small for gestational age* (SGA) newborns at less than 10% percentile, preterm deliveries, and newborn mortality (Ward & Hisley, 2016).

Pharmacology

The U.S. Preventive Services Task Force has recommended that all women during their reproductive years should take a 400 to 800 mg supplement of folic acid daily to reduce the potential for neural tube defects. Current research has determined that the same intervention of folic acid will also reduce the risk of gestational diabetes in pregnancy, including subsequent pregnancies. This low-cost intervention could be a method of reducing the risk of a mother's gestational diabetes and both maternal and fetal complications during and after pregnancy (Li et al., 2019).

The recommended first line treatment for gestational diabetes, according to ACOG (2019), is lifestyle alterations to include nutritional and exercise adjustments based on an individualized assessment and plan, with weight management included. These changes have been shown to be effective in improving perinatal outcomes and controlling maternal and fetal glucose levels in pregnancy.

Insulin is the first line pharmacological agent recommended for the treatment of uncontrolled glucose levels in gestational diabetes. This medication is preferably administered via an insulin pump for optimal glucose control if blood glucose control is not achieved with the implementation of nonpharmacological treatments. The use of a pump can also decrease the number of injections needed to decrease blood glucose levels. Short-acting or regular insulin is used in insulin pumps because the pump can deliver small amounts of insulin every few minutes when the use of longer-acting insulins is not needed.

If cost, cultural influences, or comprehension of the treatment or the injection method of administration of insulin is problematic for a pregnant patient, oral agents can be considered to treat the diagnosis. The diagnoses of hypertension, pre-eclampsia, or intrauterine growth restriction will preclude the use of oral diabetic agents due to the potential for additional complications regardless of personal choice related to insulin use.

Oral hypoglycemic agents can cross the placenta and are to be prescribed with caution. Long-term studies have not been completed to determine whether complications can occur within the fetus with the use of oral agents and so routine first line pharmacological use is uncertain; however, these medications are still prescribed in pregnancy and have been found to be associated with a decrease in maternal weight gain during pregnancy. All of these medications (and insulin) are used to treat diabetes in pregnancy and control blood glucose levels by lowering glucose levels.

The class of oral medication known as sulfonylureas is used to lower maternal blood glucose levels, but these can cross the placenta and are associated with significantly lowering fetal blood glucose levels and causing hypoglycemia. Another class of oral medication prescribed in pregnancy for gestational diabetes is biguanides. This class includes metformin, a common medication for blood glucose control. These medications are associated with a decreased risk for fetal hypoglycemia and maternal weight gain, but have been found to cross the placenta at higher levels than other oral agents. Table 7-3 provides the most common medications administered to patients diagnosed with gestational diabetes. The table includes dosage information and Safe and Effective Nursing Care (SENC) practices.

TABLE 7–3   Pharmacology for Diabetes in Pregnancy

Class	Example	Action	Dosage	Adverse Effects	SENC
Insulin	Lispro, aspart: Short-acting analogues with rapid onset of action. NPH, glargine, detemir: Long-acting coverage.	Stimulates uptake of glucose by the cells to reduce blood glucose levels. Activates enzymes phosphofructokinase and glycogen synthase to promote glycogen synthesis.	0.7–1.0 units/kg/day. Doses should be divided. Long- or intermediate-acting insulin should be combined with short-acting insulin.	Assess for hypoglycemia.	Dosage should be individualized based on patient's blood glucose patterns. Insulin pump is the preferred method of administration.
Biguanides	Metformin, Glucophage Glumetza, Riomet, Fortamet	Inhibits production of glucose in liver.	500 mg nightly for 1 week with an increase to 500 mg twice a day. Maximal dosage of 2,500–3,000 mg/per day in 2–3 divided doses.	Can cross over placenta. Preterm labor and birth. Abdominal pain, diarrhea, nausea, gastric distress, and bloating. Assess baseline creatinine level. Assess for hypoglycemia.	No long-term studies have been completed related to fetal effects. Take with meals.

TABLE 7–3 Pharmacology for Diabetes in Pregnancy—cont'd

Class	Example	Action	Dosage	Adverse Effects	SENC

Sulfonylurea	Glyburide, Glynase, Diabeta, Glynase PresTab	Increases the release of insulin from the pancreas.	2.5–20 mg/day in divided doses.
			  Maintenance 1.25–20 mg/day once per day or every 12 hours.
				Macrosomia, birth injury, hives, rash, itching, heartburn, photosensitivity, vasculitis, blurred vision, joint pain, nausea and vomiting, early satiety, diuretic effect, numbness and tingling.
				  Assess for hypoglycemia.
					Do not exceed 20 mg/day dosing.
					  Use in pregnancy if benefits outweigh risks.

(ACOG, 2019)

Summary

The incidence of diabetes in pregnancy has increased in combination with the rising rates of obesity in women. The frequency of type 1 and 2 diabetes diagnoses has increased in women of childbearing age in addition to the rising rates of the diagnosis of gestational diabetes. These diagnoses carry risks for both mother and newborn based on blood glucose alterations, associated complications, and comorbidities.

Preconception counseling is recommended, beginning at puberty and continuing throughout the childbearing years. Education related to lifestyle modifications—including nutrition, exercise, and weight loss—should be employed, and screening for all types of diabetes should occur annually and with any related symptoms of hypoglycemia or hyperglycemia. Family planning should be encouraged with the implementation of effective long-acting reversible contraception. Gestational diabetes can be controlled with appropriate management and early referral to maternal–fetal medicine specialists. Nonstress testing and assessment of the fetal biophysical profile should be included in the management and ongoing pregnancy surveillance.

Key Points

- It is estimated that up to 70% of patients diagnosed with gestational diabetes will progress to a diagnosis of type 2 diabetes mellitus post-delivery.
- All pregnant patients should be screened for gestational diabetes.
- Uncontrolled diabetes during pregnancy can result in both maternal and fetal complications.
- The recommended medication for diabetes in pregnancy is insulin.

Review Questions

1. **The pathophysiology of gestational diabetes includes which of the following? (Select all that apply.)**

   a. Placental resistance to insulin delivery

   b. Insulin resistance secondary to the hormones of pregnancy

   c. Increased glomerular filtration rate of insulin

   d. Increased hepatic insulin degradation

2. **Which of the following patients are at risk for gestational diabetes? (Select all that apply.)**

   a. Overweight patients

   b. Physically inactive patients

   c. Patients who had gestational diabetes in a previous pregnancy

   d. Patients with a diagnosis of hypertension

3. **Which of the following can be used to control glucose levels in pregnancy? (Select all that apply.)**

   a. Diet

   b. Exercise

   c. Metformin

   d. Insulin

4. **Which of the following complications can occur in a pregnancy complicated by gestational diabetes?**

   a. Macrosomia in the newborn

   b. Microsomia in the newborn

   c. Reduced maternal weight gain

   d. Multiples

5. **Which of the following is the most effective method for insulin administration in pregnancy?**

   a. Insulin pump

   b. IV insulin

   c. Intramuscular insulin

   d. Subcutaneous insulin

See the appendix for answers to review questions.

References

American College of Obstetricians and Gynecologists. (2019a). Pregestational and gestational diabetes: A resource review. Retrieved from https://www.acog.org/clinical/clinical-guidance/practice-bulletin/articles/2018/02/gestational-diabetes-mellitus

American College of Obstetricians and Gynecologists. (2019b). Frequently asked questions related to gestational diabetes. What are risk factors for diabetes? Retrieved from https://www.acog.org/womens-health/faqs/diabetes-and-women

American Diabetes Association. (2019). Hypoglycemia. Retrieved from http://www.diabetes.org/living-with-diabetes/treatment-and-care/blood-glucose-control/hypoglycemia-low-blood.html

Centers for Disease Control and Prevention. (2019). Gestational diabetes. Retrieved from https://www.cdc.gov/diabetes/basics/gestational.html

Li, M., Li, S., Chavarro, J. E., Gaskins, A. J., Ley, S. H., Hinkle, S. N., . . . Zhang, C. (2019). Prepregnancy habitual intakes of total, supplemental, and food folate and risk of gestational diabetes mellitus: A prospective cohort study. *Diabetes Care, 42*(6), 1034–1041.

National Institute of Diabetes and Digestive and Kidney Diseases. (2018). The A1C test & diabetes. https://www.niddk.nih.gov/health-information/diabetes/overview/tests-diagnosis/a1c-test

Ward, S. L., & Hisley, S. M. (2016). *Maternal-child nursing care*. Philadelphia, PA: F.A. Davis.

Chapter 8

High-Risk Conditions in Pregnancy

LEARNING OBJECTIVES

Upon completion of this chapter the student will be able to:

- Integrate knowledge of the physiology, pathophysiology, assessment, and nonpharmacological and pharmacological management of high-risk conditions in pregnancy.

- Incorporate the current standards of care for mothers diagnosed with high-risk conditions in pregnancy.

Introduction

The processes of pregnancy and birth are routinely considered to be normal extensions of health and wellness for female patients. The onset or the progression of pregnancy can at times deviate from normal. Such a deviation leads to the patient being considered and diagnosed with a high-risk pregnancy. This diagnosis results when actual or potential complications arise for the mother and/or the baby, and it requires immediate involvement of a maternal–fetal medicine specialist.

According to Ward and Hisley (2016), complications experienced during pregnancy can be serious for both the mother and fetus and can result in morbidity or even death for a mother and baby. It is essential for all pregnant women to receive early, accessible prenatal care. Early detection and treatment of complications can provide for the best possible outcomes for mother and baby throughout the pregnancy delivery and postpartum processes. Monitoring of the pregnancy is necessary to reduce the secondary effects of any pregnancy complications. Understanding the risk factors and treatment plan specific to each diagnosis will provide the patient with the knowledge necessary to care for both the mother and baby. This chapter highlights the most common high-risk pregnancy conditions, some of which are discussed more fully in other chapters in this section.

A pregnancy can be diagnosed as high-risk for many causes, including those listed below. These causes are detailed in the following Physiology section.

- Maternal age
- Existing conditions diagnosed prior to pregnancy
- Conditions diagnosed during a pregnancy
- Pregnancy specific conditions

- Fetal complications
- Lifestyle factors
- Personal history of preterm labor
- Pregnancy with multiples
- Family history
- Elevation in blood pressure

In addition to these causes, pregnancy history is a factor in complications. A maternal history of miscarriage or high-risk pregnancy conditions or a family history of genetic complications can cause problems in subsequent pregnancies. A thorough review of previous conditions and complications should always be assessed to prepare for potential complications in current and future pregnancies.

Physiology

The physiology of a normal pregnancy is outlined in Chapters 6, 7, and 9, with emphasis respectively on cardiovascular, hematological, and coagulation issues (Chapter 6); blood glucose regulation (Chapter 7); and the gastrointestinal system (Chapter 9). This section outlines the physiological causes of pregnancy complications, including many not covered in other chapters.

Maternal Age

The age of a mother at conception is significant and can contribute to a higher risk of pregnancy-related complications. Teenage pregnancies are commonly associated with the development of pregnancy-related hypertension, anemia, and preterm labor and birth. This population is often diagnosed with sexually transmitted infections and is less likely to receive early, adequate, or any prenatal care. Teen pregnancies can also result in cesarean deliveries due to *cephalopelvic disproportion* (CPD) or failure to progress during the labor process.

Women experiencing pregnancy after the age of 35 are at a higher-than-normal risk for pregnancy complications. Age-related complications specific to this age-group can include the following:

- Genetic and teratogen factors
- Delayed/prolonged labor processes
- Post-delivery complications
- Cesarean delivery
- Ectopic pregnancy
- Perinatal loss
- Cervical incompetence/insufficiency
- Gestational trophoblastic disease (Ward & Hisley, 2016)

According to Ward and Hisley (2016), *genetic factors* can cause genetic defects and congenital anomalies, in conjunction with environmental hazards or in isolation. Women are born with a fixed number of eggs within their ovaries and as they age, the risk increases for the remaining eggs to have abnormal chromosomes. One third of all birth defects are initiated by a level of genetic factors either before or after fertilization and embryo development. Maternal genetic susceptibility can also play a role in combination with chromosomal alterations in the mother, the father, or both parents. *Teratogens* can affect the developing fetus in specific ways, based on the timing and duration of exposure and genetic predisposition. The higher the exposure is early in fetal development, the more significant are the effects.

Delayed labor processes and *prolonged progression of labor* can complicate normal delivery development. Women may experience problems associated with uterine dysfunction or overstimulation, fetal malpresentation and malposition, placental placement, cephalopelvic disproportion, maternal or fetal conditions, and inadequate analgesic and anesthetic administration (Ward & Hisley, 2016).

The fourth stage of labor occurs directly after delivery until 1 to 2 hours post-delivery. This time requires frequent maternal and newborn monitoring for potential *post-delivery complications*. Excessive postpartum bleeding, alterations in vital signs, or uncontrolled pain can signify maternal complications. Vital sign or blood glucose alterations or respiratory difficulties can indicate potential newborn post-delivery complications (Ward & Hisley, 2016).

Cesarean birth accounts for one-third of all deliveries and is the most common surgical procedure performed. The procedure is performed when complications related to the pregnancy or labor occur. This surgery can itself result in complications for both the mother and newborn; it is considered a major surgical procedure with the potential for additional risks and complications when compared to a vaginal birth (Ward & Hisley, 2016).

An *ectopic pregnancy* occurs when a fertilized egg implants outside of the uterus. The majority of ectopic pregnancies implant in the fallopian tube; on the ovary, cervix, or fallopian tube; or on the bowel or abdominal wall, as shown in Figure 8-1. These pregnancies are nonviable and require treatment upon diagnosis (Ward & Hisley, 2016).

Perinatal loss can occur at any point in a pregnancy and can be caused by multiple factors. According to Ward and Hisley (2016), 12% to 15% of all pregnancies result in a loss with 22% occurring before any symptoms are present. Early pregnancy losses are considered to be prior to 12 weeks' gestation, and late pregnancy losses can occur between 12 and 20 weeks.

Cervical incompetence or *insufficiency* is the inability of a woman's cervix to maintain a pregnancy and deliver a term newborn. This condition can be congenital or result from trauma or surgical procedures of the cervix. Patients often have a history of second trimester miscarriage, which occurs in approximately 15% of all pregnancies.

Gestational trophoblastic disease is recognized as an abnormal development of the placenta in pregnancy, which produces fluid filed clusters instead of the normal placental tissue. This abnormal tissue growth, shown in Figure 8-2, leads to a loss of the

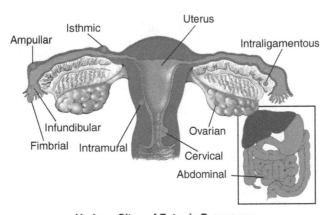

Various Sites of Ectopic Pregnancy

FIGURE 8–1 Sites of ectopic pregnancy *(From Ward, S. L., & Hisley, S. M. (2016). Maternal-child nursing care (2nd ed.). Philadelphia, PA: F.A. Davis.)*

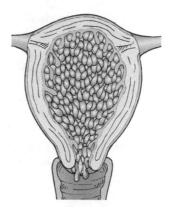

FIGURE 8–2 Gestational trophoblastic disease *(From Ward, S. L., & Hisley, S. M. (2016). Maternal-child nursing care (2nd ed.). Philadelphia, PA: F.A. Davis.)*

anticipated pregnancy, as the growth of trophoblastic tissue supplants normal placental tissue. The fluid filled clusters within the uterus will be treated by surgical removal, and chemotherapy or radiation therapy if indicated (Ward & Hisley, 2016).

Existing Conditions Diagnosed Prior to Pregnancy

A pregnant woman may have pre-existing conditions that can complicate her pregnancy and delivery. These can include many diagnosed conditions with the key ones presented here.

- Hypertension
- *Polycystic ovary syndrome* (PCOS)
- Diabetes
- Kidney disease
- Autoimmune disease
- Thyroid disease
- Obesity
- Viral infections (HIV/AIDS, Zika, COVID-19)

A diagnosis of *hypertension* can affect a pregnancy if left uncontrolled. Hypertension can cause damage to the maternal kidneys and increase the newborn's risk of a low birth weight and a diagnosis of *small for gestational age* (SGA). A newborn with SGA is at risk for hypoglycemia, hypothermia, difficulty with breastfeeding, and jaundice.

PCOS can lead to increased rates of miscarriage (typically prior to 20 weeks' gestation), gestational diabetes, pregnancy-induced hypertension, and cesarean births. Type 1, type 2, or gestational *diabetes* can affect a pregnancy if blood glucose levels are not controlled within normal ranges. Hyperglycemia can lead to birth defects, increased birth weight, or *large for gestational age* (LGA) newborns. Hyperglycemia in pregnancy can also cause significant hypoglycemia in the newborn after delivery, with resulting admission to the *neonatal intensive care unit* (NICU) for management. *Renal disease* can cause difficulties with maintaining a pregnancy and lead to preterm delivery before 37 weeks' gestation, decreased birth weight, and gestational hypertension.

Autoimmune diseases such as lupus erythematosus and Graves' disease can increase a woman's chances for miscarriage and preterm delivery. The medications prescribed to reduce symptoms of autoimmune disease can also be considered teratogenic (harmful) to a fetus, and both the mother and pregnancy must be monitored closely. There is potential for a reduction in medication dosages or complete cessation of medications. These decisions, made by the provider, can be determined as an alternative to ongoing treatment for the disease during the pregnancy.

Thyroid disease can manifest as either over- or underproduction of thyroid hormones, which are responsible for many complex functions throughout the mother's body. Thyroid disease that is left uncontrolled can cause many fetal complications, including cerebral development problems, cardiac complications or failure, and low birth weight. Maternal laboratory values should be monitored throughout the pregnancy. *Maternal obesity* can increase the risk for maternal gestational diabetes, LGA newborns, cardiac anomalies, and cesarean deliveries.

There are many types of infections that can cause pregnancy complications to occur. *HIV* can pass to the fetus through the placenta during pregnancy, delivery, and with breastfeeding. Maternal *Zika* infections can cause fetal cerebral and neurological complications. Testing is available for mothers who have been exposed before or during pregnancy. The coronavirus *COVID-19* is a new virus that has produced an increased risk of severe illness among pregnant women. There has also been an increased risk of adverse pregnancy outcomes reported in pregnancy, including preterm delivery. Newborns who test positive may have been exposed before, during, or after delivery (Centers for Disease Control and Prevention [CDC], 2020, June 25).

Pregnancy-Related Issues

A pregnant woman may begin to exhibit symptoms of newly diagnosed conditions or pregnancy-related circumstances that can complicate her pregnancy and delivery. Pregnancy-related issues occur secondary to the pregnancy and are diagnosed as high risk due to their effects on the pregnancy and fetus. The common conditions include the following:

• Gestational diabetes
• Pre-eclampsia and eclampsia
• Premature delivery
• Fetal genetic conditions or birth defects
• Multiple gestation
• Placenta previa/abruption

Gestational diabetes can occur in a pregnant woman with no history of diabetes prenatally and can increase the risk for a diagnosis of future type 2 diabetes mellitus in the mother by 50%. *Pre-eclampsia* and *eclampsia* can occur after the 20th week of pregnancy, developing when maternal blood pressure increases to a critical level.

The risk of *premature delivery* before 37 weeks increases in a pregnant patient with a history of previous preterm delivery or a pregnancy within the previous 12 months. Maternal infections and alterations in the cervix can also contribute to early labor. *Multiple gestation* pregnancies with twins, triplets, or more fetuses can increase the maternal risk for premature birth, cesarean section delivery, SGA newborns, and newborn respiratory and cardiac complications with the potential for NICU admissions.

The placenta is essential to the maintenance of pregnancy. Complications can include a *placenta previa*, which occurs when the placenta is in an abnormal position and can advance to fully cover the cervical opening. A *placental abruption* occurs when a portion of or the entire placenta detaches prematurely from the uterine wall. Both conditions may result in vaginal bleeding, which increases if accompanied by uterine contractions, and are considered obstetrical emergencies (Ward & Hisley, 2016).

Fetal Complications

Fetal conditions can be initially evaluated on ultrasound or through maternal blood testing. Fetal abnormalities can increase based on family history or may be unrelated and occur without warning. Approximately 2% of all pregnancies result in a fetal developmental complication that can be diagnosed as either a minor or major structural problem. *Fetal genetic conditions* or suspected birth defects can be diagnosed during pregnancy. The diagnosis can provide the time needed to prepare for early treatment in utero or immediately after birth, as required.

Lifestyle Factors

A woman's lifestyle choices can significantly affect a pregnancy and place the fetus at risk for complications. The most common maternal lifestyle risk factors include the following:

• Alcohol misuse
• Tobacco misuse
• Marijuana misuse
• Drug misuse

Alcohol is the most commonly abused drug during pregnancy. It has been determined that any amount of fetal alcohol exposure during pregnancy can increase the risk for *fetal alcohol spectrum disorders* (FASD), *sudden infant death syndrome* (SIDS), and a myriad of other disorders. The fetal effects of maternal alcohol consumption can range from mild to severe and are entirely preventable. Newborns may exhibit lifelong intellectual and developmental complications, behavioral problems, abnormal facial features, and cardiac, renal, orthopedic, attention span, communication, vision, and hearing complications. Women who consume alcohol are also at risk for miscarriage and stillbirths, and it has been determined that no amount of exposure is safe for a developing fetus at any stage of pregnancy (Townsend, 2019). Figure 8-3 shows facial features of *fetal alcohol syndrome* (FAS).

Tobacco and marijuana use during pregnancy puts a fetus at risk for preterm delivery, birth defects, SIDS, stillbirth, decreased blood supply to the fetus, and alterations in a newborn's immunity. The effects of secondhand smoke have also been demonstrated to cause complications for both the

> **HIGH YIELD FACT FOR TESTING**
>
> Any drug ingested in pregnancy, whether prescribed, over the counter, or illegal, can have the potential to be teratogenic to a developing fetus. All medications taken during pregnancy and breast-feeding should be discussed with a provider to reduce the potential for fetal complications.

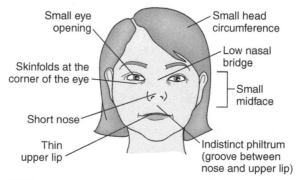

FIGURE 8–3 Facial features of fetal alcohol syndrome *(Townsend, M. C. (2019). Psychiatric mental health nursing (9th ed.). Philadelphia, PA: F.A. Davis.)*

mother and developing fetus. Marijuana is the second-most commonly abused drug, and maternal use during pregnancy can interfere with brain development and create the potential for long-term neurological and developmental complications for the newborn.

Pathophysiology

The pathophysiology of common high-risk pregnancy conditions can be extremely complicated, as two patients are involved in the reproductive process and treatment plan. This section details the pathophysiology of common complications of pregnancy. Table 8-1 summarizes those complications.

TABLE 8–1   High-Risk Conditions in Pregnancy by Trimester

Condition	Onset	Symptoms	Potential Pregnancy Outcome
Ectopic pregnancy	1st trimester	Waves of abdominal pain. Light to heavy vaginal spotting or bleeding. Dizziness, fainting, rectal pressure.	Fetal demise in 1st trimester.
Cervical insufficiency/ incompetence	Pre-pregnancy	Sensation of pelvic pressure. Backache. Abdominal cramps. A change in vaginal discharge (volume, color, or consistency). Light vaginal bleeding/spotting. Braxton Hicks–like contractions.	Premature labor and delivery in 2nd or 3rd trimester. Fetal demise in 1st, 2nd, 3rd trimester.
Gestational trophoblastic disease	1st trimester	Abnormal vaginal bleeding during or after pregnancy. Larger-than-expected uterus in the pregnancy. Severe nausea or vomiting during pregnancy. High blood pressure early in pregnancy; may include edema. Decreased fetal movement. Pain or pressure in the pelvic area. Abdominal swelling. Anemia, which can cause fatigue, dizziness, shortness of breath, or irregular heartbeat. Anxiety, irritability, feeling shaky, or severe sweating. Sleep problems. Unexplained weight loss.	Miscarriage in 1st trimester.
PCOS	Pre-pregnancy	Irregular periods or no periods. Difficulty getting pregnant (because of irregular ovulation or failure to ovulate). Excessive hair growth (hirsutism)—usually on the face, chest, back or buttocks. Weight gain. Thinning hair and hair loss from the head. Oily skin or acne.	Miscarriage in 1st or 2nd trimester.

Continued

TABLE 8–1 High-Risk Conditions in Pregnancy by Trimester—cont'd

Condition	Onset	Symptoms	Potential Pregnancy Outcome
Diabetes (gestational)	1st–2nd trimester	Sugar in urine. Unusual thirst. Frequent urination. Fatigue, nausea. Frequent vaginal, bladder, and skin infections. Blurred vision.	Large for gestational age fetus 2nd or 3rd trimester. Preterm labor and delivery 2nd or 3rd trimester.
Renal disease	Pre-pregnancy	Weight loss and poor appetite. Swollen ankles, feet, or hands. Shortness of breath. Tiredness. Hematuria. Nocturia. Insomnia. Itchy skin.	Preterm labor and delivery in 2nd or 3rd trimester.
Autoimmune disease	Pre-pregnancy	Fatigue. Joint pain and swelling. Skin problems. Abdominal pain or digestive issues. Recurring fever. Swollen glands.	Preterm labor and delivery 2nd or 3rd trimester. Fetal demise.
Thyroid disease	Pre-pregnancy	Feeling cold. Constipation. Muscle weakness. Weight gain. Joint or muscle pain. Feeling sad or depressed. Feeling very tired. Pale, dry skin.	Preterm labor and delivery 2nd or 3rd trimester. Fetal demise.
HIV/AIDS	Pre-pregnancy	Rapid weight loss. Recurring fever or profuse night sweats. Extreme and unexplained tiredness. Prolonged swelling of the lymph glands in the armpits, groin, or neck. Diarrhea that lasts for more than a week. Sores of the mouth, anus, or genitals. Pneumonia.	Preterm labor and delivery 1st, 2nd, or 3rd trimester. Newborn born with HIV.
Zika virus	Pre-pregnancy	Fever. Rash. Headache. Joint pain. Conjunctivitis (red eyes) Muscle pain.	Preterm labor and delivery 1st, 2nd, or 3rd trimester. Newborn born with Zika.
COVID-19 virus	Pre-pregnancy or pregnancy any semester	Fever or chills. Cough. Shortness of breath or difficulty breathing. Fatigue. Muscle or body aches. Headache. New loss of taste or smell. Sore throat.	Preterm labor and delivery 1st, 2nd, or 3rd trimester. Newborn born with COVID.

TABLE 8-1 High-Risk Conditions in Pregnancy by Trimester—cont'd

Condition	Onset	Symptoms	Potential Pregnancy Outcome

Pre-eclampsia/ eclampsia	3rd trimester	Excess protein in urine (proteinuria) or additional signs of kidney problems.
		Severe headaches.
		   Changes in vision, including temporary loss of vision, blurred vision, or light sensitivity.
		   Upper abdominal pain, usually under the ribs on the right side.
		Nausea or vomiting.
		Decreased urine output.
			Preterm labor and delivery 1st, 2nd, or 3rd trimester.
			Fetal demise.

Eclampsia	3rd trimester	Elevated blood pressure.
		Swelling in face or hands.
		Headaches.
		Excessive weight gain.
		Nausea and vomiting.
		   Vision problems, including episodes with loss of vision or blurry vision.
		Difficulty urinating.
		   Abdominal pain, especially in the right upper abdomen.
			Preterm labor and delivery 1st, 2nd, or 3rd trimester.
			Fetal demise.

Placenta previa	2nd trimester	Bright red bleeding from the vagina during the second half of pregnancy.
		   Range from light to heavy, and painless.
		   Contractions and bleeding. Cramping or tightening that increases with contractions, or back pressure.
			Preterm labor and delivery 1st, 2nd, or 3rd trimester.
			Fetal demise.

Placenta abruption	3rd trimester	Vaginal bleeding.
		   Discomfort and tenderness or sudden, ongoing abdominal or back pain.
		   Symptoms may occur without vaginal bleeding due to blood trapping behind the placenta.
			Preterm labor and delivery 1st, 2nd, or 3rd trimester.
			Fetal demise.

Ectopic pregnancies are those that implant in abnormal locations outside of the uterus, commonly in the fallopian tube. According to Ward and Hisley (2016), ectopic pregnancies occur secondary to multiple risk factors. Sexually transmitted infections or pelvic inflammatory disease can cause scarring in the reproductive system and lead to abnormal implantation. A history of an ectopic or surgical procedure increases the chance for subsequent ectopic pregnancies, as does hormone use, *intrauterine device* (IUD) birth control method, in vitro fertilization, and endometriosis.

Cervical incompetence or insufficiency can be secondary to cervical surgery, trauma, or infection, or it can be congenital. The condition causes the cervix to dilate prematurely with subsequent pregnancy loss, usually in the second or third trimester, without contractions, rupture of membranes, or presence of an infection. Cervical length assessments can be used to predict cervical incompetence, and the placement of a cervical cerclage in a patient with a history or high risk of loss can be used to treat and anticipate delivery. Figure 8-4 shows placement of a cervical cerclage.

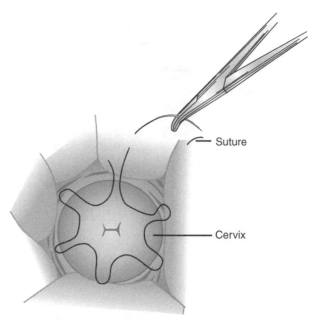

Suture

Cervix

FIGURE 8–4 Cervical cerclage *(From Ward, S. L., & Hisley, S. M. (2016). Maternal-child nursing care (2nd ed.). Philadelphia, PA: F.A. Davis.)*

Polycystic ovarian syndrome occurs secondary to a woman's insulin resistance and obesity. Insulin resistance stimulates an increased level of male hormones (androgens), which results in PCOS. PCOS is associated with hirsutism, acne, and dysmenorrhea, which are secondary to decreasing levels of progesterone. The decreased levels of progesterone can cause infertility and increase the risk for a future diagnosis of endometrial cancer (Ward & Hisley, 2016). As noted earlier, it also increases risk of miscarriage, cesarean birth, gestational diabetes, and pregnancy-induced hypertension.

Diabetes mellitus and gestational diabetes can cause pregnancy complications if blood glucose levels are not controlled. Type 1 diabetes is caused by autoimmunity that is focused on the beta cells in the pancreas; as a result, there is no insulin produced. Type 2 diabetes is the most common type and is a mixture of reduced insulin and insulin resistance. Gestational diabetes diagnosed in pregnancy is an alteration in the metabolism of carbohydrates; the diagnosis can include women with previously undiagnosed type 1 or 2 diabetes. Each of these types involves glucose metabolism and insulin production in response to the increase in metabolic processes and the movement of glucose into cells with corresponding levels of elevated circulating glucose. The developing fetus can move glucose across the placenta from maternal stores but cannot access maternal insulin, as it does not cross through the placenta. The fetus then increases its production of insulin in response to elevated maternal glucose levels. This increase supports augmented fetal development and size and leads to pulmonary complications related to a decrease in lung surfactant (CDC, 2020 June 25). Gestational diabetes is covered in detail in Chapter 7.

The elevation in blood pressure from pre-eclampsia or eclampsia can affect placental fetal blood flow; increase the potential for maternal liver, brain, and renal damage; and lead to seizures and possible death. A diagnosis of pre-eclampsia is made when an elevation in pre-pregnancy blood pressure readings occurs in conjunction with elevated levels of proteinuria. Pre-eclampsia and eclampsia are covered in detail in Chapter 6.

Renal alterations during pregnancy can range from nocturia to renal failure. Nocturia is common during the first and third trimesters and is related to the increase in the glomerular filtration rate by as much as 50%. Urinary tract infections occur frequently in pregnancy and are related to the increased production and level of residual urine secondary to ureter dilation from the increase in pregnancy-related circulating hormones. Increased levels of protein in the urine are associated with eclampsia and gestational hypertension and should be evaluated with a 24-hour urine collection. Acute renal failure to end-stage renal disease are potential but rare complications in pregnancy and may require dialysis treatment throughout the pregnancy.

Autoimmune diseases can each affect pregnancy differently, and the maternal effects will depend on the severity of the disease, treatment regimen prescribed to control the disease, and state of remission. In autoimmune disorders, the immune system's functioning is altered, and the actions of the system conflict with normal immune function. The woman's system initiates a negative response and attacks the functioning of different body systems. Based on the system involved, the pregnant patient will exhibit symptoms related to the destructive processes occurring. Lupus erythematosus, or lupus, patients have symptoms secondary to the inflammation and tissue damage that occurs. Graves' disease patients experience symptoms of increased metabolism secondary to the overproduction of thyroid hormones, resulting in hyperthyroidism or overactive thyroid. Thyroid diseases in pregnancy can range from under- to overproduction of thyroid hormone, with secondary symptoms related to the level of circulating thyroid hormones.

According to Ward and Hisley (2016), 66% of adults are overweight or obese. Overweight women have a *body mass index* (BMI) of 25 to 29.9; a condition of obesity is defined as a BMI of 30 or greater. Obesity is a common pregnancy-related condition that can contribute to and exacerbate pregnancy complications. The rate of complications increases as the woman's BMI is increased. These can include gestational hypertension, eclampsia, gestational diabetes, sleep apnea, LGA newborns, increased incidence of congenital defects, preterm birth, cesarean section deliveries, and adverse fetal outcomes to include miscarriage and stillbirths.

HIV is the virus that causes the conditions associated with AIDS. The virus alters the immune system and the woman's ability to fight infection and disease processes. The extent of illness depends on exposures, viral loads, and adherence to prescribed treatments. The virus can spread to the fetus in three ways, including during pregnancy, during delivery, or with breastfeeding. The risk of transmissions can be low with adequate maternal treatment and decreased exposure. Antiviral medications can be prescribed to significantly reduce the potential for transmission from mother to newborn; however, these medications must be taken as prescribed in order to be effective at reducing the maternal viral load.

The Zika virus is a mosquito-borne virus that is spread to mothers through the bite of an infected *Aedes* genus mosquito. In the majority of situations there are no reported symptoms, but in pregnancy there have been reports of birth defects due to transmission to the fetus. The specific birth defects reported have been microcephaly (smaller-than-normal head and brain) and severe brain defects (CDC, 2020, June 26).

The COVID-19 virus is a new virus, and the data are currently evolving to include the fact that pregnant women may be at higher risk for severe illness compared to nonpregnant women. The increased adverse pregnancy risks include preterm delivery of the newborn and severe maternal disease requiring intensive monitoring and methods of stabilization (CDC, 2020, June 26).

Placental abnormalities range from mild to severe and can include placenta previa and placental abruption. A placenta previa is a complication in which the placenta implants in an abnormal area of the uterus. A condition of placenta previa involves an implantation in the lower region of the uterus near or covering the cervical os. The previa can be diagnosed as total, partial, or marginal. A total implant is considered the greatest risk due to the potential for significant blood loss; a partial implant only partially covers the cervical os; and a marginal implant is close to but does not cover the os. The incidence is associated with multiple gestations, uterine scarring, diabetes, a history of previa or close pregnancies, or the use of cocaine, marijuana, or cigarettes (which cause a decrease in circulation and oxygen levels). Placental abruption occurs when a portion of or the entire placenta detaches prematurely from the uterine wall, and this also may cause vaginal bleeding. These hemorrhagic disorders are a primary cause of maternal deaths. Bleeding in the third trimester of pregnancy can occur in approximately 4% of pregnant patients and can be either obstetric or nonobstetric in nature. Placental abnormalities can also contribute to postpartum hemorrhage, preterm delivery, or miscarriage (Ward & Hisley, 2016).

CLINICAL PEARLS

High-risk pregnancies require close surveillance and ongoing provider monitoring for the best possible outcome for a mother and baby.

Assessment

A head-to-toe assessment with auscultation of heart, lung, breath, bowel sounds, assessment of edema, and fetal heart tones should be performed at every patient encounter. Maternal weights should be monitored to determine whether excessive weight gain or loss is occurring. Normal weight gain during pregnancy is 25 to 35 pounds. Physical and emotional stress may be present with a diagnosis of high-risk pregnancy and may interfere with a family's daily life and routines. It is essential to assess a pregnant patient for any alterations in the pregnancy or her emotional state with each prenatal visit (Dillon, 2016).

It is also important for a provider to have a complete understanding of the patient's high-risk diagnosis, management plan, and the potential for further complications for mother and baby associated with the diagnosis. The diagnosis, treatment plan, and all related information should be shared with the patient to promote an understanding of the process and expectations for the pregnancy and delivery (Ward & Hisley, 2016).

The following diagnostics may be ordered to appropriately diagnose and manage any high-risk pregnancy diagnosis:

- Complete blood count with differential
- Blood type and Rh factor
- Rubella titer for rubella virus antibodies
- *Rapid plasma reagin* (RPR)
- Hepatitis and HIV
- Urinalysis
- Electrolytes
- *Glucose tolerance test* (GTT) for blood glucose
- *Blood urea nitrogen* (BUN)
- Thyroid function testing to evaluate thyroid functioning
- PAP smear for cervical changes

- Nuchal translucency test—fluid level thickness at back of fetus's developing neck
- Prenatal *cell-free DNA* (cf DNA) screening—DNA from the mother and fetus is screened for chromosomal abnormalities
- Amniocentesis—amniotic fluid is assessed for genetic abnormalities
- *Chorionic villus sampling* (CVS)—placental cells are tested for genetic conditions
- Targeted ultrasound scanning to determine gestational age, abnormal development, and structural defects
- Ultrasound to assess cervical length and determine risk for preterm labor caused by cervical incompetence/insufficiency
- *Biophysical profile* (BPP)—assess fetal well-being by determining heart rate, muscle tone, movement, breathing, and level of amniotic fluid
- Non-stress test—assess fetal heart rate monitoring (Ward & Hisley, 2016)

It is essential to provide a pregnant mother with complete information about her high-risk diagnosis. This should include related signs and symptoms, when to contact the provider, any medications or treatments prescribed, and the importance of attending all prenatal appointments for ongoing assessments and monitoring. The importance of delivering in a hospital setting is emphasized with any high-risk diagnosis and should be discussed with the woman early in her pregnancy due to the potential for early labor, a cesarean section delivery, and transfer of the newborn to a NICU.

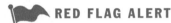 **RED FLAG ALERT**

Any alteration in the pregnancy process requires an assessment from a provider during pregnancy.

Nonpharmacological Management

Nonpharmacological management of pregnancy diagnoses will vary depending on the condition. All treatments should be discussed with the patient's provider to determine the safety of the proposed care prior to initiating any treatments.

High-risk pregnant mothers should be advised to speak with their health-care provider(s) about their diagnosed conditions during pregnancy, their long-term management plan, and how any conditions or complications may affect their labor and delivery process and their ability to "room in" with their newborn after delivery. They should be encouraged to maintain a nutritious diet and attempt to obtain adequate rest and exercise to promote ideal growth and development of the fetus throughout the pregnancy. They should also be instructed to include an adequate amount of fluid intake to prevent premature contractions, which can occur with inadequate intake and dehydration.

The diagnosis of a high-risk pregnancy necessitates an immediate referral to a maternal–fetal medicine specialist. These physician specialists are obstetricians with additional education in high-risk pregnancy management who concentrate on the supervision and care of high-risk pregnancies. The goal of a maternal–fetal medicine referral is the reduction of complications for mother and baby or babies with optimal pregnancy outcomes. This specialist should be part of the patient's medical team, which may also include other physician specialists depending on the patient's diagnosed conditions, the patient's primary care provider, at-home caregivers, and the obstetrical nurse. The nurse provides patient monitoring, support, and education, including instructing the patient to contact their provider for follow-up if they experience any of the following symptoms during their pregnancy:

- Vaginal bleeding or vaginal discharge
- Extreme headaches
- Any abdominal cramping or pain
- A decrease in fetal movement

- Burning or pain upon urination
- Vison alterations
- Increased or sudden onset of swelling
- Chills or elevated temperature
- Persistent nausea or vomiting
- Dizziness
- Any altered thoughts of harming self or baby

Pregnancy complications can require long-term therapy, including inpatient admission to the hospital or at-home care as needed to support the patient and pregnancy. Home care can be a viable alternative to costly inpatient hospital care, reducing the potential for nosocomial infections, family isolation, and onset of anxiety or depression. In many cases, visits by a community health nurse in a patient's home is the optimal choice for the patient and family.

The organization Sidelines provides support to assist pregnant patients who have been diagnosed with a high-risk pregnancy. This group can be accessed through the organization's Web site at www.sidelines.org. Support from outside sources can help alleviate fear of the unknown, isolation, stress, and disruption of the mother's normal routines (Ward & Hisley, 2016).

 CLINICAL PEARLS

Patients can obtain additional information and support related to pregnancy, maternal–fetal medicine, and other prenatal health issues from the High-Risk Pregnancy Center at the following Web site: https://www.hrpregnancy.com /patient-resources/online-resources.

Pharmacology

Any medications for pre-existing conditions taken during pregnancy should be shared with the provider to determine that the risks outweigh the benefit of continuing the medications. Many medications can have adverse effects on a developing fetus and during breastfeeding. It is important to discuss the continued use of all medications, including *over-the-counter* (OTC) medications and herbal supplements or alternative mediations uses.

Table 8-2 provides information about medications used for high-risk conditions, including normal dosages and Safe and Effective Nursing Care (SENC) practices. These medications fall into the following classes (listed in order of first appearance in Table 8-2).

Phenothiazine antiemetic—A dopamine antagonist that has an effect on the serotonergic, histamine, adrenergic, and cholinergic neurotransmitter systems.

Antihistamine—Histamine-1 receptor antagonist that blocks receptor sites and histamine-binding ability. First generation antihistamines have a central effect.

Vitamin B_6—Supplement that increases levels of vitamin B_6 in the bloodstream.

Prokinetic agent—A gut motility stimulator and antiemetic.

Central alpha-adrenergic inhibitor—A centrally active sympatholytic agent that reduces the concentration of epinephrine, norepinephrine, dopamine, and serotonin to dilate blood vessels.

Calcium channel blocker—Agent that blocks calcium from entering the cells of heart and arteries.

Peripheral arteriolar vasodilator—Agent that lowers blood pressure by exerting a peripheral vasodilating effect by relaxing vascular smooth muscle.

TABLE 8–2 Pharmacology for High-Risk Conditions in Pregnancy

Class	Example	Dosage	Indication	Adverse Effects	SENC
Phenothiazine antiemetic	Prochlorperazine, promethazine, chlorpromazine	5–10 mg PO tid or qid. Maximum dose of 40 mg/day. IM 5–10 mg IM, repeat 3–4 hours prn, maximum 40 mg/day. Rectal 25 mg rectally bid.	Treatment of nausea and vomiting in pregnancy and to promote sleep.	Dizziness, drowsiness, anxiety, insomnia, strange dreams, dry mouth, stuffy nose, blurred vision, sedation, extrapyramidal effects, hypotension.	Dosage should be individualized based on patient's nausea and vomiting patterns. Begin treatment with the lowest dose and titrate to effect. Crosses into breast milk.
Antihistamine	Diphenhydramine	25–50 mg PO tid or qid. IM/IV 10–50 mg up to 400 mg/day.	Treatment of nausea and vomiting in pregnancy and to promote sleep. General antihistamine.	Usage has been associated with cleft palate. Drowsiness, constipation, blurred vision, dry mouth, confusion, difficulty urinating, tachycardia, mood changes.	May interact with monoamine oxidase inhibitors (MAOIs). OTC cough and cold allergy or insomnia medications; anxiety or sleep medications. IV rates should not exceed 25 mg/min.
Vitamin B$_6$	Pyridoxine, Nestrex	25–75 mg once daily.	Maintain the health of nerves, skin, and red blood cells. Treats peripheral neuropathy.	Decreased folic acid, decreased sensation, headache, loss of appetite, nausea, vomiting, numbness and tingling, sensory nerve damage, sleepiness, unstable gait.	Take with meals. May interact with other medications. Safe for use with breastfeeding.
Prokinetic agent	Metoclopramide, Reglan	10–15 mg PO qid, 30 min before meals and at bedtime. Maximum dose 60 mg/day and use is limited to 12 weeks of therapy.	Treat gastroesophageal reflux disease (GERD), gastroparesis, and nausea and vomiting in pregnancy.	May cause neural development defects. Chills, clay-colored stools, dark urine, difficulty breathing, dizziness, tachycardia or irregular heart rate, fever, headache, hypertension, loss of balance and bladder control, loss of appetite, nausea, sore throat, yellow skin or eyes, vomiting, pallor.	Avoid use in first and third trimesters. Can increase postpartum depression. Avoid in patients with a history of depression. Can cause extrapyramidal syndrome of the newborn. Crosses into breast milk and the effects are unknown.
Central alpha-adrenergic inhibitor	Alpha-methyldopa, Aldomet	0.5–3 g PO per day in 2–3 divided doses.	Treats severe hypertension in pregnancy.	Sedation, hypotension, elevated liver function tests, depression, dry mouth, lethargy, hemolytic anemia.	Dosage should be individualized based on patient's blood. Begin treatment with the lowest dose and titrate to effect. Safe with breastfeeding.

Continued

TABLE 8–2 Pharmacology for High-Risk Conditions in Pregnancy—cont'd

Class	Example	Dosage	Indication	Adverse Effects	SENC
Vasodilator	Hydralazine hydrochloride	50–300 mg PO per day in 2–4 divided doses.	Treatment of severe hypertension in pregnancy.	Dizziness, tachycardia, headache, palpitations, neonatal thrombocytopenia, sedation, hypotension.	Dosage should be individualized based on patient's blood. Begin treatment with the lowest dose and titrate to effect. Safe with breastfeeding.
Alpha-/beta-adrenergic blocker	Labetalol hydrochloride (Normodyne, Trandate)	20 mg IV, then 20–80 mg every 5–15 minutes, up to a maximum of 300 mg; or constant infusion of 1–2 mg/min.	Treatment of severe, acute hypertension in pregnancy.	Dizziness, tachycardia, headache, palpitations, neonatal thrombocytopenia, sedation, arrhythmias, neonatal bradycardia, hypotension.	Dosage should be individualized based on patient's blood. Begin treatment with the lowest dose and titrate to effect. Safe with breastfeeding. Avoid with maternal asthma or heart failure.
Peripheral/ arterial vasodilator	Hydralazine	5 mg IV or IM, then 5–10 mg every 20–40 min; or constant infusion of 0.5–10 mg/hr.	Treatment of severe hypertension in pregnancy.	Dizziness, tachycardia, headache, palpitations, neonatal thrombocytopenia, sedation, hypotension.	Dosage should be individualized based on patient's blood. Begin treatment with lowest dose and titrate to effect. Safe with breastfeeding.
Calcium channel blocker	Nifedipine, Adalat, Procardia	10–30 mg PO, repeat in 45 min as needed.	Treatment of severe, acute hypertension in pregnancy.	Dizziness, tachycardia, headache, palpitations, neonatal thrombocytopenia, sedation, arrhythmias, neonatal bradycardia, hypotension. Can interfere with uterine contractions.	Dosage should be individualized based on patient's blood. Begin treatment with lowest dose and titrate to effect. Safe with breastfeeding. Avoid with maternal asthma or heart failure.
Peripheral/ arterial vasodilator	Sodium nitroprusside, Nitropress	0.25 mcg/kg/min (increase by 0.25 mcg/kg/min every 5 min to a maximum of 5 mcg/kg/min).	Treatment of severe hypertension in pregnancy.	Dizziness, tachycardia, headache, palpitations, neonatal thrombocytopenia, sedation, hypotension.	Reserved for extreme emergencies and used for shortest time possible due to the concern of cyanide toxicity. Dosage should be individualized based on patient's blood. Begin treatment with the lowest dose and titrate to effect.

(Woo & Robinson, 2020)

Summary

A diagnosis of a high-risk pregnancy can have significant effects on a mother, fetus, and family. The complications associated with a diagnosis can be severe for both the mother and fetus. These effects can lead to considerable morbidity and death.

High-risk pregnancies can include pre-existing medical diagnoses that can cause pregnancy complications or diagnoses that occur secondary to pregnancy. Pre-existing diagnoses or choices must be fully evaluated to determine the potential for complicating a pregnancy based on the effects of the diagnosis, further complications arising from the condition, and any medications prescribed for the diagnosis. A woman's age at the time of conception, family history of genetic disorders, lifestyle choices, and maternal health problems—including hypertension, diabetes, thyroid disease, obesity, asthma, clotting disorders, and infections—can cause pregnancy and delivery complications. These pre-existing diagnoses must be treated and controlled during pregnancy to reduce the potential for further pregnancy-related maternal and fetal complications, which can have lifetime effects.

A high-risk pregnancy can also include any history of previous pregnancy-related complications or current pregnancy-related complications derived from the pregnancy. Complications can include abnormal placental positioning in the uterus (to include placenta previa or abruption), alterations in fetal growth, multiples, gestational diabetes, pre-eclampsia and eclampsia, genetic conditions or birth defects, and premature labor and delivery of the newborn. These complications are associated with effects that range from alterations in blood glucose levels with resultant fetal growth pattern alterations, to cesarean delivery, delivery of a premature newborn requiring admission to the NICU, and even the potential for a fetal demise.

A high-risk diagnosis in pregnancy can affect the activities of daily living in addition to the mother's ability to continue with employment and provide ongoing care for the family throughout the pregnancy. It is important to maintain regularly scheduled provider and specialist appointments to ensure the best possible short- and long-term outcomes for the mother, pregnancy, and fetus. All medication should be taken only under the provider's supervision and with ongoing monitoring for side effects. A pregnant woman should avoid potentially harmful substances or environments to decrease the potential for harm to the fetus during the pregnancy. These include environmental and occupational exposures in addition to maternal ingestion of potentially harmful substances, such as those involved in smoking or alcohol and/or any illegal drug use. Over-the-counter medications and supplements should be discussed with the provider before continuing use.

Key Points

- Fetal exposure to any amount of alcohol during pregnancy increases risk for fetal alcohol spectrum disorders (FASD), sudden infant death syndrome (SIDS), and other disorders.
- Obesity is a common contributing or exacerbating factor in many pregnancy complications.
- Providers need to have a complete understanding of the high-risk patient's diagnosis, management plan, and potential for further complications for mother and baby.
- Physical and emotional stress often accompany a high-risk pregnancy and need to be assessed and monitored.
- Pregnancy complications may require long-term treatment, including inpatient admission to the hospital or at-home care.

Review Questions

1. **The pathophysiology of pre-eclampsia includes which of the following? (Select all that apply.)**

   a. Hypertension
   b. Edema
   c. Proteinuria
   d. Nausea and vomiting

2. **Which of the following patients are at risk for a diagnosis of high-risk pregnancy? (Select all that apply.)**

   a. Gestational diabetes
   b. Premature delivery
   c. Pre-eclampsia
   d. Multiple gestation

3. **Any medications taken for pre-pregnancy conditions should be:**

   a. Discussed with the provider.
   b. Continued at the same dosage.
   c. Discontinued.
   d. Taken at a reduced dosage.

4. **Which of the following complications can occur in a pregnancy complicated by a placental abnormality? (Select all that apply.)**

   a. Vaginal bleeding
   b. Miscarriage
   c. Premature delivery
   d. Postpartum hemorrhage

5. **Which of the following is a complication associated with maternal obesity in pregnancy? (Select all that apply.)**

   a. Cesarean section
   b. Large for gestational age (LGA) newborn
   c. Gestational diabetes
   d. Fetal cardiac anomalies

See the appendix for answers to review questions.

References

Centers for Disease Control and Prevention. (2020, June 25). Pregnancy, breastfeeding, and caring for newborns. Retrieved from https://www.cdc.gov/coronavirus/2019-ncov/need-extra-precautions/pregnancy-breastfeeding.html

Centers for Disease Control and Prevention. (2020, June 26). Facts about microcephaly. Retrieved from https://www.cdc.gov/ncbddd/birthdefects/microcephaly.html

Dillon, P. M. (2016). *Nursing health assessment*. Philadelphia, PA: F.A. Davis.

Townsend, M. C. (2019). *Psychiatric mental health nursing* (9th ed.). Philadelphia, PA: F.A. Davis.

Ward, S. L., & Hisley, S. M. (2016). *Maternal-child nursing care* (2nd ed.). Philadelphia, PA: F.A. Davis.

Woo, T. M., & Robinson, M. V. (2020). *Pharmacotherapeutics for advanced practice nurse prescribers* (5th ed.). Philadelphia, PA: F.A. Davis.

Hyperemesis Gravidarum

Upon completion of this chapter the student will be able to:

- Integrate knowledge of the physiology, pathophysiology, assessment, and nonpharmacological and pharmacological management of hyperemesis in pregnancy.
- Incorporate the current standards of care for mothers diagnosed with hyperemesis in pregnancy.

Introduction

According to Ward and Hisley (2016), nausea is one of the initial symptoms a woman experiences during her pregnancy. This nausea, and sometimes-associated emesis, is often referred to as "morning sickness," but the symptoms may occur at any time in a day. Indications and research support early nausea and vomiting associated with satisfactory fetal development due to sufficient circulating levels of pregnancy hormones present. Of all pregnancies, 70% to 85% are affected by nausea and vomiting that usually resolve after the first trimester.

A pregnant patient may be diagnosed with *hyperemesis gravidarum* (HG), which is a pregnancy complication that is characterized by excessive nausea, vomiting, weight loss, acute starvation with ketonuria, and dehydration. Syncope may be associated with this diagnosis due to the level of dehydration and fluid shifting within the body. This diagnosis is more serious than the common "morning sickness" appreciated in a majority of pregnancies, which classically ends after the first trimester of a woman's pregnancy and does not exhibit the same severity of symptoms. Hyperemesis gravidarum may diminish by 20 weeks' gestation, but frequently the diagnosis continues into both the second and third trimesters, ending after delivery. This persistent hyperemesis can result in fluid, electrolyte, and nutritional deficits; weight loss; and possible premature labor and delivery.

A diagnosis of hyperemesis gravidarum is routinely made based on the mother's signs and symptoms and the effects of nausea and vomiting during pregnancy. The definition of this diagnosis includes three or more episodes of nausea and emesis per 24-hour period with an initial loss of 5% of total body weight or 3 kg from previous pre-pregnancy weights. There is also a new onset of ketones in the urine when tested. The diagnosis can be made if there are no additional signs and symptoms indicating other maternal diagnoses.

There are many perceived causes of hyperemesis gravidarum, but the exact cause is debated. The most common perceived causes include a combination of maternal factors, with genetics often a primary cause, and a record of family members diagnosed with hyperemesis gravidarum as a common history.

The diagnosis of hyperemesis gravidarum can affect up to 2% of all pregnancies and in the past was considered a potential cause of mortality in pregnancy due to the effects of key electrolyte imbalances, dehydration, and a reduction in total circulating blood volume. This reduction in overall volume can also affect the placental circulation and fetal growth. Currently, the rate of miscarriage has been significantly reduced due to accurate diagnoses and effective treatments. The risk of premature labor and delivery (earlier than 37 weeks) persists when the nausea, vomiting, and other symptoms continue throughout the entire 9 months of a woman's pregnancy. This diagnosis is responsible for the majority of early pregnancy admissions and is the most common cause of related inpatient maternity care.

Physiology

According to Ward and Hisley (2016), several hormones are responsible for the alterations that occur with pregnancy and are present to maintain the pregnancy. The corpus luteum secretes both progesterone and estrogen, while the trophoblast that is present post-implantation secretes *human chorionic gonadotropin* (HcG). The key hormones produced by the growing placenta are estrogen and progesterone for both growth and maintenance of the pregnancy and fetus. Figure 9-1 provides the effects of the major pregnancy hormones on the reproductive system.

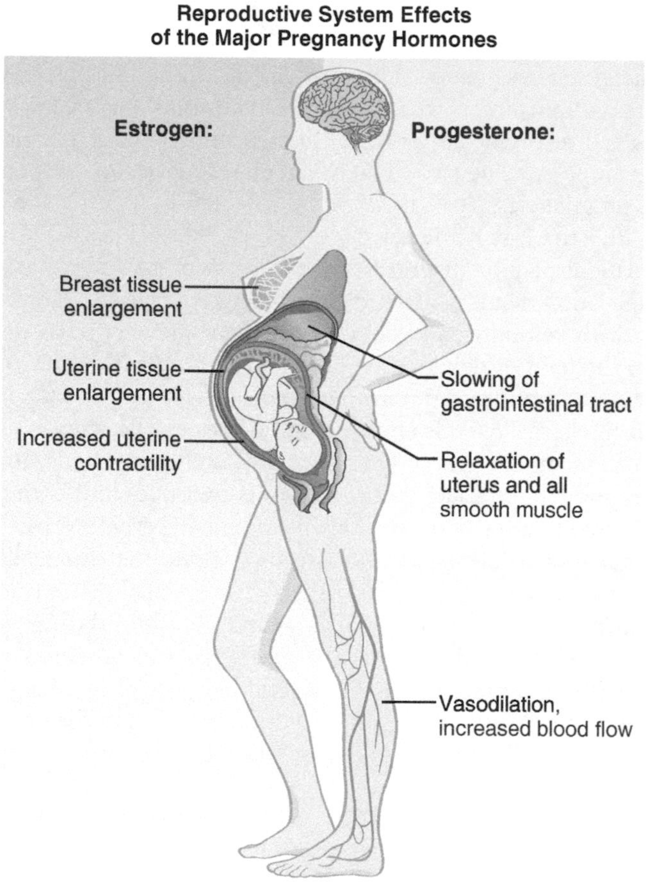

Reproductive System Effects of the Major Pregnancy Hormones

Estrogen:
- Breast tissue enlargement
- Uterine tissue enlargement
- Increased uterine contractility

Progesterone:
- Slowing of gastrointestinal tract
- Relaxation of uterus and all smooth muscle
- Vasodilation, increased blood flow

FIGURE 9–1 Effects of major pregnancy hormones on reproductive system *(Ward, S. L., & Hisley, S. M. (2016). Maternal-child nursing care. Philadelphia, PA: F.A. Davis.)*

The gastrointestinal system of a pregnant woman causes the majority of complaints during pregnancy. Nausea and vomiting, changes in taste and smell sensations, and changes in the oral and nasal mucous membranes contribute to the discomforts experienced. There also may be an alteration in carbohydrate metabolism, which contributes to the effects of nausea and emesis.

The esophagus, stomach, and cardiac sphincter increase in laxity due to the progesterone effects, which in turn decreases gastric motility and gastric emptying time. These effects intensify the symptoms and increase the potential for heartburn, gastric reflux, and additional nausea and vomiting. The intestines decrease their content movement, which increases bloating, constipation, and the potential for hemorrhoids due to decreased peristalsis and maternal straining with daily bowel movements (Ward & Hisley, 2016).

Progesterone relaxes the smooth muscles in a pregnant woman's body, which relaxes the gastrointestinal system. The esophagus becomes relaxed, as does the gastroesophageal sphincter at the top of the stomach. Due to the relaxation, gastric contents are able to reflux back into the esophagus, causing pyrosis and esophageal irritation (Ward & Hisley, 2016).

The gallbladder is also considered to be a smooth muscle and can be affected by pregnancy hormones. The emptying time can be decreased, which leads to inflammation and bile stagnation. This process can lead to the development of cholestasis, cholecystitis, or cholelithiasis. The liver can also be affected by stagnation of bile with resultant pruritus gravidarum. This is exacerbated by the ingestion of meals that contain a high fat content (Ward & Hisley, 2016).

CLINICAL PEARLS
Small, frequent meals during pregnancy can decrease the potential for the nausea and vomiting associated with the increase in pregnancy hormones.

Pathophysiology

Vomiting is a common symptom in the first trimester of pregnancy when HcG levels are at their highest. These symptoms begin at 4 to 6 weeks of pregnancy and continue until the peak of HcG at weeks 9 to 13. It has been suggested that over 60% of pregnant women experience some vomiting and 25% of woman experience isolated nausea. According to Ward and Hisley (2016), approximately 70% to 85% of pregnant women experience some level of morning sickness. The diagnosis of hyperemesis gravidarum, conversely, is second only to preterm labor as a serious complication of pregnancy that often requires admission into the hospital for further treatment (American Pregnancy Association, 2019). The differences between morning sickness and hyperemesis gravidarum are outlined in Table 9-1.

The precise cause of a diagnosis of hyperemesis gravidarum is unknown, but several risk factors have been identified that contribute to the diagnosis. According to Ward and Hisley (2016), these can include the following:

- Female child pregnancies
- Elevated levels of estrogen or HcG
- Transient elevation of thyroid hormone
- Pregnancy with multiples
- A maternal history of motion sickness or migraines
- A family history of hyperemesis gravidarum
- A maternal history of or current molar pregnancy/gestational trophoblastic disease

The effects of maternal hormones cannot be excluded as causes and the elevated levels of beta HcG are seen as the primary cause. The levels of HcG naturally decrease

TABLE 9–1 Distinguishing Between Morning Sickness and Hyperemesis Gravidarum

Morning Sickness	Hyperemesis Gravidarum
Nausea sometimes accompanied by vomiting	Nausea accompanied by severe vomiting
Nausea that subsides at 12 weeks or soon after	Nausea that does not subside
Vomiting that does not cause severe dehydration	Vomiting that causes severe dehydration
Vomiting that allows patient to keep some food down	Vomiting that does not allow patient to keep any food down

(American Pregnancy Association, 2019)

TABLE 9–2 Pathophysiological Processes Associated With Hyperemesis Gravidarum

Source	Cause	Pathophysiology

Placenta	Beta HcG	Gastrointestinal distention.
		    Interaction with thyroid stimulating hormone (TSH).
		    Can cause gestational thyrotoxicosis.

Placenta Corpus luteum	Estrogen Progesterone	Decreases gastrointestinal movement. Causes an increase in lever enzymes. Decreases esophageal sphincter pressure. Increases levels of sex steroids in the hepatic portal system.
Gastrointestinal tract	*Helicobacter pylori*	Increases circulating steroid levels.

(American Pregnancy Association, 2019)

after the first trimester of pregnancy and the majority of women experience a decline in their nausea and vomiting symptoms unless they are diagnosed with hyperemesis gravidarum (Kosus, Kosus, Hizli, & Turhan, 2014).

A secondary cause of hyperemesis relates to the increased levels of estrogen and progesterone in pregnancy. These elevated hormone levels often cause a decrease in gastric emptying time and intestinal motility leading to nausea and vomiting. Leptin is another hormone that may be involved as it controls hunger symptoms and acts as an appetite suppressant (Kosus et al., 2014). Table 9-2 outlines the hormonal contributors to hyperemesis gravidarum and the pathophysiological processes associated with each.

The signs and symptoms of hyperemesis gravidarum are associated with many other clinical diagnoses that must be ruled out in both the mother and fetus before a determination of the final diagnosis of hyperemesis gravidarum is made. The other potential diagnoses can lead to significant problems if they are not investigated and ruled out.

HIGH YIELD FACT FOR TESTING

Elevations in beta HcG levels are primarily responsible for early nausea and vomiting symptoms in pregnancy.

 CLINICAL PEARLS

A family history of hyperemesis gravidarum is common in patients diagnosed with this condition.

Assessment

A head-to-toe assessment with auscultation of heart, lung, breath, and bowel sounds should be performed with every pregnant patient encounter. Maternal weights should also be monitored at each visit to determine whether excessive weight loss has occurred with associated nausea and vomiting. It is essential to assess a pregnant patient for any weight loss, dehydration, ketonuria, and a state of alkalosis, which are symptoms often reflective of a diagnosis of hyperemesis gravidarum. The diagnosis is appreciated during pregnancy and is accompanied by the continuous symptoms of nausea and emesis often associated with dry, uncomfortable retching (Ward & Hisley, 2016).

The symptoms of hyperemesis gravidarum can be intensified by hunger, fatigue, ingestion of prenatal vitamins containing iron, and altered nutrition. The presence of certain odors can also aggravate symptoms and lead to additional nausea and emesis. An increase in coughing and sialorrhea gravidarum, or "increased salivation," are often associated with nausea symptoms and frequently precede vomiting. Constipation can be a complication, along with the ketones present in the patient's urine. Signs and symptoms of hyperemesis gravidarum can include the following (American Pregnancy Association, 2019):

- Severe nausea and vomiting
- Food aversions
- Weight loss of 5% or more of pre-pregnancy weight
- Decrease in urination
- Dehydration
- Headaches
- Confusion
- Fainting
- Jaundice
- Extreme fatigue
- Low blood pressure
- Rapid heart rate
- Loss of skin elasticity
- Secondary anxiety and or depression

Electrolyte levels should be monitored to assess for deficiencies, and replacements should be provided to reduce the risk of extended complications associated with extended maternal malnutrition. Ongoing assessments of nutritional intake, electrolytes, weight, and symptoms should continue due to the potential for enduring cycles of hyperemesis with resultant dehydration and weight loss. Nausea may be persistent without the effects of continuous emesis episodes, but this isolated symptom can prove to be debilitating to a pregnant patient during the 9 months of pregnancy. Nutritional disorders related to vitamin B deficiency may manifest and can be related to a decreased intake or absorption of thiamine (B_1), pyridoxine (B_6), or cobalamin (B_{12}). These disorders and their physiological effects can also intensify with the increased nausea and vomiting associated with a diagnosis of hyperemesis gravidarum.

The following diagnostics should be ordered to appropriately diagnose and manage hyperemesis gravidarum (American Pregnancy Association, 2019):

- Complete blood count with differential, as hematocrit levels can increase.
- Electrolytes
- *Blood urea nitrogen* (BUN)

- Thyroid function testing
- Ultrasound scanning, to determine gestational age or molar pregnancy

Before a diagnosis of hyperemesis gravidarum is made, the following related diagnoses should be ruled out (American Pregnancy Association, 2019):

- Molar pregnancy
- Urinary tract infection
- Appendicitis
- Cholecystitis
- Peptic ulcer
- Fatty liver disease
- Small bowel obstruction
- Gastroenteritis
- Thyroid disorders

Table 9-3 provides further information on diagnoses that may present with symptoms similar to hyperemesis gravidarum.

It is important to have a full understanding of the patient's diagnosis, their management plan, and the potential for complications associated with the continuation of hyperemesis gravidarum, along with any pharmacological agents ordered, their effects, and any potential side effects (Ward & Hisley, 2016).

 ASSESSMENT PEARLS

Women who are diagnosed during pregnancy should have complete resolution of all symptoms after hormone levels decline post-delivery, but some continue to have persistent nausea and vomiting.

TABLE 9–3   Differential Diagnoses in Hyperemesis Gravidarum

Etiology	Differential Diagnoses
Infections Fever or neurological symptoms	• Urinary tract infection • Hepatitis • Meningitis • Gastroenteritis
Gastrointestinal disorders Abdominal pain	• Appendicitis • Cholecystitis • Pancreatitis • Fatty liver • Peptic ulcer • Small bowel obstruction
Metabolic	• Thyrotoxicosis • Addison's disease • Diabetic ketoacidosis • Hyperparathyroidism
Drugs	• Antibiotics • Iron supplements
Gestational trophoblastic diseases	• Molar pregnancy • Choriocarcinoma

(American Pregnancy Association, 2019)

Nonpharmacological Management

It is essential for providers not only to assess the pregnant patient's ability to retain food and liquid, but also to provide suggestions for decreasing the symptoms of hyperemesis gravidarum. A patient with minor symptoms may be treated with dietary alterations, rest, and antacids by mouth. Pregnant patients should be encouraged to increase their fluid and fiber intake and decrease their fatty food intake to decrease the potential for constipation and resulting hemorrhoids. Straining with bowel movements can exacerbate these conditions and should be avoided by altering nutritional intake.

While treatment for hyperemesis gravidarum includes increasing the amounts of both fluid and nutritional intake, these amounts should be ingested in smaller meals. This may include fluids that contain electrolyte replacements, thiamine, and high-protein, bland foods. Small, frequent meals allow patients to avoid an empty stomach and decrease gastric and abdominal distention. Oral rehydration is initiated first and is considered to be a first line treatment option. Dry crackers and peppermint have been associated with a reduction in symptoms if ingested prior to rising in the morning or throughout the day as needed. Separating solids and liquids when eating and avoiding acidic food and beverages have also been shown to reduce both nausea and vomiting. Other approaches to contribute to decreasing nausea and vomiting include the avoidance of "trigger foods" and restrictive clothing that place pressure on the pregnant abdomen (Ward & Hisley, 2016).

If hyperemesis continues, the patient may require IV therapy to replace both fluids and electrolytes. Nasogastric feeding may also be needed to restore nutrition or, in extreme hyperemesis situations, a gastrostomy tube may be inserted. The gastrostomy tube is a surgical procedure and should be reserved for extreme hyperemesis gravidarum that is not relieved by either conservative or invasive measures (American Pregnancy Association, 2019).

Long-term therapy may include an inpatient admission to the hospital or home care with total parenteral nutrition through *peripherally inserted central* catheter (PICC) IV access until delivery is possible. If hospitalization is required, thromboembolic stockings will be ordered to reduce the potential for blood clot formation related to immobility. Home care and treatment are regularly available and should be considered due to the high cost of inpatient hospital care and the potential for nosocomial infections.

Both physical and emotional stress can manifest with this diagnosis and may cause patients and their families to struggle with completing normal activities of daily living. Psychotherapy has been implemented with success to reduce the symptoms and severity of hyperemesis gravidarum. There have been multiple reports of depression, feelings of isolation, and posttraumatic stress disorder in patients with this condition due to the symptoms and debilitating effects imposed by it on pregnant woman.

According to Ward and Hisley (2016), maternal depression, hypochondriasis, or excessive worrying about having a serious illness in addition to somatization can be problematic for some pregnant patients. Somatization is the process of converting mental thoughts and experiences to actual physical symptoms. These patients may require behavioral therapy throughout the pregnancy to reduce these complications. Behavioral therapy techniques may include relaxation methods, hypnosis, and psychotherapy.

Relaxation methods may be implemented to decrease symptoms and can include slow, measured breathing techniques and guided imagery. A reduction in the activities of daily living and an increase in rest and sleep may provide symptom relief for some patients. Acupuncture has also been used in attempts to reduce symptoms. The use of medication-free wristbands, which support acupressure methods and have been utilized for more than 5,000 years, are a popular method for symptom reduction. The use of either acupressure or acupuncture, treatments associated with traditional Chinese medicine, may possibly be effective in symptom reduction, but research has not found this method to provide successful relief from nausea and vomiting in all pregnant patients (Ward & Hisley, 2016).

Long-Term Management

In the past, bedrest was implemented for women experiencing obstetrically related complications including hyperemesis gravidarum. This practice has been long been associated with the potential for muscle wasting, bone loss, inability to gain weight, and cardiovascular, respiratory, and psychological complications. Extended bedrest also contributes to abnormal alterations in blood pressure maintenance, syncopal episodes, and dizziness. This practice is not first line treatment for hyperemesis gravidarum and should be reserved for patients experiencing chronic unresolved symptoms.

Ordered bedrest can be accomplished in both an inpatient and outpatient setting. An outpatient setting in a patient's private home with home-care visits by a community health nurse is the optimal choice for both the patient and their family. Outpatient care can be provided at a lower cost than inpatient care and allows for family involvement and reduced maternal feelings of isolation. Each patient must be assessed individually to determine the best long-term course of treatment if hyperemesis gravidarum is diagnosed and adversely affecting the pregnant patient.

The national support group Sidelines provides resources to assist pregnant patients who have been advised to maintain bedrest due to their diagnosis and high-risk pregnancy. Their Web site is www.sidelines.org. Support from outside sources can help to alleviate feelings of maternal isolation and stress and the disruption of normal family routines (Ward & Hisley, 2016). Patients can also obtain additional information and support from the Hyperemesis Educational Research (HER) Foundation at the following Web site: https://www.hyperemesis.org/ (American Pregnancy Association, 2019).

⟨ CLINICAL PEARLS

Any time a pregnant patient gets out of bed or up from a sitting position, they should rise slowly to reduce the effects of hypovolemia, fluid shifts, and the syncopal symptoms that can occur with rapid position changes when pregnant.

Pharmacology

Medications taken during pregnancy must be assessed to determine whether any risks outweigh the benefit of ingesting the medications. Many medications can have adverse effects on a developing fetus and should be discussed with a health-care provider, whether prescription or *over the counter* (OTC). Nausea and vomiting are common symptoms during pregnancy and typically are related to the pregnancy and the accompanying physiological changes.

Antiemetic medications can be ordered if conservative measures fail to decrease the symptoms of nausea and vomiting in hyperemesis gravidarum. This classification of drugs may be ordered to provide relief from the symptoms in addition to reducing the risk of fluid and electrolyte imbalances and nutritional deficiencies (Woo & Robinson, 2020). Antiemetics work by blocking specific neurotransmitters that trigger nausea and vomiting. Certain antihistamines may also be used to treat nausea and vomiting symptoms. A prokinetic agent that combines a gut motility stimulator and antiemetic may be prescribed to treat *gastroesophageal reflux disease* (GERD), gastroparesis, and symptoms of nausea and vomiting, although these medications are not advised during the first and third trimesters.

If IV fluids are ordered, they will often contain thiamine (vitamin B) to replace the deficiencies and volume associated with pregnancy symptoms and decreased volume. Vitamin B maintains the health of nerves, skin, and red blood cells. It also treats peripheral neuropathy and may reduce symptoms of nausea and vomiting.

Patients with a history of hyperemesis gravidarum are advised to take daily multivitamins prior to subsequent pregnancies to alleviate further complications associated with future hyperemesis gravidarum. Finally, low-molecular-weight anticoagulants can be initiated to reduce the potential for complications of blood clot formation if a patient is placed on bedrest or is experiencing a period of decreased ambulation from long-term IV therapy. Table 9-4 provides information on the most common medications administered to pregnant patients diagnosed with hyperemesis gravidarum. The table includes details about the normal dosages, along with possible side effects and Safe and Effective Nursing Care (SENC) practices.

Summary

Hyperemesis gravidarum can have debilitating effects for a pregnant woman. The symptoms may affect activities of daily living, ability to continue with employment, and ability to provide care for the family. The fetus can also be affected, largely due to maternal electrolyte imbalances, nutritional deficiencies, and lower-than-recommended maternal weight gain. Mothers who gain less than the suggested 25 to 35 pounds will often have further complications. Hyperemesis gravidarum predisposes a woman to the potential of delivery that is premature at less than 37 weeks' gestation; delivery of a newborn of lower weight than normal; and a small for gestational age newborn.

The ability to control hyperemesis gravidarum and accompanying complications can improve a pregnant woman's quality of life while decreasing problems in the newborn. The reduction of symptoms can also prevent the extraordinary associated health-care costs, which may be incurred.

The postpartum period can be affected by a diagnosis of hyperemesis gravidarum and may be complicated by physical and emotional alterations. These ongoing complications are intensified if hospitalization or bedrest is experienced during pregnancy. The ability to provide care for the newborn can be affected and may be significantly altered if the newborn must be admitted to the neonatal intensive care unit. A history of hyperemesis is strongly associated with a future diagnosis and associated potential pregnancy complications.

Key Points

- The gastrointestinal system is the source of most complaints during pregnancy, including problems with nausea and vomiting and changes in taste and smell.
- Hyperemesis gravidarum differs from morning sickness in both duration and severity and often requires hospitalization.
- The patient with HG should be monitored throughout pregnancy for nutritional intake, electrolytes, weight, and symptoms to avoid dehydration, excessive weight loss, and further complications.

TABLE 9–4   Pharmacology for Hyperemesis Gravidarum in Pregnancy

Class	Example	Action	Dosage	SENC
Antiemetic	Ondansetron, Zofran orally disintegrating tablet (ODT). Dissolved on tongue.	Serotonin 5-HT3 receptor antagonist that blocks serotonins function.	8 mg tablet PO or 10 mL of liquid bid.	Do not take with liquid, as this may increase chance of headache. Take with or without food. Do not take with medications containing serotonin; this can increase potential for serotonin syndrome. Unknown if medication crosses into breast milk. Contains phenylalanine. Side effects may include headache, light-headedness, dizziness, drowsiness, tiredness, constipation, chest pain, irregular heart rate, fainting, and QT prolongation. Increased risk of cleft palate or cleft lip.
Phenothiazine antiemetic	Prochlorperazine, promethazine, chlorpromazine	A dopamine antagonist that has an effect on the serotonergic, histamine, adrenergic, and cholinergic neurotransmitter systems.	5–10 mg PO tid or qid. Maximum dose of 40 mg/day. IM 5–10 mg IM, repeat 3–4 hr prn, maximum 40 mg/day. Rectal 25 mg rectally bid.	Dosage should be individualized based on patient's nausea and vomiting patterns. Begin treatment with the lowest dose and titrate to effect. Crosses into breast milk. Side effects may include dizziness, drowsiness, anxiety, insomnia, strange dreams, dry mouth, stuffy nose, blurred vision, sedation, extrapyramidal effects, and hypotension.
Antihistamine	Diphenhydramine	Histamine 1 receptor antagonist. First generation antihistamine. General antihistamine.	25–50 mg PO tid or qid. IM/IV 10–50 mg up to 400 mg/day.	May interact with monoamine oxidase inhibitors (MAOIs). OTC cough and cold allergy or insomnia medications; anxiety or sleep medications. IV rates should not exceed 25 mg/min. Usage has been associated with cleft palate, drowsiness, constipation, blurred vision, dry mouth, confusion, difficulty urinating, tachycardia, and mood changes.
Vitamin B_6	Pyridoxine, Nestrex	Increases levels of Vitamin B_6 in the bloodstream.	25–75 mg once daily.	Take with meals. May interact with other medications. Safe for use with breastfeeding. Side effects may include decreased folic acid, decreased sensation, headache, loss of appetite, nausea, numbness and tingling, sensory nerve damage, sleepiness, vomiting, and unstable gait.
Prokinetic agent	Metoclopramide, Reglan	Gut motility stimulator and antiemetic.	10–15 mg PO, IV, IM or rectally qid, 30 min before meals and at bedtime. Maximum dose 60 mg/day and use is limited to 12 weeks of therapy.	Avoid use in 1st and 3rd trimesters. Can increase postpartum depression. Avoid in patients with a history of depression. Can cause extrapyramidal syndrome of the newborn. Crosses into breast milk and the effects are unknown. May cause neural development defects. Side effects may include chills, clay-colored stools, dark urine, difficulty breathing, dizziness, tachycardia or irregular heart rate, fever, headache, hypertension, loss of balance and bladder control, loss of appetite, nausea, sore throat, yellow skin or eyes, vomiting, and pallor.

(Woo & Robinson, 2020)

- If treatment involves extended bedrest, home care is often available to reduce costs and minimize feelings of isolation.
- Certain antiemetic and antihistamine medications may reduce HG symptoms that resist more conservative approaches.

Review Questions

1. **The pathophysiology of hyperemesis gravidarum includes which of the following? (Select all that apply.)**

   a. An *Escherichia coli* urinary tract infection

   b. Elevated levels of human chorionic gonadotropin in pregnancy

   c. An eversion to prenatal vitamins

   d. Increased gastric emptying time

2. **Those patients with which of the following are at greatest risk for hyperemesis gravidarum? (Select all that apply.)**

   a. A personal history of hyperemesis gravidarum

   b. Pregnancy with multiples

   c. A family history

   d. Molar pregnancy

3. **Which of the following can be used to control the symptoms of hyperemesis gravidarum in pregnancy? (Select all that apply.)**

   a. Small, frequent meals

   b. Antiemetics

   c. IV fluids

   d. Vitamin B

4. **Which of the following complications can occur in a pregnancy compounded by hyperemesis gravidarum? (Select all that apply.)**

   a. Small for gestational age newborn

   b. Macrosomia in the newborn

   c. Excessive maternal weight gain

   d. Gestational diabetes

5. **Which of the following should be ordered to reduce complications associated with long-term IV therapy for hyperemesis gravidarum?**

   a. Anticoagulants

   b. Regular insulin

   c. Estrogen and progesterone therapy

   d. Antihypertensives

See the appendix for answers to review questions.

References

American Pregnancy Association. (2019). Seven common discomforts of pregnancy. Retrieved from https://americanpregnancy.org/your-pregnancy/7-common-discomforts-pregnancy/

Kosus, N., Kosus, A., Hizli, D., & Turhan, N. O. (2014). Appetite hormones and hyperemesis gravidarum. *OA Medical Hypothesis, 2*(1), 2. Retrieved from http://www.oapublishinglondon.com/images/article/pdf/1405806297.pdf

Ward, S. L., & Hisley, S. M. (2016). *Maternal-child nursing care*. Philadelphia, PA: F.A. Davis.

Woo, T. M., & Robinson, M. V. (2020). *Pharmacotherapeutics for advanced practice nurse prescribers* (5th ed.). Philadelphia: F.A. Davis.

Case Study 2 (Maternity): Vaginal Bleeding

LEARNING OBJECTIVES

Upon completion of this case study the student will be able to integrate knowledge of the physiology, pathophysiology, assessment, and management of obstetrical vaginal bleeding, with a focus on abruptio placentae.

Introduction to Obstetrical Vaginal Bleeding

When a pregnant patient experiences vaginal bleeding, it is a frightening occurrence that necessitates an immediate assessment to determine the cause, the status of the fetus, and the effects on the mother. Vaginal bleeding can be caused by either an obstetric or nonobstetric condition and can result in severe complications for both the mother and fetus if it is found to be obstetric related. Nonobstetric causes of vaginal bleeding can include *dysfunctional uterine bleeding* (DUB), varices, lacerations, malignant neoplasms, and cervicitis (Ward & Hisley, 2016).

According to Goolsby and Grubbs (2019), abnormal vaginal bleeding can occur in a pregnant or nonpregnant patient and may be a sign of a malignancy, more specifically, endometrial cancer. Endometrial cancer is the most common genital cancer in women. It can occur in women as young as 20 years, but is more common in women over the age of 60. Occurrences in European American women are as much as double the frequency of occurrences in African American women. Early detection following a complaint of vaginal bleeding, along with early diagnosis and treatment, sets the stage for a good survival rate and minimal complications.

Multiple issues with the placenta, or placentas in the case of multiples, can cause obstetric-related vaginal bleeding. These diagnoses include the different types of *placenta previa* and *placental abruption* and can be associated with symptoms of abdominal or back pain, an altered fetal heart rate (bradycardia or tachycardia), and intermittent or extended decelerations in fetal heart rate assessed on a fetal monitor. Uterine contractions may also occur with increasing tenderness and rigidity secondary to cumulative uterine bleeding (Ward & Hisley, 2016).

Placenta previa is an implantation of the placenta into the lower area of the uterus, near the cervical os or completely covering the cervical os. A placenta previa typically accounts for 20% of all antepartum hemorrhages. Placenta previa characteristically presents in one of three different patterns:

• Total or complete placenta previa
• Partial placenta previa
• Marginal placenta previa

A complete or total previa classically covers the entire cervical os and can be associated with the highest amount of potential blood loss and the greatest risk for both maternal and neonatal morbidity and mortality. A complete previa also requires a cesarean section for delivery of the neonate. A partial placenta previa partially covers a pregnant patient's cervical os and can also cause a substantial level of vaginal bleeding, with increased risk for maternal and neonatal complications. A marginal previa is diagnosed when the placenta reaches to the edge of the cervical os or when a placenta that is lying low in the uterus encroaches on the cervical os but does not completely cover the area (Ward & Hisley, 2016).

Another cause of obstetrical vaginal bleeding that is appreciably more severe and is associated with added complications is a placenta accreta. This diagnosis can involve multiple layers within the uterus and may include one or all of the following diagnoses, in addition to a diagnosis of placenta previa:

- Placenta accreta
- Placenta increta
- Placenta percreta

An accreta, increta, or percreta is regarded as an abnormally attached placenta that grows into the mother's uterine wall; it may also be associated with a placenta previa. Figure CS2–1 illustrates the three types of placenta previa and Figure CS2–2 illustrates the three types of placenta accreta (Ward & Hisley, 2016).

A placental abruption is another potential and serious obstetrical diagnosis, which presents with or without vaginal bleeding, abdominal and back pain, irregular uterine contractions, late fetal heart rate decelerations, which occur after a uterine contraction has subsided, and fetal bradycardia at a rate less than 110 per minute (Ward & Hisley, 2016).

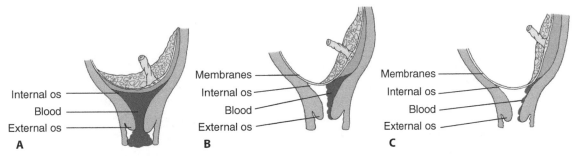

FIGURE CS2–1 ABC types of placenta previa A. Complete (total) B. Partial C. Marginal *From Ward, S. L., & Hisley, S. M. (2016). Maternal-child nursing care. Philadelphia, PA: F.A. Davis. Used with permission*

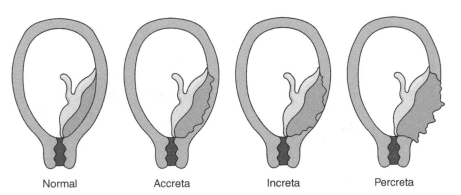

FIGURE CS2–2 Types of placenta accreta

Vaginal bleeding can also be a symptom of preterm labor (before 37 weeks' gestation) and must be thoroughly assessed to determine the etiology, the quantity and color, and any further potential problems associated with the bleeding (American College of Obstetricians and Gynecologists [ACOG], 2019).

It is essential to remember that a pregnant patient's blood volume increases by approximately 50% over pre-pregnancy blood volume with a single fetus and can be higher with multiple fetuses. This increase in blood volume provides a cushion for maternal blood loss, but can mask for a longer time period the signs and symptoms of blood volume depletion. A decrease in maternal blood pressure is a late sign of extreme blood loss. The heart rate of both mother and fetus is considered to be a better predictor of maternal hemorrhage and its fetal effects (Ward & Hisley, 2016).

Meet TM

TM is 30 weeks pregnant with twins, and is Gravida 1 Para 0 Abortion 0 (G1P1A0). She is 42 years old and smokes two packs of cigarettes daily. She is experiencing a new onset of bright red vaginal bleeding with uterine contraction and substantial onset of abdominal and back pain, which began this morning. She calls her obstetrician's office where she has received minimal prenatal care due to missed and cancelled appointments. TM is advised by CF, the triage nurse at the obstetrician's office, to call 911 and to go immediately to the nearest emergency department for an assessment. TM calls 911 for an ambulance and is transported to the closest emergency department. She is triaged by the emergency department clinical staff and is quickly taken up to labor and delivery by the paramedics. TM is transported to a room in labor and delivery, per hospital policy, because she is past 20 weeks' gestational age and is pregnant with twins. She is immediately placed on an electronic fetal monitor (EFM) to assess the fetal heart rates of the twins and to determine the presence of uterine contractions. The paramedics deliver a patient report to the staff and provide evidence of the vaginal bleeding that the patient has experienced since the patient was transported from her home.

Physiology and Pathophysiology

A placental abruption, or abruptio placentae, is a diagnosis wherein the placenta prematurely separates from the uterine wall. The placenta is implanted in the uterus in a normal manner and position prior to the abrupt separation. This separation of the placenta from the uterine wall can result in a partial or total separation with abnormal bleeding occurring between the uterine wall and the placenta location.

Half of all placental abruptions occur prior to the 30th week of pregnancy with an additional 30% diagnosed after delivery, upon the delivery attendant's inspection of the placenta post-delivery. In an abruptio placentae, the placenta partially or fully detaches from the uterine wall either before delivery or during the delivery process. Figure CS2–3 illustrates the three types of abruptio placentae.

There are also three classifications of placental abruption (Box CS2–1) (Cunningham, Leveno, Bloom, Spong, & Dashe, 2014; Ward & Hisley, 2016):

There are multiple risk factors for a placental abruption. These include cigarette smoking, methamphetamine and cocaine use, abdominal trauma, fibroids, premature rupture of membranes, maternal hypertension, multiples, or a shortened fetal umbilical cord. A history of a previous cesarean delivery or an abortion with curettage can contribute to this diagnosis (Ward & Hisley, 2016). An abruption can cause grave complications if not diagnosed quickly and early. The fetus may not receive an adequate oxygen supply to sustain life and the mother may lose a significant amount of blood. This bleeding may be hidden and not externally visible based on the containment of

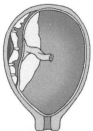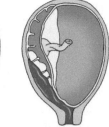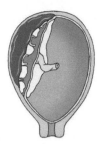

Partial separation
(concealed hemorrhage)

Partial separation
(apparent hemorrhage)

Complete separation
(concealed hemorrhage)

FIGURE CS2–3 Types of abruption placentae *From Ward, S. L., & Hisley, S. M. (2016).* Maternal-child nursing care. *Philadelphia, PA: F.A. Davis. Used with permission*

BOX CS2–1   Classifications of Placental Abruption

Grade 1: Slight vaginal bleeding and some uterine irritability are usually present. Maternal blood pressure is unaffected, and the maternal fibrinogen level is normal. The fetal heart rate pattern is normal.

Grade 2: External uterine bleeding is absent to moderate. The uterus is irritable and tetanic, or very frequent contractions may be present. Maternal blood pressure is maintained, but the pulse rate may be elevated, and postural blood volume deficits may be present. The fibrinogen level may be decreased. The fetal heart rate pattern often shows signs of fetal compromise.

Grade 3: Bleeding is moderate to severe but may be concealed. The uterus is tetanic and painful. Maternal hypotension is frequently present, and fetal death has occurred. Fibrinogen levels are often reduced or are less than 150 mg/dL; other coagulation abnormalities (e.g., thrombocytopenia and factor depletion) are present.

From Ward, S. L., & Hisley, S. M. (2016). *Maternal-child nursing care.* Philadelphia, PA: F.A. Davis. Used with permission.
    Source: Cunningham, F., Leveno, K., Bloom, S., Spong, C., & Dashe, J. (2014). *Williams Obstetrics* (24th ed.). New York, NY: McGraw-Hill Professional.

---

blood between the uterus and placenta layers. Excessive amounts of blood can also be lost through vaginal bleeding. Excess vaginal bleeding is a serious symptom, which often points to a problem originating within the placental implantation or detachment site.

Gathering Information

The receiving labor and delivery nurse initiates a pregnancy and health history on TM to determine the onset and color of the bleeding, vital signs, and any accompanying symptoms or pregnancy complications. The prenatal records are obtained from the obstetrician's office and verified with TM.

The *electronic fetal monitor* (EFM) reveals fetal bradycardia in both fetuses at rates of 90 and 90. A normal fetal heart rate is 110 to 160 per minute. There are uterine contractions present on the fetal monitor, occurring every 3 to 5 minutes and with minimal fetal variability present. A vaginal examination is not done initially due to the presence of bleeding and should not be done prior to an ultrasound assessment of the placenta. TM's vital signs are obtained and reveal a normal blood pressure with a maternal heart rate of 54 beats per minute. The labor and delivery unit staff notifies TM's obstetrician and provides the information they currently have on this pregnant patient.

Assessment and Diagnosis

The techniques of inspection, auscultation, and percussion and palpation are utilized to assess the mother when vaginal bleeding occurs. A head-to-toe assessment is critical for determining the primary complaint cause and any associated complications. The color and quantity of the vaginal bleeding is assessed in conjunction with the level of tenderness and pain, the location, presence of uterine contractions, the tone of the uterus, the vital signs of both mother and fetus and heart rate of fetus, the level of variability on the EFM, and the verbalization of any change in signs or symptoms the mother is experiencing.

A definitive diagnosis is made based on clinical assessment and findings. An abdominal ultrasound assessment can be done, if equipment is available, to determine the source of bleeding, the gestational assessment of the fetus, location of the placenta or placentas, and the amount of amniotic fluid present.

Diagnosis

The obstetrician on call, Dr. JS, conducts a focused physical assessment and examination of TM, which includes a review of EFM data on the fetuses and patient information gathered by the emergency department staff. Dr. JS orders an ultrasound, which reveals a partial placental abruption with apparent hemorrhage. TM's pain has increased in severity and her abdomen is now described as "board-like" with an increase in apparent vaginal bleeding. Dr. JS determines TM's diagnosis of partial placental abruption and communicates the diagnosis to TM and her primary obstetrician, recommending an emergency cesarean section.

Treatment Options

Based on the potential for increased vaginal bleeding, hypovolemic shock, and (in cases of partial abruption) conversion to a complete abruption, an emergency cesarean section may provide the best chance for both maternal and fetal survival of a placental abruption. If bleeding is severe, the mother may require a blood transfusion. In cases of partial placental abruption where bleeding is not severe, the fetus is not in distress, and the fetus is not close to full term, inpatient or at-home bedrest may be prescribed. If a placental abruption results in preterm delivery (before 37 weeks' gestation), the newborn(s) may require treatment in a *neonatal intensive care unit* (NICU).

Treatment and Follow-Up

TM's family has arrived, and they are updated on the treatment plan. The plan to transfer the twins to the NICU after delivery is explained to both the mother and family by the neonatal nurse practitioner. TM is transferred to the operating room for the planned cesarean section.

The delivery is successful and, based on the newborns' gestational age, they are transported to the NICU for admission, monitoring, and nutrition based on facility guidelines for newborns born at less than 34 weeks' gestation. They are cared for in the NICU until reaching an age of 37 gestational ages in adjusted weeks and are discharged home with the parents at that time.

TM is given instructions to follow up with her obstetrician in 2 weeks for laboratory workups and to monitor her progress and any signs of excessive vaginal bleeding or infection. Prior to discharge, she also is provided with ongoing education related to the care of twins to include follow-up with the assigned pediatrician within 24 hours, nutrition, symptoms to monitor for, and what new signs warrant a call to the pediatrician.

Summary

TM was pregnant with twins, was of *advanced maternal age* (AMA) of 42 years, and admitted to smoking two packs of cigarettes daily. Vaginal bleeding and abdominal and back pain are classic symptoms of abruptio placentae until proved otherwise. TM's assessment and ultrasound findings confirmed the diagnosis of placental abruption with a partial separation present. An emergency cesarean section was essential to provide the best possible outcome for all three patients.

While this case study focuses on placental abruption, other forms of obstetric vaginal bleeding can result in serious complications for both the mother and fetus. Obstetric bleeding usually is related to issues with the placenta and includes, in addition to placental abruption, placenta previa (total, partial, or marginal) and placenta accreta/percreta/increta. Placenta previa occurs when the placenta is implanted in the lower area of the uterus, near or completely covering the cervical os. Placenta accreta, percreta, and increta all represent a form of abnormally implanted placenta that grows into the uterine wall. All are serious diagnoses and require cesarean delivery.

Nonobstetrical vaginal bleeding can result from a number of causes, including endometrial cancer, which most frequently occurs in European American women over 60, and is often successfully treated if detected early.

Key Points

- The potential for grave consequences of a complete placental abruption exists if actions are not implemented to emergently deliver the fetus or fetuses.
- There are multiple risk factors associated with a diagnosis of placental abruption, and modifiable risk factors should be considered.
- There are three classifications of abruptio placentae based on the amount and color of vaginal bleeding, uterine irritability, maternal blood pressure, and fibrinogen and platelet levels.
- The normal increase in blood volume in pregnant patients can mask the signs of severe bleeding. Monitoring the heart rate of mother and fetus is the best predictor of maternal bleeding.

Review Questions

1. **Which of the following types of placenta previa completely cover the cervical os of a pregnant patient?**

   a. Marginal/low-lying previa

   b. Partial placenta previa

   c. Complete placenta previa

   d. Accreta placenta previa

2. **Which of the following can be a cause of obstetrical vaginal bleeding? (Select all that apply.)**

   a. Placenta increta

   b. Placental abruption

   c. Marginal placenta previa

   d. Partial placenta previa

3. **Which of the following are causes or conditions that may cause a placental abruption? (Select all that apply.)**

   a. Previous cesarean birth

   b. Previous abortions with curettage

   c. Multiple gestations

   d. Cigarette smoking

4. **Advanced maternal age during pregnancy can increase the risk for a placenta previa.**

   a. True

   b. False

5. **Which of the following conditions warrants a cesarean section for the safest method of delivery? (Select all that apply.)**

   a. Cervicitis

   b. Partial placenta previa

   c. Marginal placenta previa

   d. Complete placenta previa

See the appendix for answers to review questions.

References

American College of Obstetricians and Gynecologists. (2019). Bleeding during pregnancy (FAQ038). Retrieved from https://www.acog.org/Patients/FAQs/Bleeding-During-Pregnancy?

Cunningham, F., Leveno, K., Bloom, S., Spong, C., & Dashe, J. (2014). *Williams obstetrics* (24th ed.). New York, NY: McGraw-Hill Professional.

Goolsby M. J., & Grubbs, L. (2019). *Advanced Assessment: Interpreting findings and formulating differential diagnoses* (4th ed.). Philadelphia, PA: F. A. Davis.

Ward, S. L., & Hisley, S. M. (2016). *Maternal-child nursing care*. Philadelphia, PA: F.A. Davis.

Newborn

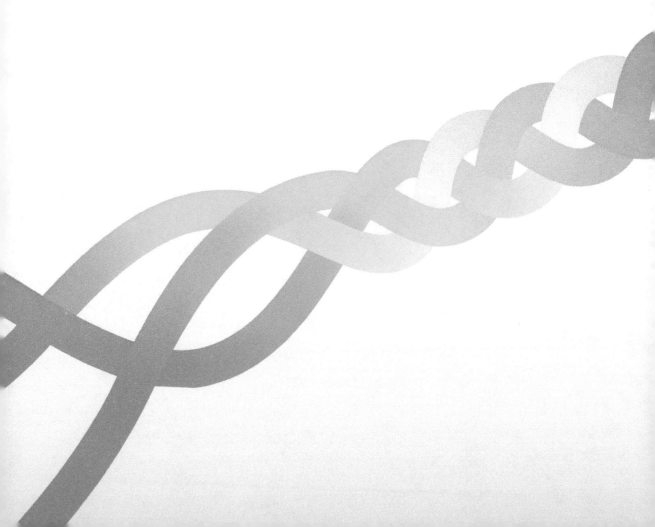

Chapter 10

Hyperbilirubinemia in the Newborn

LEARNING OBJECTIVES

Upon completion of this chapter the student will be able to:

- Integrate knowledge of the physiology, pathophysiology, assessment, and nonpharmacological management of hyperbilirubinemia in the newborn.

- Incorporate the current standards of care for newborns with hyperbilirubinemia.

Introduction

The word "jaundice" is derived from the French *jaune*, which means "yellow," and is caused by the deposit of pigmented bilirubin. Jaundice is also known by the term "icterus," which is derived from the Greek *ikteros*, which means "jaundice" (Pan & Rivas, 2017). Hyperbilirubinemia, also known as icterus or jaundice, is a yellow discoloration of the skin and mucous membranes; this condition is caused by an elevation of either the conjugated or unconjugated bilirubin in a newborn's blood. Conjugated hyperbilirubinemia, which is the more common of the two, is characteristically caused by impairment in hepatic excretion or an extra hepatic obstruction. The cause of unconjugated hyperbilirubinemia, which is less common, includes either an elevation in bilirubin production that can occur with specific hemolytic disorders or impairment in bilirubin uptake. Hemolytic disorders can also be associated with inherited disorders in the newborn. Regardless of the cause, jaundice or hyperbilirubinemia may be the only initial presenting symptom of what is considered to be a severe underlying disease process that can occur in newborns (Goolsby & Grubbs, 2015).

Hyperbilirubinemia is the most common assessment finding during the newborn period and affects more than 80% of all newborns. The healthy newborn's jaundice patterns often present with a clinical appearance that characteristically includes a yellow discoloration of the skin, conjunctiva, and palate in addition to the mucous membranes. The pattern of jaundice normally follows a classic sequencing that initially appears on the face and subsequently progresses in a cephalocaudal manner toward the newborn's trunk and lower extremities to the toes. The cephalocaudal progression of jaundice positively correlates with the serum bilirubin concentration levels. If an assessment of jaundice is made on the lower extremities of a newborn, the bilirubin level and degree of jaundice will be higher (Snell & Gardner, 2017).

Jaundice may occur in newborns of any race or ethnicity, regardless of their skin color. Low levels of bilirubin based on gestational age and hours of life are not considered to be a significant problem or require any treatment. At a minimum, all newborns should be assessed for jaundice every 8 to 12 hours in the first 48 hours of life. The exception to this guideline is in cases of ABO blood type incompatibility or hemolytic diseases of the newborn, which require more frequent assessments of bilirubin levels. The bilirubin level should additionally be assessed with the newborn's first outpatient visit prior to 3–5 days of age (Centers for Disease Control and Prevention [CDC], 2020.

The CDC has previously called for the systematic detection and management of hyperbilirubinemia in all newborns. It has been determined that breastfed newborns less than 38 weeks' gestation and who are exclusively breastfed are at a significantly higher risk than other newborns for the development of jaundice requiring interventions (Dillon, 2007).

Terminology Related to Hyperbilirubinemia

Bilirubin	The yellow, brown, or orange pigment in bile with a pH of 7.4. It is derived metabolically from hemoglobin.
Conjugated bilirubin	Bilirubin bound to glucuronic acid. It has been made soluble in water, excreted in the bile via the duodenum, and eliminated from the body through the bowel.
Unconjugated bilirubin	Unbound bilirubin. Not water soluble and difficult to excrete.
Jaundice	Yellow staining of body tissues and fluids due to excessive levels of bilirubin in the bloodstream.
Physiological jaundice	A gradual rise in total serum bilirubin that occurs after the first 24 hours of life. Benign, self-limiting, and requires surveillance.
Pathological jaundice	Jaundice is considered pathological if it occurs within the first 24 hours of life, after the first week of life, or lasts longer than 2 weeks. Infants with potentially damaging levels of bilirubin in the blood are treated with phototherapy (bili lights).
Severe hyperbilirubinemia	A total serum bilirubin that is greater than the 95th percentile for the newborn's age and requires the initiation of phototherapy for treatment of the elevated bilirubin levels.
Kernicterus	A life-threatening buildup of bilirubin in the brain and spinal cord.
Acute bilirubin encephalopathy (ABE)	Early bilirubin toxicity that may be transient and reversible. Symptoms include the following: • Early stage: hypertonia lethargy, poor sucking and decreased feedings. • Intermediate stage: Fever, high-pitched cry, moderate stupor, irritability and hypertonia characterized by backward neck arching and trunk, alternating drowsiness, and hypertonia
Chronic bilirubin encephalopathy (CBE)	A state of chronic and permanent effects of bilirubin toxicity. Symptoms may include retrocollis, opisthotonos, a shrill cry, and deficient feeding periods, episodes of apnea, fever, deep stupor or even coma, seizures, or death.

(Kaplan, Wong, Sibley, & Stevenson, 2015; Venes, 2017)

Physiology

The production of bilirubin is normally accelerated in a newborn when compared to adults. Beginning in the first day of life, the bilirubin production is two to three times the rate of an adult with the average at 8 to 10 mg/kg of a newborn's weight each day. In addition, at birth newborns experience both a development of polycythemia and an accelerated rate of heme breakdown; these processes are both affected by the reduced life of newborns' red blood cells. The newborn's elevated levels of both hemoglobin and hematocrit may also impact bilirubin levels; these higher levels of both hemoglobin and hematocrit that were once essential in utero with lower oxygen levels are no longer necessary after delivery, and the process of red blood cell degradation is initiated. This process increases the serum levels of bilirubin, which subsequently increases the potential for hyperbilirubinemia in the newborn (Snell & Gardner, 2017).

A newborn's red blood cell life span is 70 to 90 days when compared to the life span of 120 days in both children and adults. In addition, in utero a newborn's excess bilirubin level was removed by the mother's liver. Upon delivery, a newborn must excrete elevated bilirubin independently while experiencing a period of immature liver functioning. Hepatic functioning can also result in inadequate removal of the elevated bilirubin by excretion, with subsequent jaundice occurring (Snell & Gardner, 2017).

The rate of bilirubin excretion and elevation in serum levels can also be associated with the decreased transit time through a newborn's intestines as well as the decreased enterohepatic circulation time. The conjugation process of bilirubin occurs within the hepatocytes, with the subsequent conversion of conjugated bilirubin into bile and excreted into the intestines. Bilirubin is then absorbed from the bowel and returns to the liver. Any change in the rate of a newborn's transit time has the potential to break down bilirubin's conjugation and cause unconjugated bilirubin to be further absorbed, thus leading to hyperbilirubinemia (see Figure 10-1) (Snell & Gardner, 2017).

HIGH YIELD FACT FOR TESTING

Hyperbilirubinemia is multifactorial, and its treatment is dependent on normal functioning of multiple body systems, including the gastrointestinal, renal, neurological, and hematological.

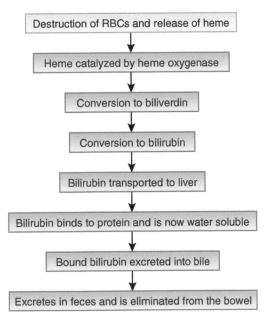

FIGURE 10-1 The metabolism of bilirubin

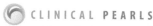
Many factors may affect a newborn's excretion of bilirubin and should be taken into consideration.

Pathophysiology

Hyperbilirubinemia is a condition caused by an excess of serum bilirubin in a newborn due to excessive hemolysis, ABO blood type incompatibility, hepatocellular injury, and bile duct obstruction or decreased excretion. Newborns initially have immature liver function and cannot break down the products of hemolysis easily. The by-product of this hemolysis is bilirubin, and due to their hepatic immaturity, newborns are unable to conjugate bilirubin or naturally break down bilirubin. The result is an excess of serum bilirubin and a decrease in bilirubin excretion through both a newborn's urine and stool. The combination of these factors can subsequently result in symptoms and a diagnosis of hyperbilirubinemia (Capriotti, 2020).

The quantity of intestinal flora within the newborn's intestines is another factor in the reduction of bilirubin to urobilinogen for excretion in the stool. The intestinal flora is normally diminished in the newborn's bowel when compared to adults, and the bilirubin level in the bowel is increased. These levels may subsequently inhibit the newborn's ability to convert bilirubin to urobilinogen for excretion. In addition, increased bilirubin levels in the intestinal tract may result in elevated levels of circulating bilirubin within the enterohepatic circulation and subsequent jaundice (Snell & Gardner, 2017).

Elevated serum levels of bilirubin subsequently can cause hyperbilirubinemia in newborns. At low levels, bilirubin is considered to be a weak acid that has antioxidant properties to provide for the ability to bind to membrane lipids. This binding limits the potential damage that occurs with elevated bilirubin levels through a process known as *peroxidation*. Lipid peroxidation occurs when a hydroxyl radical abstracts an electron from polyunsaturated fatty acids. This process creates an unstable lipid radical, which can then react with oxygen to form a fatty acid called a *peroxyl radical*. Repeated cycles of this process can cause severe damage to cell membranes and cell death. This repeated process could be the primary cause of the jaundice complications assessed in the newborn (Ayala, Munoz, & Arguelles, 2014).

Elevated levels of bilirubin, a weak acid, are toxic to the newborn and may lead to neuronal damage with subsequent neurological dysfunction. In the newborn, the clinical significance of an elevated bilirubin level is the propensity for disposition within the skin and mucous membranes. This bilirubin deposition creates the characteristic yellow skin, eye, and mucous membrane colorings that are typically associated with a diagnosis of jaundice in the newborn (Ayala et al., 2014).

Hyperbilirubinemia is often predictable in the progression of onset, from initial symptoms to potential complications. Physiological jaundice typically does not occur until after a newborn is 24 hours of age and is classically self-limiting and benign in nature when compared to pathological jaundice, which requires prompt, early interventions. Severe hyperbilirubinemia is defined as a total serum bilirubin that is greater than the 95th percentile for the newborn's age and requires the initiation of phototherapy for treatment of the elevated bilirubin levels (Figure 10-2).

A diagnosis of kernicterus in a newborn is considered to be a pathological diagnosis that is considerably more pathological than severe hyperbilirubinemia. It is characterized by brain stem nuclei and cerebellum staining due to the severely elevated levels of bilirubin. The word "kernicterus" is derived from the German *kern*, meaning "a kernel or nucleus" and the Greek *ikteros*, meaning "jaundice." This diagnosis can be avoided

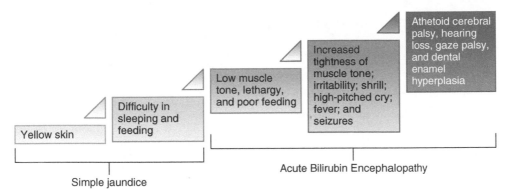

FIGURE 10–2 Predictable trajectory of hyperbilirubinemia

by prompt treatment and resolution of a diagnosis of hyperbilirubinemia. Additional diagnoses associated with untreated bilirubin levels may include *acute bilirubin encephalopathy* (ABE). This is a state of early bilirubin toxicity that may be both transient and reversible. The two stages of ABE are early and intermediate. *Chronic bilirubin encephalopathy* (CBE) is considered to be a state of both chronic and permanent effects related to bilirubin toxicity. Symptoms may include retrocollis, opisthotonos, a shrill cry, deficient feeding periods, episodes of apnea, fever, deep stupor or even coma, seizures, or death.

It is essential to recognize and promptly treat a newborn diagnosed with jaundice. The early assessment, identification, and treatment of newborns with elevated bilirubin levels will decrease the potential for long-term consequences related to the effects of hyperbilirubinemia.

HIGH YIELD FACT FOR TESTING

A visual assessment of jaundice is unreliable in dark-skinned newborns.

CLINICAL PEARLS

The visual recognition of jaundice does not always correlate with the actual severity of the jaundice.

Incidence

In both late-preterm (gestational age between 34 weeks and 36 weeks and 6 days) and pre- to full-term infants (37 weeks to 40 weeks), it is expected for the bilirubin levels to increase shortly after birth. Bilirubin levels characteristically follow an hour-specific percentile trajectory with a decline in levels by the end of the first week of life. The majority of term newborns experience a peak level of serum bilirubin between the second and fourth days of life, which commonly does not exceed 6 mg/dL. Late-preterm newborns reach their peak later, at 5 to 7 days of life and will demonstrate a higher peak bilirubin level than the majority of full-term newborns. The late-preterm newborn is also at risk for elevated levels of serum bilirubin, resulting in a higher-than-normal rate of rise in levels and a higher probability for a diagnosis of hyperbilirubinemia (Snell & Gardner, 2017).

Bilirubin levels will predictably return to normal levels by the 12th day of life in the majority of newborns (less than 1 mg/dL), but may rise to appreciably higher levels in a small percentage of preterm, late-preterm, and term newborns. This group of newborns diagnosed with hyperbilirubinemia must be appropriately treated within a

TABLE 10–1   Effects of Bilirubin Toxicity in Newborns

Early	Late	Chronic
Lethargy	Irritability	Kernicterus
Poor feeding	Opisthotonos	High-frequency hearing loss
High-pitched cry	Seizures	Paralysis of upward gaze
Hypotonia	Apnea	Dental dysplasia
	Oculogyric crisis	Mild mental retardation Athetoid cerebral palsy
	Hypertonia	
	Fever	

(Mayo Clinic, 2018a)

timely manner to prevent any irreversible complications from occurring. These complications may include severe hyperbilirubinemia, kernicterus, or bilirubin neurotoxicity (Snell & Gardner, 2017).

Jaundice that is left untreated can cause both mental and developmental delays. Untreated newborns may progress from a diagnosis of jaundice to a diagnosis of acute, reversible bilirubin encephalopathy (ABE) with further progression to chronic, irreversible bilirubin encephalopathy or kernicterus (CBE) (Kaplan, Wong, Sibley, & Stevenson, 2015) (Table 10-1). Therefore, it is important for nurses to focus on newborns who are at risk for the developing jaundice with accurate assessment, prevention, and early intervention.

Assessment

Assessment of a newborn's skin pigmentation is difficult because coloring is highly variable among newborns of all racial and ethnic backgrounds. There may be variations in skin color over a newborn's different body regions. A diagnosis of jaundice or hyperbilirubinemia indicates an elevation of bilirubin levels and can often be initially detected in the sclera of the newborn's eyes and mucous membranes before an elevation is noted on a skin assessment (Goolsby & Grubbs, 2015). A thorough newborn assessment for jaundice is essential to decrease the potential for complications related to hyperbilirubinemia. The nursing assessment includes visually assessing the newborn and obtaining diagnostic studies to assess severity and treatment success. Diagnostic studies include the measurement of bilirubin levels by transcutaneous meters, plasma levels, or both, and obtaining maternal and newborn blood typing and Rh factors to assess ABO incompatibility. An assessment of both maternal and newborn clinical factors is essential. In addition, the application of a nomogram or graphical calculating method to guide clinical practice and treatment of elevated bilirubin levels and a diagnosis of jaundice is essential (see the accompanying box, Studies for Diagnosing the Causes of Newborn Hyperbilirubinemia).

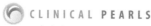 CLINICAL PEARLS

It is important to examine newborns in natural light in order to accurately assess the color of sclera, mucous membranes, and skin.

Studies for Diagnosing the Causes of Newborn Hyperbilirubinemia

ABO Incompatibility and Blood Typing: Rhesus (Rh) factor is an inherited protein found on the surface of red blood cells. If blood has the protein, then it is Rh-positive. If blood lacks the protein, then it is Rh-negative. Rh-positive is the most common blood type. The Rh factor can affect both the mother's pregnancy and the newborn after delivery if the mother is Rh-negative and the newborn is Rh-positive (Rh incompatibility).

Mother's Rh factor	Father's Rh factor	Baby's Rh factor	Precautions
Rh-positive	Rh-positive	Rh-positive	None
Rh-negative	Rh-negative	Rh-negative	None
Rh-positive	Rh-negative	Could be Rh-positive or Rh-negative	None
Rh-negative	Rh-positive	Could be Rh-positive or Rh-negative	Rh immune

Coombs Test: a positive direct Coombs test indicates antibodies that act against red blood cells. This may result in hemolytic disease of the newborn. A negative Coombs test indicates that the newborn is not affected by Rh incompatibility.

Complete Blood Count (CBC): a blood test used to detect a range of disorders. A complete blood count test measures the following:

- Red blood cells, which carry oxygen
- White blood cells, which fight infection
- Hemoglobin, the oxygen-carrying protein in red blood cells
- Hematocrit, the proportion of red blood cells to the fluid component, or plasma, in blood
- Platelets, which help with blood clotting

Reticulocyte Count: a measure of the number of red blood cells delivered by bone marrow. It is elevated with active erythropoiesis or hemolysis in the newborn.

Serum Bilirubin Level: an assessment of levels of bilirubin in the blood.

Indirect (Unconjugated) Bilirubin Level: bilirubin that is bound to the protein albumin in the blood is unconjugated, or indirect and is the difference between total and direct bilirubin.

Direct (Conjugated) Bilirubin Level: conjugated, or direct, bilirubin travels from the liver into the small Intestine and is water soluble and is the difference between total and direct bilirubin.

Transcutaneous Bilirubin Level: an indirect measurement of bilirubin through a newborn's skin.

(Mayo Clinic, 2018b)

Risk Factors/Score for Hyperbilirubinemia

Screening for newborn hyperbilirubinemia begins with an assessment of potential risk factors that may be present in the newborn. Nurses are direct client care providers and often the first to recognize the signs and symptoms of hyperbilirubinemia. The newborn assessment in addition to the evaluation of risk factors begins upon delivery and continues throughout the inpatient and outpatient encounters. See Box 10-1 for jaundice risk factors.

The risk scoring for neonatal hyperbilirubinemia is used to evaluate the need for early interventions and/or treatment. The use of risk scoring in combination with

BOX 10-1   JAUNDICE Risk Factors

- **J**aundice in the first 24 hours.
- **A** sibling with a history of jaundice.
- **U**nrecognized hemolysis (ABO or Rh incompatibility)
- **N**on-optimal suck/nursing
- **D**eficiency in G6PD
- **I**nfection
- **C**ephalohematoma/or bruising
- **E**ast Asian or Mediterranean descent

PRENATAL RISK FACTORS
- Advanced maternal age (AMA)
- Maternal diabetes
- First trimester bleeding
- Maternal blood and Rh type
- Sibling with a history of hyperbilirubinemia
- Asian, American Indian, or Greek descent
- O-positive or Rh-negative maternal blood type

NEWBORN, INTRAPARTUM, POSTNATAL RISK FACTORS
- Male newborn
- Maternal illness: gestational diabetes
- Less than 38 weeks gestation
- Operative vaginal delivery
- Birth trauma
- Excessive weight loss after birth
- TORCH infections, including:
  a. Toxoplasmosis
  b. Other infections to include parvovirus, coxsackie virus, chicken pox, chlamydia, HIV, Lyme disease, syphilis, Zika fever, and hepatitis B.
  c. Rubella
  d. Cytomegalovirus
  e. Herpes simplex type 2 or neonatal herpes simplex
- Sepsis
- Enzyme deficiency
- Liver malfunction
- Inadequate feedings
- Pitocin for induction or augmentation of labor
- Delayed meconium passage
- Internal bleeding
- Cephalohematoma/bruising
- Coombs positive

(Adapted from Snell & Gardner, 2017; CDC, 2015)

universal screenings of transcutaneous and serum bilirubin levels is the most effective method for identifying newborns at risk for hyperbilirubinemia (see Table 10-2) (Muchowski, 2014).

 CLINICAL PEARLS
Jaundice within 24 hours of life is pathological jaundice; after 24 hours, it can be considered physiological jaundice.

TABLE 10–2 Risk Score for Neonatal Hyperbilirubinemia

Variable	Score
Birth Weight:	
2,000–2,500 g (4 lb, 7 oz to 5 lb, 8 oz)	0
2,501–3,000 g (5 lb, 8 oz to 6 lb, 10 oz)	3
3,001–3,500 g (6 lb, 10 oz to 7 lb, 11 oz)	6
3,501–4,000 g (7 lb, 11 oz to 8 lb, 13 oz)	9
4,001–4,500 g (8 lb, 13 oz to 9 lb, 15 oz)	12
4,501–5,000 g (9 lb, 15 oz to 11 lb, 1 oz)	15
Oxytocin (Pitocin) use	4
Vacuum delivery	4
Breast and formula feeding	4
Exclusive breastfeeding	5
Gestational age <38 weeks	5

A score of 8 or higher suggests an increased risk of hyperbilirubinemia, and a transcutaneous and/or serum bilirubin level should be obtained.

Nonpharmacological Management and Treatment

The American Academy of Pediatrics (AAP, 2004) developed guidelines for the identification and management of hyperbilirubinemia in newborns with a gestational age of 35 weeks and above (see boxed Clinical Provider and Nursing Standards below). The guidelines are aligned with the Institute of Medicine's (IOM) position statement that includes patient safety, timely management of interventions, primary and secondary prevention and diagnostic evaluation, risk assessment, follow-up, and patient treatment (Snell & Gardner, 2017).

Unless the bilirubin level is considered to be emergent, conservative measures should be implemented initially to treat jaundice. This includes increasing the newborns intake and treatment by phototherapy, which will promote the absorption and excretion of serum bilirubin. Phototherapy will create a reaction by which unconjugated bilirubin is transformed into photoproducts that can be easily excreted by the newborn. The AAP has developed guidelines for the initiation of phototherapy that take into consideration the newborn's age, dietary intake, and any potential risk factors (Snell & Gardner, 2017).

The most commonly used phototherapy treatment tool is the nomogram (Figure 10-3), which was produced by the AAP in 2004. This tool provides guidelines for the initiation and discontinuation of phototherapy and is based on the newborn's gestational age, total serum bilirubin levels, and risk factors. The provider's assessment of these parameters places the newborn's risk and need for phototherapy at a lower, median, or higher level. The guidelines also take into consideration associated risk factors including isoimmune hemolytic disease, *glucose-6-phosphate dehydrogenase* (G6PD) deficiency, asphyxia, significant lethargy, temperature instability, sepsis, acidosis, or serum albumin levels less than 3 g/dL (AAP, 2004).

Phototherapy treatment should take into consideration the potential for newborn and mother complications, to include temperature instability due to an imbalance of the thermal environment, separation of family and newborn, interference with family bonding, and the potential for electrolyte imbalance.

Clinical Provider and Nursing Standards for the Management of Hyperbilirubinemia

Clinical nursing interventions related to the prevention and management of jaundice

1. Promote and support breastfeeding.
2. Recognize that visual estimation of jaundice can lead to errors and should be followed with bilirubin level monitoring.
3. Recognize that newborns under 38 weeks' gestation and breastfeeding are at a higher risk.
4. Perform a jaundice assessment daily and upon discharge on all newborns.
5. Provide families with discharge instructions related to the recognition of jaundice in newborns.

Clinical provider interventions related to the prevention and management of jaundice

1. Establish protocols for the identification and evaluation of hyperbilirubinemia.
2. Measure *total serum bilirubin* (TSB) or *transcutaneous bilirubin* (TCB) levels of infants within the first 24 hours of life and prior to discharge.
3. Interpret bilirubin levels according to the infant's gestational age in hours.
4. Treat newborn jaundice as indicated based on the serum bilirubin levels and gestational age.

(Adapted from AAP, Subcommittee on Hyperbilirubinemia, 2004)

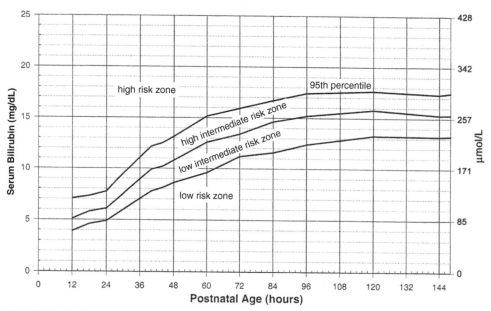

FIGURE 10–3 Information provided by nomogram *Reproduced with permission from* Pediatrics, Vol. 114 (1), 297–316, Copyright © 2004 by the AAP

If the initial phototherapy treatment is ineffective, the newborn may require exchange blood transfusions or the administration of *IV immunoglobulin G* (IVIG) therapy. Exchange transfusions may be indicated if the serum bilirubin levels are greater than 25 mg/dL and symptoms of hyperbilirubinemia and acute bilirubin encephalopathy are present in the newborn. These procedures are completed in the neonatal intensive care unit with close cardiac and respiratory monitoring and personnel in place (Snell & Gardner, 2017).

Dietary Changes

Decreased caloric intake, decreased stooling, and/or mild dehydration associated with a newborn's insufficient intake from breast or formula feedings may contribute to higher levels of unconjugated bilirubin and a diagnosis of hyperbilirubinemia. The newborn will need to increase their intake in order to promote the excretion of elevated bilirubin levels. This intervention may require more frequent breast or formula feedings or the addition of the supplementation of formula to exclusively breastfed newborns for a period of time. Supplementation with formula is not ideal for exclusively breastfed newborns but may be medically necessary. Newborns with a weight loss over 10%, signs of dehydration, decreased excretion of both urine and stool, or any clinical signs of jaundice or associated risk factors should be provided with an increase in oral intake by both breastfeeding from the mother or donor milk and/or formula feeding.

Discharge Instructions

Discharge instructions should be provided to all families related to the symptoms, potential effects, and treatment of jaundice in their newborn. The following symptoms require the parents to contact the newborn's provider:

- New or worsening yellow skin or eyes
- Decreased voiding or stooling
- Pale, chalky-colored bowel movements
- Dark urine that stains the diaper
- Trouble with feeding
- Inconsolable crying
- Vomiting
- Fever

Summary

Jaundice or hyperbilirubinemia is the development of an elevation in bilirubin levels in newborns during the first days to weeks of life. The immaturity of a newborn's liver and the breakdown of red blood cells contribute to the development of elevated bilirubin levels and a diagnosis of jaundice. The level of bilirubin and the gestational age of a newborn determine the type and duration of treatment needed. The majority of newborns will not require any treatment and the diagnosis will be self-limiting, as in a diagnosis of physiological jaundice. In some cases, the elevated level of bilirubin will require treatment and surveillance to prevent long-term complications. These long-term, preventable complications could include deafness, cerebral palsy, or other forms of permanent damage to a newborn's brain.

The nursing management of hyperbilirubinemia should be focused on decreasing both serum conjugated and unconjugated bilirubin levels though ordered interventions. This can be accomplished by initiating conservative measures early in the newborn's life with the onset of moderate bilirubin level elevations. Each newborn should be systematically monitored for hyperbilirubinemia based on their gestational age, intake and output, bilirubin levels, and individual response to jaundice treatment. The judicious monitoring of bilirubin levels will lead to a decrease in the most common cause of readmission in the newborn period. Measures to decrease bilirubin levels should also be supervised by nursing personnel to assess the effectiveness of the initiated interventions and prevent further complications.

Key Points

- Maternal and newborn risk factors for the potential development of jaundice should be identified early.

- All newborns should be assessed for jaundice at 24 hours and prior to discharge, and with the first newborn outpatient appointment.

- Breastfed newborns with less than 38 weeks' gestation and exclusively breastfed are at a significantly higher risk of jaundice than formula-fed newborns with over 38 weeks' gestation.

- Visual estimation of hyperbilirubinemia may lead to errors in appropriate management. Skin color is highly variable among newborns of all racial and ethnic backgrounds; therefore, serum bilirubin levels are recommended for accurate level assessment.

- Conservative measures should be initiated first for elevated bilirubin levels in physiological jaundice.

- Diagnostic testing for hyperbilirubinemia should include blood typing, complete blood count, reticulocyte count, and direct, indirect, and total bilirubin levels.

- The AAP nomogram should be utilized to determine the need for phototherapy.

- Adverse short-term effects of phototherapy including temperature instability, maternal separation, and bonding interference should be assessed.

- Parents should be provided with discharge instructions related to the assessment of jaundice and when to call their provider.

Review Questions

1. **Late preterm infants will have peak bilirubin levels at how many days?**

   a. Day 2 of life

   b. Day 3 of life

   c. Upon delivery

   d. Day 5 of life

2. **As the nurse performs the initial assessment of a newborn, which finding would be a cause for concern and warrant prompt provider follow-up?**

   a. Vernix caseosa

   b. Lanugo hair

   c. Mongolian spots

   d. Jaundice

3. **Jaundice is caused by an excess of which of the following in a newborn's blood?**

   a. Uric acid

   b. Bilirubin

   c. Hemoglobin and hematocrit

   d. Sodium and potassium

4. **If hyperbilirubinemia is not treated, which of the following may occur?**

   a. Damage to the brain and hearing

   b. Inability to breastfeed adequately

   c. Weight loss.

   d. Alteration in newborn growth

5. **The newborn's plan of care should include which of the following to limit the development of hyperbilirubinemia?**

   a. Monitor for the passage of stool.

   b. Substitute breastfeeding with formula feeding.

   c. Initiate phototherapy at 24 hours of life.

   d. Supplement breastfeeding with formula feeding.

See the appendix for answers to review questions.

References

American Academy of Pediatrics, Subcommittee on Hyperbilirubinemia. (2004). Management of hyperbilirubinemia in the newborn infant 35 or more weeks of gestation. *Pediatrics, 114*(1), 297–316.

Ayala, A., Munoz, M., & Arguelles. S. (2014). Lipid peroxidation: Production, metabolism, and signaling mechanisms of malondialdehyde and 4-hydroy-2-nonenal. *Oxidative Medicine and Cellular Longevity, 2014*, 360438. Retrieved from http://dx.doi.org/10.1155/2014/360438

Capriotti, T. (2020). *Pathophysiology: Introductory concepts and clinical perspective* (2nd ed.). Philadelphia, PA: F.A. Davis.

Centers for Disease Control and Prevention. (2020). What are Jaundice and Kernicterus. Retrieved from https://www.cdc.gov/ncbddd/jaundice/facts.html

Dillon, P. M. (2016). *Nursing health assessment*. Philadelphia, PA: F.A. Davis.

Goolsby, M. J., & Grubbs, L. (2015). *Advanced assessment: Interpreting findings and formulating differential diagnoses*. Philadelphia, PA: F.A. Davis.

Kaplan, M., Wong, R., Sibley, E., & Stevenson, D. (2015). Neonatal jaundice and liver diseases. In R. Martin, A. Fanaroff, & M. Walsh (Eds.), *Fanaroff & Martins' neonatal-perinatal medicine* (pp. 1618–1673). Philadelphia, PA: Elsevier.

Mayo Clinic. (2018a). Infant jaundice. Retrieved from https://www.mayoclinci.org/diseases-conditions/infant-jaundice/symptoms-causes/syc-20373865

Mayo Clinic. (2018b). Tests and procedures. Retrieved from https://www.mayoclinic.org/tests-procedures

Muchowski, K. E. (2014). Evaluation and treatment of neonatal hyperbilirubinemia. *American Family Physician, 89*(11), 873–878.

Pan, D. H., & Rivas, Y. (2017). Jaundice: Newborn to age 2 months. *Pediatrics in Review, 38*(11), 499–510. doi:10.1542/pir.2015-0132

Snell, B. J., & Gardner, S. L. (2017). *Care of the well newborn*. Burlington, MA: Jones & Bartlett Learning.

Venes, D. (Ed.). (2017). *Taber's cyclopedic medical dictionary* (23rd ed.). Philadelphia, PA: FA Davis.

Chapter 11

Congenital Heart Disease

LEARNING OBJECTIVES

Upon completion of this chapter the student will be able to:

* Integrate knowledge of the physiology, pathophysiology, assessment, and nonpharmacological and pharmacological management of congenital heart disease.

* Incorporate the current standards of care for newborn patients with congenital heart disease.

Introduction

The majority of newborns transition from intrauterine to extrauterine life without any complications. The transition involves significant alterations in both the anatomy and physiology of the newborn during the first few minutes to hours of life. Preparation for birth should include an assessment of the mother's perinatal course and any fetal or maternal factors that may alter the delivery and resuscitation processes. Nurses providing care during the delivery process and transition period must have the skills essential to both identify and provide treatment for any compromised newborn undergoing an abnormal transition.

Congenital heart disease (CHD), or congenital heart defects in the newborn population, falls under the category of structural complications. A defect occurs when the heart or blood vessels near the heart do not develop normally before birth and the circulation pattern is impaired (American Heart Association [AHA], 2018). CHD is divided into two principal categories: cyanotic and acyanotic cardiac lesions. The cyanotic cardiac lesions are characterized as cardiac defects that cause all deoxygenated blood to be shunted away from the pulmonary circulation and directed toward the systemic circulation. The shunting of blood is considered complete shunting when mixing of oxygenated and deoxygenated blood transpires. This is typically secondary to a parallel circulation with reduced resistance to blood flow or open fetal shunting. In contrast, with incomplete shunting with CHD, there is a partial mixture of both oxygenated and unoxygenated blood through the fetal shunts that remain patent in the newborn (Snell & Gardner, 2017).

In comparison, the acyanotic cardiac lesions of CHD are characteristically less threatening at birth and may not even be diagnosed or detected on assessment during maternal prenatal testing. Newborns born with acyanotic lesions tend to become symptomatic only after post-delivery changes occur within the pulmonary and systemic systems. These vascular alterations typically cause several resistance conversions during the first several hours post-delivery (Snell & Gardner, 2017). The resistance conversions involve the pulmonary removal of lung fluid, the secretion of surfactant, and the coordination of breathing. In addition, the low-pressure placenta is delivered, and the cardiovascular system responds by altering blood flow, cardiac pressures, and vessel dilation and constriction.

Cyanotic cardiac lesions require maintenance of the patency of the newborn's *ductus arteriosus* (DA). The patency of the DA is essential for survival of these newborns with cyanotic lesions post-delivery and has resulted in the designation *ductal-dependent lesions*. It is essential to recognize the presence of cyanotic cardiac lesions, as they require early diagnosis and treatment. Stabilization of the newborn is essential prior to any planned medical and/or surgical interventions (Snell & Gardner, 2017).

Physiology

Newborns in utero are dependent on their mothers for survival. The mother delivers both oxygen and nutrients to the fetus and removes all stored wastes at the uterine insertion site. Gas exchange occurs at the placental intervillous space where maternal uterine venous blood enters the uterus, and the umbilical vein carries all oxygenated blood from the placenta to the fetus in utero (Snell & Gardner, 2017).

The fetal pulmonary system is unable to participate in fetal oxygenation prior to birth. The amount of cardiac output circulating to the fetal lungs in utero is minimal because of the elevated pressures and resistance created by the pulmonary circuit. The fetal anatomic shunting that occurs in utero facilitates the movement of blood from right to left side of the heart instead of left to right; this movement enhances the distribution of both nutrients and oxygen directly to the fetal tissues (Fraser, 2014).

The newborn's heart has four chambers: the upper two chambers (atria) and the lower two chambers (ventricles). These chambers are separated by tissue called a septum and blood is pumped through the four chambers with the guidance of heart valves, which open and close to provide one-direction blood flow. Congenital cardiac disease can involve the newborn's valves, chambers, septum, arteries, or circulation or blood flow complications (AHA, 2018).

As shown in Figure 11-1:

- The *ductus venosus* guides oxygenated fetal blood from the umbilical vein to the fetus's inferior vena cava.
- The *ductus arteriosus* guides fetal blood from the pulmonary artery to the descending aorta.
- The *foramen ovale* guides the fetus's intra-arterial oxygenated blood from the umbilical vein to bypass the pulmonary circulation through the right to left atria.

At birth, a newborn's lungs and pulmonary system begin to exchange gases, a process previously handled by the mother's placenta in utero. The newborn's previously fluid-filled alveoli begin to fill with air. This gas exchange occurs upon initiation of the newborn's independent breathing. As the blood flow changes and pressures increase, the foramen ovale and ductus arteriosus begin to close and the maternal placenta ceases to function. The changes in ambient temperature and the chemical, mechanical, and sensory stimuli from intrauterine to extrauterine life also assist in initiating the first newborn respirations. The pulmonary vascular resistance is decreased, and pulmonary blood flow is increased, with resulting increases in both the left atrial volume and pressures. The newborn's circulation redistributes blood flow with increasing systemic vascular resistance and subsequent decreases in right atrium pressures; this process then generates the permanent left-to-right circulation pattern needed for independent extrauterine life (Snell & Gardner, 2017).

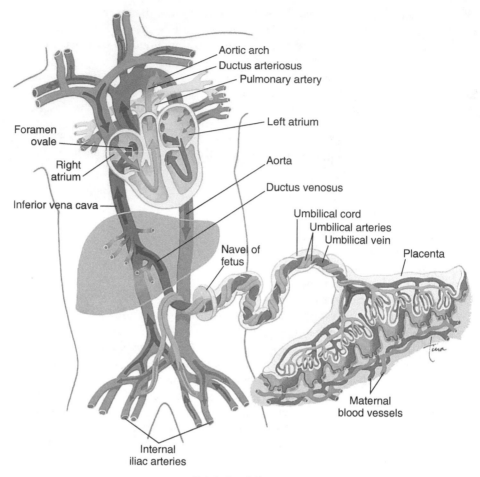

Aortic arch
Ductus arteriosus
Pulmonary artery
Left atrium
Foramen ovale
Right atrium
Aorta
Ductus venosus
Inferior vena cava
Umbilical cord
Umbilical arteries
Umbilical vein
Placenta
Navel of fetus
Maternal blood vessels
Internal iliac arteries

Fetal circulation

FIGURE 11–1 Fetal circulation patterns *From Dillon:* Nursing health assessment, *2nd edition. Philadelphia, PA: FA Davis.*

Pathophysiology

Congenital cardiac disease or defects are differentiated from cardiac dysfunction based on the etiology. Congenital disease occurs secondary to structural complications that are present at birth and may alter the normal circulatory flow of blood through the heart and throughout the body. Cardiac dysfunction or inability of the newborn heart to function normally by pumping blood and providing oxygen and removing wastes may occur resultant to clinical disorders. These may include disorders related to pulmonary disease, cardiac arrhythmias, shock, surgical procedures, infections, or intravenous catheter placement. Approximately 10% of all newborns will not accomplish successful intrauterine-to-extrauterine transition and may require assistance to initiate or sustain their independent self-regulating circulation and respirations (Snell & Gardner, 2017).

According to the AHA (2018), a congenital heart defect is a structural problem within the heart that is present at delivery in a newborn. These defects occur during development in the fetus close to the time of conception. CHD can have an effect on both cardiac functioning and circulation, and the diagnosis may also increase the risk of developing secondary medical diagnoses.

Table 11-1 details the specific cardiac defects originally described in the chapter introduction, along with the associated symptoms. The pathology of the newborn defects is further designated broadly as either cyanotic or acyanotic defects.

Acyanotic cardiac defects can be secondary to obstructive lesions. These lesions lead to stenosis, narrowing, or left-to-right shunting of blood, with resulting

TABLE 11–1 Congenital Cardiac Defects

| Cardiac Defect | Cyanotic Heart Diseases | |
	Pathology	Assessment Findings

Tetralogy of Fallot (ToF)	Opening between the lower chambers of the heart.
	    Obstruction from the heart to the lungs.
	    The aorta (blood vessel) lies over the opening in the lower chambers.
	    The muscle surrounding the lower right chamber becomes overly thickened.
		Cyanosis
		Arrhythmias

Transposition of the great arteries (TGA)	The two main arteries carrying blood away from the heart are reversed.	Arrhythmias Decreased heart muscle or valve function
Total anomalous pulmonary venous return (TAPVR)	Defect in the pulmonary vein from the heart to lungs.	Cyanosis Tachypnea
Tricuspid atresia	No tricuspid valve with abnormal blood flow from the right atrium to right ventricle.	Cyanosis
Ebstein's anomaly	Malformed heart valve that improperly closes with blood leakage from lower to upper chambers.	Cyanosis Heart failure Arrhythmias Fatigue Edema
Single ventricle	Compromised blood flow to either the body or the lungs.	Cyanosis
Pulmonary atresia	No pulmonary valve with abnormal blood flow from the right ventricle into the pulmonary artery into the lungs.	Cyanosis Risk of infection Decreased energy Arrhythmias Edema Blood clots
Coarctation of the aorta (severe)	Left-to-right shunting from narrowing of the aorta with the potential for left-sided heart failure.	May have no symptoms present at birth. Can cause elevated blood pressure, heart failure, or heart damage.
	Acyanotic Cardiac Diseases	
Ventricular septal defect (VSD)	Abnormal opening between ventricles.	Harsh systolic murmur heard at lower left sternal border.

Atrial septal defect (ASD)	Left-to-right shunting of blood between an abnormal opening in the atria.
	    Pulmonic valve closes late.
	    Common in the foramen ovale site.
		May have a wide split S2.
		    Murmur heard in pulmonic area.

Continued

TABLE 11-1   Congenital Cardiac Defects—cont'd

	Acyanotic Cardiac Diseases	
Patent ductus arteriosus (PDA)	Ductus fails to close after birth.	Bounding pulses Wide pulse pressure Active PMI Machine-like murmur heard at fourth intercostal space.
Arteriovenous canal defect (AVC)	A large hole in the center of the heart affecting all four chambers where there is normally a division. Allows blood to mix and chambers and valves do not route blood properly.	Tachypnea, poor feeding and growth. Symptoms may occur weeks after birth.
Coarctation of aorta (mild–moderate)	Left-to-right shunting from narrowing of the aorta with the potential for left-sided heart failure.	Systolic murmur with an S3. Unequal, weak lower versus upper extremity pulses and blood pressure. Preductal oxygenation higher than post-ductal levels. Poor feeding and growth.

(Adapted from AMA, 2018; Ashwath & Snyder, 2015)

decreased levels of circulating oxygen. Heart failure or the inability to pump adequate circulating levels of blood is the most common symptom. Based on the levels of circulating oxygen, a newborn may exhibit varying levels of cyanosis, or blue skin discoloration, with both acyanotic and cyanotic cardiac defects.

Cyanotic cardiac defects can be caused by abnormalities within the heart valves, aorta, or blood vessels surrounding the newborn's heart. These defects cause a right-to-left shunting, resulting in low circulating oxygen levels and cyanosis secondary to the presence of one or more defects. A decrease in the oxygen saturation will cause cyanosis around lips, nose, and mouth of newborns (Ward & Hisley, 2016).

Cardiac failure, or congestive heart failure, is another potential cardiac complication in newborns diagnosed with congenital or acquired cardiac conditions. This occurs when the newborn's heart cannot perform adequately to move blood forward through circulation. The newborn's blood becomes "congested" in the opposite direction, with resultant loss of the cardiac pumping action required for adequate circulation. The subsequent problem of decreased circulation is peripheral edema secondary to excess fluid buildup in the lungs and liver (Ward & Hisley, 2016).

Newborns exposed to high levels of glucose or significant shifts in maternal glucose in utero are also at risk for cardiac failure and congenital cardiac disease secondary to the development of cardiac hypertrophy or cardiomegaly. Hypertrophy is an abnormal enlargement or thickening of the cardiac muscle, and cardiomegaly is considered to be an enlarged heart with secondary ineffective pumping and decreased circulation. At birth, the newborn may exhibit symptoms of cardiac failure and resulting neonatal distress as described in the Assessment section. These symptoms increase the potential for both newborn morbidity and mortality.

Early and frequent monitoring of fetal growth and cardiac function in utero, in addition to maintaining normal maternal glucose levels in pregnancy, is essential to reduce the risk of complications in newborns. The continuance of normal glucose levels may also reduce the potential for congenital cardiac disease, cardiomegaly, and cardiomyopathy in the newborn. Additional risk factors include a low newborn birth weight, maternal comorbidities, a family history of congenital cardiac disease, and the presence of a first-born child (Snell & Gardner, 2017).

CLINICAL PEARLS

It is important to recognize and treat congenital cardiac disease early in the life of a newborn.

Assessment

A complete assessment of the newborn's transition from intrauterine to extrauterine life is essential immediately after delivery and should take place in the delivery area. Symptoms of newborn distress related to congenital cardiac disease (shown in the accompanying Assessment boxes) should be observed for, noted, and treated as necessary. The newborn's signs and symptoms are considered to be serious based on the timing and continuation of them post-delivery. The symptoms are similar, but the key differences are related to the severity, persistence, and effects of the symptoms on the newborn.

The initial assessment of the newborn should include a full head-to-toe physical examination and gestational age assessment in addition to the measurement of Apgar scores (see Figure 11-2). Apgar assessments and scoring should occur at 1 and 5 minutes of life and up to 10 and 20 minutes if initial low scores are obtained. The newborn should continue to have ongoing support and surveillance of their physiological transition and adaptive behaviors of transitioning from intrauterine to extrauterine life. Every newborn assessment should include the parents, if appropriate, to initiate and provide ongoing education and support related to their newborn's transition process and continuing care (Snell & Gardner, 2017).

Assessment of Abnormal Newborn Transitioning Immediately After Delivery

Tachypnea: More than 60 breaths/minute. Can be an early symptom of newborn cardiac conditions.
Vital Signs: Unequal pulses, higher in the upper extremities and lower in the lower extremities.
Blood Pressure: A difference in blood pressures of 15–20 mm Hg is significant between upper and lower extremities.
Grunting: Forced expiration through a partially closed glottis, which increases transpulmonary pressure to increase gas and air exchange and attempts to stabilize alveoli opening by delaying expiration.
Retractions: Inward pulling of the chest wall on inspiration. Reported as substernal (below), suprasternal (above), intercostal (in-between), supracostal (above), or subcostal (below).
Nasal Flaring: An attempt on inspiration to increase the nares size and decrease the resistance of the airway.
Hypoxia: Lowered concentration of O_2 in circulation and tissues.
Skin Color Assessment:

  Pink: Occurring later than delivery.
  Pallor: Pale skin color with poor peripheral circulation may be associated with systemic hypotension.
  Central Cyanosis: Blue discoloration on the core of newborn's body.

(Adapted from Gardner, Enzman-Hines, & Nyp, 2016; Pramanik, Rangaswamy, & Gates, 2015)

Assessment Signs/Symptoms of Abnormal Newborn Transitioning After 1 Hour of Life Post-Delivery

- Persistent tachypnea, nasal flaring, grunting, and retractions lasting more than 1 hour of life, with bradycardia.
- Persistent lung rales with retractions, flaring, and grunting more than 1 hour of life.
- Persistent peripheral and central cyanosis with an O_2 saturation <90% and on room air (21% oxygen) and prolonged need for O_2 supplementation after 3 hours of life.
- Prolonged apnea >20 seconds with bradycardia <80 heart rate.
- Significant skin pallor or ruddiness.
- Low body temperature <97.7°F after 3 hours of life.
- Slow capillary refill >3 seconds.
- Unstable blood pressure continues.
- Abnormal neurological behavior, including lethargy, decrease in activity, hypotonia, irritability, tremors, and jitteriness.
- Increased oral secretions, drooling, choking, and coughing, with associated cyanosis.

(Adapted from Gardner & Hernandez, 2016; Hernandez & Thilo, 2005)

Apgar Score

Gestational age_____ weeks

Sign	0	1	2	1 minute	5 minute	10 minute	15 minute	20 minute
Color	Blue or pale	Acrocyanotic	Completely pink					
Heart rate	Absent	<100 minute	>100 minute					
Reflex irritability	No response	Grimace	Cry or active withdrawal					
Muscle tone	Limp	Some flexion	Active motion					
Respiration	Absent	Weak cry: hypoventilation	Good, crying					
			Total					

Comments:	Resuscitation					
	Minutes	1	5	10	15	20
	Oxygen					
	PPV/NCPAP					
	ETT					
	Chest compressions					
	Epinephrine					

FIGURE 11–2 Apgar scoring in the newborn

The Apgar score describes the condition of the newborn immediately after birth and, when applied, is a tool for an initial newborn assessment. The scoring measures appearance (skin color), pulse (heart rate), grimace response (reflexes), activity (muscle tone), and respirations (breathing rate and effort). Scoring range is between 0 and 10, with 10 the highest possible score. This measurement provides a mechanism to record the newborn's intrauterine-to-extrauterine transition and provides a scoring method to initiate immediate care as needed. The score can be affected by the newborn's gestational age, a high-risk pregnancy, any maternal medications, a cesarean section delivery, any complication during the delivery process, and cardiac and respiratory conditions (American College of Obstetricians and Gynecologists and the American Academy of Pediatrics, 2015).

The cardiac examination of a newborn should include a minimum of a 1-minute assessment of the heart rate and rhythm at the *point of maximal impulse* (PMI), which is located at the third intercostal space mid-clavicular line. The normal resting heart rate is between 120 and 160 beats per minute to a high of 180 per minute with the newborn crying. Auscultation of the chest should include the aortic, pulmonic, Erb's point, tricuspid, and mitral areas in addition to S1 and S2 heart sounds and S3 and S4 if warranted. Murmurs should be followed up with a referral to and a consultation with pediatric cardiologist prior to discharge from the hospital or birthing center (Snell & Gardner, 2017). Murmurs may be accompanied by shortness of breath or alterations in blood pressures and should be followed up with diagnostic testing (Ward & Hisley, 2016).

Prompt assessment and screening for congenital cardiac disease or congenital heart defects is essential to prevent newborn disability or death (see the accompanying Diagnostic Studies box). Newborn congenital cardiac screening with pulse oximetry may provide the information necessary to diagnose a newborn with cardiac defects before signs and symptoms are present and prior to discharge from the hospital or birthing center. This includes an assessment after 24 hours of life of the newborn's right hand (preductal reading or the portion of the aorta proximal to the ductus arteriosus opening) and right foot (post-ductal reading or the portion of the aorta distal to the opening of the ductus arteriosus opening). This congenital cardiac screening is considered to be normal if the oxygen saturations of the newborn's hand and foot are greater than 95% and a difference of no more than 3% oxygen saturation exists between the two right-sided newborn areas. A difference greater than 3% oxygen saturation between the two areas requires a prompt referral to a pediatric cardiologist for follow-up and additional diagnostic testing (Snell & Gardner, 2017).

Diagnostic Studies for Congenital Cardiac Defects and Disease Diagnosis in the Newborn

Chest Radiography: This is a noninvasive medical test and the most commonly performed x-ray. A chest x-ray yields an image of the heart, lungs, blood vessels, airways, and the bones of the chest and spine. Chest x-rays can also reveal fluid in or around lungs or air surrounding a lung.

Extremity Blood Pressures: Total blood pressure readings are determined by measuring the systolic and diastolic blood pressures. Systolic blood pressure measures the force the heart exerts on the walls of the arteries each time it beats. Diastolic blood pressure measures the force the heart exerts on the walls of arteries in between beats. Assessing all extremities provides additional information in diagnosing congenital cardiac disease.

Arterial Blood Gas Measurement: Hypoxemia or hypercapnia is determined by measuring the oxygen and carbon dioxide levels in a blood sample taken from an artery (arterial blood gas). Normal arterial oxygen is approximately 80 to 100 millimeters of mercury (mm Hg). Values below 60–80 mm Hg usually indicate the need for supplemental oxygen. Normal carbon dioxide levels are from 27–40 mm Hg, and levels lower or higher require interventions to maintain respirations.

Electrocardiogram: An EKG is a noninvasive, painless test that records the electrical signals or activity in the heart on paper or digitally. It is a common test used to detect heart problems and monitor the heart's status. Sensors or electrodes that can detect the electrical activity of the heart are attached to the chest and limbs to determine the heart rate, rhythm, or other pertinent information related to the heart's condition.

Echocardiogram: An echocardiogram uses high-frequency sound waves to produce images of the heart. This test allows for visualization of the heart's beating; the heart chambers, valves, and walls; and the blood vessels pumping blood.

Continued

Diagnostic Studies for Congenital Cardiac Defects and Disease Diagnosis in the Newborn—cont'd

Cardiac Catheterization and Angiography: This combined procedure is used to diagnose and treat cardiovascular conditions and cardiac functioning. The cardiac muscle, valves, and coronary arteries can be visualized to assess functioning and pressures within the heart. During cardiac catheterization, a long, thin tube called a *catheter* is inserted in an artery or vein in the groin, neck, or arm and threaded through the blood vessels to the heart. Additional diagnostic tests may be performed as part of a cardiac catheterization.

Cardiovascular Magnetic Resonance Imaging or Computed Tomography: An MRI or CT scan is used to diagnose and evaluate congenital heart defects. Either can be used to create images of and evaluate cardiac chambers, septal defects, and anomalous (abnormal) connections. They can also be used to diagnose defects related to blood flow through the cardiac valves, outflow tracts, and shunts.

(Mayo Clinic, 2018c)

HIGH YIELD FACT FOR TESTING

Assessment of central cyanosis in a newborn is considered to be a late symptom of a serious problem.

Additional diagnostic studies may be indicated to determine the cause of any cardiac decompensation signs and symptoms in the newborn. A referral to a pediatric cardiologist could include the tests outlined in the Diagnostic Studies box to measure cardiac functioning and the need for further testing and treatment.

 CLINICAL PEARLS

Prone positioning of the newborn onto a parent's chest enhances respirations and improves lung oxygenation, mechanics, and volume.

Nonpharmacological Management

A congenital heart defect may range from mild to severe, and the treatment is dependent on the type, effects, and severity of the defect. The initial and ongoing management of a newborn with congenital cardiac disease depends on the specific diagnosis and symptoms. Congenital heart disease may have no long-term effects and may self-correct as a pediatric patient ages or may go untreated. These diagnoses may only require an initial pediatric cardiology referral with ongoing future observation.

Nutrition. Breast or formula feeding can be used for newborns with cardiac diagnoses. A feeding schedule is best for these newborns with feeding supplementations as needed for weight gain. Newborns with cyanotic cardiac disease or related cardiac failure may require a slower weight gain schedule to provide for additional feeding times and smaller volumes. Fortification of both breast and formula may be necessary to provide additional calories in order to prevent the newborn from experiencing failure to thrive or insufficient weight gain or inappropriate weight loss.

Activity Restrictions. Specific newborn patients may require limitations on the amount and types of activities based on their diagnosis, but most are able to participate fully or near fully in activities throughout their lives.

Medical Care. Routine pediatrician or family physician follow-up is essential for newborns with congenital cardiac disease to assess for complications and the need for further evaluations by the pediatric cardiologist.

Infection Prevention. Prevention of infection is critical for newborns with congenital cardiac disease. This includes proper hygiene, avoidance of crowded areas, appropriate nutrition practices, frequent hand washing, and assessment of the option of daycare.

Pharmacology

The treatment for congenital cardiac defects is dependent on which area of the newborn's heart is affected and the severity of the cardiac defect. Medications to treat the effects of the newborn's defect are considered, based on the size and weight of the newborn and associated conditions and or complications related to the cardiac defect.

The gold standards of therapy for congenital cardiac defects include stabilization of the newborn, administration of oxygen as needed, and the administration of *prostaglandin therapy* (PgE2) to maintain the patency of the ductus arteriosus if required for the diagnosed cardiac defect.

Many congenital heart defects can be effectively treated with medications and other treatments that assist the heart to work more effectively. Table 11-2 outlines commonly used cardiac medications for both congenital cardiac disease and defects.

> **HIGH YIELD FACT FOR TESTING**
>
> Stabilization of newborns with diagnosed congenital cardiac disease may involve the administration of PgE2.

Surgical Management

There are certain heart defects that are considered to be serious, even life threatening. These defects require a rapid diagnosis and immediate treatment. Alternative treatments for congenital heart defects may involve a surgical procedure immediately after birth or later when the newborn has gained weight, has been feeding well, and is further stabilized to tolerate the procedures. Surgical repair may be a palliative repair or a complete repair of an anatomical deformity. The palliative surgeries are performed when the newborn is young and may not be able to tolerate the complex procedures. Complete cardiac surgical repairs are performed as a remedy or definitive complete treatment for a diagnosed cardiac anomaly (Ward & Hisley, 2016). Surgical management of a newborn born with congenital cardiac disease or defects may include the following procedures:

Cardiac Catheterization Repair. An invasive cardiac catheterization can be performed to determine pressures within the cardiac vessels and to provide a radiological view of the cardiac anatomy. The cardiac catheterization procedure can be used to obtain a cardiac biopsy, or a defect may be repaired utilizing heart catheterization techniques to restore openings or narrowed areas within the heart. The risks related to these procedures are kept to a minimum but may include bleeding, infection, thrombus formation, arrhythmias, cardiac perforation, stroke, or, rarely, death of the patient.

Closure Devices. Congenital abnormal cardiac communications or shunts can be repaired in the cardiac catheterization laboratory. Examples of defects that can be repaired with this method include atrial septal defects, patent foramen ovale, and patent ductus arteriosus.

Opening Devices. Abnormal narrowed areas within the heart, including vessels or valves, can be opened, dilated, or have a stent placed in the narrowed area during a cardiac catheterization procedure.

Angiography. This procedure allows for visualization of the valves, blood vessels, ventricles, and septal defects. A catheter is placed in the heart and a contrast dye is injected to highlight any abnormalities present.

TABLE 11–2   Medications Used to Treat Congenital Heart Defects

Class	Examples	Action	Dosage	SENC
Sodium channel blockers (class 1A)	Procainamide Disopyramide phosphate	Myocardial depressant that decreases myocardial excitability and conduction.	Supraventricular tachycardia and ventricular tachycardia, 15 mg/kg/min. 10–30 mg/kg/day in divided doses every 6 hr.	Fatigue, fever, arrhythmias, diarrhea, nausea, vomiting, excess salivation, rash, decreased hemoglobin, hematocrit, and platelets.
Sodium channel blockers (class 1B)	Lidocaine Mexiletine	Restores normal heart rhythms by stabilizing the neuronal membrane by inhibiting the neuronal fluxes required for impulse conduction. Inhibits the inward sodium current and reduces the action potential.	Ventricular fibrillation and ventricular tachycardia, 1 mg/kg once followed by 20 to 50 mcg/kg/min. 1.4–5.1 mg/kg/dose every 8 hr. May increase to 8 mg/kg/dose in infants.	Bradycardia, hypotension, cardiac arrest, arrhythmias, tachycardia, ventricular fibrillation. Nausea, vomiting, rash, dry mouth, diarrhea, constipation, tingling, and tremors.
Sodium channel blockers (class 1C)	Propafenone Flecainide	Antiarrhythmic action is to stabilize the myocardial membrane action to decrease SVT, and ventricular arrhythmias. Slow nerve impulses to the heart to decrease supraventricular tachycardia (SVT), ventricular arrhythmias, atrial flutter, and fibrillation arrhythmias.	Use and dose determined by medical provider. 1 mg/kg/dose every 8–12 hr to 2 mg/kg/day every 12 hr.	Nausea, vomiting, constipation, weakness, dyspnea, bradycardia, diarrhea. Bradycardia, dizziness, fainting, edema, weight gain, and tachycardia.
Angiotensin-converting enzyme (ACE) inhibitors	Captopril Enalapril	Assist in relaxing blood vessels and prevent the body from producing angiotensin II, which constricts blood vessels	2.5–6 mg/kg/day PO divided every 6–12 hr; start 0.15–0.3 mg/kg/dose; maximum 6 mg/kg/day. Test dose: 0.01–0.05 mg/kg/dose, Monitor blood pressure carefully for 1–2 hr; if tolerated, give 0.01–0.05 mg/kg 2–3 times daily, increased as necessary to maximum 2 mg/kg daily in divided doses.	Monitor for dry cough, hyperkalemia, fatigue, dizziness, headache, angioedema, teratogenicity, and loss of taste. Feeding problems may result from changes in taste.

Class II antiarrhythmics: Beta-adrenergic blocking agents	Propranolol Atenolol	Reduce blood pressure, heart rate and force of cardiac contraction by blocking epinephrine and for SVT prophylaxis.	Arrhythmias: 0.5–1 mg/kg/day in divided doses every 6–8 hr; titrate dosage upward every 3–5 days; usual dose: 2–4 mg/kg/day; higher doses may be needed; do not exceed 16 kg/day. Hypertension: 0.5–1 mg/kg/day in divided doses every 6–12 hr; increase gradually every 5–7 days. 0.3–1.3 mg/kg daily.	Fatigue, weight gain, cool extremities, shortness of breath, increased triglycerides, hypoglycemia, and difficulty sleeping. A regular sleep/wake schedule may help the newborn to achieve adequate sleep. Do not abruptly discontinue this medication.
Class III antiarrhythmics: Prolong repolarization	Amiodarone	Suppress or prevent abnormal cardiac arrhythmias by slowing nerve impulses in the heart.	Loading dose of 25 mcg/kg/min for 4 hr, then 5–15 mcg/kg/min not to exceed 1,200 mcg/24 hr.	Prolong QT interval, edema, tachycardia, bradycardia, angina, rash.
Class IV antiarrhythmics: Calcium channel blockers	Verapamil Diltiazem	Block calcium from entering cardiac cells to lower blood pressure.	0.1–0.3 mg/kg, not to exceed 5 mg over 2 min with a second dose not to exceed 10 mg after 30 min. Then maintenance of 4–8 mg/kg/day. 1.5–2.0 mg/kg/day divided tid-qid Maximum 3.5 mg/kg/day.	Constipation, headache, dizziness, edema, flushing, nausea, and dizziness.
Angiotensin II receptor blockers (ARBs)	Losartan	Treat elevated blood pressure and heart failure by blocking angiotensin II and causing blood vessel dilation.	0.7–1.4 mg/kg PO every day; Start: 0.7 mg/kg PO qd up to 50 mg/day; Maximum 1.4 mg/kg/day up to 100 mg/day.	Dizziness, hyperkalemia, angioedema, GI upset, teratogenicity. The risk of cancer as an adult can be addressed with genetic testing.
Diuretics	Thiazide: Chlorothiazide Hydrochlorothiazide Loop: Furosemide Potassium sparing: Spironolactone	Reduce blood pressure and edema by assisting to excrete sodium and fluid. Thiazide Loop Potassium sparing	c-20–40 mg/kg/day divided bid. h-2–3.3 mg/kg/dose bid. f-1–4mg/kg/dose, 1–2 × per day. s-1.5–3.5 mg/kg/day divided q 6–24 hr.	Hyponatremia, dehydration, muscle cramps, hyperbilirubinemia, ototoxicity. Teach parents to monitor number of wet diapers daily for normal fluid status. Monitor renal function, blood pressure, and electrolytes.

Continued

TABLE 11–2 Medications Used to Treat Congenital Heart Defects—cont'd

Class	Examples	Action	Dosage	SENC
Prostaglandins		Administered to maintain the patency of the ductus arteriosus until surgical ligation is performed.	Initial dose: 0.05–0.1 mcg/kg/min continuous infusions. May advance to 0.2 mcg/kg/min.	Apnea, fever, flushing, hypotension, hypoglycemia.
Cardiac glycoside Class IV antiarrhythmics: Endogenous Nucleoside/antiarrhythmic	Digoxin Adenosine	Reduce heart rate, increases force of cardiac contraction, prolongs refractory period of atrioventricular (AV) node and decreases conduction through the sinoatrial (SA) and AV nodes. Conversion of abnormal cardiac rhythms to normal sinus rhythm by impairing conduction through the AV node.	20–30 mcg/kg given as 50% of the dose initially and 25% of the dose in each of 2 subsequent doses every 6–12 hours daily. 0.05 mg/kg and increased in increments of 0.05 mg/kg every 1–2 min to a maximum of 0.25 mg/kg.	Bradycardia, arrhythmias, edema, pulmonary rales and crackles, altered electrolyte levels, vomiting. Atrial fibrillation or flutter, bradycardia, dyspnea, flushing, chest pain, and apnea.

(Adapted From Mayo Clinic, 2018a; Vallerand & Sanoski, 2019; Ward & Hisley, 2016)

Myocardial Biopsy. A biopsy is performed in the heart catheterization laboratory to assess for causes of myocardial issues and the potential for rejection in pediatric patients who have received a cardiac transplant.

Minimally Invasive Cardiac Surgery (Closed Heart Surgery). This surgical procedure involves a small incision between the ribs with the insertion of instruments through the small incision to repair any cardiac defects present.

Open-Heart Surgery. An open-heart surgical repair requires the chest to be opened to repair the defect and often the patient is placed on heart-lung bypass during the procedure. The use of heart-lung bypass provides the opportunity to repair the cardiac muscle, valves, or blood vessels.

Cardiac Transplant. If surgical repair is not an option, then a heart transplant may be warranted. This procedure is reserved for life-threatening cardiac diagnoses. A progressive cardiac transplant program may be implemented to attempt to correct cardiac conditions, but a transplant is often necessary in the child's future (Ward & Hisley, 2016).

The decision by the cardiologist or cardiothoracic surgeon to diagnose and repair a cardiac defect takes into consideration multiple variables related to the newborn. These can include the gestational age and weight, nutritional status, associated comorbidities, and signs and symptoms. Depending on the cardiac defect diagnosis and the procedure used to repair the defect, patients may also require additional infection prevention support. A congenital cardiac defect or repair can increase the risk for future infections, particularly in defects that were repaired with a prosthetic material or device. These infections can typically affect the heart valves or lining and can be prevented by the prophylactic administration of antibiotics prior to any future surgical procedures (Mayo Clinic, 2018a).

Nurses can support the newborn and family by reinforcing information presented by the cardiologist and surgeon during both the pre- and postoperative periods. The inclusion of assessments, support of positive outcomes, timely patient interventions, and evaluation of ongoing care are essential for the nurse providing care to a patient with a cardiac defect. The care for post–cardiac surgery patients is complex and requires a collaborative team effort to ensure a progressive recovery. The postoperative care involves the concepts of assessment, nutrition, hygiene, a gradual increase in activities, and physiological and psychosocial care (Ward & Hisley, 2016).

All parents of newborns diagnosed with a congenital cardiac defect who are discharged from the hospital should be provided with extensive discharge instructions. These should include information related to medications; vital sign assessments to include respirations, heart rate, blood pressure, and temperature; follow-up appointments; future diagnostic testing and procedures; short- and long-term care; anticipated and unanticipated complications; and contact information for all questions and concerns (Ward & Hisley, 2016).

Complementary Therapies: Long-Term Management

Pediatric patients with congenital cardiac defects may require multiple procedures and surgeries throughout their lives based on their initial cardiac diagnosis. The continuing interventions will require ongoing medical and surgical care for this unique population. In addition, monitoring of the patient's physical tolerance and adaptation to the symptoms of the cardiac diagnosis will be necessary.

Throughout these patients' childhood years, a pediatrician in collaboration with a pediatric cardiologist will monitor their progress and developmental milestones, with an eventual transfer of care to an adult physician and adult cardiologist occurring around 18 years of age.

The physical and emotional development of a patient with a cardiac defect can be affected secondary to the extended recoveries from either initial or ongoing medical or surgical procedures. These treatment regimens and associated restrictions may cause a lag in physical and emotional development and cause a noticeable delay when compared to other children their size and age. These complications can last through the school years and may affect their ongoing ability to read, write, and learn effectively.

Emotional challenges associated with developmental complications are often evident in patients with a history of a congenital cardiac defect and may affect their ability to effectively cope, feel secure about their abilities, and assimilate into school and social and peer groups. Support groups are often recommended for these children, their siblings, and their families so they may meet and interact with other families with the same types of issues, medical and surgical histories, medication regimens, and diagnoses. The groups are very effective in creating relationships that provide both emotional support and ongoing supportive relationships (Mayo Clinic, 2018a).

Summary

The current care of newborns with congenital cardiac defects is focused on providing the least invasive, most effective medical and surgical treatments based on the patient's diagnosis. Early maternal obstetrical care and diagnosis of fetal cardiac disease provides the newborn with the best chance for survival and ongoing optimal care. Each newborn should be monitored during the prenatal, intrapartum, and postpartum periods to ensure early intervention and essential treatment is initiated when necessary.

The implementation of congenital cardiac screening as a requirement for all newborns has provided information for earlier referrals to a pediatric cardiologist. Cardiac defects are not always diagnosed prenatally or at birth. Approximately 18 of every 10,000 newborns are diagnosed with a congenital cardiac defect. The American Academy of Pediatrics (2018) recommends that all newborns be universally screened for congenital cardiac disease, and the screening should be added to the uniform newborn screening panel.

Key Points

- All newborns should be assessed for congenital cardiac disease in the delivery area, again prior to discharge from the hospital, and at the first and ongoing outpatient or home visits.

- Maternal and newborn risk factors for congenital cardiac disease should be identified.

- Diagnostic testing for congenital cardiac disease includes congenital heart screening, EKG, echocardiogram, chest x-ray, arterial blood gas tests (ABGs), and blood pressure assessment.

- Parents should be provided with discharge instructions related to the diagnosis of congenital cardiac disease and treatments.

- Newborns with a diagnosis of congenital cardiac disease will require lifelong evaluations by a cardiologist.

- There is a potential for developmental delays in a child diagnosed with a congenital cardiac defect.

- Infection prevention is necessary for a patient with a congenital heart defect.

Review Questions

1. **Which of the following defects are associated with tetralogy of fallot?**

   a. Aorta exits from the right ventricle, pulmonary artery exits from the left ventricle, and two noncommunicating circulations present.

   b. Ventricular septal defect, overriding aorta, pulmonic stenosis, and muscle surrounding the lower right chamber becomes overly thickened.

   c. Coarctation of aorta, aortic and mitral valve stenosis, and patent ductus stenosis.

   d. Tricuspid valve atresia, atrial and ventricular septal defect, and hypoplastic right ventricle.

2. **When creating a teaching plan for the parents of a newborn diagnosed with pulmonary atresia, the nurse should include a description of the diagnosis which is:**

   a. A single vessel arising from both ventricles.

   b. Obstruction of blood flow from the left ventricle to the pulmonary artery.

   c. Abnormal blood flow from the right ventricle into the pulmonary artery into the lungs.

   d. Return of blood to the heart without entering the right atrium.

3. **A newborn is to undergo a surgical repair for a *ventricular septal defect* (VSD). Performing the procedure may prevent which of the following?**

   a. Ventricular arrhythmias   c. Respiratory acidosis

   b. Failure to thrive   c. Complete heart block

4. **A newborn diagnosed with coarctation of the aorta may exhibit which of the following symptoms?**

   a. Difficulty feeding   c. Ruddy skin color

   b. Hyperglycemia   d. Hypotonia

5. **The ductus arteriosus is a fetal structure that functions to guide:**

   a. Blood from the pulmonary artery to the descending aorta.

   b. Intra-arterial blood flow from right to left in the fetus.

   c. Unoxygenated blood from the umbilical vein to the fetus's inferior vena cava.

   d. Cardiac output from the aorta to the right ventricle.

See the appendix for answers to review questions.

References

American Academy of Pediatrics. (2018). Program to enhance the health & development of infants and children (PEHDIC). Retrieved from https://www.aap.org/en-us/advocacy-and-policy/aap-health-initiatives/PEHDIC/Pages/Newborn-Screening-for-CCHD.aspx

American College of Obstetricians and Gynecologists and the American Academy of Pediatrics. (2015). The Apgar score. Committee Opinion No. 644. *Obstetrics & Gynecology, 126*(4), e52–e55.

American Heart Association. (2018). About congenital heart defects. Retrieved from http://www.heart.org/en/health-topics/congenital-heart-defects/about-congenital-heart-defects

Ashwath, R., & Snyder, C. S. (2015). Congenital defects of the cardiovascular system. In R. J. Martin, A. A. Fanaroff, & M. C. Walsh (Eds.), *Neonatal-perinatal medicine* (10th ed., pp. 1230–1249). St. Louis, MO: Mosby-Year Book.

Fraser, D. (2014). Newborn adaptation to extrauterine life. In K. R. Simpson & P. A. Creehan (Eds.), *Perinatal nursing* (4th ed., pp. 581–596). Philadelphia, PA: Wolters Kluwer.

Gardner, S. L., Enzman-Hines, M., & Nyp, M. (2016). Respiratory diseases. In S. L. Gardner, B. S. Carter, M. Enzman-Hines, & J. A. Hernandez (Eds.), *Merenstein and Gardner's handbook of neonatal intensive care* (8th ed., pp. 565–643). St. Louis, MO: Elsevier-Mosby.

Gardner, S. L., & Hernandez, J. A. (2016). Initial nursery care. In S. L. Gardner, B. S. Carter, M. Enzman-Hines, & J. A. Hernandez (Eds.), *Merenstein and Gardner's handbook of neonatal intensive care* (8th ed., p. 84). St. Louis, MO: Elsevier-Mosby.

Hernandez, J. A., & Thilo, E. (2005). Routine care of the full-term newborn. In L. C. Osborn, T. G. Dewitt, L. R. First, & J. Zenel (Eds.), *Pediatrics*. St. Louis, MO: Elsevier-Mosby.

Mayo Clinic. (2018a). Congenital heart defects in children. Retrieved from https://www.mayoclinic.org /diseases-conditions/congenital-heart-defects-children/diagnosis-treatment/drc-20350080

Mayo Clinic. (2018b). Medications. Retrieved from https://www.mayoclinic.org/diseases-conditions /high-blood-pressure/in-depth/ace-inhibitors/art-20047480

Mayo Clinic. (2018c). Tests and procedures. Retrieved from https://www.mayoclinic.org/tests-procedures

Pramanik, A. K., Rangaswamy, N., & Gates, T. (2015). Neonatal respiratory distress: A practical approach to its diagnosis and management. *Pediatric Clinics of North America, 62*(2), 453–469. doi:10.1016 /j.pcl.2014.11.008

Snell, B. J., & Gardner, S. L. (2017). *Care of the well newborn*. Burlington, MA: Jones & Bartlett Learning.

Vallerand, A. H., & Sanoski, C. A. (2019). *Davis's drug guide for nurses* (16th ed.). Philadelphia, PA: F.A. Davis.

Ward, S. L., & Hisley, S. M. (2016). *Maternal-child nursing care with women's health companion: Optimizing outcomes for mothers, children, and families* (2nd ed.). Philadelphia, PA. F.A. Davis.

Chapter 12

Respiratory Conditions

LEARNING OBJECTIVES

Upon completion of this chapter the student will be able to:

- Integrate knowledge of the physiology, pathophysiology, assessment, and nonpharmacological and pharmacological management of respiratory conditions.

- Incorporate the current standards of care for newborn patients with respiratory conditions.

Introduction

The newborn's adaptation to extrauterine life is a complex process requiring all systems to function normally throughout the birth and transitional progression. During these initial hours and days after delivery, all newborns and their families need substantial emotional, physical, and spiritual care provided to them as a foundation for the rest of their lives.

A small proportion (10%) of newborns require additional assistance to transition from intrauterine life and initiate and maintain independent respiratory efforts at birth. This assistance is often required for only a short duration, with the majority of newborns quickly maintaining self-regulating respiratory efforts. A diagnosis of respiratory distress is one of the complications that can be realized in the very early period following delivery. Respiratory complications in newborns can be a significant cause of mortality and morbidity if not quickly recognized or treated. Each delivery must have a minimum of two attendants capable of performing the initial neonatal resuscitation efforts and one attendant capable of delivering advanced care related to intubation and vascular access per newborn as required (Snell & Gardner, 2017).

The American Academy of Pediatrics (Warren & Phillipi, 2012) sets the standards for neonatal care, and these standards require providers to be available to care for newborns both during and after the birth. Newborns are to be cared for and observed until they have successfully completed their post-delivery transition. All providers who attend deliveries must be competent to distinguish normal transition and any deviations from the normal transition of newborns. This assessment includes the evaluation and recording of the newborn's general condition, respiratory and cardiac functioning, color, muscle tone, and vital signs.

Certain newborns may require resuscitation and should be identified prior to delivery. The risk factors are recognized based on the perinatal history and status of both the mother and fetus during the labor process. Upon delivery, the initial assessment is made based on the newborn's gestational age, muscle tone, and the presence of unassisted breathing and or crying. The reasonable window to assess and make a newborn resuscitation determination is the first minute of life, also known as the "Golden Minute" of a newborn's life (Snell & Gardner, 2017).

A newborn's progress after delivery is closely related to both the fetal and maternal history during pregnancy and delivery. A full assessment of the maternal records can provide information and planning for the prevention of unfavorable birth outcomes. Genetic and family histories are also important aspects of medical record evaluations and can provide information related to potential newborn complications post-delivery (Snell & Gardner, 2017).

Physiology

Normal physiological transitioning at birth requires the advancement of the newborn from the birth process through successful transitioning to extrauterine life. The significant physiological change for the exchange of gases is the transfer from the placenta in utero to the newborn's lungs immediately upon delivery. The fluid-filled lungs quickly transition to air-filled with each of the newborn's breaths. The ventilation of the newborn's lungs decreases the pulmonary vascular resistance with an increase in pulmonary blood flow. As described in Chapter 11, the increase in pulmonary flow subsequently increases left atrium pressures and volume with a closure of the foramen ovale and ductus venosa. The functional closure of the other fetal shunt, the ductus arteriosus, occurs within a few weeks after birth (Snell & Gardner, 2017).

The transitional period for the newborn involves three stages: the first stage from 0 to 30 minutes (first period of reactivity), the second stage from 30 minutes to 2 hours (period of decreased responsiveness), and the third period from 2 to 8 hours (second period of reactivity). These predictable stages cover the first 8 hours of life and the changes in vital signs, including respiratory rates and breath sounds, motor activity, color, bowel sounds, and responsiveness of the newborn (Snell & Gardner, 2017).

The basic physiological functioning of the newborn's respiratory tract is the process of air exchange from the upper to lower airways. The respiratory system also protects the lungs from foreign substances and is responsible for warming, filtering, and humidifying any oxygen entering the lungs. The lower respiratory tract is involved in the air exchange process of oxygenating the newborn's blood and eliminating carbon dioxide at the alveolar level (Capriotti, 2020).

The normal respiratory system of a newborn undergoes significant changes at birth as it begins the adaptation process for extrauterine life. In utero, the mother's placenta functions to support oxygen and carbon dioxide exchanges through the blood in the placenta. At the moment of delivery, the newborn's collapsed lungs are filled with amniotic fluid. The first breath of the newborn occurs quickly as the central nervous system reacts to the new external environment and rapid ambient temperature change. The initial respiratory efforts of the newborn activate significant physiological changes within both the respiratory and circulatory systems, including the following:

- Circulatory resistance to the lungs decreases, with a subsequent increase in oxygenation levels.
- Blood vessel resistance increases.
- Amniotic fluid is absorbed by the body or drains from the respiratory system.
- Inflation of the lungs occurs with independent respiratory movement of breathing oxygen inward to the bloodstream (inhalation) and removal of carbon dioxide by breathing outward (exhalation) (Capriotti, 2020).

An important element of the lung development of a fetus is the production of pulmonary surfactant. This substance, made by type II alveolar cells, is considered to be a surface-active lipoprotein complex (phospholipoprotein). This protein consists of both phospholipids and proteins, which contain both hydrophilic and hydrophobic regions for alveoli support. The fetus begins to produce quantities of surfactant at approximately 35 weeks of gestational development. This early production helps to support the respiratory functioning of newborns that are born early, between 35 to 40 weeks of gestation. Surfactant is responsible for lowering the airway surface tension in the alveoli and is released directly into the lung tissues for this purpose. This action supports the initial lung alveoli expansion and maintenance of expansion through respirations. The reduction in surface tension increases lung compliance, which allows for adequate lung inflation and a reduction in the workload of the newborn's breathing (Capriotti, 2020). Newborns born before 35 weeks of gestation do not have sufficient levels of pulmonary surfactant. These newborns may not be able to support their respiratory function independently and may present at delivery with respiratory difficulty to respiratory distress (Capriotti, 2020).

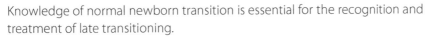

CLINICAL PEARLS
Knowledge of normal newborn transition is essential for the recognition and treatment of late transitioning.

Pathophysiology

The etiology of newborn respiratory distress is variable, but the end result is impairment in the oxygenation to the newborn's vital organs due to inadequate ventilation. This impairment in oxygenation can cause retention and elevations of carbon dioxide and decreased oxygen levels. Carbon dioxide increases can lead to a state of acidosis due to alterations in the delicate acid–base balance of a newborn. Respiratory distress may be a single diagnosis, or it may be associated with a multitude of other contributing medical disorders. These conditions can range from structural to functional to acquired problems within the pulmonary system. Acquired problems may be related to an injury that developed in the newborn while in utero or during or after the process of delivery (Snell & Gardner, 2017).

During the process of fetal development, the newborn may experience malformations of the bronchopulmonary system or congenital pulmonary abnormalities. These may result in a life-threatening pulmonary diagnosis for the newborn. A diagnosis of upper airway complications can also affect newborn transitioning and optimal airway functioning. A diagnosis of choanal atresia or nasal occlusion; obstructions in the glottis, larynx, or thorax; weakness in the trachea or larynx; or abnormally underdeveloped lung tissue may also occur. Any newborn who requires support for respirations is at risk for the development of a chronic lung disease diagnosis. This may occur due to the required treatment and resulting alterations that occur in lung tissue. This can cause long-term pulmonary fibrosis with secondary atelectasis and hyperinflation within the newborn's pulmonary system (Snell & Gardner, 2017).

The immediate and ongoing care of a newborn requires the provider to have knowledge about the mother's health and medication history, the course of the pregnancy and any related complications, the labor and birth process, any required resuscitation methods, the postpartum period, and any risks or concerns related to the mother's and fetus's course of treatment. Table 12-1 provides some of the potential factors that can affect the newborn's birth and transition from intrauterine to extrauterine life.

Knowledge about normal versus abnormal newborn transitioning is essential for health-care providers involved in the care of mothers and newborns in the delivery process. Early recognition of complications or the need for interventions during the birth or delivery process will provide the newborn with the resources necessary

TABLE 12–1   Maternal, Obstetric and Neonatal Factors That Increase Abnormal Newborn Transitioning

Maternal factors	Chronic hypertension Pregnancy-induced hypertension Diabetes mellitus Gestational diabetes Renal disease Infectious process Tobacco, alcohol, or illegal substance abuse Collagen vascular diseases Hemoglobinopathies Maternal medications
Obstetric factors	Rh or other isoimmunization Intrauterine growth restriction Decrease in fetal movement Multiples Oligohydramnios Polyhydramnios Vaginal bleeding during third trimester Cesarean delivery
Neonatal factors	<37 weeks' gestation: prematurity >42 weeks' gestation: post-maturity Small for gestational age Large for gestational age Infectious process Abnormalities with metabolism Birth-related trauma Fetal malformations Anemia Needed resuscitation at delivery Apgar score of 0–4 at 1 minute of life

(Adapted from Hernandez & Thilo, 2005; Snell & Gardner, 2017)

for successful transition. For example, newborns born before 35 weeks' gestation, with insufficient levels of pulmonary surfactant, normally require supplementary respiratory support to include both oxygen delivery and monitoring upon delivery. In addition, the administration of artificial surfactant for the promotion of complete lung expansion is often required. This support may be necessary in the first hours to months of life, depending on the severity and gestational age of the newborn. The assessment of a newborn continues throughout the postpartum period with careful attention paid to the newborn's ability to maintain normal ventilation and vital signs. Any alteration in these measurements should be investigated further to prevent irreversible complications in the newborn.

HIGH YIELD FACT FOR TESTING

Stabilization of preterm newborns may require the installation of intratracheal surfactant therapy.

Assessment

A complete assessment of the newborn's transition to extrauterine life is essential immediately after the newborn is born in the delivery area. This initial assessment should include vital sign measurement in conjunction with a full head-to-toe physical examination and assessment of the newborn's definite gestational age. As shown in Chapter 11, the measurement of Apgar scores at 1 and 5 minutes of life and up to 20 minutes (if applicable) is also essential to determine the ability of the newborn to transition from intrauterine to extrauterine life. The newborn should continue to have ongoing support as needed and surveillance of their physiological transition and adaptive behaviors of transitioning. Each newborn assessment should include the parents if appropriate in order to provide ongoing support and education related to the transition, management, and care of their newborn (Snell & Gardner, 2017).

An assessment of the newborn's respiratory system includes an evaluation of chest symmetry and movement and a determination of the respiratory rate and depth and effort with breathing. Respiratory patterns and any use of accessory muscles should be noted. Lung auscultation is conducted both anteriorly and posteriorly. Patterns of irregular breathing may be accompanied by short periods of apnea for up to 20 seconds in the newborn. This is considered a normal variation and should be communicated to the parents. Ongoing education should also be provided to parents related to the recognition of respiratory distress upon discharge. The accompanying box defines the specific clinical indicators that may be assessed in a newborn who is experiencing any degree of respiratory difficulty or distress during the transition process, while under hospitalization, and after discharge. These symptoms are indicative of potential complications and warrant close observation of the newborn and appropriate management and treatment as needed.

Table 12-2 describes the etiology, incidence, signs and symptoms, mortality, and management for the most common causes of respiratory distress in the newborn. These diagnoses are considered to be the characteristic diagnoses experienced by delivery unit personnel related to newborn transitioning and should be anticipated and prepared for in any newborn delivery and setting.

The observation of abnormal respirations and associated symptoms in any newborn warrants further exploration, assessment, and diagnostic testing to guide their treatment. Diagnostic studies can provide a baseline for the newborn and stipulate guidelines to determine the extent of a newborn's distress and the potential for worsening

---

Assessment Symptoms of Abnormal Newborn Transitioning After Delivery

- Persistent tachypnea, nasal flaring, grunting, and retractions lasting over 60 minutes of life with bradycardia.
- Hypoxemia/hypoxia by pulse oximetry or arterial blood gas.
- Persistent lung rales with retractions, flaring, and grunting over 60 minutes of life.
- Persistent cyanosis with an O_2 saturation <90 and on room air and prolonged O_2 supplementation after 3 hours of life.
- Central cyanosis of skin, nails, and mucous membranes (a late sign of distress).
- Prolonged apnea >20 seconds with bradycardia <80 beats per minute heart rate.
- Significant skin pallor or ruddiness.
- Low temperature <97.7°F after 3 hours of life.
- Slow capillary refill >3 seconds.
- Unstable blood pressure.
- Abnormal neurological behavior: lethargy, decrease in activity, hypotonia, irritable, tremors, and jitteriness.
- Increased oral secretions, drooling, choking, or coughing with associated cyanosis.

(Adapted from Gardner & Hernandez, 2016; Hernandez & Thilo, 2005)

TABLE 12–2   Causes of Respiratory Distress in the Newborn

Diagnosis	Etiology	Incidence	Symptoms	Mortality Rate	Management
Transient tachypnea of the newborn (TTN)	Presence of lung fluid not cleared by normal mechanisms (absence of labor, cesarean section, or deficient sodium transport at the cellular level; Snell & Gardner, 2017).	0.3%–0.5% of term and late-preterm infants with onset at birth.	Tachypnea present and lasting 12–72 hours until lung fluid is absorbed.	Low	NPO. Oxygen, warmth, IV fluids for hydration and calories until tachypnea has resolved and newborn able to take PO feeding.
Meconium aspiration syndrome (MAS)	Meconium aspiration that causes inflammation and obstruction, which interferes with surfactant action (Pramanik, Rangaswamy, & Gates, 2015).	2%–10% of term and post-term newborns exposed to MSAF, 5%–30% of these births occur with MSAF present (Snell & Gardner, 2017).	Symptoms progressing from inflammation to poor oxygenation & ventilation with tachypnea, grunting, flaring, retractions, hypoxia, acidosis. Risk for pneumothorax and PPHN.	Up to 40%.	Oxygen, CPAP to improve oxygen levels. Ventilator for continued acidosis, hypoxia; may require surfactant, ECMO, and iNO therapy (Edwards et al., 2013; Pramanik et al., 2015).
Respiratory distress syndrome (RDS)	Inadequate surfactant, which acts to lower alveoli surface tension and prevent alveoli collapse upon expiration. Maintains FRC.	Related to newborn's gestational age, <28 weeks: 60%, <34 weeks: 5% and can occur in <39 weeks— late and <37 weeks— preterm newborns.	Tachypnea, grunting, nasal flaring, hypoxia, acidosis, and hypercarbia at delivery.	10%	Oxygen by hood, nasal cannula, CPAP or ventilation, warm environment, and surfactant therapy.
Persistent pulmonary hypertension in the newborn (PPHN)	Pulmonary vasculature fails to relax after newborn's initial breaths at delivery. Hypoxia occurs causing pulmonary constriction with subsequent >PVR and <SVR.	1:500–1:1500 deliveries. Can affect term and post-term newborns. Caused by both pulmonary and nonpulmonary disorders.	Tachypnea, grunting, nasal flaring, retracting, hypoxia, acidosis, and hypercarbia. Acidosis and hypoxia are persistent and life threatening.	High. Reversible if identified and treatment is initiated early.	Oxygen, CPAP to improve oxygen levels. Ventilator for continued acidosis, hypoxia, may require surfactant, ECMO, and iNO therapy (Snell & Gardner, 2017).

(Gardner, Enzman-Hines, & Nyp, 2016; Smith & Carley, 2014)

CPAP, continuous positive airway pressure; ECMO, extracorporeal membrane oxygenation; FRC, functional residual capacity; iNO, inhaled nitric oxide; MSAF, meconium-stained amniotic fluid; PVR, peripheral vascular resistance; SVR, systemic vascular resistance.

symptoms. The following diagnostic studies are the most commonly utilized methods to analyze the newborn's condition (Ward & Hisley, 2016):

Arterial Blood Gas Measurement. Hypoxemia is determined by measuring the oxygen level in a blood sample taken from an artery (*arterial blood gas*, ABG). Normal arterial oxygen is approximately 75 to 100 millimeters of mercury (mm Hg). Values under 60 mm Hg usually indicate the need for supplemental oxygen. Carbon dioxide levels and acid–base balance are measured.

Cardiac Ultrasonography. This imaging is used to rule out any cardiac anomalies and visualize right-to-left shunting.

Chest Radiography. Chest x-rays produce images of the heart, lungs, blood vessels, airways, and the bones of the chest and spine. Chest x-rays can also reveal fluid in or around lungs or air surrounding the lungs.

Oxygen Saturation. This test assesses the level of oxygen in the capillaries. This is the best method to ensure adequate oxygenation with oxygen usage.

HIGH YIELD FACT FOR TESTING

Assessment of central cyanosis in a newborn is considered a late symptom.

Serum Blood Tests. Blood glucose levels, complete blood count, and electrolytes are measured to assess for any abnormalities specifically, hypoglycemia, hyperglycemia, hypomagnesemia, and hypocalcemia.

CLINICAL PEARLS

All delivery unit personnel must receive adequate education and training to resuscitate any newborn experiencing respiratory distress.

Nonpharmacological Management

Nonpharmacological management of newborns diagnosed with respiratory distress and conditions may include some or all of the following to reduce the pulmonary workload and the potential for long-term complications for the newborn:

- Warm, humidified oxygen delivery by nasal cannula, mask, oxygen hood, or endotracheal tube and ventilator to increase and maintain normal oxygen levels.
- *Inhaled nitric oxide* (iNO) therapy to reduce muscle tone, which reduces pulmonary artery pressures and causes vasodilation and increased ventilation of the lungs.
- *Nothing per os* (NPO) to reduce the energy required to feed by mouth and decrease respiratory compromise
- *Extracorporeal membrane oxygenation* (ECMO), a cardiopulmonary bypass treatment implemented to provide heart–lung bypass outside of the newborn's body for life-threatening cardiac or pulmonary diagnoses. Can be utilized for extended periods while treatment is initiated for underlying diagnoses. ECMO can be venovenous for isolated pulmonary conditions or venoarterial for combined cardiac and pulmonary diagnoses.

Long-Term Management

Depending on the type of pulmonary defect and any concurrent diagnoses, the newborn's family will require specific discharge education related to the diagnosis, care at home, prescribed and over-the-counter medications, and follow-up with their pediatrician and pediatric pulmonologist. Depending on the newborn's nutritional status, a referral may also be made to a lactation consultant and nutritionist to ensure the newborn is receiving adequate caloric intake and nutrition sufficient for ongoing growth and development.

Emotional issues associated with developmental complications often surface in patients with a history of both congenital cardiac and pulmonary defects, and these may affect their ability to effectively cope, feel secure about their abilities, and assimilate into school and peer groups. Support groups are often recommended for these children and their families in order to meet other families with similar clinical issues and diagnoses. The groups are effective in creating relationships that can provide both emotional support and ongoing connections for both the child and the family (Mayo Clinic, 2018).

Pharmacology

The management of a newborn with respiratory difficulty or distress often requires pharmacological intervention. The purpose of the administration of medications to newborns diagnosed with pulmonary disease and complications is to support, enhance, and sustain optimal pulmonary functioning while decreasing the potential for long-term pulmonary complications. Table 12-3 lists the most common medications administered and provides information about the normal dosages and Safe and Effective Nursing Care (SENC) practices. These medications fall into five classifications, including alkalinizing agents, antibiotics, *central nervous system* (CNS) stimulants, corticosteroids, and sterile nonpyrogenic pulmonary surfactants.

The newborn's diagnoses and associated complications will determine which classification of medications will be initiated and continued, and the length of time these medications will be necessary for optimum lung functioning. Medications are optimally administered either by intravenous (umbilical vein, *peripherally inserted central catheter* [PICC], or central line) or intratracheal (through an endotracheal tube) routes.

The specific diagnoses, pathology, and diagnostic results will determine the appropriate treatment and the potential for both acute and chronic long-term outcomes for the newborn. The early recognition of potential and actual pulmonary complications in the newborn will guide diagnosis and treatment modalities, while providing the best outcome.

Summary

The period of transitioning after delivery is a critical time for the nurse to carefully assess the newborn for any signs and symptoms of potential complications. Early recognition and management of any respiratory compromise are essential for the newborn to reduce further complications, morbidity, and mortality. The initial and ongoing support provided to a newborn will help to prevent any additional problems related to extrauterine transitioning.

The first 1 to 24 hours are a critical time for all newborns' conversion to extrauterine life and include the maintenance of a warm environment, blood glucose monitoring, adequate nutrition, and observation for adequate and normal fetal-to-newborn adaptation. Any deviation from normal transitioning requires ongoing support and nursing observation to reduce potential acute and chronic complications in the newborn.

A newborn may require an extended stay in the hospital to stabilize and maintain adequate respirations, ventilation, and oxygenation. Any pulmonary diagnosis has the potential for both acute and chronic symptoms in the newborn and requires support, treatment, and family preparation for discharge to the community.

TABLE 12–3   Medications Used to Treat Newborn Respiratory Complications

Class	Examples	Action	Dosage	S/NC
Alkalinizing agent	Bicarbonate	Reduction in acidosis to decrease pulmonary resistance.	IVP 1–2 mEq/kg to a maximum concentration of 0.5 mL.	Monitor serum potassium levels for hyperkalemia and ABGs for alkalosis.
Antibiotics	Ampicillin Gentamycin	Reduction of bacterial pathogens.	IV 100 mg/kg/dose Age in weeks | Postnatal (days) | Dose (mg/kg) | Interval (hr) ≤29 | 0 to 7 | 5 4 | 48 36 24 30 to 34 | 0 to 7 ≥8 | 4.5 4 | 36 24 ≥35 | ALL | 4 | 24	
CNS stimulants	Caffeine	Stimulates the respiratory center in apnea to reduce the frequency of apnea, hypoxemia, and ventilator weaning failures.	IV loading dose: 20 mg/kg/dose over 30 min, then 5 mg/kg/dose every 24 hr.	Failure to gain weight, hyper- or hypo-glycemia, sleeplessness, arrhythmias, diuresis, tachypnea, seizures, hypertension, irritability.
Corticosteroids	Dexamethasone	Anti-inflammatory agent to decrease inflammation and improve ventilation and oxygenation.	IV 1–3 days: 0.075 mg/kg/dose, 4–6 days: 0.050 mg/kg/dose, 7–8 days: 0.025 mg/kg/dose and 9–10 days: 0.01 mg/kg/dose.	Hyperglycemia, glycosuria, electrolyte disturbance, impaired wound healing, leukocytosis.
Sterile nonpyrogenic pulmonary surfactants	Survanta	Reduces minimum surface tension and increases pulmonary compliance and oxygenation in newborns.	IT (intratracheal) 4 mL/kg q 6 hr × 4 doses in the first 48 hr of life.	Monitor heart and respiratory rates. Bradycardia, hypotension, oxygen desaturation, endotracheal tube blockage, pulmonary hemorrhage, and nosocomial infection. Give within 15 min of birth in prematurity.

(Epocrates, 2018; Ward & Hisley, 2016)

Discharge instructions from an acute care facility should include instructions on the signs and symptoms to assess for in acute respiratory compromise and deterioration in the newborn. These should include an increase in respiratory rate; noisy respirations including grunting, stridor, or wheezing; chest retractions, including subcostal, intercostal, or suprasternal; cyanosis; excessive secretions; elevation in temperature; difficulty eating; a decrease in voiding and stool patterns; lethargy; or excessive crying or inconsolability.

Key Points

- All newborns should be assessed for respiratory distress at delivery and throughout their transitional period. A key component of the initial nursing assessment of the newborn includes a thorough assessment of the respiratory system.

- Maternal and newborn risk factors for potential respiratory complications should be identified when possible prior to delivery.

- Diagnostic testing for respiratory compromise and complications includes vital sign assessment, skin color, chest x-ray, oxygen saturation, and ABG.

- Assessment for respiratory complications will determine whether further treatment and management are required.

- Parents should be provided with discharge instructions related to the diagnosis of respiratory disease and ongoing treatments and follow-up.

Review Questions

1. **The physiological effect of artificial pulmonary surfactant is to:**
   a. Increase alveolar surface tension.
   b. Decrease alveolar surface tension.
   c. Promote a normal respiratory rate.
   d. Decrease alveolar expansion.

2. **At how many weeks of gestation is pulmonary surfactant initially produced in the fetus?**
   a. 40
   b. 24
   c. 35
   d. 12

3. **Inadequate ventilation in the newborn may result in which of the following?**
   a. Respiratory alkalosis
   b. Respiratory acidosis
   c. A decrease in surfactant production
   d. Hyperoxemia

4. **Which of the following is considered to be a late sign of distress in a newborn?**
   a. Central cyanosis
   b. Circumoral cyanosis
   c. Tachycardia
   d. Tachypnea

5. **Which of the following occurs secondary to newborn transitioning?**
   a. Fetal shunts close.
   b. Surfactant production decreases.
   c. Carbon dioxide levels increase.
   d. A cardiac murmur is heard upon auscultation.

See the appendix for answers to review questions.

References

Capriotti, T. (2020). *Pathophysiology: Introductory concepts and clinical perspectives* (2nd ed.). Philadelphia, PA: F.A. Davis.

Epocrates. (2018). Retrieved from https://online.epocrates.com/drugs

Gardner, S. L., Enzman-Hines, M., & Nyp, M. (2016). Respiratory diseases. In S. L. Gardner, B. S. Carter, M. Enzman-Hines, & J. A. Hernandez (Eds.), *Merenstein and Gardner's handbook of neonatal intensive care* (8th ed., pp. 565–643). St. Louis, MO: Elsevier-Mosby.

Gardner, S. L., & Hernandez, J. A. (2016). Initial nursery care. In S. L. Gardner, B. S. Carter, M. Enzman-Hines, & J. A. Hernandez (Eds.), *Merenstein and Gardner's handbook of neonatal intensive care* (8th ed., p. 84). St. Louis, MO: Elsevier-Mosby.

Hernandez, J. A., & Thilo, E. (2005). Routine care of the full-term newborn. In L. C. Osborn, T. G. DeWitt, L. R. First, & J. Zenel (Eds.), *Pediatrics*. St. Louis, MO: Mosby.

Mayo Clinic. (2018). Tests and procedures. Retrieved from https://www.mayoclinic.org/tests-procedures.

Pramanik, A.K., Rangaswamy, N., & Gates, T. (2015). Neonatal respiratory distress: A practical approach to its diagnosis and management. *Pediatric Clinics of North America, 62*(2), 453–469. doi:10.1016/j.pcl.2014.11.008

Smith, J. R., & Carley, A. (2014). Common neonatal complications. In K.R. Simpson & P.A. Creehan (Eds.), *Perinatal nursing* (4th ed., pp. 662–698). Philadelphia, PA: Wolters Kluwer.

Snell, B. J., & Gardner, S. L (2017). *Care of the well newborn*. Burlington, MA: Jones & Bartlett Learning.

Ward, S. L., & Hisley, S. M. (2016). *Maternal-child nursing care with women's health companion: Optimizing outcomes for mothers, children, and families* (2nd ed.). Philadelphia, PA: F.A. Davis.

Warren, J. B., & Phillipi, C. A. (2012). Care of the well newborn. Pediatrics in review. *Journal of the American Academy of Pediatrics, 33*(1), 4–18. doi: 10.1542/pir.33-1-4

Chapter 13

Prematurity and Newborn Complications

LEARNING OBJECTIVES

Upon completion of this chapter the student will be able to:

- Integrate knowledge of the physiology, pathophysiology, assessment, and nonpharmacological and pharmacological management of prematurity in the newborn.
- Identify common complications associated with prematurity in the newborn.
- Incorporate the current standards of care for newborns born premature at less than 37 weeks' gestation.

Introduction

Prematurity is diagnosed in any newborn born at less than 37 of 40 weeks' gestational age. The care of this specialized population has evolved over the past years to include a technology-enhanced specialty of current newborn care and the nursing profession. The survival rate of this high-risk population has been increasing, but the mortality and morbidity rates continue to remain elevated when compared to full-term newborns born without the need for resuscitation, or without any complications related to prematurity (Ward & Hisley, 2016).

Premature birth and its complications are the largest contributors to infant death in the United States and a major cause of long-term health problems in the children who survive post-resuscitation and neonatal care. The mission of the March of Dimes is to reduce preterm birth rates and increase equity among families in every state. Each state is assigned an annual grade for preterm birth rates based on its reportable numbers. The goal is to decrease annual premature birth rates to less than 8.1% and provide continued progress toward solutions that help all mothers and babies have healthy, full-term deliveries with minimal to no complications (March of Dimes Foundation, 2019).

The risk for complications in premature newborns can occur at any time in their intrauterine stage, during the labor and delivery process, or post-delivery during the extrauterine stage. Complications in the high-risk premature newborn born at less than 37- and 0/7-weeks' gestation may be predicted based on the prenatal course or may occur suddenly without any forewarning. The potential for complications in a premature newborn must be anticipated and prepared for in any facility providing maternal and newborn care. In the event that a delivery complication precipitously develops or quickly progresses, the health-care delivery team must be prepared to provide optimal newborn care based on the current standards of maternal and newborn care (Capriotti, 2020).

The level of care provided during the delivery process can have lifelong implications for the newborn's growth and development as well as the family's developmental processes. The newborn's care during the prenatal period, the delivery process, any required resuscitation, and the health-care team's attention to appropriate, timely treatment must be well organized and focused on evidence-based clinical decisions (Capriotti, 2020).

Newborn resuscitation begins immediately after delivery. The resuscitation team is responsible for quickly assessing the newborn's respiratory and circulatory transition status and intervening as appropriate. The majority of premature newborns will require some assistance to initiate and sustain breathing. This can include blow-by oxygen or *positive pressure ventilation* (PPV). A lesser number of newborns will require extensive resuscitation interventions including *cardiopulmonary resuscitation* (CPR) and emergency medications. The need for newborn resuscitation cannot always be projected during the labor process; therefore, a resuscitation team must always be available in the event a newborn requires emergent interventions (Weiner & Zaichkin, 2016).

The nursing care specific to the care of this high-risk population of newborns focuses on the promotion of healthy growth and development while decreasing the potential for further complications related to the diagnosis of prematurity in the newborn. The newborn should be assessed frequently to determine milestone and growth achievement, as minimal to serious developmental delays are common in these high-risk newborns (Ward & Hisley, 2016).

Physiology

The neonate experiences multiple body system processes during the intrauterine, intrapartum, and extrauterine post-delivery phases. The systems most affected in the newborn by a premature birth include the respiratory, circulatory, and neurological systems. The goal in the provision of care for a premature newborn is to promote healthy growth and development while diminishing the potential for further complications related to the diagnosis of prematurity in the newborn and the affected body systems.

A normal term newborn has the ability to mature their fetal lungs continually in utero until the time of delivery. Lung maturity can be determined by assessing the *lecithin-to-sphingomyelin* (L/S) ratio and *phosphatidylglycerol* (PG) levels. These components are essential for the promotion of pulmonary oxygenation, maintaining open functioning alveoli, and decreasing lung surface tension. Alveolar ducts and alveoli increase in number, size, and shape in conjunction with the pulmonary vasculature until approximately 40 weeks of gestation. A birth that occurs prior to this normal growth time frame exposes the newborn to the potential for ongoing pulmonary complications (Ward & Hisley, 2016).

The circulatory system provides the blood supply to the neonate's organs in utero, and this system increases in force and resiliency along with the growing fetus until reaching term gestation. At the time of a term birth, the newborn has three fetal circulatory shunts (the ductus arteriosus, ductus venosus, and foramen ovale) that convert the newborn from neonatal to adult circulation. This conversion occurs to provide for the normal flow of oxygen to the lungs and blood filtering by the liver in the absence of the placenta, whose role in utero provided the needed oxygenation and circulation. (Ward & Hisley, 2016).

Complications of inadequate circulatory system functioning related to prematurity can range from unequal, diminished pules, uneven extremity blood pressure readings, increased capillary refill time, cardiac murmurs, pulmonary hypertension, and congestive heart failure. Each cardiac complication must be assessed to establish the etiology and symptom severity prior to determining treatment options.

The neurological system in a newborn is composed of both the peripheral and central nervous systems in conjunction with the sympathetic and parasympathetic systems. It is normal for term newborns to be born with immature neurological systems. The premature newborn is at a significantly higher risk of complications associated with the neurological system based on their gestational age and the high level of neurological immaturity associated with a diagnosis of prematurity. The term newborn already has an underdeveloped system that includes a decrease in synapses and dendrite connections, in addition to a decrease of nerve cell myelination necessary for the conduction of impulses. This underdevelopment is markedly increased in the premature newborn (Ward & Hisley, 2016).

During the initial post-delivery period and the first year of life, both term and preterm newborns experience significant physiological changes. These include periods of both rapid growth and development. Preterm newborns may experience these normal physiological changes at a different pace than term newborns based on their determined gestational age at birth and any subsequent complications that may occur post-delivery (Ward & Hisley, 2016).

 CLINICAL PEARLS

It is essential for health-care providers to be able to recognize and treat complications in both term and premature newborns as they transition after delivery.

Pathophysiology

Prematurity in the newborn can lead to a myriad of complications, ranging from low birth weight, temperature instability, and nutritional and body system complications to jaundice and sepsis. These complications may not be discernible and may be nonspecific initially, but subtle indicators that mimic other common newborn illnesses frequently manifest in a newborn born with a diagnosis of prematurity. A heightened assessment sense is essential when providing care to newborns born prematurely.

Low birth weight and fetal distress during the labor process and delivery can be predictors for immediate and future complications in premature newborns. The labor process, maternal complications, and labor medications can contribute to or exacerbate the potential for problems in the premature newborn.

The pulmonary system is particularly vulnerable in a premature newborn and is the most common complication of this high-risk group. The gestational age and levels of L/S and PG determine the newborn's ability to breathe spontaneously and independently without any type of ventilation support. Newborns born prematurely are specifically at risk for *respiratory distress syndrome* (RDS), which can require an extended stay in a *neonatal intensive care unit* (NICU) for the purpose of providing pulmonary support and treating complications associated with this diagnosis.

The circulatory system is also susceptible to complications in the premature newborn. Based on the normal physiology in a term newborn, this system increases in strength and resiliency as the gestational age advances. Any reduction of the increased blood flow to the brain and heart compromises the fetus and high-risk newborn. Normal cardiac shunt closure is dependent and based on extrauterine oxygen and pressure changes. If the premature newborn's heart does not respond to the normal physiological closure mechanisms, a structural abnormality may exist and must be investigated. This abnormality will place the newborn at an increased risk for both circulatory compromise and further damage to their fragile blood vessels (Ward & Hisley, 2016).

Temperature instability is common in the premature newborn and must be prevented beginning at delivery. The newborn's temperature can decrease in response to exposure to extrauterine cool surfaces, room temperature, or fluid and oxygen administration. The newborn's exposure to a decreased temperature results in a breakdown of the brown adipose tissue responsible for maintaining heat production in newborns. This response can lead to a condition known as *cold stress* with a secondary increase in the newborn's metabolism and further heat loss. The thin skin of a premature newborn also contributes to the potential for hypothermia through the process of evaporation or evaporative heat loss (Ward & Hisley, 2016).

The high-risk newborn is furthermore at an increased risk for immaturity of the neurological system, which decreases their ability to manage the external stimuli to which they are exposed, commencing at delivery. Neurological deficits in the newborn may be experienced on both a short- and long-term basis due to the disruption of neuron development and subsequent ongoing complications associated with prematurity (Ward & Hisley, 2016).

A high-risk newborn is extremely vulnerable to complications during both the intrauterine and extrauterine periods, based on their level of prematurity as determined by their gestational age. Newborns can be exposed to a host of complications and toxins that can affect their intrauterine growth and development. These exposure factors may compromise a newborn's ability to continue the maturation process in utero until reaching the full-term gestational age of 37 weeks or greater.

All newborns have a degree of immaturity related to their immune system, but preterm newborns are more susceptible to adverse outcomes secondary to infections related to their immature and ineffective functioning immune systems. The underdeveloped immune system in a preterm newborn is unable to provide the protection necessary to fully reduce the newborn's risk for infections. In addition, premature newborns are appreciably more likely to require pharmacological support to prevent or treat infections until their immune systems are fully functioning. Both early- and late-onset sepsis in premature newborns are potential significant risks and must be assessed. It is essential that sepsis be treated using a judicious approach in order to reduce the potential for ongoing further complications and morbidity in the newborn. The accompanying boxed list provides risk factors for infections in premature newborns that may compromise a newborn during any of the stages of pregnancy, from implantation to delivery.

The most common causative organisms in premature newborn infections include bacteria, viruses, and fungi. These organisms are the primary causes of early-onset infections (within the first 72 hours of life). These infections are associated with a higher degree of mortality and morbidity with late-onset infections (72 hours of life and beyond) or sepsis, which is considered a serious systemic bacterial infection contained within the newborn's bloodstream. Based on the current trend of encouraging earlier maternal and newborn discharges, these serious infections may manifest once an infant is discharged home and before adequate follow-up with their health-care provider has occurred. The accompanying boxed list provides causative agents of early-onset and late-onset neonatal infections.

Risk Factors for Infections in Premature Newborns

- Immature immune system based on gestational age:
  - Decreased inflammatory immunity
  - Decreased humoral immunity
  - Decreased passive immunity
- Lack of local inflammatory reactions at portal of infection entry
- Non-specific signs and symptoms
- Higher risk in male newborns
- Lower risk with breastfeeding
- Sources: transplacental, perinatal, postpartum
- Administration of antibiotics
- Low socioeconomic status
- Intrauterine growth restriction
- Low birth weight
- Underweight
- Decreased nutritional intake
- Intrapartum complications
- Use of instruments in delivery
- Maternal elevated temperature
- Maternal infection
- Group B streptococci
- Chorioamnionitis
- Premature or prolonged rupture of membranes
- Decreased Apgar scoring
- Use of an internal monitor electrode
- Any resuscitation at delivery
- Congenital newborn malformations
- Invasive maternal or newborn procedures
- Intravenous access
- Lumbar puncture
- Surgical procedures

(Adapted from Gardner, 2009; Gardner & Snell, 2016)

Causative Agents of Early- and Late-Onset Newborn Infections and Sepsis

EARLY-ONSET INFECTIONS AND SEPSIS ORGANISMS
- Group B streptococci (GBS)
- *Escherichia coli*
- Coagulase-negative staphylococci
- *Staphylococcus aureus*
- *Neisseria meningitides*
- *Streptococcus pneumoniae*
- *Haemophilus influenzae*, type B and non-typeable
- *Klebsiella pneumoniae*
- *Pseudomonas aeruginosa*
- *Enterobacter* species
- *Serratia marcescens*
- Group A streptococci
- Anaerobic species

Causative Agents of Early- and Late-Onset Newborn Infections and Sepsis—cont'd

LATE-ONSET SEPSIS INFECTIONS AND SEPSIS ORGANISMS
- Coagulase-negative staphylococci
- *Escherichia coli*
- *Klebsiella* species
- *Enterobacter* species
- *Candida* species
- *Malassezia furfur*
- Group B streptococci (GBS)
- Methicillin-resistant *Staphylococcus aureus* (MRSA)

(Adapted from Gardner & Snell, 2016 and reproduced from Pammi, Brand, & Weisman, 2016; Snell & Gardner, 2017).

It is essential to prevent infections in this newborn population as much as possible. If infections do occur, the health-care team must have the ability to recognize and treat these infections promptly. Newborns often present with atypical signs and symptoms when an infection is manifesting. These symptoms are often subtle and can resemble other diagnoses including hypothermia, hypoglycemia, respiratory problems, and cardiac and neurological complications. In fact, an infection in a newborn may not have any apparent signs or symptoms present, but a subtle change in behavior may occur. In a premature newborn, by the time definite, apparent symptoms are present, overwhelming sepsis may be in place and cause significant problems for the neonate. The accompanying boxed list describes the signs and symptoms of neonatal infections.

It is essential for health-care providers to be able to recognize the potential for and the symptoms associated with infections in both newborns and infants. The ability to treat promptly and with appropriate medications is fundamental to preventing a devastating outcome on the pediatric patient.

HIGH YIELD FACT FOR TESTING

Preterm newborns may be at risk for complications at any time in their intrauterine or extrauterine growth.

CLINICAL PEARLS

The implementation of hand hygiene is a critical step in the reduction of infections and must be enforced with any direct contact with newborns, especially those born prematurely (Snell & Gardner, 2017).

Signs and Symptoms of Neonatal Infections

- Temperature instability: hypothermia of hyperthermia
- Respiratory distress: tachycardia, bradycardia, hypotension, pallor, poor peripheral perfusion (capillary refill time >3 seconds), weak pulses, decreased urine output
- Neurological changes: irritability, lethargy, seizures, apnea as a manifestation of seizure
- Feeding abnormalities: change in feeding behaviors, poor feeding, vomiting, abdominal distention, diarrhea
- Jaundice: progression of jaundice from head to toe; increase in direct or indirect bilirubin levels
- Skin changes: rash, purpura, erythema, petechiae
- Metabolic changes: acidosis (metabolic and/or respiratory), hypoglycemia, hypoxia

(Data from Gardner, 2007, 2016; Pammi, Brand, & Weisman, 2016)

Assessment

Premature newborns frequently require some level of resuscitation at delivery related to their immature systems, specifically the respiratory and circulatory systems. Every attempt should be made with each premature delivery to identify the prospective for newborn resuscitation and to be equipped to respond to any complications that occur prior to and in the immediate post-delivery phases. All potential identifiable risk factors must be recognized and anticipated for based on the maternal and fetal history, including if prenatal care was established and followed through during the pregnancy.

A number of specific factors place a mother at risk for experiencing a preterm birth, including the factors listed below:

- Maternal smoking
- Maternal age (older than 35 years or younger than 20 years)
- Maternal drug abuse
- Female partner abuse
- Multiple gestations
- Maternal uterine abnormalities
- Fetal anomalies
- Maternal infection (especially chlamydia, gonorrhea, and bacterial vaginosis)
- Maternal cervical anomalies
- History of previous preterm births (carries twice the risk)
- African American descent
- Genetic susceptibility (Ward & Hisley, 2016)

At the time of delivery, the health-care delivery team will determine the level of resuscitation required based on their initial and ongoing assessments. Apgar scoring is utilized to both determine and assess fetal well-being after delivery. Dr. Virginia Apgar, who was a practicing anesthesiologist, developed the Apgar scoring tool for initial newborn evaluation in 1952. This scoring method is used to guide the delivery team in determining immediate care for a newborn. This is particularly critical for any premature newborn that may require supplementary cardiac, respiratory, and neurological post-delivery support (Dillon, 2016).

The Apgar scoring is established at both 1 and 5 minutes from the time of birth. Continued 5-minute newborn assessments are made as needed to determine further resuscitation efforts until the newborn is approximately 20 minutes of age. The Apgar scoring evaluates the newborn's skin color, heart rate, reflex irritability, muscle tone, and respirations on a 0 to 2 scale for each area. The lowest total Apgar score that can be applied to a newborn is 0, with the highest application score possible a 10. Table 13-1 provides specific guidelines related to the newborn Apgar scoring available for all health-care providers (Snell & Gardner, 2017).

TABLE 13-1 Apgar Scoring of Newborns

Heart rate	0 = Absent	1 = <100 BPM	2 = >100 BPM
Respirations	0 = Absent	1 <30, irregular	2 = Strong cry, regular
Muscle tone	0 = Flaccid	1 = Some flexion in arms and legs	2 = Full flexion, active movement
Reflex irritability	0 = No response	1 = Grimace, weak cry	2 = Vigorous cry
Color*	0 = Pale, blue	1 = Body pink, extremities blue	2 = Totally pink

(Adapted from Dillon, 2016)

BPM, beats per minute

* During the assessment and Apgar scoring of the newborn with darker skin, the health-care team will assess the soles of the feet, palms of the hand, and roof of the mouth before assigning the score for color.

In addition to Apgar assessments, high-risk premature newborns are categorized based on two specific criteria: birth weight recorded in grams in addition to pounds and ounces, and the gestational age or length of time in utero. The weight and gestational age are plotted on a gestational age assessment graph and the newborn is classified according to their placement (Ward & Hisley, 2016). This graph is shown in Figure 13-1.

The newborn age classifications include the following:

- *Small for gestational age* (SGA): Infants that are at or below the 10th percentile in birth weight.
- *Average for gestational age* (AGA): A birth is considered to be appropriate for gestational age if the birth weight is between the 10th and 90th percentiles for the infant's gestational age and sex.
- *Large for gestational age* (LGA): Infants that are at or above the 90th percentile in birth weight.

These categories provide a foundation on which to initiate care after delivery. The gestational age predetermines the interdisciplinary care necessary for the newborn and the determination for newborn classification based on these criteria. Weight may be the only criterion for classifying premature newborns with low birth weights. These newborns are at an elevated risk of mortality based on their newborn weight and potential complications. These at-risk weights include the following:

- *Low birth weight* (LBW) at less than 2,500 g
- *Very low birth weight* (VLBW) at less than less than 1,500 g
- *Extremely low birth weight* (ELBW) at less than 1,000 g

The Ballard gestational age by maturity rating tool provides an additional method to assess a newborn's gestational age. This tool measures the newborn's neuromuscular and physical maturity, which is plotted onto a scale to determine the newborn's gestational age in weeks. This measurement should be conducted within the first 12 hours of life to ensure accuracy. There are six areas of both neuromuscular and physical maturity that are rated on a scale of –1 to 5. The scores are totaled to achieve a score that determines gestational age. Figure 13-2 shows the Newborn Ballard Gestational Age Assessment Tool (Ward & Hisley, 2016).

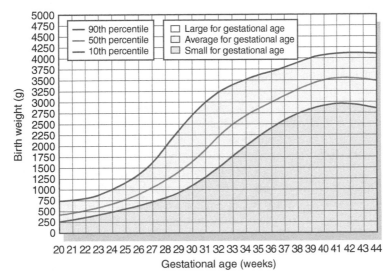

FIGURE 13–1 Newborn Gestational Age Assessment Graph *Courtesy of Mead Johnson Nutritionals.*

Neuromuscular Maturity

	-1	0	1	2	3	4	5
Posture							
Square Window (Wrist)	-90°	90°	60°	45°	30°	0°	
Arm Recoil		180°	140°-180°	110°-140°	90°-110°	<90°	
Popliteal Angle	180°	160°	140°	120°	100°	90°	<90°
Scarf Sign							
Heel to Ear							

Physical Maturity

								Maturity Rating	
								Score	Weeks
Skin	Sticky Friable Transparent	Gelatinous Red Translucent	Smooth pink Visible veins	Superficial Peeling or rash, few veins	Cracking Pale areas Rare veins	Parchment Deep cracking No vessels	Leathery Cracked Wrinkled	-10	20
Lanugo	None	Sparse	Abundant	Thinning	Bald areas	Mostly bald		-5	22
								0	24
Plantar Surface	Heel-toe 40–50 mm:-1 <40 mm:-2	>50 mm No crease	Faint red marks	Anterior transverse crease only	Creases ant. 2/3	Creases over entire sole		5	26
								10	28
Breast	Imperceptible	Barely perceptible	Flat areola No bud	Stippled areola 1–2 mm bud	Raised areola 3–4 mm bud	Full areola 5–10 mm bud		15	30
								20	32
Eye/ear	Lids fused loosely:-1 tightly:-2	Lids open Pinna flat Stays folded	Sl. Curved pinna; soft; slow recoil	Well-curved pinna; soft but ready recoil	Formed and firm Instant recoil	Thick cartilage Ear stiff		25	34
								30	36
Genitals (Male)	Scrotum flat, smooth	Scrotum empty Faint rugae	Testes in upper canal Rare rugae	Testes descending Few rugae	Testes down Good rugae	Testes pendulous Deep rugae		35	38
								40	40
Genitals (Female)	Clitoris prominent Labia flat	Prominent clitoris Small labia minora	Prominent clitoris Enlarging minora	Majora and minora equally prominent	Majora large Minora small	Majora cover clitoris and minora		45	42
								50	44

FIGURE 13–2 Newborn Ballard Gestational Age Assessment Tool *From Ballard, J. L., et al. (1991). New Ballard Score, expanded to include extremely premature infants. Journal of Pediatrics, 19(3), 417–423. Used with permission.*

The assessment of a neonate requires a systematic approach, which is followed by a head-to-toe evaluation. The initial and ongoing assessments may be performed with the family present if the newborn's condition warrants, while under a radiant warmer, in an isolette, or in an open crib as warranted for proper maintenance of the newborn's body temperature. The techniques of auscultation, inspection, and light to deep palpation are utilized to obtain information on the newborn's condition. The skin, head, and chest, and the cardiac, pulmonary, gastrointestinal, musculoskeletal, urological, neurological, and sensory systems are included in a complete newborn assessment. The newborn assessment process is an excellent time for family education related to the newborn, if possible, as they begin their initial bonding or ongoing bonding process.

All normal and abnormal observations and assessments should be documented to provide a baseline related to the newborn's condition to be used as a point of comparison for ongoing future assessments. Normal newborn reflexes are assessed

HIGH YIELD FACT FOR TESTING

Accurate initial assessments of premature newborns are essential to provide the appropriate initial care and timely treatment of complications.

and newborn serum metabolic and congenital cardiac screening tests, hearing assessments, and car seat testing are performed on each premature newborn in the hospital setting, prior to their discharge home.

ASSESSMENT PEARLS
All delivery unit personnel must receive adequate education and training to assess and provide care for any newborn born prematurely.

Nonpharmacological Management

The care needed for premature newborns is complicated and multifactorial and may require a transfer to a facility that provides a higher level of care specific to the newborn's needs. This specialized care involves a team approach that promotes holistic, safe developmental care that aims to promote growth while reducing the potential for further complications. The following areas are important to support and maintain in the clinical setting in order to encourage newborn growth and decrease the potential for further newborn complications:

• Maintenance of nutrition with reduction in complications
• Supportive environment
• Skin and developmental care
• Sleep promotion
• Reduction of overstimulation
• Positions of comfort
• Prevention of infection
• Temperature maintenance by providing a *neutral thermal environment* (NTE)
• Reduction of pain
• Maintenance of normal blood glucose levels
• Reduction in the effects of jaundice
• Maintenance of optimal system functioning
• Maintenance of normal calcium and magnesium levels
• Maintenance of breathing with apnea reduction
• Maintenance of heart rate with bradycardia reduction
• Reduction of the potential for *retinopathy of prematurity* (ROP)
• Reduction of the potential for intracerebral bleeding
• Assessment and care related to newborn screening results
• Assessment and care related to other complications of the premature newborn
• Ongoing family education and preparation for discharge (Ward & Hisley, 2016)

The premature newborn is often admitted to the NICU for their initial stabilization and ongoing care. Appropriate developmental care is provided in the NICU and transitional nurseries to decrease the potential for any long-term developmental disabilities in the newborn. The objective of NICU care is to simulate an intrauterine environment as much as possible in order to promote as normal as achievable growth and development in the high-risk newborn. The length of stay in the hospital depends on both the mother's and premature newborn's conditions. The mother is often discharged from the hospital prior to the newborn due to the complexity of the diagnoses associated with the early delivery of a premature high-risk newborn.

This experience can be particularly frightening for families, and the nursing staff should pay particular attention to providing support to and educating these families about the immediate care and goals for their newborn, as well as the care that will be provided in this intensive environment. Family-centered care and primary nursing are paramount in the care of any premature newborn, to provide support and consistency throughout the potential extended inpatient stay (Ward & Hisley, 2016). This education may include environmental and sleep safety measures; recognition of potential complications and their symptoms; medication and oxygen administration as needed; skin care; and nutritional instructions related to appropriate age and weight, and calorie formula administration or breast feeding. The family of a newborn who receives care in the NICU are required to complete a CPR class in order to provide this procedure in the event it is needed after the newborn's discharge from the hospital

Long-Term Management

The care and management of newborns diagnosed with both short- and long-term complications often include intensive long-term care and follow-up. A newborn that has been in a NICU is often termed a "NICU graduate" upon discharge from the unit. This history of a premature newborn requiring care in a NICU setting often necessitates intensive management and care. The follow-up can include long-term, ongoing follow-up appointments with an ophthalmologist, physical and occupational therapists, a developmental specialist, a neurologist, cardiologist, pulmonologist, a dietician, orthopedics specialist, pediatrician, case manager, social worker, and speech pathologist.

Alternative Treatments

A family's cultural and spiritual practices and beliefs should be acknowledged and supported if possible, throughout the hospitalization, based on the newborn's condition. It is important for families to have the opportunity to preserve their customs and traditions related to the pregnancy, delivery, and newborn care if possible. These customs support family attachment and bonding and encourage breastfeeding practices in the immediate post-delivery phase and throughout the mother's and newborn's care (Ward & Hisley, 2016).

Pharmacology

The pharmacology regimen ordered will be specific to each neonate depending on the high-risk newborn's diagnoses and management plan. Medications to treat the effects of prematurity in a newborn are based on the size and weight of the newborn and associated conditions and/or complications related to prematurity. The pharmacological management of a premature newborn depends on systems and symptoms. A premature newborn experiencing respiratory complications will require medication to lower pulmonary surface tension and increase compliance and oxygenation of the lung's alveoli. The medication often administered includes a pulmonary surfactant, which is ordered to prevent and treat a diagnosis of respiratory distress syndrome in newborns. The class of methylxanthine may also be ordered to support a newborn's respiration and to prevent apnea of prematurity, based on the medication's action of central nervous system and respiratory stimulation. These classes of medication are first line, essential medications to enhance pulmonary functioning in a premature newborn. Respiratory complications are the most commonly observed complications in a premature newborn and require both monitoring and pharmacological interventions.

The provider should prescribe the safest medication at the lowest appropriate dosage initially and monitor the premature newborn for the onset of any associated complications with the medication before any modifications are made to the dosage. The effectiveness of all medications prescribed in newborns should be closely supervised to determine the value of the medication versus the onset of any detrimental effects. Table 13-2 provides information related to premature newborn pharmacology.

TABLE 13-2 Premature Newborn Pharmacology

Class	Example	Action/Indication	Dosage	Adverse Effects	SENC
Macrolides	Erythromycin, Ilotycin	Suppresses protein synthesis at the level of the 50S ribosome. Prophylaxis prevention of ophthalmia neonatorum in infants.	Apply a ribbon of ointment to each eye from the inner to outer eye canthus.	Eye irritation.	Administer within 1 hr after delivery.
Fat-soluble vitamins	Vitamin K	Required for hepatic synthesis of blood coagulation factors II (prothrombin), VII, IX, and X. Prevention and treatment of hypoprothrombinemia and hemorrhagic disease of the newborn.	0.5–1.0 mg IM.	GI: gastric upset, unusual taste. Dermatological: flushing, rash, urticaria. Hematological: hemolytic anemia. Local: erythema, swelling, pain at the injection site.	Give within 1–2 hr after birth, may repeat in 6–8 hr if needed and at 2–3 weeks if indicated.
Sterile nonpyrogenic pulmonary surfactants	Beractant, Survanta	Lowers surface tension of alveoli level. Lowers surface tension and increases pulmonary compliance and oxygenation in newborns. Given for surfactant deficiency. Prevents and treats RDS in newborns.	100 mg/kg of birth weight. 4 doses within the first 48 hr of life every 6 hr.	Transient bradycardia, hypotension, oxygen desaturation, endotracheal tube blockage, pulmonary hemorrhage, and possible increased nosocomial infections.	Give within 15 min of birth. Perform a naso-oral suction before administration. Warm vial 20 min to room temperature before administration. Do not suction for 1 hr after administration. Do not refrigerate vial once warmed. Discard contents.
Methylxanthines	Caffeine citrate, Cafcit	Central nervous system stimulant. Respiratory stimulant. Prevention and treatment of apnea in newborns.	20 mg/kg IV, PO. Maintenance. Therapeutic level is 5–20 mcg/mL.	Complications related to abrupt withdrawal.	Therapeutic caffeine level should be assessed once weekly. Withdraw medication slowly.

(Adapted from Ward & Hisley, 2016)

Summary

In summary, early and prompt recognition and assessment of potential and actual complications in a premature newborn can lead to a reduction in current and long-term health problems for the newborn and their family. Early birth patterns and subsequent complications are the largest contributors to infant mortality and a key cause of long-term health problems in the pediatric population of newborns who survive post-resuscitation and initial and ongoing neonatal care

The goal of the care provided to a high-risk newborn includes the initial and ongoing stabilization of the newborn, recognition of the gestational age and weight to determine the classification of the newborn and any related complications, and the prevention and reduction of prospective complications in the acute care setting. The recognition of complications provides the health-care provider with the essential information needed to consult with and appropriately refer newborns and their families to specific providers.

Discharge planning commences on admission of the high-risk newborn and every intervention should be initiated to stabilize and support both the newborn and their family during initial and ongoing required care. Family education is a vital aspect of the high-risk premature newborn's care and should include clear instructions on symptoms of a sick newborn. Families should be encouraged to contact and follow up with their outpatient providers for any questions or concerns upon discharge. The education provided in the hospital can effectively reduce the potential for additional complications once the newborn has been discharged home with their family members (Ward & Hisley, 2016).

Key Points

- All newborns should be assessed for gestational age and weight at delivery to determine appropriate care.
- The more premature a newborn is, the greater the risk for mortality in this population.
- An important factor of the initial nursing assessment of the premature newborn includes a thorough assessment of all systems.
- Maternal risk factors for prematurity should be identified prior to delivery.
- An admission of a premature newborn to a NICU is a significant stressor for emerging families.

Review Questions

1. **The effects of prematurity in a newborn may include which of the following? (Select all that apply.)**
    a. An alteration in family bonding
    b. An underdeveloped neurological system
    c. An increase in the potential for infection
    d. The inability to maintain an adequate body temperature

2. **When is a newborn diagnosed with prematurity?**
    a. At 40 weeks' gestation
    b. At 24 weeks' gestation
    c. Below 37 weeks' gestation
    d. Below 40 weeks' gestation

3. **A newborn diagnosed as large for gestational age (LGA) is at what percentile on the growth curve?**

   a. Less than the 10th percentile

   b. Over the 90th percentile

   c. Between the 10th and 90th percentile

   d. Less than the 50th percentile

4. **Which of the following are factors to be considered in any preterm newborn? (Select all that apply.)**

   a. Nutrition

   b. Skin care

   c. Reduction of apnea and bradycardia

   d. Promotion of family bonding

5. **A newborn's classification is based on which of the following?**

   a. Birth weight and gestational age

   b. Mother's estimated date of delivery

   c. Lecithin-to-sphingomyelin ratio

   d. Prostaglandin levels

   See the appendix for answers to review questions.

References

Capriotti, T. (2020). *Pathophysiology: Introductory concepts and clinical perspectives* (2nd ed.). Philadelphia, PA: F.A. Davis.

Ballard, J. L., Khoury, L. C., Wedig, K., Wang, L., Eilers-Walsman, B. L., & Lipp, R. (1991). New Ballard Score, expanded to include extremely premature infants. *Journal of Pediatrics, 19*(3), 417–423.

Dillon, P. M. (2016). *Nursing health assessment*. Philadelphia, PA: F.A. Davis.

Gardner, S. L. (2007). Late-preterm ("near-term") newborns: A neonatal nursing challenge, *Nurse Currents, 1*(1), 1–7.

Gardner, S. L. (2009). Sepsis in the neonate. *Critical Care Clinics of North America, 21*(1), 121–141.

Gardner, S. L., & Snell, B. J. (2016). Care of the well newborn. How will I know my newborn is sick? *Nurse Currents, 2*(2), 1–8.

Pammi, M., Brand, M. C., & Weisman, L. E. (2016). Infection in the neonate. In S. L Gardner, B. S. Carter, M. Enzman-Hines, & J. A. Hernandez (Eds.), *Merenstein and Gardner's handbook of neonatal intensive care* (8th ed., pp. 537–563). St. Louis, MO: Mosby-Elsevier.

Snell, B. J., & Gardner, S. L. (2017). *Care of the well newborn*. Burlington, MA: Jones & Bartlett Learning.

Ward, S. L., & Hisley, S. M. (2016). *Maternal-child nursing care*. Philadelphia, PA: F.A. Davis.

Weiner, G. M., & Zaichkin, J. (Eds.). (2016). *Textbook of neonatal resuscitation* (7th ed.). Elk Grove Village, IL: American Academy of Pediatrics.

Case Study 3 (Newborn): Nutrition

LEARNING OBJECTIVES

Upon completion of this case study the student will be able to integrate knowledge of the physiology, pathophysiology, assessment, and medical and surgical management of altered nutrition in a newborn.

Introduction to Newborn Nutrition

According to Goolsby and Grubbs (2019), the assessment of a newborn's diet and feeding tolerance is essential for each well-child assessment and evaluation appointment. It is critical for health-care providers to be familiar with the normal intake, output, and weight alteration of each newborn patient being assessed. Parents should be asked about the frequency and amount of the newborn's feedings, the tolerance of these feedings by the newborn, and the type and consistency of any PO feeds they are providing to the newborn.

Nutrition is a delicate balance between the newborn's nutritional intake and the current physiological requirements necessary for the developing child. An assessment of nutritional status achieves multiple objectives. These can include the following (Dillon, 2016):

- Identification of nutritional deficiencies
- Assessment of current dietary patterns that are improving or aggravating other health diagnoses
- A baseline evaluation of current nutrition
- A point in which to plan and educate on changes in nutrition for future nutritional intake

A nutritional assessment in a newborn is critical to complete during every provider visit in order to identify promptly any prospective nutritional risks, the presence of medical or surgical conditions contributing to any nutritional imbalance, and the potential for medical or surgical interventions to support optimal nutritional intake.

Nutritional risk can be assessed in newborns that exhibit any of the following during a nutritional assessment:

- Unintentional weight loss of 10% of most recent or ideal weight
- History of illness, surgical procedures, or trauma
- Signs of nutritional insufficiency or depletion
- Economic influences associated with decreased nutritional intake or absorption of nutrient
- Symptoms of nausea, vomiting, or diarrhea
- Diminished sucking attempts or interest in eating (Dillon, 2016)

If parents are supplementing breast milk feedings with formula feeds, the type of formula and caloric content should also be documented. If the parents have initiated solid foods in a newborn, the amount of liquid ingested is important to ascertain in addition to the solid intake amounts. It is recommended that solid foods not be initiated until a child is 4 to 6 months of age. At this point in a child's development, solids should only be a complement to breastfeeding or formula feeding. Some parents whose intention is to increase the newborn's sleeping periods may have initiated solid foods earlier than recommended by the American Academy of Pediatrics (2019). A newborn needs to be fed every 2 to 4 hours and on average every 3 hours. Initiating solids earlier may essentially increase complications related to anemia and allergies and potentially increase the chances of future obesity.

Newborns require 110 to 120 kcal/kg/day with breastfeeding or bottle feeding every 2.0 to 3.0 hours. The total intake for each 24-hour period should be approximately a total of 20 to 24 ounces combined feeding types. The recommended intake for a newborn should provide adequate calories for a weight gain of 0.5 to 1 ounce per day. This intake should be adequate until a newborn reaches approximately 2 months of age. The caloric content and required daily fluid ounce intake should increase to accommodate the growing baby with an anticipated normal weight gain at the same rate as a newborn of 0.5 to 1 ounce per day. It is not until 4 months of age that the weight gain begins to increase to a daily gain of 1 ounce per day or up to 8 ounces per week (Goolsby & Grubbs, 2019).

A food intake recorded history of nutritional intake and output can be implemented to accurately determine the feeding patterns and amounts a newborn is ingesting for a suggested period of time ranging from 3 to 5 days. The importance of recording intake and output is essential in the first few months of a newborn's life. Well newborn visits with a health-care provider can monitor a newborn's weight and growth pattern in conjunction with the nutritional information and feeding tolerances provided by the parents. Any alteration in nutritional patterns should be documented and monitored by a health-care provider to determine whether underlying pathology exists.

Meet Female Newborn DB

Baby DB is a 6-day-old Mexican American female newborn who has presented at her health-care provider's office for an appointment post-discharge from the newborn nursery at the local hospital. She was born at 37 weeks' gestation at 7 pounds 6 ounces. She was discharged from the newborn nursery with her mother at 36 hours of age and received a visit from a lactation consultant prior to discharge. Newborn DB experienced a 5% weight loss during her inpatient stay in the hospital, but her parents insisted on an early discharge due to their self-pay status. DB was weighed in the provider's office, and it was determined she had lost 1 pound and 2 ounces since her date of birth 6 days prior to the visit, which was a 15% weight loss.

The parents voice a concern that DB has been "spitty" with every feeding with both breast milk and 20-calorie formula supplementation. The "spitty" episodes of emesis have increased since her discharge, and these episodes have the parents "concerned about her health." The "spitty" periods have been followed by episodes of clear to formula-colored emesis, which has since converted in the past 24 hours to a bright green color.

Upon taking the health history of the newborn, Nurse CF learns that DB has not voided or stooled in the past 24 hours and has had limited PO intake. The newborn's mother had a history of gestational diabetes, diet controlled, and pregnancy-induced hypertension with this pregnancy. The mother's blood pressure was controlled in the hospital with both intravenous magnesium sulfate and labetalol.

According to Dillon (2016), maternal health problems such as gestational diabetes and cardiac or renal disease may cause potential risk factors in a newborn. In addition, the duration of the pregnancy and any pregnancy complications can cause problems in a newborn and should be observed and assessed for in them.

Physiology and Pathophysiology

Adequate nutrition in a newborn can be altered by the presence of feeding difficulties, inadequate intake, or inability to retain feedings. Any ongoing symptoms related to nutritional alterations warrants further examination to rule out the presence of *gastrointestinal* (GI) pathology. The presence of any green emesis is a significant concern in any patient, but it is specifically concerning in a newborn who is eating poorly, has experienced significant weight loss, and who is not voiding or stooling sufficiently.

An intestinal malrotation in a newborn is a congenital anomaly that results from an abnormal rotation of the gut as it returns to the neonate's abdominal cavity during embryogenesis. Most newborn patients with a midgut malrotation develop a volvulus, or twisting of the small or large intestines, within the first week of life. (See Figure CS3-1.) The twisting of the bowel can lead to a bowel obstruction and a decreased blood supply to the twisted areas. This may include the surrounding tissues in combination with GI ischemia or death of the intestinal tissue. The newborn may experience unstable hemodynamics, metabolic acidosis, and necrosis with intestinal perforation. These conditions put the newborn at critical risk for further complications.

Complications of a volvulus can include a severe blood infection called *sepsis*. A volvulus must be treated as soon as possible to lessen the risk of complications, which may include the following:

- A malabsorption disorder called *short bowel syndrome*, which results from a decrease in the amount of small intestines
- An infection of the abdomen, known as *secondary peritonitis*

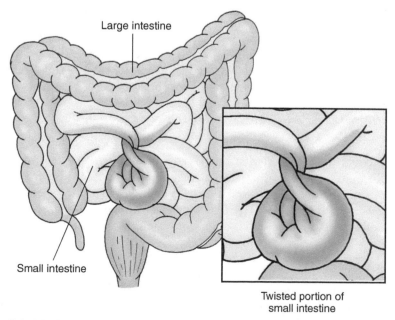

FIGURE CS3–1 Volvulus *(Finnegan & Eagle, 2016)*

This diagnosis can be commonly associated with other newborn abdominal anomalies, including a diaphragmatic herniation, gastroschisis, omphalocele, or choanal atresia (https://www.aap.org/en-us/advocacy-and-policy/aap-health-initiatives/HALF -Implementation-Guide/Age-Specific-Content/Pages/Infant-Food-and-Feeding.aspx).

Gathering Information

Nurse CF assesses DB's medical and social history. The parents are asked about their newborn's feeding patterns, duration and amounts of feedings, symptoms, and history. The parents state their newborn does not seem interested in feeding and "she has not really been eating well since discharge." They have been concerned about her intake, but they did not have transportation to come to the provider's office sooner. Upon further discussion, the parents describe the green emesis and show the staff a baby blanket they brought in with a large amount of the green emesis on it.

Assessment and Diagnosis

The techniques of inspection, auscultation, and percussion and palpation are utilized to assess the nutritional and hydration state of the newborn. A head-to-toe assessment is critical for determining any nutritional problems and associated complications. It is abnormal to have weight loss occur within a short period of time associated with alterations in the mucosa, skin turgor, intake, and urine and stool output. This alteration can have a profound effect on all of the newborn's body systems.

Symptoms of a complication, including a volvulus or malrotation, can include sudden stretches of crying, the newborn drawing their legs up as if in pain, lethargy or decreased activity, and an elevation in both breathing and heart rates. Bilious vomiting is often the initial symptom and abdominal distention may or may not occur.

During the full assessment of the newborn, all body systems should be monitored for associated complications. A weight is obtained with all clothing removed, and a measurement tape is used to determine length for a weight-for-length percentile. Head and chest circumferences are obtained to determine head and chest circumference-for-age percentages.

Newborn reflexes should be evaluated during a newborn assessment, including the rooting, sucking, and palmar grasp and Moro reflexes. The absence of newborn reflexes may indicate a problem or complication in the newborn (Dillon, 2016).

The information obtained during the assessment is plotted on a gender-specific growth chart for birth to 24-month-old patients to determine the precise distribution of body measurements as determined by the WHO Child Growth Standards (http:// www.who.int/childgrowth/en).

Diagnosis

A focused physical examination of DB reveals a quiet appearing newborn with no evidence of urine or stool in the diaper. The health-care provider, JH, places the newborn on an NPO status, then assesses DB's abdomen, finding it to be soft and distended with hypoactive bowel sounds. The concern for a GI complication related to the signs and symptoms verbalized by the parents and the incidence of green emesis is discussed and the need for immediate follow-up is presented to the parents. DB is urgently referred to the radiology department at the local hospital for an abdominal x-ray test to rule out an acute abdominal obstruction. The parents are informed of provider JH's immediate concern for the newborn. The decision is made to transfer newborn DB to the hospital, and an ambulance is called for transport because of the provider's high suspicion of a surgical emergency diagnosis.

The radiologist calls provider JH's office after the abdominal x-rays are read and requests an order for an upper GI contrast study for confirmation of the suspected diagnosis. The upper GI study confirms an abdominal obstruction. A nasogastric tube and intravenous access are placed in radiology and a pediatric surgical consultation is made for a diagnosis of malrotation.

Treatment Options

A prompt diagnosis is essential to timely medical or surgical interventions, which support enhanced outcomes for the newborn. A volvulus can be life threatening if not recognized or treated promptly by a surgical intervention.

An upper GI contrast study may show an obstruction at the second portion of the duodenum. Emergency surgical intervention should be considered once this diagnosis is established in a newborn. Midgut volvulus can be associated with a mortality rate of 28%. Elective surgery may also be performed in patients who have been diagnosed by an x-ray study performed for other symptoms or for a suspected diagnosis.

Abdominal surgery is needed to correct a volvulus by "untwisting" the malrotated areas of the intestines. If an area of the intestine has a reduced blood supply with subsequent ischemia, a portion of the intestines may need to be removed. This procedure may leave a newborn's appendix in a different location in the abdomen and an appendectomy may also be performed to reduce the potential for future complications associated with the appendix.

Treatment and Follow-Up

Newborn DB was admitted to the pediatric unit from the radiology department, and an order for NPO was written. Intravenous fluids were initiated to prevent dehydration, and a pediatric surgeon assessed DB and evaluated the diagnostic tests.

The decision was made to take DB to the operating room for a surgical repair as soon as possible to prevent further damage to the intestines by restoring circulation after untwisting the malrotation. The surgical procedure to repair the intestinal twisting was a success, and circulation was restored to the intestinal area. An appendectomy was performed to prevent future potential complications of this organ.

The newborn was discharged home without incident after a 2-day hospitalization, to a positive long-term outlook. No further treatment or follow-up was needed for this diagnosis and surgical treatment.

Summary

A nutritional assessment in a newborn is an essential component of every provider visit, so that possible nutritional risks can be quickly identified and corrected. Adequate nutrition in a newborn can be affected by the presence of feeding difficulties, inadequate intake, or inability to retain feedings. Sources of these problems can include medical or surgical conditions that can require medical or surgical interventions. Any ongoing symptoms related to nutritional alterations warrant further examination to rule out the presence of gastrointestinal pathology. The presence of green emesis, in particular, is concerning in a newborn who is not eating well, has lost significant weight over a short period of time, and who is not voiding or stooling sufficiently. Additional symptoms can include sudden periods of crying, an accelerated heart rate and respirations, a decrease in movement, and failure to thrive. These symptoms can indicate the congenital anomaly of intestinal malrotation, which often leads to the development of a volvulus (twisting of the small or large intestines) within the first year of life. The outlook for volvulus varies and depends largely on the speed of diagnosis and treatment. Early diagnosis and treatment of volvulus can help prevent future serious gastrointestinal complications and nutritional deficiencies.

Key Points

- It is important for parents to maintain records of a newborn's intake and output to establish adequate nutritional patterns.
- A timely assessment of a newborn with a gastrointestinal malrotation is essential to reduce the potential for complications.
- The signs and symptoms of a newborn gastrointestinal surgical emergency can be subtle and may mimic other diagnoses.

Review Questions

1. **The nurse is reviewing the health history of a 5-day-old newborn. The nurse understands that a newborn's nutrition should consist of which of the following at 5 days of age? (Select all that apply).**
   a. Soft foods
   b. Breast milk
   c. Formula
   d. Steamed vegetables

2. **When explaining the normal weight gain of a newborn to parents, which of the following statements made by the nurse is correct?**
   a. "You should expect a weight gain of 0.5 to 1.0 ounce daily for the next 2 months."
   b. "Breast milk and formula should be alternated with each feeding."
   c. "You can expect to feed your newborn until they are full each feeding."
   d. "It is acceptable to let your newborn sleep through the night without feedings."

3. **Which of the following symptoms are suggestive of a gastrointestinal volvulus? (Select all that apply).**
   a. Distended abdomen
   b. Hypoactive bowel sounds
   c. Increased stooling
   d. An increase in breast milk or formula intake

4. **A gastrointestinal malrotation is considered to be a surgical emergency.**
   a. True
   b. False

5. **The nurse understands that a normal newborn reflex associated with feeding is which of the following?**
   a. Moro
   b. Palmar grasp
   c. Babinski
   d. Rooting

See the appendix for answers to review questions.

References

American Academy of Pediatrics. (2019). Infant food and feeding. Retrieved from https://www.aap.org/en-us/advocacy-and-policy/aap-health-initiatives/HALF-Implementation-Guide/Age-Specific-Content/Pages/Infant-Food-and-Feeding.aspx

Dillon, P. M. (2016). *Nursing health assessment*. Philadelphia, PA: F.A. Davis.

Finnegan, L., & Eagle, S. (2016). *Medical terminology in a flash! A multiple learning styles approach* (3rd ed.). Philadelphia, PA: F.A. Davis.

Goolsby, M. J., & Grubbs, L. (2019). *Advanced assessment: Interpreting findings and formulating differential diagnosis*. Philadelphia, PA: F.A. Davis.

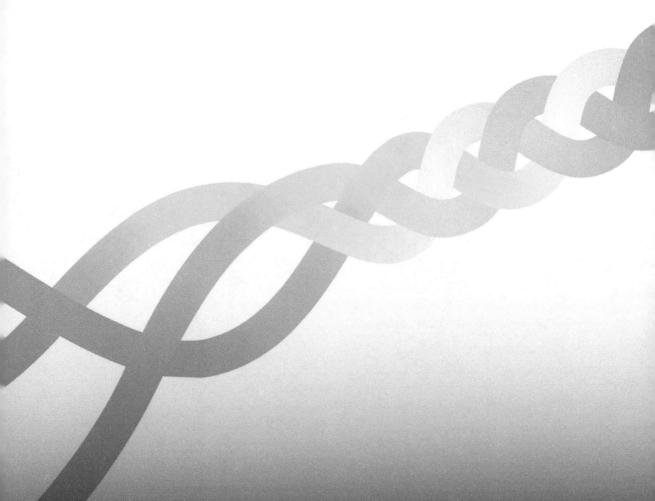

Section **4**

Pediatrics

Chapter 14

Asthma

LEARNING OBJECTIVES

Upon completion of this chapter the student will be able to:

- Integrate knowledge of the physiology, pathophysiology, assessment, and nonpharmacological and pharmacological management for care of a pediatric patient with asthma.
- Appraise current standards of care for pediatric patients with asthma.

Introduction

Asthma is the most common chronic pediatric illness, affecting over 6.2 million (8.4%) of U.S. children and their families (American Lung Association [ALA], 2020; Centers for Disease Control and Prevention [CDC], 2017). Globally, it is estimated that 235 million people of all ages have asthma (World Health Organization [WHO], 2017); although it is a public health problem in all countries, over 80% of asthma deaths occurs in low-income and lower-middle-income countries.

Asthma's associated breathing problems are usually episodic, inferred by the term *asthma attack*; however, the underlying causative inflammation is a continuous and chronic condition. Airway obstruction that occurs with acute attacks may be prevented with vigilant asthma management and is usually reversible with medication(s). With early identification and treatment, acute asthma attacks may be prevented, and there are no permanent changes to the lungs. Many pediatric patients and their families are not aware of the necessity of daily management of inflammation caused by asthma (ALA, 2020; Global Initiative for Asthma [GINA], 2017). Because the illness may not manifest itself on a daily basis, adherence to a daily regimen of preventive care may be very difficult.

Healthy People 2020 Guidelines for asthma management include recommendations for children to have current asthma action plans and to receive quality patient education in order to improve outcomes (U.S. Department of Health and Human Services, 2017). Improved asthma symptom control is associated with positive outcomes in children, specifically better school attendance and fewer emergency room visits and/or hospitalizations (ALA, 2020; National Asthma Education and Prevention Program [NAEPP], 2007). It is important to facilitate an optimal asthma management plan for each child. Many nurses are in daily contact with children who have asthma and may have multiple opportunities to influence the management of this condition.

Physiology

Certain specific physical factors contribute to asthma severity in children. There is significant airway resistance in children due to the following characteristics of child physiology as opposed to the physiology of adults: (1) larger tongue, (2) smaller airways due to predominantly nose breathing, (3) decreased pharyngeal muscle tone, (4) increased airway compliance, and (5) less elastic recoil (NAEPP, 2007). The respiratory muscles, especially the diaphragmatic muscles, are not as efficient and also have less endurance in children than in adults. Children have fewer alveoli and collateral channels of ventilation, which negatively affects resting respiratory function. This is especially significant when compensatory increased respiratory capacity is required, such as during exercise. Children also have high resting metabolic rates and oxygen consumption, resulting in less capacity to adapt to deficits and often leading to an acute asthma attack. Immature neurological breathing control increases the risk of apnea (ALA, 2010a; Asthma and Allergy Foundation of America [AAFA], 2020; NAEPP, 2007).

In 2007, the National Heart, Lung, and Blood Institute (NHLBI) released recommendations for treatment based on the frequency of symptoms, which are still considered the standard of care. Asthma is classified as (1) mild intermittent, (2) mild persistent, (3) moderate persistent, or (4) severe persistent (GINA, 2017; NAEPP, 2007). This classification is based on the frequency of events in the following categories: (1) asthma symptoms, (2) nighttime awakenings, (3) short-acting beta agonist use, (4) interference with activities, (5) lung function, and (6) exacerbations (NAEPP, 2007). For the child with intermittent asthma, there may be rare interferences with activities, and asthma symptoms are present fewer than 2 days per week. At the other end of the continuum, the child with severe asthma has persistent symptoms, and activities are extremely limited. As asthma severity increases, there is the potential for a greater negative impact on the child and family. Fortunately, most asthma in children is categorized as mild to moderate, and only 10% of asthma in children is considered severe, based on the new criteria (ALA, 2020). However, these severe cases represent a disproportionate amount of the mortality and cost statistics related to this condition (ALA, 2020; NAEPP, 2007).

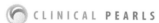

CLINICAL PEARLS
Asthma must be viewed by the child and family as a chronic illness, rather than merely occasional acute exacerbations.

Pathophysiology

Asthma is a condition characterized by an ongoing, underlying inflammatory process, with periods of latency and exacerbations (ALA, 2020). Asthma is the result of a complex interaction of changes at the cellular level leading to chronic inflammation in the airways and hyper-responsiveness of the bronchioles (ALA, 2020; NAEPP, 2007). At the cellular level, inflammation may be mediated and increased by the presence of *platelet-activating factor* (PAF), which also causes bronchoconstriction. PAF initiates an inflammatory response in the bronchioles. The levels of PAF are regulated by *PAF acetylhydrolases* (PAF-AH), which are enzymes that break down PAF and convert it into an inactive compound. When there are high concentrations of PAF in the lungs due to an allergic response, there will be more inflammation and bronchoconstriction. While the levels of PAF-AH can be measured and a child with low PAF-AH levels identified as high risk for anaphylaxis after exposure to an allergic trigger, the physiological mechanisms related to regulating PAF-AH have not yet been identified (ALA, 2020). Although no medications increase the PAF-AF enzymes levels, pediatric massage has been effective in reducing both PAF and prostaglandin levels with an accompanying improvement in clinical symptoms in children with asthma (Wu, Yang, & Zhang, 2017).

After initial diagnosis, children may experience a latent phase of asthma and be asymptomatic; however, the inflammatory condition remains active, especially in the lower airways. With exposure to a trigger, such as secondhand smoke, the airways constrict due to hyper-responsiveness, causing coughing and wheezing (ALA, 2020). The airways in children are very small, so a small degree of increased inflammation and/or bronchoconstriction can cause significant respiratory impairment (ALA, 2020; NAEPP, 2007).

Physiological Factors

There are four physiological factors that interact to cause asthma: bronchoconstriction, airway edema, airway hyper-responsiveness, and airway remodeling. Airway narrowing, caused by acute or chronic bronchoconstriction, occurs and results in interference with airflow. In an acute asthma attach, this bronchoconstriction occurs quickly in response to a trigger. When an allergen is the trigger, bronchoconstriction results from an IgE-dependent release of mediators (histamine, tryptase, leukotrienes, and prostaglandins) from mast cells that contract airway smooth muscle. Medications, including aspirin and other NSAIDs, may cause bronchoconstriction in some children. Environmental triggers, such as exercise, cold air, air pollution, and stress, can also cause bronchoconstriction; these responses are less well understood but may be related to pro-inflammatory cytokines (GINA, 2017; NAEPP, 2007).

Airway edema occurs with the progression of asthma and includes inflammation, increased mucus production and the formation of mucus plugs. Also, airway hyper-responsiveness occurs in more severe asthma and is due to the bronchioles' constriction in response to methacholine and inflammation. Airway remodeling occurs when there are permanent structural airway changes, which is particularly ominous when it occurs in children because the long-term effects are serious (NAEPP, 2007).

Age

The child's age and developmental level also are indicative of the amount of independence in self-management that the child may safely assume. Because over half of all cases of asthma begin before the age of 10, the family may incur years of daily stress related to managing a chronic illness with a complicated medication regimen (Ezzell, 2017). Asthma classification in children 12 years and older is the same as for adults and is based on criteria described earlier (NAEPP, 2007). Because a child's age is usually directly correlated to their size (except in conditions with growth retardation, cardiovascular conditions that impair growth, and/or musculoskeletal diseases that affect stature and growth), the bronchioles and related structure grow as the child ages. With the small bronchioles of an infant, minimal inflammation or constriction may impede airflow and result in asthma symptoms, while larger bronchioles are often less hyper-responsive and have a larger lumen that is not as easily affected by these factors (GINA, 2017; NAEPP, 2007).

Sex

There are disparities between the sexes in asthma prevalence. Historically, boys were more likely to have asthma; however, CDC data reveal a shift with a rate of 6.2% among boys, as compared to a 9.1% rate among girls (ALA, 2020; CDC, 2018). From a social perspective, boys are less likely than girls to accept asthma as a part of their personal identity (GINA, 2017), and thus may have more difficulty incorporating necessary asthma management into daily routines and treating themselves in public settings. However, because boys often minimize the effect of asthma, they may be more likely to participate in physical activities, especially sports, and therefore experience higher levels of normalization as compared to girls (GINA, 2017).

Genetics

Recent research into intergenerational asthma has investigated the association between parental and child asthma (Clancy & Blake, 2013; Valerio, Andreski, Schoeni, & McGoagle, 2010). Those researchers found that children with a parent with asthma were almost twice as likely to have asthma, as compared to children who did not have a parent with asthma. Also, in a longitudinal study by Tai (2016) that followed children with asthma into adulthood, most children with mild intermittent asthma achieve remission and do not have ongoing symptoms into adult life. In this study, the main risk factors for persistent asthma into adulthood were female sex, parental history of asthma, and atopy in allergic rhinitis. Specifically, atopy refers to the genetic predisposition to develop any allergic disease and is usually associated with a heightened immune response to common allergens, especially inhaled allergens (e.g., perfumes, pollution, pollen) and/or food allergens. In addition, a French study identified the following factors that increase susceptibility to adverse respiratory effects of asthma: parent history of allergies, stressful event, and male sex (Ranciere, Bougas, Viola, & Momas, 2017).

It is accepted that asthma is a complex disorder, with both genetic and environmental factors responsible for its expression in children.

Race and Environment

According to the CDC, African Americans have higher morbidity and mortality due to asthma (CDC, 2017). Fortunately, asthma rarely leads to death in children, and only 185 children died of asthma in 2017, which corresponds to a death rate of 2.5/million; the death rate for asthma in adults is 13.4/million (CDC, 2017). However, a comparison of asthma by racial groups has the following results: European American (8.1/million), African American (22.7/million), and Hispanic American (7.1/million) (CDC, 2017). Similarly, in the CDC 2018 statistics, there are disparities among asthma prevalence based on race: European American (7.6%), African American (10.6%), and Hispanic American (6.4%). African American children age 10 years and younger had the highest risk of increased asthma prevalence, morbidity, and potential mortality (CDC, 2018).

Exposure to poor air quality is also an environmental asthma trigger, and African Americans are more likely to live in urban areas that have poor air quality (ALA, 2020; CDC, 2017). There is a disproportionate burden of exposure to air toxins in the African American population. Specifically, 68% of African Americans live within 30 miles of a coal-fired power plant, as compared to 56% of European Americans. Also, ozone exposure increases the mortality rates among African Americans at a higher rate than for European Americans, which is an example of racial disparities in the response to poor air quality (AAFA, 2020).

Assessment

A diagnosis of asthma is based on assessment findings; however, a diagnosis of asthma is also age dependent. According to the American Association of Pediatrics, for children 5 years of age and older, doctors diagnose asthma with the same tests used to identify the disease in adults. However, in younger children, a definitive diagnosis may be difficult because symptoms, especially wheezing, may be related to other causes and diagnostic tests aren't as accurate (Mayo Clinic, 2017). On inspection, the pediatric patient with asthma may have no visible signs of their chronic illness (Dillon, 2017).

If the child has concomitant allergies, they may exhibit darkness under their eyes (e.g., *allergic shiners*) and/or a horizontal nasal crease (e.g., from frequent *allergic salute*). During an acute attack, the patient will often appear anxious and may have peripheral cyanosis. However, careful observation of the child's breathing may reveal increased respiratory rate and use of accessory muscles (Dillon, 2017; Goolsby & Grubbs, 2015).

Asthma does not usually result in any abnormal findings on palpation, nor is palpation an effective assessment tool during an acute attack. Percussion findings are also normal unless there is hyper-resonance due to air trapping. However, with a child's thin chest wall, hyper-resonance may be difficult to determine (Dillon, 2017). Wheezing on auscultation is the hallmark objective finding of asthma. However, wheezing may be due to inflammation from any causative agent and is not limited to asthma. These continuous (as compared to intermittent, such as rhonchi) musical tones are most commonly heard at end inspiration or early expiration. They are a result of an obstructed airway lumen that gradually opens during inspiration or gradually closes during expiration. As the airway lumen becomes smaller, the air flow velocity increases, resulting in vibration of the airway wall.

Wheezes can be classified and/or described as either high-pitched or low-pitched wheezes. It has been inferred that high-pitched wheezes are associated with disease of the small airways and low-pitched wheezes are associated with disease of larger airways; however, this relationship between sounds and the size of airways has not been confirmed (ALA, 2020; GINA, 2017). Wheezes may be monophonic (a single pitch and tonal quality heard over a focal area) or polyphonic (multiple pitches and tones heard over a multiple areas of the lung).

Wheezes are due to decreased airway lumen diameter related either to inflammation or thickening of reactive airway walls or to collapse of airways. It is important to note in which lung field(s) the wheezing occurs, which provides an estimate of the extent and severity of bronchoconstriction. However, with a child's thin chest wall, wheezing is often audible throughout lung fields. The nurse should also note if wheezing occurs on inspiration and/or expiration; while either type of wheezing may occur in asthma, it is the high-pitched inspiratory wheeze of stridor that occurs with significant airway resistance (Dillon, 2017; NAEPP, 2007). Finally, when airways are very inflamed, air movement is so impaired that wheezes may actually decrease while the condition worsens; the nurse must take into account all assessment findings in order to correctly evaluate the child's condition as it changes (Goolsby & Grubbs, 2015).

HIGH YIELD FACT FOR TESTING

A written asthma action plan should always accompany an asthma diagnosis.

Diagnostic Tests

Pulmonary function tests are performed to measure lung function. With asthma, there may be diminished *forced expiratory volume* (FEV) and decreased *forced vital capacity* (FVC) due to diminished expiration and outflow. Chest x-ray of a child with asthma is usually normal unless there is significant air trapping and is therefore not useful enough to warrant risk to the child (Goolsby & Grubbs, 2015).

Peak flow measurements are a simple, inexpensive, and noninvasive way to monitor a child's asthma management. It is recommended for children in all asthma classifications, but especially for children who have frequent symptoms. Based on the NHLBI guidelines for asthma management, a child with severe asthma will require multiple daily assessments of peak flow with medication adjustments based on their status (NAEPP, 2007). Teaching points for patient and family education on using peak flow meter measurements effectively are provided in SENC Box 14-1.

SENC BOX 14–1 Safe and Effective Nursing Care for Patient Education on Using a Peak Flow Meter

1. Place the marker at the bottom of the scale on the flow meter.
2. Have the child stand up or sit up so there is maximum diaphragmatic expansion.
3. Instruct the child to:
   - Take a deep breath
   - Close lips around the mouthpiece
   - Blow (not huff or cough) out as hard and as fast as possible.
4. Write down the number from the meter.
5. Obtain a total of three measurements and document the best in the child's journal. Follow the asthma action plan based on the reading.

Nonpharmacological Management

Self-management is an important coping mechanism for both the child and their family. Necessary changes for the family who has a child with asthma may include making alterations to the environment to decrease asthma triggers, learning daily asthma management techniques (see SENC Box 14-1), and living with the possibility of an asthma attack that will require emergent intervention (ALA, 2020; NAEPP, 2007). When using any self-management technique, it's important that the child learn and use good technique, and make best efforts, so cooperation is key.

Asthma Education Programs

When the child and family have adequate information and skills to successfully manage the illness, they are empowered and feel less stressed and overwhelmed. Asthma education programs have been implemented in partnerships with school systems to provide information to children with asthma about how to better manage their condition. In general, these programs have been successful in providing asthma education in the school setting but have encountered difficulties in outcome measurement. There are many factors that impact a child's asthma management, and education is only one aspect of a multifaceted condition.

Asthma camps are innovative interventions that allow children with asthma to safely participate in activities that may otherwise be discouraged for them (AAFA, 2020; ALA, 2020). Additionally, asthma camps are effective in increasing self-efficacy among the children and their ability to manage asthma, along with helping to decrease the stigma of having a chronic illness by creating support among children with asthma (NAEPP, 2007).

Asthma Care Coordination

In this model of care coordination, a nurse makes a home visit to assess the child's asthma triggers and help the family address challenges with asthma management. Then, the asthma care navigators connect the child and family with care providers to encourage continuity of care and decrease *emergency department* (ED) care utilization. The navigator role developed in oncology nursing but has subsequently been used in a variety of care areas. It carries the following responsibilities: coordination of care, communication, education, and expertise in knowledge and experience (Baileys et al., 2018). According to the American Association for Respiratory Care (AARC), respiratory therapists are also fulfilling the navigator role and promoting better outcomes (AARC, 2020). With asthma, the care coordination aspect can be a valuable deterrent to fragmented care and resulting frequent ED visits with inadequate follow-up care. For example, in a multi-site study, Janevic and colleagues used structured asthma care coordination programs to improve outcomes for children in urban, low-income African American and Hispanic American communities. Children enrolled in these programs experienced fewer asthma symptoms and had fewer asthma-related ED visits as compared to a control group (Janevic et al., 2016). Similarly, a study by Smith, Clayton, Woodell, and Mansfield (2017) found that navigators helped parents understand and manage their child's asthma primarily by helping them identify potential asthma triggers and individualize the asthma management plan.

Environmental Changes

Nurses teach families how to identify the specific triggers for their child's asthma, such as viral infections, allergies, and exercise, and then how to make environmental changes to avoid these triggers. While asthma attacks are often unpredictable and unpreventable, parents can be armed with knowledge and skills to reduce the environmental triggers and manage acute attacks. Infections are the main trigger of acute asthma in children of all ages, followed by allergies in school-age children (Dondi et al., 2017).

There is also evidence that early intervention when a child develops a viral infection, with increased asthma medication, will decrease potential exacerbations and potential complications, such as pneumonia. Because children who are in day care settings are often exposed to more illnesses, it is important to identify signs and symptoms of a respiratory infection early.

Exposure to air toxins such as those emitted by coal-fired power plants and ozone is associated with asthma exacerbations, particularly among African American children, as noted earlier. The relationship between *traffic-related air pollution* (TRAP) and the incidence of asthma in preschool children is well supported. Parents can protect their children from air pollution by limiting their time outside when air quality is poor, keeping windows closed when traveling in a car, and ensuring older school buses are replaced or retrofitted to decrease emissions. Laws that restrict air pollution will help prevent acute asthma attacks in sensitive children and may result in better asthma outcomes (U.S. Environmental Protection Agency [EPA], 2020).

In order to determine specific allergens and/or sensitivities, skin or in vitro testing is indicated for patients with asthma. Once the asthma triggers are identified, a multifaceted approach is most effective. All children with asthma should avoid exposure to tobacco smoke, including secondhand exposure on clothing, hair, and furniture. Allergen immunotherapy may be indicated when there is a clear connection to symptom exacerbation with exposure (NAEPP, 2007). With individualized care based on the classification of the child's asthma and the child's response to treatment, the child and entire family can lead active lives (NAEPP, 2007).

Exercise

While exercise may be a trigger for asthma, it may also be beneficial for children with asthma when it is well controlled and not too strenuous. If indicated, it is important for children to use an inhaler prophylactically before exercising. If cold weather is a trigger, the child should not exercise in the cold, thus paring two triggers and potentiating a synergistic effect. But when approached within guidelines, exercise can result in improved lung function, which may decrease asthma symptoms (GINA, 2017; Mayo Clinic, 2017).

ASSESSMENT PEARLS

Children and families should be taught how to monitor asthma control using a peak flow meter at home.

Pharmacology

Evidence supports using a full assessment of the patient in order to individualize pharmacological treatment for asthma. The step method is used as a guide, but the patient's regimen should always be based on current lung function measured by peak flow. The step treatment is based on age and has established age categories as follows: 0 to 4 years, 5 to 11 years, and 12 years and older (see Table 14-1).

The steps are implemented when nonpharmacological interventions, such as trigger removal, are not effective and the child experiences symptoms. A child is usually started on step 1, which is a short-acting beta-adrenergic inhaler unless symptoms are more severe than mild intermittent. Steps 1 and 2 are the same, regardless of the child's age. At step 3 there are differences in medication for the 0 to 4 age-group as a *long-acting beta agonist* (LABA) or low-dose *inhaled corticosteroid* (ICS) may be used with older children. Children are started on step 1 whenever possible, and reevaluated monthly with an initial diagnosis and then usually every three months, so there is a balance of optimal symptom control with lowest medication usage (NAEPP, 2007).

When a child is stable at a step for at least 3 months, the provider may choose to decrease by a step, after taking into consideration other factors such as comorbidities, seasonal allergies, and environmental triggers. An evaluation of the appropriateness of the current step, and whether to increase, maintain, or decrease it, should be performed at each primary care visit (NAEPP, 2007). When a child has an asthma exacerbation and/or other illness, it is not considered a safe time to make changes to their asthma step regimen (ALA, 2020).

In a study of 600 parents with asthma, it was noted that parents had incorrect perceptions regarding their child's illness, including (1) that asthma is solely hereditary, and (2) that children may become dependent on asthma medications (Abu-Saheen, Nofal, & Heena, 2016; Woo & Robinson, 2020). The more that parents understand the importance of the medications prescribed for their child, and are involved in

TABLE 14–1   Pharmacological Treatment for Patients with Asthma Based on Age

Step	0–4 Years	5–11 Years	12 Years and Over
1	SABA as needed	SABA as needed	SABA as needed
2	Low-dose ICS OR Cromolyn or montelukast	Low-dose ICS OR Cromolyn or theophylline	Low-dose ICS OR Cromolyn or theophylline
3	Medium-dose ICS	Low-dose ICS + either LABA or theophylline OR Medium-dose ICS	Low-dose ICS + LABA OR Medium-dose ICS
4	Medium-dose ICS + either LABA or montelukast	Medium-dose ICS + LABA	Medium-dose ICS + LABA
5	High-dose ICS + either LABA or montelukast	High-dose ICS + LABA	High-dose ICS + LABA and consider omalizumab
6	High-dose ICS + either LABA or montelukast + oral corticosteroids	High-dose ICS + LABA or montelukast + oral corticosteroids	High-dose ICS + LABA + oral corticosteroids and consider omalizumab

(NAEPP, 2007; Woo & Robinson, 2020)
  ICS, inhaled corticosteroid; LABA, long-acting beta agonist; SABA, short-acting beta agonist

decision making, the more likely they are to adhere to the step method of pharmaco-logical treatment for asthma (Ezzell, 2017). It is important to have open communica-tion with parents and to negotiate how they can best make environmental changes and incorporate medication regimens into their families' lives (Wallinger & Hucker, 2012).

Short-Acting Beta Agonists (SABA)

These medications stimulate beta$_2$-adrenergic receptors in the lungs, which results in bronchodilation, which in turn results in smooth muscle relaxation. As the name implies, a SABA has both a fast onset and short duration of action, making them the preferred treatment for an acute attack and/or exacerbation. These medications are first line for asthma management as long as the asthma is classified as mild inter-mittent and the inhaler isn't needed more than twice a week (NAEPP, 2007; Woo & Robinson, 2020). It is important for parents to realize that even though their child rarely has asthma symptoms that are well controlled with a SABA, they are at risk for a more severe asthma attack (GINA, 2017). Guidelines for teaching children and their families to use a SABA are presented in SENC Box 14-2.

Long-Acting Beta Agonists (LABA)

These medications also stimulate beta$_2$-adrenergic receptors in the lungs and result in bronchodilation. However, they have both a slower onset of action with a longer effec-tive duration, as compared to the SABA group, and are effective as a preventive treat-ment in asthma management. When the child experiences asthma more frequently and has reached step 3 (if 5 years or older) or step 4 (if up to 4 years old), a LABA may be added to an ICS for symptom control. According to current NHLBI guidelines, a LABA is added to another medication and is not used alone (GINA, 2017; NAEPP, 2007; Woo & Robinson, 2020).

Inhaled Corticosteroids (ICS)

This category of medications is often necessary for long-term control of persistent asthma and is implemented at step 2 or 3, depending on age. Because ICSs are inhaled, they have a direct anti-inflammatory effect in the lungs. They are usually administered as a daily maintenance dose, which may be once a day for increased convenience and compliance. Children and their parents need education on administration to ensure that maximum benefit is obtained from the lowest dose and that side effects are mini-mized (NAEPP, 2007; Woo & Robinson, 2020). Because the ICS class of medications is critical to maintaining asthma control and preventing exacerbations, it is necessary for children and parents to adhere to the regimen (Ezzell, 2017). (See SENC Box 14-3.)

SENC BOX 14-2 Safe and Effective Nursing Care for Patients on SABA for Asthma Exacerbations and Prophylaxis

1. Use of a SABA depends on severity of symptoms. Clarify what specific symptoms should prompt SABA use (coughing, wheezing, respiratory infection).
2. If administering SABA via nebulizer treatments, usually 3 treatments (1 every 20 minutes) are adequate to resolve an asthma attack. If not, consult your health-care provider.
3. A short course of oral systemic corticosteroids (1–2 mg/kg/day × 3–5 days) taken with a SABA may also be needed to resolve an asthma exacerbation, especially if there are comorbidities, such as a respiratory infection.
4. If a child uses a SABA more than 2 days/week for symptom relief, treatment may need to move to the next step.

> **SENC BOX 14–3**   Safe and Effective Nursing Care for Patients on Inhaled Corticosteroids for Asthma
>
> 1. To decrease the potential for mouth irritation and yeast infection:
>   - Use lowest effective dose.
>   - Rinse mouth after administration.
>   - Use inhaler device and rinse after use.
> 2. ICS use may slow a child's growth rate slightly. This effect on linear growth is not predictable and is generally small (about 1 cm), appears to occur in the first several months of treatment, and is not progressive.
> 3. Systemic side effects may occur but are much less than with oral steroids.
> 4. Emphasize that this medication is for prevention and will not be effective in an acute attack.

Combination Inhalers

These medications combine in a single inhaler an ICS and a LABA, both of which are preventive or maintenance asthma treatments. When a child is at step 3 or 4 (depending on age), the combination of these two maintenance medications can be administered in this manner. Patients are able to administer two maintenance medications, usually twice daily with a dose dependent on asthma severity. It is crucial that the child and family understand that these are two separate medications and that they are both preventive and not for an acute asthma attach. With proper education, this can be an effective method to increase convenience and compliance with the plan of care (NAEPP, 2007; Woo & Robinson, 2020).

Leukotriene-Receptor Antagonists

By binding to IgE receptors on the surface of mast cells and basophils, the leukotriene-receptor antagonists inhibit the release of inflammatory mediators and are effective as a treatment for asthma as well as for chronic allergic conditions (see Chapter 15). Leukotrienes are considered more important than prostaglandins in the inflammatory response, so blocking their activity prevents bronchoconstriction and mucus production due to allergens. Montelukast is approved for use in children over age 12 months both for prophylaxis and acute treatment of allergic rhinitis (American Academy of Allergy Asthma and Immunology [AAAAI], 2020; Woo & Robinson, 2020).

Mast Cell Stabilizers

Cromolyn is the medication in this classification that is used to treat asthma in children. It exerts an anti-inflammatory effect by inhibiting the activation and release of mast cells (inflammatory mediators) for early- and late-phase asthma response. It is thought to work by decreasing the neural response to irritation of sensory nerve fibers in the airways and decreasing the release of cytokines from pre-formed eosinophils (Sharma, Hashmi, & Chakraborty, 2020). It is especially effective when the asthma triggers are allergens or exercise. This medication is administered by metered-dose inhaler or nebulizer and has fewer side effects than inhaled steroids. It must be used daily for at least 3 to 4 weeks before its maximum effect is achieved. Its four times a day dosing is a barrier to compliance, especially for a school-age child. Cromolyn is useful in asthma prevention and is not for acute attacks even though it can be administered via nebulizer (Woo & Robinson, 2020). The major side effects include coughing, flushing, palpitation, pruritus, dysphagia, esophageal spasm, tinnitus, polycythemia, pancytopenia, wheezing, bronchospasm, throat irritation, nasal congestion, and anaphylaxis (Sharma et al., 2020; Woo & Robinson, 2020).

Biological Response Modifier/Monoclonal Antibody

These medications, such as omalizumab (Xolair), are usually introduced only with persistent asthma symptoms in steps 5 and/or 6. These medications bind to IgE receptors on the surface of mast cells and basophils, which decrees the release of inflammatory mediators. Administration is via the subcutaneous route and requires close monitoring for anaphylaxis. Due to the immunosuppressive properties of the medication, exposure to viral infections and live vaccines should be avoided (NAEPP, 2007; Woo & Robinson, 2020). These and all other asthma medications are detailed in Table 14-2.

> **HIGH YIELD FACT FOR TESTING**
>
> Many children do not use proper technique when administering an inhaler; have the child bring their inhaler to office visits and demonstrate how they use it.

TABLE 14–2 Medications for Treating Asthma

Class	Example	Action	Indication	Adverse Effects	SENC
Short-acting beta agonists	Albuterol 1–2 inhalations q 4–6 hr. Administered via nebulizer if child cannot use inhaler.	Activates adrenergic (primarily beta$_2$) receptors in lungs to promote bronchodilation.	Treatment of an acute asthma attack and/or prophylactically when exposure to an asthma trigger is anticipated.	Arrhythmias, tachycardia, hypertension, hyperactivity, insomnia dizziness, vertigo.	Close monitoring of cardiac rate/rhythm, blood pressure, pulse oximetry.
Long-acting beta agonists	Formoterol Inhale contents of 1 capsule q 12 hr.	Stimulates production of intracellular cyclic adenosine monophosphate (AMP), which relaxes smooth muscle and inhibits release of mediators from mast cells in lungs.	Treatment of asthma and prevention of exercise-induced asthma.	Headache, bronchitis, dyspnea, fatal asthma exacerbation.	Best administered 12 hr apart to ensure adequate coverage over 24 hr.
Inhaled corticosteroids	Mometasone 1 inhalation 100 mcg qd	Decrease inflammation in lung tissue, especially bronchioles.	Treat asthma and decrease inflammation.	Oral candidiasis, sore throat, hoarseness.	Distinguish between oral and nasal inhalers.
Leukotriene receptor antagonists	Montelukast 4 mg qd for child 12 mo–5 yr 5 mg qd for child older than 6 yr.	Inhibit bronchoconstriction and mucus production by blocking leukotrienes.	Prophylaxis and treatment of asthma.	Dizziness, headache, nasal congestion.	Chewable tablets contain phenylalanine. Administer at bedtime.
Mast cell stabilizers	Cromolyn Inhaled nasally qid or 2.5–10 mg/kg/day in 3–4 doses.	Inhibits release of bronchoconstrictors; histamine and slow-reacting substance of anaphylaxis (SRS-A).	Prevention of mild to moderate asthma and allergic rhinitis.	Angioedema, anaphylaxis, bronchospasm.	Administer oral dose with food to decrease gastrointestinal (GI) irritation.

Asthma Action Plan

Undergirding the use of the above medications, is the child's asthma action plan. Based on the child's symptoms and peak flow measurements, medications may be adjusted by the parent in the short-term until seen by a provider (ALA, 2020; GINA, 2017; NAEPP, 2007; Woo & Robinson, 2020). An asthma action plan is usually developed by the child's primary care provider (physician, nurse, or physician assistant) or an asthma specialist and is based on the step management approach; it uses a traffic light analogy to guide parents in the management of their child's chronic illness. Once established and implemented, an asthma action plan can be used across many settings (home, school, camp, etc.), by both medical personnel (school nurses) and others (teachers, coaches, family members), to safely mange a child's asthma symptoms and provide for a more active life (ALA, 2020; NAEPP, 2007). While children vary in their development and associated abilities to manage their asthma, it is reasonable to expect an older child (age 12 and above) to be an active participant in their asthma management (AAFA, 2020; ALA, 2020).

In the green zone, the child achieves 80% to 100% of predicted peak flow and is without asthma symptoms such as cough, wheeze, shortness of breath, or chest tightness. The plan for the child should be maintained; no changes are needed.

In comparison, when the child is in the yellow zone, the peak flow is 50% to 80% and the child may be experiencing asthma symptoms. The yellow zone plan may include increasing dosage and/or frequency of a current medication or adding a medication. If these medication changes do not result in improved symptoms within 12 to 24 hours, parents are instructed to call the provider.

Finally, a child in the red zone achieves less than 50% of their peak flow predicted number and is in an emergency situation. Parents are instructed to call the child's provider and prepare to seek emergent treatment. In addition to the asthma action plan, parents should be educated to seek emergent care under the conditions presented in SENC Box 14-4 (ALA, 2020; GINA, 2017; NAEPP, 2007; Woo & Robinson, 2020).

▶ RED FLAG ALERT

Nurses should know their state laws for a child's right to carry and self-administer asthma medication at school.

Complementary and Alternative Therapies (CAT)

Complementary therapies may be used as an adjuvant to traditional asthma management using the step guidelines, but there is limited evidence that these therapies are effective. Because the stress of managing a chronic illness may be improved by most types of relaxation and/or exercise (Ezzell, 2017), it is reasonable that these

---

SENC BOX 14–4 Safe and Effective Nursing Care to Instruct Parents When the Child Is in a Red Zone

SEEK EMERGENT CARE WHEN A CHILD:
- Has to stop talking to catch their breath
- Uses abdominal muscles to breathe
- Has enlarged nostrils (flaring)
- Is trying so hard to breathe that the abdomen is sucked under the ribs with breathing (retractions)

interventions may improve the child's asthma and assist in its control. However, massage and acupressure/acupuncture may provide measurable physiological changes for an improved lung function (*Acupuncture for Kids*, 2015; Wu et al., 2017). Depending on the age of the child, the child (or parent) should be asked in an accepting and non-judgmental manner if they use CAT, and these therapies should be considered as part of SENC.

Supervised Progressive Exercise

Physical training has been shown to benefit children for several reasons. First, the physical changes that occur with conditioning help to increase lung vital capacity and improve peak flow measurements. Exercise is also an effective method for managing stress, which may be an asthma trigger. Even when children require premedication with a SABA to participate in exercise, there are benefits to their increased activity (AAFA, 2020; ALA, 2020; NAEPP, 2007). Exercise that gradually challenges a child and requires increasingly greater effort, especially respiratory effort, is considered to be progressive and beneficial. Notably, this type of exercise may need to be initially established and supervised in a medical setting, such as an outpatient rehabilitation center, as there are potential initial risks of asthma exacerbation. Once the child has demonstrated a sustained and increasing tolerance to exercise (e.g., respiratory rate remains in a safe range for age, shortness of breath resolves quickly with rest, no audible wheezing), they can safely exercise independent of medical supervision. However, any child with asthma should notify an adult or peer when engaging in activity that may result in an asthma exacerbation as a safety precaution.

Breathing and Movement Techniques

There is limited evidence that qi gong and tai chi are effective in improving symptoms and possibly decreasing asthma severity by helping the body to maintain higher dehydroepiandrosterone (DHEA) levels, which are protective against allergic responses. The focus on deep breathing in each of these exercise forms may also improve lung function via increased vital capacity (ALA, 2020).

Buteyko is a method of controlled breathing that is based on the premise that asthma is worsened by rapid and/or mouth breathing, which is not supported by evidence. In comparison, qi gong and yoga breathing both use deep, slow breaths, while Buteyko uses breath holding and the controlled decrease of ventilation and respiratory rate. This slower respiratory rate may affect the role of carbon dioxide in body physiology, carbon dioxide levels being the stimulus for effective respirations. While emphasizing nasal breathing may have benefits because it humidifies, warms, and cleans air before it enters the lungs, strict nasal breathing during physical exercise may lead to decreased vital capacity, especially when there is inflammation and bronchoconstriction present due to asthma. Because the safety of this method is not supported by evidence, it is not recommended for children (National Asthma Council Australia, 2017).

Acupuncture

Researchers at the Cleveland Clinic have used acupuncture successfully with children for many disorders, including asthma and allergies, with few side effects. Evidence from a study with a sample of 450 children (age 0 to 17 years) showed that those children who had acupuncture experienced safe and effective symptom relief. In acupuncture, local, regional, or global points are either stimulated or calmed to

TABLE 14–3   Dietary Supplements for Asthma with Evidence to Support Efficacy

Supplement	Dose	Action and Side Effects (SEs)
Caffeine	3–9 mg/kg	Increases resting lung capacity and decreases exercise-induced asthma. SEs: Agitation, tachycardia, arrhythmias, withdrawal headaches, insomnia, diarrhea.
Vitamin D	500 units	May decreases risk of asthma exacerbations by increasing ration of T2 to T1 helper cells and promoting early immune response.

reduce symptoms (*Acupuncture for Kids*, 2015). If children are reluctant to be exposed to needles, acupressure may be used effectively initially and may lead to gently inserting needles; laser and/or electrical stimulation are also methods of delivering acupuncture.

Dietary Supplements

While dietary supplements may not be used regularly for children with asthma, there are two that have support in the literature: caffeine and vitamin D (see Table 14-3). These are not, however, without potential side effects, adverse reactions, and potential drug interactions (National Asthma Council, 2017; Woo & Robinson, 2020).

Massage

In a meta-analysis of the effect of massage therapy on asthma outcomes by Wu and colleagues (2017), the authors concluded that massage had the following positive effects: improved pulmonary function, decreased PAF and prostaglandin levels, and increased PAF-AH and Prostaglandin D_2 Receptor 1 (DP_1). However, they questioned the methodological rigor of some of the studies that were included, and they recommend more randomized controlled studies be performed (Wu et al., 2017). While massage should not be used in place of a step approach to medication, it may be an effective nonpharmacological adjuvant to an asthma management plan and has no potential side effects (Wu et al., 2017).

Summary

The consequences of having a child with asthma may be negative for both the child and other family members. Several potential negative consequences relate to childhood asthma. First, each school absence is a missed opportunity for a child to learn and develop (NAEPP, 2007). A child who has frequent illnesses is at risk for problems with school performance and delays in normal development because school provides a supportive environment for a child to meet developmental milestones (ALA, 2020; NAEPP, 2007). Next, children who have asthma frequently require care from EDs and inpatient care settings, which has implications related to cost of care, coordination of care, school absences, and parents' lost work time and wages (ALA, 2020). Last, stress levels for the entire family are often increased when a child has asthma; it is vital that the nurse plans family-centered care that addresses this stress and connects families with the necessary resources. Living with asthma is a changing, and often unpredictable environment; the child and family must be equipped to cope with this highly dynamic, chronic condition and benefit from information that is individualized and responsive (Smith et al., 2017).

Key Points

- Current knowledge of asthma is essential because it is the most common chronic illness in primary care settings.
- Asthma triggers may include cold air, stress, pet dander and other allergens, exercise, air pollution, ozone, and respiratory infection.
- Accurate peak flow measurement is necessary for correct medication regimens.
- Treatment for children with asthma is based on their age and frequency of symptoms.
- It is important to involve family members in the management of a child's asthma, including environmental alterations.
- Older children must understand their asthma action plan and be able to administer medication in an acute attack.

Review Questions

1. **The nurse anticipates that the patient will be placed on an inhaled corticosteroid. Select all of the following that apply to taking this medication, no matter which dose (low, medium, or high).**

   a. Use inhaler on an empty stomach.
   b. Use a spacer with this medication.
   c. Rinse your mouth after the inhalation.
   d. Take medication at same time each day, preferably in the morning.
   e. This medication may be inhaled orally or nasally.

2. **The family asks you, the nurse, if there's anything they can do in addition to giving their child medication for asthma. The nurse's best response is:**

   a. "Stop smoking in the house or car with your child."
   b. "Consider replacing shag carpets with wood floors."
   c. "If you have a pet, it could live outside."
   d. "Understand your child's asthma action plan."

3. **The 13-year-old patient has had asthma since she was 3 years old. She wants to go to asthma camp. What responses from the nurse are appropriate to help her and her family make a decision that will have the most benefit? (Select all that apply.)**

   a. "You have had asthma for 10 years; you know everything you need to know about asthma."
   b. "We need to make sure your asthma is in the mild category before you are away from home."
   c. "Let's make sure you understand your current asthma action plan."
   d. "This will be a great opportunity to have some freedom from asthma."
   e. "Evidence supports that these camps have positive outcomes for children and their families."

4. **A 6-year-old child is diagnosed with mild intermittent asthma. According to step pharmacological management, what is the appropriate anticipated plan of care?**

   a. Trigger identification and environmental alterations.
   b. Short-acting beta agonist (SABA) as needed.

c. SABA q 12 hours.

d. Low-dose inhaled corticosteroid q 12 hours and SABA as needed.

5. **The parent asks when to take their child with asthma for emergency care. The nurse provides education that includes which of the following signs and symptoms? (Select all that apply.)**

a. Stopping mid-sentence to catch breath

b. Paleness of the extremities

c. Audible wheezing

d. Nasal flaring

e. Chest retractions

See the appendix for answers to review questions.

References

Abu-Shaheen, A. K., Nofal, A., & Heena, H. (2016). Parental perceptions and practices toward childhood asthma. *BioMed Research International, 2016.* doi:10.1155/2016/6364194

Acupuncture for kids. (2015). Cleveland, OH: Cleveland Clinic. Retrieved from https://health.clevelandclinic.org/2013/02/acupuncture-for-kids/

American Academy of Allergy Asthma and Immunology (AAAAI), (2020). *Leukotriene modifiers.* Retrieved from: https://www.aaaai.org/conditions-and-treatments/drug-guide/montelukast

American Association for Respiratory Care. (2020). An RT is navigating the way. Retrieved from https://www.aarc.org/careers/career-advice/professional-development/an-rt-navigator-is-navigating-the-way/

American Lung Association. (2020). *Asthma & children* [Fact sheet]. Retrieved from http://www.lung.org/lung-health-and-diseases/lung-disease-lookup/asthma/learn-about-asthma/asthma-children-facts-sheet.html.

Asthma and Allergy Foundation of America. (2020). Asthma overview. Retrieved from http://www.aafa.org

Baileys, K., McMullen, L., Lubejko, B., Christensen, D., Haylock, P. J., Rose, T., . . . Srdanovic, D. (2018). Nurse Navigator Core Competencies: An update to reflect the evolution of the role. *Clinical Journal of Oncology Nursing, 22*(3), 272–281. Retrieved from https://doi.org/10.1188/18.CJON.272-281

Centers for Disease Control and Prevention. (2017). Most recent national asthma data. Retrieved from https://www.cdc.gov/asthma/most_recent_national_asthma_data.htm

Centers for Disease Control and Prevention. (2018). Asthma surveillance data. Retrieved from https://www.cdc.gov/asthma/asthmadata.htm

Clancy, J., & Blake, D. (2013). Pathophysiology and pharmacological management of asthma from a nature-nurture perspective. *Primary Health Care, 23*(7), 34–41.

Dillon, P. (2017). *Nursing health assessment: A critical thinking, case studies approach* (2nd ed.). Philadelphia, PA: F.A. Davis.

Dondi, A., Calamelli, E., Piccinno, V., Ricci, G., Corsini, I., Biagi, C., & Lanari, M. (2017). Acute asthma in the pediatric emergency department: Infections are the main triggers of exacerbations. *BioMed Research International, 2017.* doi:10.1155/2017/9687061

Ezzell, K. G. (2017). Strategies to guide medication adherence discussions with parents of children with asthma. *Pediatric Nursing, 43*(5), 219–222.

Global Initiative for Asthma. (2017). *Pocket guide for asthma management and prevention.* Fontana, WI: Author. Retrieved from http://ginasthma.org/pocket-guide-for-asthma-management-and-prevention

Goolsby, M., & Grubbs, L. (2015). *Advanced assessment: Interpreting findings and formulating differential diagnoses.* Philadelphia, PA: F.A. Davis.

Janevic, M. R., Stoll, S., Wilkin, M., Song, P. K., Baptist, A., Lara, M., . . . Malveaux, F. J. (2016). Pediatric asthma care coordination in underserved communities: A quasi-experimental study. *American Journal of Public Health, 106*(11), 2012–2018. doi:10.2105/AJPH.2016.303373

Mayo Clinic. (2017). Childhood asthma. Retrieved from https://www.mayoclinic.org/diseases-conditions/childhood-asthma/symptoms-causes/syc-20351507

National Asthma Council Australia. (2017). Asthma and complementary therapies. Retrieved from https://www.nationalasthma.org.au/living-with-asthma/resources/patients-carers/brochures/asthma-complementary-therapies

National Asthma Education and Prevention Program. (2007). *The Expert Panel Report 3: Guidelines for the diagnosis and management of asthma.* Bethesda, MD: National Heart, Lung, and Blood Institute, National Institutes of Health. Retrieved from http://www.nhlbi.nih.gov/guidelines/asthma/

Rancière, F., Bougas, N., Viola, M., & Momas, I. (2017). Early exposure to traffic-related air pollution, respiratory symptoms at 4 years of age, and potential effect modification by parental allergy, stressful family events, and sex: A prospective follow-up study of the PARIS birth cohort. *Environmental Health Perspectives, 125*(4), 737–745. https://doi.org/10.1289/EHP239

Sharma, S., Hashmi, M., & Chakraborty, R. (2020). *Asthma medications.* StatPearls [Internet]. Retrieved from https://www.ncbi.nlm.nih.gov/books/NBK531455/

Smith, L., Clayton, M., Woodell, C., & Mansfield, D. (2017). *The role of patient navigators in improving caregiver management of childhood asthma*. Research Triangle Park, NC: RTI Press.

Tai, A. (2016). Strengths, pitfalls, and lessons from longitudinal childhood asthma cohorts of children followed up into adult life. *BioMed Research International, 2016*. doi:10.1155/2016/2694060

U.S. Department of Health and Human Services. (2017). *Healthy People 2020*. Retrieved from: https://www.healthypeople.gov/2020/

U.S. Environmental Protection Agency. (2020). *Replacing old school buses*. Retrieved from https://www.epa.gov/cleandiesel/clean-school-bus-replacement

Valerio, M., Andreski, P., Schoeni, R., & McGonagle, K. (2010). Examining the association between childhood asthma and parent and grandparent asthma status: Implications for practice. *Clinical Pediatrics, 49*, 535–540. doi:10.1177/0009922809356465

Wallinger, C., & Hucker, J. (2012). Caring for a child with asthma: Pre-registration education. *Nursing Children & Young People, 24*(3), 26–28.

Woo, T., & Robinson, M. (2020). *Pharmacotherapeutics for the advanced practice nurse prescribers* (5th ed.). Philadelphia, PA: F.A. Davis.

World Health Organization. (2017). *Chronic respiratory diseases: Asthma*. Retrieved from http://www.who.int/respiratory/asthma/ooope/en/

Wu, J., Yang, X., & Zhang, M. (2017). Massage therapy in children with asthma: A systematic review and meta-analysis. *Evidence-Based Complementary & Alternative Medicine*, 1–8. doi:10.1155/2017/5620568

Chapter 15

Allergic and Hypersensitivity Disorders

Upon completion of this chapter the student will be able to:

- Integrate knowledge of the physiology, pathophysiology, assessment, and nonpharmacological and pharmacological management for care of a pediatric patient with an allergic disorder.

- Appraise current standards of care for pediatric patients with allergic disorders.

Introduction

This chapter will focus on allergic disorders, which include local responses to allergens, such as allergic rhinitis and conjunctivitis, along with life-threatening systemic hypersensitivity reactions, such as food, Hymenoptera, and latex. The pathophysiological processes are similar in these responses; however, the overall outcomes may vary greatly among children. The common response is that the body mounts a protective reaction to a substance that it identifies as foreign. While the underlying mechanism is an effective defense against infection and other potential harmful substances, when the body's reaction is to generally innocuous substances (e.g., food) and the response itself interferes with quality of life (e.g., allergic rhinitis) and/or is potentially lethal (e.g., anaphylaxis), the child and family need an effective plan of care (Capriotti, 2020; "Hypersensitivity Reactions," 2020).

According to the American Academy of Allery, Asthma, & Immunology (AAAAI, 2020a), allergic disorders affect up to 30% of children globally. The most common allergic disorder, allergic rhinitis, is present in 10% to 30% of the world's children. It may be difficult to discern between frequently occurring viral respiratory infections and allergic rhinitis in young children (younger than 3 years), so accurately capturing prevalence in this age-group is difficult. Also, children frequently have multiple allergic conditions that develop over the first years of life. For example, they often have atopic dermatitis before an episode of allergic rhinitis, and allergic conjunctivitis frequently occurs with rhinitis (Solomon, Wheatley, & Togias, 2015). When there are several allergic conditions present, definitive diagnoses of allergic disorder(s) may be more likely.

Globally, the rise in prevalence of allergic diseases has continued in the industrialized world for more than 50 years, with sensitization rates (defined by *immunoglobulin E* [IgE] antibodies) to one or more common allergens among school children currently approaching 40% to 50% of the population. In 2012, 9%, or 6.6 million children, reported allergic rhinitis (i.e., hay fever) in the previous 12 months. From 2017 data, 5.6%, or 5.9 million U.S. children, have either current or a history of food allergy (Mahr & Hernandez-Trujillo, 2017). In 2010, black children in the United States were more likely to have skin allergies (17%) than white (12%) or Asian (10%) children, whereas globally, urticaria occurs with lifetime prevalence above 20% across races. Also, from 2012 data, 12%, or 8.8 million children, reported skin allergies in the past 12 months (AAAAI, 2020a). Based on these statistics, it is evident that allergies are a major health concern for many children and their families. Nurses need current knowledge about managing both acute and chronic conditions that arise from the immune system (National Institute of Allergy and Infectious Diseases [NIAID], 2020).

Physiology

The immune system is composed of multiple structures that act together to protect the body against foreign substances. First, the immune system must accurately distinguish these foreign substances from the body's own tissue. Then there are two types of immune responses—innate/adaptive immune responses and humoral/cell-mediated responses—both of which are responsible for the body's immune responses (Baiu & Melendez, 2018; Capriotti, 2020; "Hypersensitivity Reaction," 2020; NIAID, 2020). Initially, when the body encounters a pathogen, the innate immune system is responsible for the immediate, yet nonspecific, response. Then, the adaptive immune system activates a subsequent response, in which a previously encountered pathogen is recognized, by a process known as *immunological memory*. Therefore, the adaptive immune system has a more focused and rapid response with each subsequent exposure (Baiu & Melendez, 2018; Farbman & Michelson, 2016). The innate responses are essentially the initial and less complex response that then calls the adaptive immune responses to join them; these two responses work in tandem to more effectively eliminate the pathogens. The innate and adaptive immune systems use cell-mediated and humoral responses and are dependent on the ability to distinguish *self* versus *non-self* molecules. The *non-self* molecules, antigens, are foreign to the body and bind to specific receptors, eliciting an immune response (AAAAI, 2020b; Capriotti, 2020; NIAID, 2020; Solomon et al., 2015; World Allergy Organization [WAO], 2020).

Lymphocytes, both T cells and B cells, work within distinct processes in the immune system. First, T cells (also known as killer T cells, or cytotoxic T-lymphocytes), identify and kill cells that are abnormal, due to infection or other processes. Naive cytotoxic T cells have not encountered a foreign substance; however, they are activated when they interact with the foreign molecule and form a bond. At this point, the T cell produces multiple *effector* cells that circulate and destroy the same pathogen wherever it is encountered. Then, after resolution of the infection, a few effector cells survive as memory cells; these cells are able to identify a subsequent exposure to the same foreign substance (antigen) and initiate a rapid and effective immune response (Baiu & Melendez, 2018; Capriotti, 2020). Another type of T cell, CD4 lymphocytes, or *helper* T cells, are important in the adaptive immune response. While the CD4 lymphocytes are not cytotoxic or phagocytic, they direct other cells to perform these important functions within the immune system (AAAAI, 2020b; "Hypersensitivity Reactions," 2020; NIAID, 2020).

The B lymphocytes are an integral part of the humoral immune response. Like the T cell, B cells have unique receptors that bind with one specific antigen once they are activated. When a B cell encounters an antigen, it is urged by a helper T cell to differentiate into an effector cell, or plasma cell, which lives 2 to 3 days and secretes antibodies. Similar to T cells, a small percentage of B cells survive to become antigen-specific memory B cells (Farbman & Michelson, 2016; NIAID, 2020). Because both B and T memory cells can react via different pathways to an antigen, a subsequent exposure to an antigen should produce a stronger and faster immune response. These subsequent responses are considered *adaptive* because the immune system has improved effectiveness; but these responses may also become *maladaptive* if the receptors react to the body's own substances in addition to foreign ones (AAAAI, 2020b; Baiu & Melendez, 2018; NIAID, 2020).

Immunological memory may be *passive* when it is acquired via maternal transmission administration of *immunoglobulin G* (IgG), or *active* when the child has had the disease or (preferably) through immunization, especially when it relates to life-threatening disease. Passive immunity, while usually only short term, is especially important in an infant, as it is the only type of immunity that is available at birth. Maternal passive immunity is provided primarily by two mechanisms: maternal IgG, which is transported directly across the placenta, and through breast milk, which contains antibodies (predominantly IgA) (Capriotti, 2020; NIAID, 2020). With active immunity via immunization, an antigen stimulates the immune system to develop protective immunity against that specific organism via an adaptive immune response, which is long term. Most viral vaccines (e.g., varicella; *measles, mumps, rubella* [MMR]) use live attenuated viruses, so it is important that the child is not immunosuppressed or in contact with people who are immunosuppressed when receiving the immunization. However, bacterial vaccines (*Haemophilus influenzae* type B [Hib]; diphtheria, tetanus, pertussis [DTaP]) are inactivated versions of the microorganisms, so the same precautions do not apply. These bacterial vaccines often require adjuvants to activate the antigen-presenting cells of the immune system (AAAAI, 2020; Centers for Disease Control and Prevention [CDC], 2018).

Children's immune systems develop as they age. This is reflected in infants' increased susceptibility to infections and also their hypersensitivity to potential allergens as their bodies develop the ability to discern *self* from *non-self* molecules. Infections may be life threatening in an infant because the immature immune system does not respond effectively. As the child matures, so does the immune system, and once the child is an adolescent their functioning should be comparable to that of an adult (AAAAI, 2020b; Capriotti, 2020; Farbman & Michelson, 2018).

> **HIGH YIELD FACT FOR TESTING**
>
> The child's age significantly affects the expected normal function of the immune system.

 CLINICAL PEARLS

Infants are susceptible to infection because their only source of immunity is *passive* immunity.

Pathophysiology

As discussed in the previous section, the nurse must account for the age of the child when deciding if there is a pathological process occurring versus a normal age-appropriate immune response. Once the child reaches adolescence, the adaptive system response is usually effective in destroying pathogens and their associated toxins. Sometimes the adaptive system incorrectly responds to a harmless foreign substance or does not recognize a molecule as *self*. When this occurs, the child may experience environmental allergies, asthma, atopic dermatitis, or another allergic condition (AAAAI, 2020b; Capriotti, 2020).

Regardless of age, when an allergic reaction occurs, there is an acute and a late-stage response. In a type I hypersensitivity reaction, the child encounters the allergen for the first time, and an antigen-presenting cell causes a response in a T helper type 2 (Th2) lymphocyte. These immune cells are a type of T cell and produce a cytokine, interleukin-4. As Th2 cells interact with other lymphocytes, B cells make IgE, which is an antibody. IgE then circulates and binds to specific IgE receptors, which are located on the surface of mast cells and basophils. Both types of immune cells are part of the inflammatory response; IgE-coated cells are considered sensitized to the specific allergen (Baiu & Melendez, 2018; "Hypersensitivity Reactions," 2020; NIAID, 2020).

Inflammation occurs as one of the first responses of the immune system to a pathogen; the increased blood flow of inflammation results in redness, swelling, heat, and pain. Eicosanoids and cytokines are chemicals released by cells due to infection. Prostaglandins are a type of eicosanoid that causes fever and vasodilation; leukotrienes, another type of eicosanoid, attract leukocytes into the area of infection (AAAAI, 2020b; Kronemeyer, 2017). Interleukins are a type of cytokine that increases white blood cell function, along with release of growth and cytotoxic factors. Cytokines and other chemicals promote movement of these immune cells to fight infection and promote healing ("Hypersensitivity Reactions," 2020; NIAID, 2020; Kronemeyer, 2017).

If the child is exposed to the same allergen again, that allergen will bind with the IgE molecules on the surface of these mast cells or basophils, which activates them. Once activated, the cells degranulate and release histamine along with other inflammatory chemical mediators, including cytokines, interleukins, leukotrienes, and prostaglandins (AAAAI, 2020b; "Hypersensitivity Reactions," 2020). These chemical mediators can cause both vasodilation and bronchoconstriction. Depending on the child, allergen, and mode of exposure, acute stage symptoms may be generalized (anaphylaxis) or localized. The predominant systemic symptoms of anaphylaxis are the following:

- Vasodilation
- Mucous secretion
- Nerve stimulation
- Smooth muscle contractions

The local effects are dependent on the site, but common ones include itching, rash, and wheezing (Baiu & Melendez, 2018; Capriotti, 2020; Farbman & Michelson, 2016).

A late phase of a type I reaction often follows the acute response within 8 to 12 hours, and symptoms that have resolved may recur or worsen, along with the development of new symptoms. In this phase, other types of leukocytes (neutrophils, lymphocytes, eosinophils, and macrophages) migrate to the initial allergen exposure site. Cytokines secreted from the mast cells are responsible for the continued long-term effects. Late phase reactions in asthma are dependent on T_H2 cells and are due to chemical mediators released from eosinophils. The helper T cells release cytokines that activate cytotoxic T cells (CD-8) and recruit macrophages. The pathophysiology of allergic contact dermatitis is a type IV hypersensitivity reaction resulting from CD8+ cells that destroy target cells and macrophages, which produce hydrolytic enzymes that increase the chemical bond based on the breakdown of H_2O into separate molecules (Capriotti, 2020; "Hypersensitivity Reactions," 2020; Nierengarten, 2017).

There is disagreement globally about the definition of anaphylaxis across age-groups. However, based on a recent review, a consensus definition of anaphylaxis was determined to be "a severe systemic hypersensitivity reaction that is rapid in onset; characterized by life-threatening airway, breathing, and/or circulatory problems; and usually associated with skin and mucosal changes" (Reber, Hernandez, & Galli, 2017, p. 335). In short, anaphylaxis is an extreme allergic response from a sudden, systemic degranulation of mast cells releasing histamine. The word *anaphylaxis* means "contrary protection" in Greek, which aptly describes the situation when the body mounts a reaction to an otherwise harmless substance (Bethel, 2013; Capriotti, 2020). The child has been exposed to the antigen previously without a reaction, but with a subsequent exposure develops a severe, and often life-threatening, response. Most episodes occur within seconds to minutes after exposure; however, a reaction can be delayed for several hours (Baiu & Melendez, 2018; Farbman & Michelson, 2016; "Hypersensitivity Reactions," 2020). Symptoms typically involve more than one organ system due to the systemic nature of the immune response. Anaphylaxis can recur even without a second exposure; one in five children has a second reaction within 24 hours of the initial episode, which is known as a *biphasic reaction*. Prompt administration of epinephrine during the initial episode of anaphylaxis is the best prevention for the complication of biphasic reaction (AAAAI, 2020b; Bethel, 2013; Farbman & Michelson, 2016; Viale & Yamamoto, 2010).

The roles of IgE and IgG antibodies, immune effector cells, and mediators were a focus of a review by Reber et al. (2017). According to Reber and colleagues, data on immunological mechanisms of anaphylaxis from human subjects are limited because of the life-threatening nature of anaphylaxis and ethical constraints. While there was evidence that children with allergic disease have elevated IgE levels, the role of IgG in anaphylaxis is not supported by current evidence. Also, mast cells, basophils, eosinophils, neutrophils, and macrophages act as inflammatory mediators during anaphylaxis. Because so many types of cells contribute to anaphylaxis, it is a complex reaction with many potential complications. Genetic factors may affect anaphylaxis presentation and severity, so it is important to assess for a family history of anaphylaxis (AAAAI, 2020b; Bethel, 2013; Capriotti, 2020).

The potential for a life-threatening anaphylactic response is highest in children who have several risk factors, including exposure to latex through instrumentation and repeat catheterization; family history of asthma, food allergy, and/or anaphylaxis; adolescents, because they may take risks to ingest a potential allergen and delay treatment; and children with both food allergies and asthma. Counseling should focus on children at increased risk for anaphylaxis, so they have adequate education about current treatment guidelines and are prescribed epinephrine for self-administration (AAAAI, 2020b; CDC, 2020; Kelly & Sussman, 2017; Sircherer et al., 2017).

The complement system is a physiological response, composed of more than 20 proteins, that releases chemicals that attack the surfaces of foreign cells. This system augments the antibodies' attack on pathogens and is the major humoral component of the innate immune response. Complement proteins bind to antibodies that are already attached to pathogens, triggering a rapid killing response. Once a complement protein binds to a pathogen, it activates further enzyme activity, which then activates other complement proteases. These peptides attract immune cells, increase vascular permeability, and cover the pathogen surface. All of these actions increase the likelihood of pathogen destruction by the immune system. Complement proteins also directly kill cells by affecting cell membrane permeability (Baiu & Melendez, 2018; Capriotti, 2020; "Hypersensitivity Reactions," 2020; Reber et al., 2017).

Assessment

Alterations in the immune system are expressed in both focused (e.g., rash) and systemic (e.g., asthma) signs and symptoms; therefore, an assessment of the child with allergies will often reveal abnormalities in multiple systems, as outlined in Table 15-1 (AAAAI, 2020b; "Hypersensitivity Reactions," 2020; NIAID, 2020). As with any assessment of a child, normal findings will vary with the age and developmental abilities of the child. Because the normal functioning of the immune system is emerging as the child develops, the nurse may encounter wide ranges of normal findings that must be discriminated from those caused by a pathological process (Dillon, 2017).

A head-to-toe approach will be used to address the effects of an altered immune system in a child. Generally, there are no manifestations on the head, unless an atopic dermatitis rash is present (Kronemeyer, 2017; Nierengarten, 2017). The eyes should be assessed for conjunctivitis that is associated with an allergic response, which will result in bilateral pink conjunctiva with clear secretions. It is important to distinguish this condition from an infectious conjunctivitis, in which the eye(s) is severely reddened and often swollen, and drainage is copious and purulent. While allergic conditions may cause altered sensations in the ear, including tinnitus and discomfort, the physical examination is usually normal (Dillon, 2017; Goolsby & Grubbs, 2015).

There are often significant abnormal findings in the child's nose, so the nurse must determine the best time and method for viewing the mucosa. With an older child, this examination can be negotiated and rewarded; whereas a smaller child may need to be held by a parent or another staff member for both the ear and nose examinations. Nasal mucosa is often pale and boggy with clear, watery drainage. The child and/or parent may complain of a frequent *runny* nose; an *allergic salute* (allergic crease), or horizontal line across the nose, may be present because the child uses a hand to resolve the associated itching and drainage. This type of drainage should be distinguished from the normal nasal congestion and associated sneezing that occurs in newborns and resolves by age 2 to 3 months. The mouth and throat of the child will usually be normal except for clear postnasal drainage that may be visible in the pharynx (AAAAI, 2020b; Dillon, 2017; Goolsby & Grubbs, 2015).

If the child is experiencing an acute allergic reaction, physical findings will be different and will include laryngeal redness and edema, which are signs of an emergent situation (Goolsby & Grubbs, 2015). The cardiac and lung assessments will reveal abnormalities, such as decreased breath sounds, wheezing, stridor, and tachycardia. The child may not be able to speak in complete sentences and may need to take a

TABLE 15-1 Allergic Signs/Symptoms by System

System	Signs/Symptom
EENT	Eyes: Redness and itching of conjunctiva, excessive watery secretions Nose: Swelling of the nasal mucosa, excessive nasal secretions, sneezing Ears: Feeling of fullness and/or pain, impaired hearing
Respiratory	Coughing, *bronchoconstriction, *wheezing, *dyspnea, *laryngeal edema, *angioedema
Integument	Rashes, specifically *hives (urticaria)
Gastrointestinal tract	*Abdominal pain, *bloating, *vomiting, *diarrhea

*Indicates signs/symptoms of anaphylaxis.

breath mid-sentence, similar to a child having an asthma attack (see Chapter 14) (Dillon, 2017).

The skin assessment will also vary greatly if there is an acute, versus chronic, allergic response. Hives are a heraldic sign of an acute reaction. The most common types of dermatitis in children are atopic on contact. Recurrent, erythematous, dry, itchy, scaly patches occur with atopic dermatitis. The rash often occurs on flexor surfaces of the extremities, along with the face and neck. Over time, these areas may become hardened with lichenification. The rash is extremely pruritic and may become secondarily infected (Dillon, 2017; Kronemeyer, 2017). This condition is most common in infants and young children and often resolves spontaneously with age. With contact dermatitis, there is usually an exposure to an allergen or irritant that is determined from the history. The lesions are usually reddened discrete papules that may form vesicles, drain, and become secondarily infected (Dillon, 2017; NIAID, 2020).

Finally, the gastrointestinal signs and symptoms noted in Table 15-1 are more common in infants and younger children, especially when they encounter a food to which they are allergic (AAAAI, 2020b; Goolsby & Grubs, 2015; Kronemeyer, 2017).

Food Allergy

Food allergy has become a global health concern and is seen in many practice settings. Food-induced anaphylaxis is the most frequent type of pediatric anaphylactic reaction and is responsible for over 30,000 visits to emergency departments and 150 deaths per year in the United States (CDC, 2020; Demkin, 2017; WAO, 2020). Food allergy may be caused by different physiological processes; allergic reactions may be due to IgE-mediated and/or non-IgE–mediated processes, with the IgE-mediated being more common and leading to anaphylaxis. IgE-mediated food allergies affect 5% to 8% of children; serum IgE levels are often evaluated as a diagnostic tool but have low predictive value (AAAAI, 2020b; CDC, 2020; Stukus, Kempe, Leber, Thornton, & Scherzer, 2016).

Children may have allergic reaction to any food, but the most prevalent and potentially serious offenders are cow's milk, hen's egg, peanuts, tree nuts, and seafood (Sicherer et al., 2017). The review of current research recommendations focused on IgE-mediated responses and included improved monitoring of prevalence and risk factors, utilizing allergy testing in concert with medical history, evidence-based prevention strategies, using intramuscular epinephrine promptly for anaphylaxis, improved food labeling, *epinephrine auto-injector* (EA) for infants, and guidelines to prevent food allergies (AAAAI, 2020b; CDC, 2018; Sicherer et al., 2017).

Parental management of a child's food allergy can be a source of stress for the entire family. Parents must be vigilant that the child does not ingest or be exposed to a potential allergen, while the child must learn impulse control about food choices early. Incomplete or improperly labeled food exists, despite the *Food Allergen Labeling and Consumer Protection Act* (FAL-CPA) of 2004, which requires all food products regulated by the U.S. Food and Drug Administration (FDA) to have a label that states whether the product contains a major food allergen. There is proposed legislation to improve food labeling guidelines, but it is the nurse's responsibility to be informed about food labeling and to educate parents and children about it (CDC, 2018; Demkin, 2017).

When children are denied their trigger food, it may result in a temper tantrum from a younger child or a much more serious depressive state in an adolescent, where there is already a high risk for depression (Beaver & Jordan, 2015). The scenario of a child going to a birthday party but not being able to enjoy all the food with their friends due to food allergy remains a common occurrence for children with allergies. It can often be difficult for children with food allergies to eat in a restaurant for fear of encountering an allergen, especially with the potential for cross contamination in the kitchen (CDC, 2018; NIAID, 2020b; WAO, 2020).

Latex Allergy

During the 1980s and 1990s, the risk of Ig-E mediated sensitization to *natural rubber latex* (NRL) was very high in certain populations, including children with atopic dermatitis, spina bifida, and/or urological disorders. Latex precautions were promoted by various professional organizations, including the American Academy of Asthma, Allergy, & Immunology; the American College of Allergy, Asthma, & Immunology; and the Association of periOperative Registered Nurses. This resulted in safer care of patients with latex allergy. Despite these initiatives, which identified and removed most sources of NRL proteins, it is recommended that patients with spina bifida continue to avoid all latex from birth. Providers—especially urologists, neurosurgeons, and orthopedic surgeons—need to remain vigilant about this principle (AAAAI, 2020b; Kelly & Sussman, 2017).

There are three types of latex allergy: irritant contact dermatitis (least serious), allergic contact dermatitis (delayed, more severe local reaction), and latex hypersensitivity (the most serious type that can lead to anaphylaxis). There are systemic signs and symptoms that only occur with latex hypersensitivity, such as nasal congestion, conjunctivitis, abdominal cramps, hive, itching, chest pain, dyspnea, hypotension, and anaphylaxis. While latex has been removed from many products because of the increased incidence of latex allergies, parents should be aware of common household sources of latex (see SENC Box 15-1) (AAAAI, 2020b; "Hypersensitivity Reactions," 2020; Kelly & Sussman, 2017; Nierengarten, 2017; WAO, 2020).

Medication Allergy

Nurses are responsible for assessing allergies to medications. Penicillin allergy is the most commonly reported medication allergy in children; however, the true incidence of penicillin allergy in children is low. These data suggest that parents incorrectly report adverse reactions, such as rash (maculopapular, rather than hives) or diarrhea as a drug allergy. With penicillin the preferred therapy for many infectious processes, it is important to identify children who can safely take this effective medication (Capriotti, 2020; "Hypersensitivity Reactions," 2020; Nierengarten & Wyles, 2017).

SENC BOX 15-1   Safe and Effective Nursing Care for Finding Potential Sources of Latex in a Child's Environment

- Rubber sink stoppers and sink mats
- Water hose
- Tub toys
- Disposable diapers
- Waterproof bed pads
- Undergarments and other clothing with elastic
- Glue, paste, art supplies, and glue pens
- Older dolls, particularly Barbie dolls
- Keyboards and calculators
- Remote controller for video games
- Eye pieces for camera, telescope, or binoculars
- Some balloons

Atopic Dermatitis

Atopic dermatitis (AD) is an inflammatory skin disease, and occurs frequently in children, especially in infants. There is a 20% prevalence rate across childhood, with 60% of those cases developing in children 1 year of age and younger. While it is not an allergic process, it is often associated with other allergic conditions, such as food allergy, asthma, and allergic rhinitis. With AD, the skin lacks certain proteins that maintain the skin's barrier to water, and the skin becomes swollen, red, and itchy ("Hypersensitivity Reactions," 2020; Kronmeyer, 2017; Nierengarten, 2017). This condition may resolve with age or may continue into adulthood. Consistent application of occlusive emollients applied after bathing promote hydration of the skin, and use of topical steroid ointments intermittently reduces inflammation; however, the chronicity and unpredictability of this condition is often frustrating to families (AAAAI, 2020b; NIAID, 2020).

Diagnostic Tests

Diagnostic tests are used in conjunction with patient/family history and physical assessment findings to confirm an allergy to a specific substance and normal functioning of the immune system. Blood testing may be preferred in the following situations:

• Patient must remain on antihistamine.
• Patient has severe eczema.
• Testing with an allergen may cause a life-threatening positive reaction.
• Infants and young children may not tolerate skin testing.

In a review of IgE testing for food allergies, the results showed that primary care providers used this method to identify food allergen panels more frequently than allergy specialists; this generated a higher cost and has not proven more accurate (Solomon et al., 2015; Stukus et al., 2016).

Generally, the most common laboratory tests that are used to diagnose allergic disorders are those for the immunoglobulins (see Table 15-2), especially IgE and IgG. Immunoglobulins are composed of two types of protein chains: a heavy and a light chain. The heavy chain determines the immunoglobulin class and is denoted by Greek letters, which correspond to IgM (μ), IgD (δ), IgG (γ), IgE (ε), and IgA (α). In a type I hypersensitivity (e.g., anaphylaxis, drug reactions, food allergies, insect venom allergies), the immune system produces specific IgE antibodies, which can recognize a specific allergen; it activates basophils and mast cells, so they release histamine, leukotrienes, and certain interleukins (Capriotti, 2020; "Hypersensitivity Reactions," 2020). The IgE antibodies are responsible for an immediate allergic reaction. Usually the child/family will know what substance, especially a food, is the trigger, but IgE testing may be confirmatory. In a type II reaction (e.g., rheumatic fever, Graves' disease, pernicious anemia), IgM and IgG antibodies bind to antigens and the complement system is activated with resulting phagocytosis of cells. Also, there is antibody-dependent cell-mediated cytotoxicity (e.g., natural killer cells), which interferes with normal cell function. By comparison, in a type III reaction (e.g., drug-induced hypersensitivity vasculitis, serum sickness, systemic lupus erythematosus), IgG antibodies bind to circulating antigens, and there is an immune complex formed in tissues that attracts neutrophils and results in phagocytosis of cells. Finally, a type IV reaction (e.g., acute and chronic transplant rejection, contact dermatitis, Hashimoto's thyroiditis, rheumatoid arthritis, and type 1 diabetes) is a cell-mediated response with presensitized T lymphocytes causing an inflammatory response that is often delayed up to 3 days after exposure (Capriotti, 2020; "Hypersensitivity Reactions," 2020; Solomon et al., 2015).

TABLE 15–2 Immunoglobulins' Function Overview

Immunoglobulin	Function in Infectious and Allergic Processes
IgA	Stops colonization by pathogens and prevents infections. Interacts with receptors to stimulate inflammatory processes.
IgD	Antigen receptor on naïve B cells (no exposure to antigens). Activates basophils and mast cells to release histamine.
IgE	Binds to allergens; activates mast cells and basophils to release histamine. IgE levels in a normal individual are 0.05% of the Ig concentration. In children with allergic conditions, IgE comprises 75% of the concentration. Essential role in type I hypersensitivity reactions, including allergic asthma, allergic rhinitis, food allergies, chronic urticarial, and atopic dermatitis. Used in desensitization immunotherapy.
IgG	Most common antibody, comprising 75% of serum antibodies. Formed and released by plasma B cells. Each IgG has two antigen binding sites. Provides antibody-based immunity and reactions against antigens. The only antibody that crosses the placenta. Associated with type II and III hypersensitivity reactions.
IgM	Active in early stages of B cell-mediated (humoral) response, before IgG is present.

When food allergies are suspected, an *oral food challenge* (OFC) is the preferred method of confirming a diagnosis because self-reported allergy is correlated with an overestimated prevalence. In an OFC, the child ingests a potentially allergenic food in a medically supervised feeding and is assessed for signs and symptoms afterward. Obviously, if the child has a history of a delayed reaction, a strong family history of food allergy, or other risk factors for anaphylaxis, the diagnostic benefit of OFC is weighed against the potential risk of anaphylaxis. (CDC, 2020; NIAID, 2020; Sircherer et al., 2017). Confirmatory testing, when possible, is recommended whenever allergens are identified. Assuming incorrectly that an allergen has been identified, either via a false negative or false positive, may result in exposure to a true allergen and a result in serious reaction (AAAAI, 2020b; Sicherer et al., 2017).

Skin testing may also be performed as a part of the diagnostic process. It is commonly used when the following diagnoses are possible: allergic rhinitis, allergic asthma, dermatitis (eczema), food allergies, penicillin allergy, Hymenoptera allergy, and/or latex allergy (AAAAI, 2020b; Mayo Clinic, 2017; Nierengarten & Wyles, 2017). While skin testing is usually considered safe for all age-groups, including infants, it is contraindicated in certain situations. First, if the child has a history of a severe anaphylactic reaction, any exposure to the antigen may be life threatening. Next, some patients must remain on medications that interfere with testing, such as antihistamines, tricyclic antidepressants, and anti-reflux (H_2 blockers), and any monoclonal antibodies, such as omalizumab. Last, when eczema affects the arms and back where testing is placed, there may not be adequate unaffected skin surface (AAAAI, 2020b; "Hypersensitivity Reactions," 2020; Mayo Clinic, 2017).

Skin testing can be accomplished by using a prick test, which uses a lancet to introduce small amounts of the antigen under the skin. Children are observed immediately and for 15 minutes after application of the antigen for a reaction, which is measured for redness and/or induration. With a skin injection test, intradermal introduction of the allergen is used, but due to the increased discomfort as compared to the prick test, is not common with children (AAAAI, 2020b; Mayo Clinic, 2017). Patch testing may also be used, especially when a delayed reaction is expected. Patches are applied to the skin and worn for 48 hours; up to 30 allergens may be tested simultaneously. Because the child is not under constant supervision during patch testing, it should not be used when there is suspected anaphylaxis for any of the allergens. Also, any of these types of skin testing may be difficult to analyze on dark skin (AAAAI, 2020b; Mayo Clinic, 2017; NIAID, 2020). While there are standards for reaction measurement, there may be subjectivity in the assessment. False negatives and false positives may also occur. Sensitivity refers to the ability to identify a true positive (i.e., a test with low sensitivity has high rate of false positives); whereas specificity refers to the ability to identity a true negative (i.e., a test with low specificity will have a high rate of false positives). However, skin testing has the advantages of being more sensitive than blood testing and also less expensive (AAAAI, 2020b; Mayo Clinic, 2017; NIAID, 2020).

RED FLAG ALERT

Penicillin is the most common cause of anaphylaxis; therefore, it is important to determine whether an allergy exists with skin testing.

HIGH YIELD FACT FOR TESTING

A written allergy action plan to be implemented with any future reactions should always accompany a diagnosis of an allergic reaction.

Nonpharmacological Management

Necessary changes for the family who has a child with allergy may include making alterations to the environment to decrease potential exposure to allergens, learning preventive measures, and living with the possibility of an allergy attack that will require emergent intervention. SENC Box 15-2 provides an overview of actions that nurses can teach parents and children to take to avoid or minimize exposure to allergy-related reactions (AAAAI, 2020b; NIAID, 2020).

SENC BOX 15–2 Safe and Effective Nursing Care for Allergy Contact and Anaphylaxis Prevention Education

TEACH THE PARENT AND CHILD TO:
- Avoid allergens.
- Communicate with other adults, especially teachers about their specific allergens if known.
- When and how to use an epinephrine auto-injector (EA).

TO PREVENT FOOD ALLERGY REACTION:
- Learn how to read food labels and avoid cross-contact.
- Read the label every time you buy a product; ingredients may change.

TO PREVENT INSECT ALLERGY REACTION:
- Wear closed-toe shoes.
- Use insect repellent when outdoors.
- Avoid loose-fitting clothing that can trap an insect between the clothing and the skin.
- Avoid bright-colored prints that resemble flowers.

TO PREVENT MEDICATION ALLERGY REACTION:
- Keep a current list of medication allergies.
- Wear a medic-alert bracelet.
- Tell providers the specific symptoms that the child experienced with allergy.

SENC BOX 15–2 Safe and Effective Nursing Care for Allergy Contact and Anaphylaxis Prevention Education—cont'd

TO PREVENT LATEX ALLERGY REACTION:
- Tell all providers (doctors, dentists, therapists, etc.) about a child's latex allergy.
- Wear medic-alert bracelet.

TO PREVENT ATOPIC DERMATITIS:
- Avoid and/or treat concomitant allergies to pollen, mold, dust mites, or animals.
- Avoid cold and dry air in the winter. Consider adding humidification to home environment.
- Avoid colds with hand hygiene and keeping away from crowds.
- Avoid flu with hand hygiene, keeping away from crowds, and a flu vaccine. (Dosing for flu vaccine is age dependent: 6–35 months: 0.25 mL for Fluzone Quadrivalent OR 0.5 ml FluLaval Quadrivalent; 36 months and older: 0.5 mL all inactivated influenza vaccines; CDC, 2018.)
- Avoid contact with irritants (perfumes, scented lotions, soap), chemicals (laundry detergents), scratchy materials (wool).
- Keep skin well lubricated.
- Avoid excessive emotional stress.
- Avoid frequent or long hot baths or showers.
- Do not swim regularly in chlorinated or salinated pools, as water is drying to the skin.

Anaphylaxis Education Programs

Self-management is an integral part of the treatment plan for a child who has experienced an anaphylactic reaction. Depending on the age of the child, the parent and/or child (AAP recommends by age 12 or 13) must be educated in how to avoid allergens and make necessary lifestyle changes, such as not eating certain foods, alerting teachers and friends of allergies, and learning how to administer epinephrine via an epi-pen (see SENC Box 15-3). In addition to administering epinephrine, there are other important considerations of treating an anaphylactic reaction, such as calling emergency medical services and following up with a primary care provider who notes the event in the health record (AAAAI, 2020b; Bethel, 2013; Mahr & Hernandez-Trujillo, 2017).

Allergy Care Coordination

Similar to asthma care coordination, a nurse may make a home visit to assess the child's allergy triggers and help the family address challenges with environmental management. Then, the child and family are connected with primary care providers and specialists, as needed, to encourage continuity of care and decrease *emergency department* (ED) care utilization. Care coordinators act as navigators to coordinate care among providers (including emergency care centers) to communicate changes in the treatment plan and to promote compliance with appointments and follow-up. In a recent review of children admitted to a large tertiary care center for food-induced anaphylaxis, the majority of patients received epinephrine auto-injector training before discharge, but 31% of patients had no plan for allergy specialty follow-up (AAAAI, 2020; Mahr & Hernandez-Trujlllo, 2017). Because allergies, especially anaphylaxis, are not necessarily daily concerns for the family, it is easy for allergy management to lose importance for a busy child and family (AAAAI, 2020b; Bethel, 2013; Mahr & Hernandez-Trujillo, 2017).

> **SENC BOX 15–3** Safe and Effective Nursing Care for Administering Epinephrine and Care Afterward
>
> - Teach parent and child (age appropriate) how to administer epinephrine.
>   - Create an individualized allergy action plan outlining symptoms that require epinephrine administration.
>   - Teach the parent and/or child how to administer and watch them perform a return demonstration.
>   - Demonstrate to parent and child how to administer promptly when anaphylaxis is probable, especially if child has asthma or a history of previous anaphylactic reaction. *Note:* AAP recommends children by age 12 to 14 are capable of self-administration.
>   - Demonstrate how the EA automatically injects a single dose as it is pressed against child's outer thigh as this is not intuitive to many parents
>   - Teach additional people (e.g., coaches, teachers) who spend time with the child how to use EA.
>   - Instruct parent to place child in position based on individual needs after epinephrine administration—usually supine on side with legs elevated. If child self-administers, have the child demonstrate the recovery supine position.
> - Instruct parent/child to ALWAYS have two EA auto-injectors accessible in case of malfunction or inadequate response to first dose.
> - Instruct parent to store EA at room temperature; discard if the liquid is not clear.
> - Instruct parent/child to check expiration date monthly and replace when expired.
> - Instruct parent/child to ALWAYS call EMS after epinephrine administration.

 RED FLAG ALERT

Nurses should know their state laws for a child's right to carry and self-administer epinephrine at school.

Environmental Changes

As with environmental changes that are effective for asthma (see Chapter 14), nurses can teach families how to use results from the skin testing or blood tests to identify and remove their child's allergy triggers. While allergen immunotherapy is often necessary to see significant decrease in symptoms, this treatment is usually much more effective in combination with alterations to the environment.

ASSESSMENT PEARLS

A thorough assessment of the home environment may include a home visit.

Pharmacology

Children with allergies are often on daily medication as a preventive measure and then also have access to medications that are given on an emergency basis. It is important that the child and their family understand the importance of each type of medication in managing their allergic condition. Topical preparations may also be used for local reaction to allergens. The primary medications used to treat allergies are discussed in the following sections and summarized in Table 15-3 at the end of the Pharmacology section.

Antihistamines

The antihistamine class of medications has been used successfully as both preventive and to treat acute allergic reactions. Antihistamines work by blocking histamine at the H_1 receptor sites; they do not decrease histamine that is already in the circulation

TABLE 15–3   Medications Used to Treat Allergic Disorders in Children

Class	Example	Action	Dosage	SENC

First generation antihistamines	Diphenhydramine	Blocks H_1 receptor sites and histamine binding ability.
		    Temporary relief of acute allergic symptoms. May be adjuvant to epinephrine in anaphylaxis.
			6.25 mg q 4–6 hr in children 2–6 yr
			    12.5–25 mg q 4–6 hr in children 6–12 yr
			    May be administered Orally, IM or IV
				*SEs: Drowsiness, cardiovascular collapse, anaphylactic reaction.
				    Observe child for excessive drowsiness and respiratory depression.

Second generation antihistamines	Loratadine	Long-acting non-sedating selective H_1 receptor blocker.
		    Relief of symptoms of allergic rhinitis and chronic urticaria.
			<30 kg: 5 mg/day
			    >30 kg: 10 mg/day
				SEs: Usually minimal, but may include arthralgia, dizziness, GI upset. Give on empty stomach.

Nasal corticosteroids	Fluticasone	Seasonal allergic rhinitis.
		    Relieves inflammation in nasal mucosa.
			27.5 mcg/inhalation
			    1–2 puffs/nostril/day for children age 2–11 yr
			    2 puffs/nostril/day for children over 12 yr
				SEs: Nasal dryness, irritation, bloody drainage, headache. Distinguish between oral and nasal inhalers.

Leukotriene receptor antagonists	Montelukast	Inhibit bronchoconstriction and mucus production by blocking leukotrienes.
		    Prophylaxis and treatment of allergic rhinitis.
			4 mg daily for child 12 mo–5 yr
			    5 mg daily for child older than 6 yr
				SEs: Dizziness, headache, nasal congestion. Nightmares/night terrors. Chewable tablets contain phenylalanine. Administer at bedtime.

Adrenergic receptor agonists	Epinephrine	Relieves bronchospasm associated with anaphylaxis.	SC: 0.1–0.5 mL/kg of 1:1,000 q 10–15 min
			    IV: 0.01 mL/kg of 1:1,000 q 10–15 min
				SEs: Tachycardia, increased blood pressure, cardiac arrhythmias.
				    If given outside hospital, call 911 for transport and follow-up care.

Topical corticosteroids	Hydrocortisone	Decreases inflammation of Atopic dermatitis.	0.1% Apply sparingly to affected area for children over 3 months old.	SEs: Hypersensitivity. Do not use if area is possibly infected. Potential for systemic toxicity is greater in small children due to greater ratio of skin surface area to body weight.

*SEs, side effects.

or prevent histamine release (AAAAI, 2020b; Woo & Robinson, 2020). Within this group of medications, there are first and second generation medications that have slightly different mechanisms of action with resulting differences in side effects. The primary difference is that the first generation antihistamines bind nonselectively to all H_1 receptors and cause both stimulation and depression in the *central nervous system* (CNS) (Woo & Robinson, 2020). These CNS side effects, especially drowsiness, can be particularly disturbing for children related to behavior and school performance. In comparison, second generation antihistamines work selectively in peripheral H_1 receptors, so they are less sedating (AAAAI, 2020b; WAO, 2020).

For acute hypersensitivity reactions, the first generation antihistamines are usually preferred for their rapid action and effectiveness; diphenhydramine is the drug of choice for a child in this situation (Woo & Robinson, 2020). As noted in Table 15-3 (end of Pharmacology section), diphenhydramine may be administered parenterally, which is necessary if there is laryngeal edema and resulting difficulty swallowing as part of the allergic reactions. While paradoxical, a child can have an allergy to this medication, and anaphylaxis to diphenhydramine has occurred (WAO, 2020; Woo & Robinson, 2020).

Nasal Corticosteroids

Because allergic rhinitis is a local IgE-mediated reaction of the nasal mucosa in response to inhaled allergens, nasal corticosteroids are used to manage the inflammatory response. These medications have a local effect in the nose without absorption into the circulation. The inhaler may be used one or two times a day during acute symptoms for 5 to 7 days or used preventively when there is potential for exposure to known allergens and/or ongoing symptoms. Fluticasone is the most commonly used nasal steroid and is not approved for children younger than 4 years old at this time (AAAAI, 2020b; NIAID, 2020; Woo & Robinson, 2020). The dosing for this medication is based both on age and symptom relief. In younger children (4 to 12 years), one puff/nostril is used initially; if this dose is effective in symptom relief, then it is used as a maintenance dose. If one puff does not resolve symptoms, it may be increased to two puffs/day. After stabilization, the dose is decreased to one puff daily if possible. Conversely, in children over 12 years of age, the higher dose of two puffs/nostril/day is usually the beginning dose (Woo & Robinson, 2020).

Leukotriene-Receptor Antagonists

As detailed in Chapter 14, leukotriene-receptor antagonists inhibit the release of inflammatory mediators and are effective as a treatment for chronic allergic conditions. Montelukast is approved for use in children over age 12 months both for prophylaxis and acute treatment of allergic rhinitis (AAAAI, 2020b; Woo & Robinson, 2020).

Topical Corticosteroids

The usual treatment for atopic dermatitis, which often accompanies allergic conditions such as asthma and rhinitis, includes steroidal preparations, which work by blocking the inflammatory reaction. Low-strength corticosteroids are used for areas of thinner skin (face, diaper area, skinfolds) and in infants. Moderate strength steroids may be used in older children. All strengths of steroid are used for the shortest time possible; usually effectiveness is assessed at 2 weeks, and then the dose is tapered. When the child experiences an exacerbation, the 2-week administration cycle is initiated (AAAAI, 2020b; Nierengarten, 2017; Woo & Robinson, 2020).

Nonsteroidal Anti-inflammatory Topical Treatment

New topical nonsteroidal anti-inflammatory medications (crisaborole) work by blocking the enzyme *phosphodiesterase 4* (PDE4). PDE4 inhibitors block release of cytokines, which cause inflammation in the skin and are approved for use in children over age 2 years. It is a petroleum-based ointment, so it has an additional emollient effect and is recommended for mild to moderate AD. Pain at the site of application is the only adverse reaction that has been reported in greater than 1% of patients aged 2 to 79. Crisaborole has the advantage that it may be used for longer than the 2-week recommended period for steroid preparations, therefore extending the time of treatment and its potential effectiveness (AAAAI, 2020b; Nierengarten, 2017; Woo & Robinson, 2020). Pimecrolimus may be used for atopic dermatitis that has responded to other topical agents; it is a *topical calcineurin inhibitor* (TCI) that works by decreasing the skin's immune response, thereby decreasing the allergic reaction (Upton, Schellack, & Motswaledi, 2016).

Desensitizing Immunotherapy

Despite the development of newer medications for treating allergies, desensitizing immunotherapy remains an effective treatment for children who have extreme hypersensitivity to identified allergens and/or cannot avoid specific allergies. It works by desensitizing children to their identified allergens, thereby lessening the severity and eliminating their reaction. Once allergens are identified, immunotherapy is developed that is based on the child's individual allergen profile. The specific allergen(s) is administered in increasing strengths in order to desensitize the child to the substance over time (CDC, 2017; Mayo Clinic, 2017). Its effectiveness varies, but 2 years of immunotherapy in childhood has been shown to provide long-term benefits for some children. While not usually indicated for food or medication allergies, immunotherapy promotes positive outcomes for children who have allergic rhinitis and/or asthma (AAAAI, 2020; CDC, 2017; Mayo Clinic, 2017).

See Table 15-3 for an overview of medications used to treat allergic disorders in children.

Allergy Action Plan

A health-care provider will initiate an allergy action plan anytime a child has a witnessed or reported anaphylactic reaction to a trigger. The action plan includes specific recommended treatment for an allergic reaction, is signed by a prescribing provider (physician, advanced practice nurse, or physician's assistant), and includes emergency contact information. Treatment for severe or mild symptoms are outlined; how to administer epinephrine is also presented in a step-by-step sequence, including who is responsible at school. The allergy action plan should be updated frequently and communicated to people who are in frequent contact with a child with a history of anaphylaxis. It should also be posted in the home (AAAAI, 2020; Mahr & Hernandez-Trujillo, 2017; WAO, 2020).

Complementary and Alternative Therapies (CAT)

These therapies can be effective adjuvants or alternatives to traditional treatments for hypersensitivity. Therapies may be allergen specific, such as those targeted at certain food allergies. Allergen-nonspecific therapies are aimed at supporting a healthy immune response and decreasing the hypersensitivity reaction to any allergen. While some children and their families benefit from CAT in the management of allergic conditions, they are not usually covered by insurance and can be quite expensive.

Allergen Specific

There are several variations of food *oral immunotherapy* (OIT), an allergen-specific therapy that promotes desensitization to the offending food allergen by ingesting small amounts at first and increasing these amounts over time. In food OIT, the child follows a detailed and highly controlled plan; the amount of allergenic food is increased over a short period of time to reach a predetermined target dose, which is then maintained every day. As long as the child is tolerating the maintenance dose, it is increased at periodic intervals. Children on OIT have been temporarily desensitized to their food allergies. However, allergic reactions during the buildup and target dose phases are common and the AAAAI has not made specific recommendations regarding its efficacy (AAAAI, 2020b; CDC, 2020).

In a similar therapy, food *sublingual immunotherapy* (SLIT), a tiny dose of the allergen in liquid form is administered to the child who holds it under the tongue to allow for absorption and then swallows it. Patients begin the process with one drop of the liquid each day and increase this over time. While the rates of desensitization are not as high as with OIT, there are fewer side effects (CDC, 2020; Saporta, 2018).

In a newer related treatment, *epicutaneous immunotherapy* (EPIT), a patch that contains the food allergen is applied to the skin, releasing small amounts of the allergen into the skin over time. With repeated exposure to the small doses, the immune system is desensitized. These therapies should be evaluated for their benefits and only implemented with highly motivated and compliant children and their families to ensure safety (AAAAI, 2020b; CDC, 2020; Saporta, 2018).

Allergen Nonspecific

There are several therapies that may improve the overall functioning of the child's immune system, thereby improving its ability to correctly identify foreign substances. First, traditional Chinese medicine using Chinese herbs has been studied in the prevention of anaphylaxis in patients with food allergies (specifically, peanut and tree nut). These herbs may change the immune system to become less sensitive, while causing few side effects. Specifically, astragalus, codonopsis, ginger, and medicinal mushrooms may promote normal immune functioning and relieve allergy symptoms. Quercetin and stinging nettle are natural substances that act to block histamine release. Acupuncture, a treatment originally from China, may improve allergy symptoms. Laser, tuning forks, and acupressure have shown the same result without using needles (AAAAI, 2020b; Beaver & Jordan, 2015; NIAID, 2020).

The ingestion of probiotics, either in food or as a supplement, results in the introduction of healthy bacteria into the gastrointestinal tract. Probiotics initiate changes in the immune system to prevent and treat atopic dermatitis (eczema) and food allergies and to promote normal immune system function. It is best to eat fiber-rich foods that encourage normal microbes in the gastrointestinal tract, but supplemental probiotics, through food and/or medication, may also be advantageous. To date, there is no conclusive evidence as to their effectiveness in children (AAAAI, 2020b; CDC, 2020).

Homeopathy has been investigated regarding its effectiveness in promoting immune health. The undergirding principle of homeopathy is the administration of micro-doses of a substance, usually herbal, to stimulate healing. Two remedies suggested for allergy symptoms are allium cepa (for sneezing, runny and irritated nose, and watery eyes) and kali bichromicum (for persistent sinus congestion with thick nasal discharge). Additional anti-inflammatory remedies that are recommended to relieve allergic disorder in children include Apis, Ars, Cham, and Nux vom (Beaver & Jordan, 2015). While there is anecdotal evidence that these treatments may be effective in children with allergies, they are not part of a standard treatment plan (AAAAI, 2020b; CDC, 2020).

Summary

The child with allergies often has difficulty participating in common activities that promote growth and development because of the potential for allergic symptoms and, for some, anaphylaxis. School attendance may be negatively impacted by an allergic reaction and its sequelae. When a child has any chronic illness that impacts regular school attendance, they are at risk for developmental delays because school provides a challenging yet supportive environment (AAAAI, 2020b; CDC, 2020). Specifically for the child with an allergic condition, they are unable to take full advantage of educational opportunities when they have constant rhinitis, are fatigued from lack of sleep, and/or are drowsy from medications. If the child requires care from the ED and inpatient care settings, there are potential complications of expensive care, fragmentation across care settings, school absences, increased risk of bullying due to preferential treatment at school, and parents' lost work time and wages (AAAAI, 2020b; Mahr & Hernandez-Trujillo, 2017). Finally, the potential for an anaphylactic reaction is a major stressor for the child and all family members. Stress may be expressed in various ways including strained relationships within and outside the family, poor school performance, substance abuse in parents and older children, and unhealthy lifestyle patterns (lack of exercise, poor dietary choices, and lack of involvement in social activities). Children may deliberately ingest a known allergen or delay seeking treatment for a potentially lethal reaction because they are stigmatized by their condition and want to "feel normal." Because these allergic disorders have both short-term and long-term implications for the child and family, they should be addressed regularly during any visits with providers for health promotion and/or acute illness.

Key Points

- Nurses need to dispel the myth that allergies are not a serious health concern among children.
- A thorough history is often the most effective assessment tool to correctly identify allergens and resulting reactions.
- The immune system works through a complex system of cells and processes to protect against infection and respond to foreign substances.
- Allergy triggers may include foods, latex, pollen, dust, dander, insect venom, and environmental chemicals.
- If a child has experienced anaphylaxis, they must carry an epinephrine auto-injector and have an allergy action plan.
- Based on skin testing and/or IgE blood tests, desensitizing immunotherapy may be initiated and have long-term results.
- Allergy medications are administered both prophylactically and for acute reactions.

Review Questions

1. **The nurse anticipates that the child will be referred to an allergy specialist for skin testing. Which of the following apply to patient education for this process? (Select all that apply.)**
   a. "Take your antihistamine medications as scheduled to prevent a severe reaction."
   b. "Do not take antihistamines for at least 24 hours before testing."
   c. "Use extra emollient on the area so itching will not occur."
   d. "You will be observed for anaphylaxis during skin testing."
   e. "This testing will be definitive in identifying specific allergens to avoid."

2. **The family who has a child with a history of an anaphylactic allergic asks you, the nurse, "Why do we have to tell everyone about our child's allergy? I'm afraid he will be bullied and treated differently if friends know he can't eat certain foods. He's old enough to avoid them." The nurse's best response is which of the following?**
   a. "Give your child several weeks to manage it on his own, but you may need an allergy action plan."
   b. "If he's very careful about what he eats, he should be safe away from home."
   c. "Because your child has had an anaphylactic reaction, a well-communicated allergy action plan is necessary. "
   d. "As long as your child understands the allergy action plan, only teachers need to know."

3. **The 13-year-old patient has had food allergies since she was 3 years old. She wants to try foods that she has previously had reactions to. What response(s) from the nurse are appropriate? (Select all that apply.)**
   a. "Your last skin testing was 10 years ago; due to immune system development, your allergies may have changed."
   b. "It would be safe to try food oral therapy to decrease sensitivity to these foods."
   c. "You will always be allergic to these foods, but we can manage it with medications."
   d. "We need to wait until you have gone through puberty to reassess your food allergies."
   e. "Evidence supports the reassessment of your food allergies periodically."

4. **A 10-month-old child is diagnosed with mild atopic dermatitis. According to current pharmacological management, what is the appropriate anticipated plan of care?**
   a. No treatment needed; very common in infants
   b. Emollient after bathing and low-dose topical steroid for 2 weeks
   c. Emollient before bathing and antihistamine
   d. Low-dose topical steroid for 4 weeks and herbal supplements

5. **The parent asks when to take their child with allergies for emergency care. The nurse provides education that includes which of the following signs and symptoms? (Select all that apply.)**
   a. After epinephrine is administered
   b. After an antihistamine is administered
   c. Audible wheezing
   d. Hives are present
   e. Swelling of tongue and lips

See the appendix for answers to review questions.

References

American Academy of Allergy, Asthma, & Immunology. (2020a). *Allergy statistics.* Retrieved from http://www.aaaai.org/about-aaaai/newsroom/allergy-statistics

American Academy of Allergy, Asthma, & Immunology. (2020b). *Allergies: Symptoms, diagnosis, treatment & management.* Retrieved from https://www.aaaai.org/conditions-and-treatments/allergies

Baiu, I., & Melendez, E. (2018). Anaphylaxis in children. *JAMA, 391*(9), 86–87.

Beaver, L., & Jordan, L. (2015). A cup of tea in the consulting room: The latest in homoeopathy about eczema and allergies. *Journal of the Australian Traditional-Medicine Society, 21*(2), 96–99.

Bethel, J. (2013). Anaphylaxis: Diagnosis and treatment. *Nursing Standard, 27*(41), 49–56.

Capriotti, T. (2020). *Pathophysiology: Introductory concepts and clinical perspectives* (2nd ed.). Philadelphia, PA: F. A. Davis.

Centers for Disease Control and Prevention. (2018, July). *Understanding how vaccines work.* Retrieved from https://www.cdc.gov/vaccines

Centers for Disease Control and Prevention. (2020, February). *Food allergies.* Retrieved from https://www.cdc.gov/healthyschools/foodallergies/index.htm

Demkin, T. P. (2017). Pediatric food allergies: Pitfalls in current food labeling regulations. *Pediatric Nursing, 43*(5), 237–240.

Dillon, P. (2017). *Nursing health assessment: A critical thinking, case studies approach* (2nd ed.). Philadelphia, PA: F.A. Davis.

Farbman, K., & Michelson, K. (2016). Anaphylaxis in children. *Current Opinions in Pediatrics, 28*(3), 294–297.

Goolsby, M., & Grubbs, L. (2015). *Advanced assessment: Interpreting findings and formulating differential diagnoses.* Philadelphia, PA: F.A. Davis.

Hypersensitivity reactions. (2020). Retrieved from https://www.amboss.com/us/knowledge/Hypersensitivity_reactions

Kelly, K., & Sussman, G. (2017). Latex allergy: Where are we now and how did we get there? *Journal of Allergy and Clinical Immunology, Practice, 5*, 1212–1216.

Kronemeyer, B. (2017). Advances in pediatric inflammatory skin disease. *Dermatology Times, 38*(2), 14–19.

Mahr, T. A., & Hernandez-Trujillo, V. P. (2017). First-ever action plan for epinephrine and anaphylaxis. *Contemporary Pediatrics, 34*(8), 16–42.

Mayo Clinic. (2017). Allergy skin testing. Retrieved from https://www.mayoclinic.org/tests-procedures/allergy-tests/about/pac-20392895.

National Institute of Allergy and Infectious Diseases. (2020). *Allergic diseases.* Retrieved from https://www.niaid.nih.gov/diseases-conditions?f%5B0%5D=disease%3A51

Nierengarten, M. B. (2017). Asthma and food allergies associated with early-onset AD: New research looked at subtypes of atopic dermatitis for clues to other allergic diseases. *Contemporary Pediatrics, 34*(9), 30–31.

Nierengarten, M. B., & Wyles, D. (2017). Allergy questionnaire determines true penicillin allergy. *Contemporary Pediatrics, 34*(5), 23–24.

Reber, L. L., Hernandez, J. D., & Galli, S. J. (2017). The pathophysiology of anaphylaxis. *The Journal of Allergy and Clinical Immunology, 140*(2), 335–348. https://doi.org/10.1016/j.jaci.2017.06.003

Saporta, D. (2016). Sublingual immunotherapy: A useful tool for the allergist in private practice. *BioMed Research International, 20*, 161–166. doi:10.1155/2016/9323804

Sicherer, S. H., Allen, K., Lack, G., Taylor, S. L., Donovan, S. M., & Oria, M. (2017). Critical issues in food allergy: A National Academies Consensus Report. *Pediatrics, 140*(2), 1–8. doi:10.1542/peds.2017-0194

Solomon, C. G., Wheatley, L. M., & Togias, A. (2015). Allergic rhinitis. *New England Journal of Medicine, 372*(5), 456–463. Retrieved from https://ezproxy.queens.edu:2048/login?url=https://search.proquest.com/docview/1650588285?accountid=38688

Stukus, D. R., Kempe, E., Leber, A., Thornton, D., & Scherzer, R. (2016). Use of food allergy panels by pediatric care providers compared with allergists. *Pediatrics, 138*(6), 83. doi:10.1542/peds.2016-1602

Upton, E., Schellack, N., & Motswaledi, M. (2016). A review of the management of childhood atopic eczema at the primary healthcare level. *Current Allergy & Clinical Immunology, 29*, 3–34.

Viale, P., & Yamamoto, D. (2010). Biphasic and delayed hypersensitivity reactions. *Clinical Journal of Oncology Nursing, 14*(3), 347–356. doi:10.1188/10.CJON.347-356

Woo, T., & Robinson, M. (2020). *Pharmacotherapeutics for the advanced practice nurse prescribers* (5th ed.). Philadelphia, PA: F.A. Davis.

World Allergy Organization. (2020). *Allergic diseases resource center.* Retrieved from https://www.worldallergy.org/adrc/

Chapter 16

Gastroesophageal Reflux Disease

Upon completion of this chapter the student will be able to:

• Integrate knowledge of the physiology, pathophysiology, assessment, and nonpharmacological and pharmacological management for care of a pediatric patient with gastroesophageal reflux disease.

• Appraise current standards of care for pediatric patients with gastroesophageal reflux disease.

Introduction

According to the clinical report of American Academy of Pediatrics (AAP), and the guidelines co-developed by the North American Society for Pediatric Gastroenterology, Hepatology, and Nutrition (NASPGHAN) and the European Society for Paediatric Gastroenterology, Hepatology and Nutrition (ESPGHAN), it is important to distinguish between *gastroesophageal reflux* (GER) and *gastroesophageal reflux disease* (GERD), especially in children. These authorities define GER as "the passage of gastric contents into the esophagus with or without regurgitation and/or vomiting" (Rosen et al., 2018, p. 519), and GERD as "when GER leads to troublesome symptoms that affect functioning and/or complications" (Rosen et al., 2018, p. 520).

When caring for all pediatric age-groups, experts agree that children diagnosed with GERD may benefit from and often require further evaluation and treatment. Children with GER usually improve over time or with conservative management (Rosen et al., 2018). While there are care guidelines for GER/GERD, a recent systematic review of 46 studies on pediatric GERD concluded that there is inconsistency among definitions and outcome measures, and recommended development of core outcomes to guide the evaluation of evidence in caring for these children (Singendonk et al., 2017). In response, NASPGHAN and ESPGHAN (2018) developed algorithms for the diagnosis and treatment of GERD after evaluating the quality of evidence in a literature review using the Grading of Recommendations Assessment, Development and Evaluation (GRADE) system. This chapter presents current standards of care for children across the spectrum of this condition.

The global prevalence of GERD is increasing across all ages; however, GERD is far less common than GER. Overall, GER/GERD affects approximately 3.3% of children and is a global health problem (Quitadamo et al., 2014). There are population-based differences; for example, the prevalence of both reflux disorders is lower in eastern Asia (8.5%), as compared with Western Europe and North America (10% to 20%). However, with the increased prevalence of obesity and the westernization of diet in Asia, the prevalence of GERD is rapidly increasing there (Quitadamo et al., 2014; Sharma, 2018). Also, there is evidence of a genetic component to GERD and its complications, including erosive esophagitis, Barrett's esophagus, and esophageal adenocarcinoma (Rosen et al., 2018). Increased prevalence of obesity and asthma in children may also be related to the increased rate of GERD. The relationship between asthma and GER is not clear, but half of children with asthma also have GERD. The symptoms of GERD and asthma worsen when they occur together (Li, 2019), and when this happens, medications are not as effective in symptom control of either condition, such as coughing, shortness of breath, wheezing, and chest pain. There are implications for nurses to advocate for screening and preventive measures for obesity and asthma, based on these potential negative outcomes. Finally, GERD is more prevalent in children who have other underlying medical conditions, such as prematurity, neurological impairment, and pulmonary problems, including cystic fibrosis; there are other guidelines that address the specific treatment needs of this patient population (Li, 2019; Rosen et al., 2018).

The 2018 guidelines published by NASPGHAN and ESPGHAN focus on improving practice consistency and promoting positive patient outcomes and specifically address the overuse of a GERD diagnosis in healthy infants who have feeding difficulties that may be bothersome but do not meet criteria for a diagnosis. Because the incidence of GER is approximately 75% in healthy infants (peaking at 4 months) and 95% of all cases resolve by age 1, a GERD diagnosis must be based on objective criteria, such as diagnostic evidence of reflux and/or esophagitis (Barnhart, 2016; Leung & Hon, 2019; National Institute of Diabetes and Digestive and Kidney Diseases [NIDDKD], 2019). Experts agree that the definitions of GER and GERD are difficult to distinguish in the pediatric population, making it difficult to quantify the incidence and prevalence of each condition; moreover, the degree of parental concern is often a significant factor in the diagnostic process (Rosen et al., 2018). To date, there is no gold standard diagnostic tool for GERD in infants and children, so a diagnosis may be based on the relationship of clinical signs and symptoms with reflux events after eliminating alternative diagnoses (NIDDKD, 2019; Quitadamo et al., 2014; Rosen et al., 2018).

Physiology

The normal physiology changes somewhat in the pediatric patient as growth and development occur throughout the gastrointestinal system. These changes in the upper gastrointestinal tract promote effective swallowing and prevent reflux. The esophagus, part of the upper gastrointestinal tract, is a tube, composed of fibrous muscles that connects the mouth with the stomach. In adults, it is approximately 12 inches long. While its length varies based on the size of the child, generally it is approximately 2 inches in an infant and grows to adult size by age 18. The epiglottis is an important structure at the top of the esophagus that prevents food from entering the larynx. Its development and functionality are usually complete as the infant enters the second year of life (at approximately 12 months), when the risk of choking and/or aspiration decreases (NIDDKD, 2019; Rosen et al., 2018; Rybak, Pesce, Thapar, & Borrelli, 2017).

The two esophageal sphincters, upper and lower, are also key in its normal function. The *upper esophageal sphincter* (UES) surrounds the upper part of the esophagus. It is composed of skeletal muscle but is not under voluntary control; swallowing triggers opening of the UES. The *lower esophageal sphincter* (LES) is between the esophagus and stomach, surrounding the lower part of the esophagus; it is also called the cardiac sphincter or cardioesophageal sphincter. Normal function of the LES prevents reflux of gastric acidic content, or GER, which can lead to GERD, with subsequent damage of the esophageal mucosa. The esophageal muscle, with a rich blood supply, consists of both striated and smooth muscles, the former innervated by lower motor neurons and the latter by sympathetic and parasympathetic nerves, both via the vagal nerve (Baird, Harker, & Karmes, 2015; Rosen et al., 2018; Rybak et al., 2017).

In order for normal digestion to occur, food must move through the upper gastrointestinal tract, from mouth to stomach, which begins with chewing (after teeth erupt) and swallowing. After food is taken in through the mouth, swallowing propels the food bolus into the pharynx and then via the esophagus into the stomach. A functioning epiglottis moves backward during swallowing to cover the larynx; simultaneously, the UES opens so food enters the esophagus. Rhythmic contractions of the muscular esophagus propel food down the esophagus toward the stomach. Food in the mouth and within the esophagus are responsible for these peristaltic movements. These movements also stimulate opening of the LES so food can empty into the stomach (NIDDKD, 2019; Rosen et al., 2018; Rybak et al., 2017).

While this opening is necessary for normal movement of food along the gastrointestinal tract it can also allow for backflow of gastric contents into the esophagus. Gastric acid is necessary for digestion, but is an irritant in the esophageal mucosa. Normally the LES muscle is tense so it contains the acidic stomach contents, remaining in a closed position unless stimulated to open by peristalsis. The LES relaxes due to peristalsis in the esophagus so liquids or solids are allowed into the stomach for digestion. Once the LES is open, closure occurs automatically due to the muscle contraction, but is also promoted by the anatomical structure of the acute angle of His and lower crura of the diaphragm (Baird et al., 2015; Rosen et al., 2018).

According to experts, GER is physiologically normal and occurs daily in healthy individuals across the life span, including infants, children, and adolescents. It usually occurs due to intermittent relaxation of the LES that occurs independent of swallowing and allows gastric contents to reflux into the esophagus (Rosen et al., 2018; Rybak et al., 2017). In infants, regurgitation is the most obvious symptom of GER, and occurs in 50% of all infants; notably, excessive irritability and pain without an associated gastrointestinal symptom (i.e., regurgitation) is likely *not* to be GERD (Baird et al., 2015; Rosen et al., 2018; Rybak et al., 2017). However, clinical symptoms in infants are not reliable indicators of GERD and often do not correlate with pH monitoring results and endoscopic findings. An infant with GERD may present with regurgitation, or *spitting up*, irritability, failure to thrive, stridor, wheezing, and/or recurrent pneumonia (Rosen et al., 2018). There is also minimal evidence of a cause-and-effect relationship between GER/GERD and infant apnea (Barnhart, 2016). Generally, GERD symptoms decrease as the age of the child increases; for adolescents, these episodes after meals tend to last less than 3 minutes and cause minimal if any discomfort (Rybak et al., 2017)

The current guidelines recognize several problems with diagnosing GER and/or GERD based solely on symptoms. First, there are wide differences in the expression of the signs and symptoms based on age. And for infants, the primary symptom of spitting up, is so prevalent that it is difficult to determine whether intervention is appropriate. Decreasing feeding volumes and frequency is the first recommendation to avoid overfeeding infants and decrease associated GER symptom (Rosen et al., 2018). However, non-symptom-based diagnostic procedures are often invasive, resulting in reluctance from providers and/or parents to pursue them. Current clinical practice guidelines developed by NASPGHAN and ESPGHAN guide the diagnosis and management of GER in infants and children, which is complicated by the widely varying symptomatology that is often age dependent (Rosen et al., 2018; Wakeman, Wilson, & Warner, 2016).

CLINICAL PEARLS

Normal growth and development are signs that GER does not have detrimental effects, despite bothersome signs and symptoms.

Pathophysiology

Normally, gastric contents pass into the esophagus in both adults and children; but, in infants, this occurrence is exacerbated by their liquid milk-based diet, recumbent position, and an immature gastro-esophageal junction (structurally and functionally) (Rybak et al., 2018).

The pathophysiology of GER and/or GERD occurs primarily in the lower esophagus and upper stomach, or fundus, and the LES that is located at the juncture between these two structures. A malfunctioning LES allows acidic gastric contents to backflow into the esophagus. The musculature of the LES may be weakened due to several factors, such as: malformation in utero, presence of a hiatal hernia, low pressure at the LES junction, intermittent LES relaxation, abnormal neurological function, and/or an increase in the angle of His (Barnhart, 2016; Capriotti, 2020; Leung & Hon, 2019). Infants are especially at risk for GER because anatomically they have round abdomens due to adipose deposits, and the gastrointestinal tract is maturing as it grows and develops. Also anatomically, it is a short distance from the mouth to the stomach so liquids and food reach the LES quickly; an immature LES may not function reliably (Leung & Hon, 2019; Rosen et al., 2018; Rybak et al., 2017).

As the infant's gastrointestinal tract matures, the motility through the tract becomes more reliable and predictable. The prevalence of GER is age-related, and normal daily reflux decreases as the child ages, with resolution of symptoms in most children by 18 months. In contrast, persistent GERD symptoms have an adverse effect on the child's well-being regardless of age (Leung & Hon, 2019; Rosen et al, 2018; Wakeman et al., 2016). Postprandial reflux occurs when there is a malfunction in the stomach's fundus and food is not able to flow into the stomach. Motility dysfunction in the lower stomach that causes delayed emptying also contributes to GER. Additionally, abnormal motility in the duodenum may also contribute to delayed stomach emptying (Ambartsumyan & Rodrigues, 2014; Capriotti, 2020). Abnormalities at any point along the gastrointestinal tract may be responsible for the development of GER and/or GERD, as shown in Table 16-1.

Without treatment for GER, the esophagus is exposed to stomach acid, which often results in damage to the esophageal lining, also known as *esophagitis*. The damage to the esophagus may include inflammation, bleeding, and ulceration. These esophageal changes may also result in strictures so the child experiences difficulty swallowing and may experience additional discomfort due to poor motility of food into the stomach. Finally, Barrett's esophagus is a serious complication of GERD that occurs when damaged esophageal cells become cancerous (Barnhart, 2016; Leung & Hon, 2019).

HIGH YIELD FACT FOR TESTING

GER may resolve over time, without intervention, if it is due to the immaturity of the gastrointestinal tract, rather than being pathological condition.

TABLE 16–1 Potential Causes of GER/GERD

GI Tract Location	Anatomical	Physiological
Oral cavity	• Infants have poorly coordinated swallowing.	• Lack of teeth leads to poorly formed food bolus that is difficult to swallow. • Under and/or over-salivation affects food bolus.
Esophagus	• UES and LES musculature are immature. • Esophagus is short so food/liquids reach LES quickly.	• LES doesn't respond consistently to peristaltic stimulus.
Stomach	• Fundal musculature and innervation are immature. • Stomach is small.	• Fundus doesn't consistently respond to esophageal peristalsis. • Stomach doesn't increase in size to accommodate input. • Delayed stomach emptying.
Duodenum	• Small size of structure.	• Inconsistent duodenal motility.

Assessment

Obtaining subjective and objective data for a comprehensive assessment of GER requires the nurse to focus on the structure and function of the gastrointestinal tract, including feeding, vomiting, abdominal and/or chest discomfort, abdominal size, and bowel habits. Depending on the age of the child, data may be obtained from the child and/or parent, along with observation. Because assessment finding analyses are often age dependent, changing as the gastrointestinal tract grows and matures, each section focuses on age-specific techniques and findings. In addition, the nurse should ask about the use of any complementary therapies for GERD in children, as their usage is increasing despite lack of evidence as to their efficacy (Dillon, 2017; Goolsby & Grubbs, 2015; NIDDKD, 2019).

During assessment of a child of any age, the nurse should be alert to the following symptoms that are indicative of another condition, and *not* GER(D). In the general survey, the child will have weight loss, lethargy, fever, excessive irritability, or dysuria. In the neurological assessment there are abnormalities in head size (i.e., micro/macrocephaly), bulging fontanels, or seizures. While abnormalities in the gastrointestinal system are expected, the following signs are not consistent with GER(D): projectile, nocturnal, and/or bilious vomiting; hematemasis; chronic diarrhea; rectal bleeding; or abdominal distension (NIDDKD, 2019; Rosen et al., 2018).

Assessment of the Infant

When performing an assessment, initial observation of an infant should occur when the infant is calm and comfortable if possible. It is also optimal to observe a feeding to assess for any difficulties, such as choking, regurgitation, grunting, or agitation. Research suggests that infants with GERD who experience frequent regurgitation and irritability during feeding often elicit maternal feelings of frustration and anger, which have the potential to negatively affect the mother–infant relationship (Neu et al., 2014).It is important, therefore, to accurately assess feeding in these mother–infant dyads. It is often difficult to distinguish GERD symptoms from normal physiological regurgitation in infants. However, typical GERD symptoms in infants include frequent regurgitation, vomiting, crying, irritability, poor weight gain, and food refusal

(Wakeman et al., 2016). Because infants cannot verbalize their symptoms, the nurse must use surrogates; irritability accompanied with back arching in infants is considered a reliable indicator of heartburn (Rybak et al., 2017). The nurse should ask the parent about the child's usual feeding behaviors and daily intake; from this information, adequacy of caloric and nutrient requirements can be calculated. An intake diary may be recommended if growth and development are not maintaining a normal trend. The oral mucosa of the infant's mouth should be moist and pink; inflammation may be normal due to tooth eruption, but red and/or white patches are abnormal findings. Mouth discomfort is a significant deterrent to normal feeding patterns and may be related to GER development (Dillon, 2017).

The infant's abdomen should be round, with equal chest and abdominal circumferences; if the abdomen is larger, abnormal distension is present. Peristaltic movements or waves may be visible across the abdomen. Accurate measurement and analysis of an infant's weight is necessary so adequacy of feeding/nutrition can be evaluated. On auscultation, bowel sounds should be present in all quadrants and the abdomen should be soft on palpation. Tympany is a normal finding on percussion, as infants swallow air, especially with feeding. The umbilicus should be flat; an enlarged or protruding umbilicus may signal a hernia. The liver edge is normally palpable at 1 to 2 cm below the right costal margin of the rib cage (Dillon, 2017; Goolsby & Grubbs, 2015).

Assessment of the Toddler and Preschooler

By the toddler stage, feeding has become an independent activity and often a source of control for the developing child. Tooth eruption continues but should not affect feeding as significantly as it did in infancy. Toddlers and preschool-age children may present with nonspecific symptoms, including intermittent regurgitation, heartburn, decreased food intake with associated poor weight gain, and wheezing (Wakeman et al., 2016). Toddlers may also have episodes of vomiting and abdominal pain with poor appetite and feeding. Abdominal girth should now be less than the chest circumference as the potbelly disappears due to increased abdominal musculature strength; the nurse should assess for hernia formation that results from weak muscles. Auscultation should reveal active bowel sounds, and the liver should remain palpable below the right costal margin. While there is wide variance in the timing of toilet training, it is usually successfully completed by the end of the preschool stage and should be assessed as part of a thorough gastrointestinal system evaluation. Delay in toilet training may be due to structural or physiological abnormalities that need further evaluation (Dillon, 2017; Goolsby & Grubbs, 2015).

Assessment of the School-Age Child and the Adolescent

School-age and adolescent children are usually amenable to sharing information about their dietary intake and elimination patterns; this information may be confirmed by the parents if necessary. Their symptom report is more reliable and usually includes typical reflux symptoms, such as heartburn and associated abdominal discomfort (they may describe *sour burps*). Respiratory presentations remain common in the age-group, including wheezing, recurrent pneumonia, and sinusitis (Dillon, 2017; Rosen et al., 2018). While abdominal pain may have a psychological component, a physiological cause for abdominal pain should always be addressed and ruled out first (Dillon, 2017).

On inspection the abdominal skin should be intact without lesions or masses. Depending on size and recent weight gain, striae may be present. Obesity is related to the development of GER, so recent weight gain may be a significant indicator that the child is at increased risk for GER and should be screened appropriately. The abdomen should appear symmetrical from costal margins to iliac crest, with a flat umbilicus centrally located. Percussion should reveal tympany and dullness, based on abdominal contents; this usually is not affected by the presence of GER. Pulsations and/or peristaltic waves may be normal observations across a thin abdomen.

When auscultating and palpating, the nurse should assess any area last that the child has reported as uncomfortable or painful. Each quadrant should be auscultated for a minimum of 5 minutes before determining that bowel sounds are absent. If GER is present, there may be increased bowel sounds due to increased motility in the *gastrointestinal* (GI) tract, but bowel sounds may also be normal. With a bowel obstruction, the bowel sounds will be absent distal to the obstruction and hyperactive proximal to it. These usually occur in the lower bowel and are not related to GER, which is an upper GI tract disorder. The nurse should then auscultate for vascular abdominal sounds (bruits and venous hums) with the stethoscope bell, while using the diaphragm for bowel sound assessment. Both light and deep palpation should be performed—light palpation to identify any areas of tenderness or superficial masses, deep palpation to assess organ size and tenderness. The liver gradually increases in size as the child grows and reaches adult size of 6 to 12 cm, 4 to 8 cm at midsternal line. An empty bladder should not be palpable, and if a distended bladder is present, it may be a source of abdominal discomfort (Dillon, 2017; Goolsby & Grubbs, 2015).

Diagnostic Testing

Physical assessment findings are often normal in the child with GER/GERD; therefore, appropriate follow-up with diagnostic tests may be necessary. Usually, pediatricians refer children to pediatric gastroenterologists for this level of evaluation. Current AAP guidelines allow for pharmacological treatment of GER based on reported symptoms, but a GERD diagnosis is usually based on objective findings from one of the tests described in the following sections (Baird et al., 2015; Rosen et al., 2018; Short, Braykov, Bost, & Raval, 2017).

Upper GI Series (Barium Swallow)

This procedure uses x-ray imaging to examine the *upper gastrointestinal* (UGI) tract. Currently, routine UGI imaging is not indicated for the diagnosis of GERD because the false-positive rate is high due to non-pathological reflux. In addition, episodes of reflux are often infrequent, brief, and difficult to capture during this type of diagnostic testing. A UGI may be used effectively to rule out anatomical abnormalities but is not recommended for screening for GERD, especially when the presenting symptoms are dysphagia and odynophagia and/or bilious vomiting (Baird et al., 2015; Barnhart, 2016). An example of a physiological abnormality is inflammation of the esophageal mucosa, caused by reflux, which results in thickening of the esophageal wall. Prolonged reflux may cause ulcerations of the esophageal wall, which are visible with this test. Structural abnormalities, such as a hiatal hernia, malrotation, or duodenal web, are also detectable. Reflux of barium into the esophagus may not correlate with the severity of GERD or associated esophageal inflammation.

An infant with persistent, forceful vomiting should have pyloric ultrasonography to evaluate and rule out pyloric stenosis. The child drinks a thick, chalky liquid contrast agent containing barium; even though the contrast is flavored, it is still not pleasant tasting and often difficult for younger children to ingest enough for testing. A tube may be placed temporarily to instill the contrast agent in pediatric patients with difficulty swallowing. The current guidelines are to use barium studies to exclude anatomical abnormalities but not to diagnose GERD in children (Rosen et al., 2018).

Upper Endoscopy

Endoscopy is a more invasive procedure for detecting GERD and especially its complications, such as inflammation, ulcers, and tumors. Because it requires sedation, there are potential associated problems that must be considered. The fiberoptic camera provides direct visualization of tissue and the ability to obtain biopsies for pathological analysis. Esophageal biopsy is beneficial to distinguish between GERD and other conditions, such as eosinophilic esophagitis, infectious esophagitis (candida and/or herpetic), Crohn's disease, or Barrett's esophagus. Endoscopy with esophageal biopsies is recommended only when complications of GERD are suspected and not for diagnosis of GERD (Baird et al., 2015; Rosen et al., 2018).

Esophageal Monitoring

This procedure is often performed with an upper endoscopy; both pH monitoring and manometry assess the esophageal functioning (NIDDKD, 2019). Esophageal pH monitoring has proved both sensitive and specific in detecting gastroesophageal reflux. A pH probe is passed transnasally or a wireless esophageal pH capsule can also be used to monitor the esophageal pH. The main limitation of esophageal pH monitoring is that it does not detect reflux episodes other than those that are acidic (Leung & Hon, 2019).

In certain situations, children with associated with respiratory symptoms, such as wheezing, often experience brief episodes of GER, but these symptoms resolve rapidly. While the GER symptoms have clinical importance in these children, the pH test may not be considered abnormal based on standard criteria. Importantly, children should be off all acid-suppression medications before pH probe testing is performed to prevent false-negative results (Wakeman et al., 2016). Based on pH monitoring, higher acid levels are indicative of reflux in the lower esophagus. The manometry measurements evaluate the strength of muscle contractions in the esophagus, including that of the LES. Increased levels are indicative of a stricture, while lower levels occur with sphincter weakness or incompetence (NIDDKD, 2019).

Multiple Intraluminal Impedance (MII)

Multiple intraluminal impedance (MII) is a newer diagnostic test that detects the movement of fluids (acidic and nonacidic), solids, and air in the esophagus, including volume, speed, and physical length of esophageal boluses. Combined with pH monitoring, MII is becoming the primary diagnostic test for evaluating reflux of all types of gastric contents; specifically, MII is effective in evaluating the relationship of GER and GERD correlate with apnea, cough, and behavioral symptoms. There is some evidence that combined MII/pH studies may more accurately correlate with duration of GERD symptoms and provide prognostic information; one catheter can be used for the MII and pH measurements. This testing is appropriate when less invasive diagnostics are inconclusive and/or the child remains symptomatic (Baird et al., 2015; Barnhart, 2016).

Gastroesophageal Scintigraphy

Gastroesophageal scintigraphy is another diagnostic test that detects the reflux of ^{99m}Tc-labeled (a radioactive isotope) solids or liquids into the esophagus or lungs from the stomach. Both postprandial reflux and gastric emptying are measured; however, there are no age-specific normal values for formulating a definitive diagnosis. Therefore, gastroesophageal scintigraphy is not recommended for evaluating pediatric patients with GER at this time, but it may be used when GERD is suspected (Barnhart, 2016; Rosen et al., 2018).

Nonpharmacological Management of GER

Nonpharmacological management strategies are age specific due to the significant changes that occur in the UGI tract as the child matures. For breastfed infants, changes in the maternal diet may result in marked improvement of GER(D) symptoms; these changes include eliminating milk and eggs for at least 2 weeks. While breastfeeding is encouraged for all infants, including those with GER(D), some infants with significant reflux need thickened feeds. Pumped breast milk can be thickened with commercial thickeners; each thickener has varying recommendations and age restrictions. Breast milk cannot be thickened with cereal, as the cereal is digested by the amylases in breast milk (Rosen et al., 2018). Changing formula is considered a nonpharmacological intervention; a 2- to 4-week trial of extensively hydrolyzed protein-based or amino acid–based formula may be recommended for infants suspected of having GER(D) because symptoms of GERD and cow's milk protein allergy are identical. A change in formula may result in symptom resolution for symptoms due to either cause. (Rosen et al., 2018).

For formula-fed infants, an extensively hydrolyzed protein or amino acid–based formula may decrease reflux. Another feeding alteration that may decrease reflux is the use of thickened feedings, either by adding dry rice cereal to formula or using commercially thickened formulas. Thickened feedings have long been a recommended treatment for GERD even though there is only limited evidence to support its effectiveness (Rosen et al., 2018). A review of 14 *randomized controlled trials* (RCTs) found that thickeners significantly decreased regurgitation and resulted in increased weight gain in infants (Barnhart, 2016). With thickened feedings, there is less regurgitation rather than a decrease in the number of reflux episodes. Potential problems are the effect on the normal resolution of reflux in infants and the risk for developing allergies to thickening agents. The esophageal musculature strengthens with development and use; with thickening agents, the muscles are not challenged to develop normally, resulting in prolonged GER symptoms and possible long-term effects. Use of thickening agents or rice cereal also increases the calories of the formula, and the relationship between thickened formulas and childhood obesity has not been determined. Finally, more frequent, smaller feedings are often recommended; however, this can be difficult to accomplish when balancing other responsibilities, such as caring for older children and/or working outside the home (Kiefer, 2015; Rosen et al., 2018).

Currently, there is insufficient evidence to support positioning therapy, but head elevation in a left lateral positioning may decrease an infant's crying and associated distress (Rosen et al., 2018). In a recent review of seven RCTs, researchers concluded that positional therapy should not be used with sleeping infants due to the risk of *sudden infant death syndrome* (SIDS). Rather, supine position is strongly recommended for sleeping infants, even though GER is diminished when the infant is prone (Baird et al., 2015). Elevation of the head has been studied and established as an effective strategy in adults but not in children (Rosen et al., 2018). Prone positioning ("tummy time") after feeding is acceptable and safe for an infant who is directly observed and awake. In a recent study, the left lateral position was associated with decreased emesis. Correctly positioning the infant during and after feeding may significantly decrease GER symptomology. After age 1, the risk of SIDS greatly decreases, and the prone position may be used effectively. While the seated position has been discouraged, it is offered as an alternative to semi-supine in current guidelines. The semi-supine position after feeding, particularly in an infant seat, frequently exacerbates GER and should be avoided. Optimally, the infant feeds with head slightly elevated and then keeps the head elevated during the immediate postprandial period to promote movement of fluids into the stomach and to prevent the risk of reflux (Baird et al., 2015; Rosen et al., 2018).

For older children and adolescents, the nonpharmacological recommendations are similar to those for adults, including weight loss if overweight. Even minor weight loss can help reduce GERD symptoms. Abdominal adipose tissue decreases patency of the LES. Similarly, tight-fitting clothing creates extra pressure in the abdominal cavity and may exacerbate GERD symptoms. Wearing looser-fitting clothing may significantly improve GERD (Kiefer, 2015). In addition, studies suggest that in a significant percentage of children with GERD, symptoms may persist throughout adolescence and continue into adulthood. It is, therefore, important to aggressively address obesity as a risk factor and support the child in a program of increased exercise and/or calorie reduction as indicated (Rybak et al., 2017).

Positioning changes (head of bed on blocks) may be effective for older children (10 years and older), although the effectiveness of positioning has not been investigated thoroughly in these age-groups. Dietary changes may also be recommended, including not overeating. Adolescents are advised to avoid the following: caffeine, chocolate, spicy or fried foods, carbonation, alcohol, and smoking. Chewing sugarless gum after a meal has been shown to be effective in decreasing reflux in these age-groups and is well accepted and tolerated (Baird et al., 2015; NIDDKD, 2019; Rosen et al., 2018).

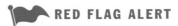

HIGH YIELD FACT FOR TESTING

Targeted assessment and genetic testing may be beneficial in discerning GER from GERD.

 RED FLAG ALERT

Without treatment, GERD can lead to serious long-term complications, including an increased risk of cancer.

ASSESSMENT PEARLS

An accurate abdominal assessment is best obtained from a child who is not in pain or anxious; implement interventions to decrease these before an assessment if possible.

Pharmacology

Medications are used to treat GER and GERD effectively in infants and children. Antacids, alginates, histamine₂ blockers, and *protein pump inhibitors* (PPIs) are the primary medications that are indicated to control symptoms, disease progression, and potential complications. For older children and adolescents who can accurately describe their symptoms of heartburn and chest pain, the short-term use of a pharmacological agent may be used to diagnose and treat GER; however, diagnostic testing may be required in younger children to identify the condition before such medications are prescribed. The goal for any pharmacological intervention for GER(D) is to use the lowest doses of medication for the shortest time possible to minimize potential side effects (Leung & Hon, 2019).

Antacids

In mild GER(D), antacids may be effective in short-term management of symptoms but are not recommended for chronic use (Rosen et al., 2018). Antacids buffer the acidic stomach contents but are not recommended in children younger than 1 year, due to the potential for milk-alkali syndrome (Baird et al., 2015). Generally, antacids work by the following actions:

- Neutralizing hydrogen ions in gastric secretion
- Protecting gastric mucosa
- Absorbing and inactivating pepsin-binding bile salts
- Increasing lower esophageal sphincter pressure
- Inhibiting gastric emptying rate (Woo & Robinson, 2020)

Antacids may be administered every 30 to 60 minutes for relief of acute symptoms and also 1 and 3 hours after meals for prophylaxis. Antacids have varying, *acid-neutralizing capacity* (ANC), which may be used to guide the choice of antacid. Aluminum hydroxide and magnesium hydroxide have the highest ANC and are often the choice when there is severe hyperacidity. Constipation often occurs as a side effect of aluminum- and calcium-based antacids. Magnesium-based antacids are the only antacid recommended for infants and often cause diarrhea as a side effect (Baird et al., 2015; Woo & Robinson, 2020). The child's normal bowel habits and whether they are prone to constipation may also affect the decision to treat with a specific antacid. Various antacids and their pediatric dosing are included in Table 16-3 at the end of the Pharmacology section.

Alginates

The composition of alginates varies widely, but generally these medications contain an alginic acid, which forms a viscous foam when it comes in contact with the esophageal mucosa. Compared to antacids, the alginates float and are selectively retained in the fundus, forming a protective *raft* that floats above gastric contents. Using this unique mechanism, alginates create a mechanical barrier that displaces the postprandial acid pocket in the proximal stomach where it is most likely to reflux into the esophagus and cause symptoms (Leung & Hon, 2019; NIDDKD, 2019; Rosen et al., 2018). Alginates may be used as an alternative to thickening infants' feeding but are not recommended as a chronic treatment (Rosen et al., 2018). Dosing timing is needed for maximum effectiveness. When an alignate is taken before a meal, it does not float on the meal; thus, it is diluted with fluid from the meal and emptied ahead of the meal. Anti-foaming agents also decrease the surface tension of gas bubbles, so the bubbles are able to move through the digestive tract. Therefore, both agents should be given 30 minutes after a meal, similar to the administration of antacids (Woo & Robinson, 2020).

Histamine$_2$ Blockers

These medications, also known as *histamine H_2 antagonists* (H_2RAs), block acid secretion by gastric parietal cells by initiating a reversible blockade of histamine at the histamine$_2$ receptors. They are effective in preventing and managing GERD, along with gastric and duodenal ulcers (Leung & Hon, 2019). Medications in this class have varying effects on the following: volume and acidity of gastric acid, gastric emptying time, and LES pressure. If a patient does not respond to a histamine H_2 blocker, it is rare that another medication from this class will be effective (NIDDKD, 2019; Rosen et al., 2018; Woo & Robinson, 2020).

As part of the Best Pharmaceuticals for Children Act, these medications have been studied extensively (Leung & Hon, 2019; NIDDKD, 2019). Famotidine is the preferred H_2 blocker for infants and children; the dosage for famotidine is presented in Table 16-3 and is usually administered once or twice a day, either with food or immediately after food and at bedtime. The dosage must be decreased when there is concomitant renal impairment as evidenced by increased creatinine levels (Woo & Robinson, 2020).

Proton Pump Inhibitors

PPIs are used to treat GERD by reducing hydrogen ion secretion at the secretory surface of the parietal cells. They inhibit gastric acid secretion through selective blockade of the gastric parietal cell H⁺K⁺ *adenosine triphosphatase* (ATPase; also referred to as the proton pump), an enzyme that is necessary for gastric acid secretion (Kierkas et al., 2014; Leung & Hon, 2019). Gastric acid is reduced by 90% and occasionally there is achlorhydria, or a complete lack of hydrochloric acid, which may affect digestion as it is a necessary component of the digestive process. The effect of a dose lasts up to 72 hours after ingestion. With the decreased gastric acid, there is decreased blood flow to the antrum, pylorus, and duodenal bulb, which may negatively affect digestion. There is also increased serum pepsinogen levels and decreased pepsin secretion, which will decrease GER(D) symptoms but may also affect digestion (Leung & Hon, 2019; Woo & Robinson, 2020).

Use of PPIs is approved for the short-term treatment of GERD in infants and children. PPIs are first line treatment for erosive esophagitis in infants with GERD; if PPIs are contraindicated, then H₂RAs are recommended. Unless a complication is present, pharmacological treatment of infants with GERD is not recommended (Leung & Hon, 2019; Rosen et al, 2018). There is concern that growing children experience an increased rate of respiratory and gastrointestinal infections when on PPIs (Woo & Robinson, 2020). Specifically, recent studies have suggested an association between long-term PPI use and pneumonia, *Clostridium difficile* colitis, and gastrointestinal bacterial overgrowth (Rosen et al., 2018). When children are treated with PPIs, cellular changes can occur that may be related to the development of gastric cancers in later life so there should be vigilant screening and monitoring for this complication. PPIs should be taken regularly and can be taken safely with antacids (except with infants). Data also suggest that pharmacokinetics of PPIs in children 1 to 6 years of age differs from that of adults; children need to take higher doses of these medications to achieve acid suppression (Winter, 2020).

If PPIs don't result in GERD symptom relief within 3 months of initiating treatment, they should be discontinued and other diagnoses considered (Kung et al., 2017; Quitadamo et al., 2015; Woo & Robinson, 2020). There are many potential reasons for failure of a PPI to improve symptoms, which are presented in Table 16-2 (Kung et al., 2017). According to recent research, when GERD does not respond to PPI treatment, genetic factors related to PPI metabolism by the CYP2C19 enzyme should be considered (Franciosi et al., 2018). Experts agree that longitudinal long-term studies on the benefits and risks of PPIs in the pediatric population are needed

TABLE 16–2 Potential Reasons for PPI Failure

Non-Reflux-Related	Reflux-Related
• Esophageal motility dysfunction • Esophagitis • Functional heartburn caused by anatomical malformation • Genetic factors that affect CYP2C19 enzyme activity	• Compliance with medication dosing and administration time • Nocturnal acid secretion • Gastric acid hypersecretion • Hiatal hernia • Acid pocket (a short zone of acidic gastric acid that accumulates after meals) at gastro-esophageal junction • Poor esophageal clearance • Delayed gastric emptying • Weakly acidic reflux • Duodenal reflux resulting in bile reflux • Impaired esophageal mucosal integrity • Concomitant functional bowel disorder

and there is no conclusive evidence of their efficacy in infants (Franciosi et al., 2017; Kierkus et al., 2014; Quitadamo et al., 2015; Rosen et al., 2018; Woo & Robinson, 2020).

Specifically, the use of esomeprazole for infants has been studied in a multisite double-blind, placebo-controlled study in which 81 of the 98 children experienced symptom improvement in the open label phase on the medication. When children were moved to the double-blind phase, there wasn't a statistically significant difference in the symptom improvement between groups (Winter et al., 2015). One of the primary goals of using a PPI for acid suppressive therapy is to relieve symptoms that are associated with esophageal inflammation and to prevent complications. The only PPI approved by the U.S. Food and Drug Administration (FDA) for treating children 1 to 11 months old for erosive esophagitis due to GERD is esomeprazole, so it is important to understand its effectiveness and potential side effects (Winter et al., 2015; Woo & Robinson, 2020).

Another specific situation is the use of dexlansoprazole 30 mg delayed-release capsule daily for adolescents with symptomatic *nonerosive gastroesophageal reflux disease* (NERD). Gold and colleagues (2017) conducted a study across 71 sites, with a sample size of 104 adolescents. The medication was well tolerated; 73 of the 805 subjects reported decreased symptoms of heartburn, gastric pain, and acid regurgitation. The subjects maintained an electronic dairy of symptoms and also completed the *Pediatric Gastroesophageal Symptom and Quality of Life Questionnaire-Adolescents-Short Form*, which showed increased quality of life during the 4-week study. Approximately 5% of the sample experienced diarrhea and headache as side effects of dexlansoprazole (Gold et al., 2017).

Prokinetic Agents

These medications are generally not used to treat children with GERD because the potential side effect and adverse effects outweigh the benefits. However, a prokinetic, which increases gastrointestinal motility, may be an adjuvant pharmacological agent in the treatment of GERD if there is concurrent delayed gastric emptying. Potential advantages of prokinetics include the following:

• Increased esophageal peristalsis
• Accelerated esophageal acid clearance
• Increased gastric emptying
• Increased LES pressure

Prokinetics are usually used as an adjunct to PPI therapy (Kung et al., 2017). When a prokinetic may be beneficial for a child with GERD, erythromycin is the first line recommendation (Ambartsumyan & Rodriguez, 2014). Data are not available about the effectiveness of other macrolides to improve gastric emptying and antral motility in children. Metoclopramide, a dopamine receptor antagonist, is not recommended for long-term use due to the risk of central nervous system adverse effects, such as acute dystonic reactions and tardive dyskinesia. Domperidone has less potential for these neurological side effects but is not approved for use in children due to the potential cardiac complications (prolonged QT syndrome, arrhythmias, and sudden death) (Ambartsumyan & Rodriguez, 2014; Woo & Robinson, 2020).

See Table 16-3 for an overview of medications used for treating GER/GERD in children.

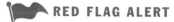
HIGH YIELD FACT FOR TESTING

Antacids are not administered to infants.

RED FLAG ALERT

Timing of medication administration related to feeding greatly affects effectiveness in symptoms relief.

TABLE 16–3   Medications for Treating GER/GERD in Children

Class	Example	Action	Indication	Adverse Effects	SENC
Antacids	Aluminum hydroxide; 300–900 mg/dose after meals and qh; over 1 yr of age. Aluminum hydroxide/magnesium hydroxide combination; 0.5 mL/kg: 2 hr after meals and qh. 10–20 mL orally 4 × a day. Maximum dose: 80 mL/day over 1 and <12 yr.	Neutralizes gastric acidity and increases LES tone. Neutralizes gastric acidity and increases LES tone.	Mild GER/GERD. Moderate to severe GER/GERD.	Slows gastric motility and causes constipation. Diarrhea.	Contraindicated with severe abdominal pain of unknown origin. Contraindicated in impaired renal function.
Histamine₂ blockers	Famotidine; 0.5 mg/kg/day, Age 1 yr and less. 1 mg/kg/day in 2 doses. Up to 40 mg/day. Ages 1 yr and up.	Reduces gastric acid secretion by 30%–35%.	GER/GERD.	Vomiting, irritability in infants; jaundice, hepatitis, liver enzyme abnormalities, vomiting, nausea, abdominal discomfort, anorexia, dry mouth in children.	Begin if lifestyle changes are not effective.
Proton pump inhibitors	Esomeprazole 0.7–3.33 mg/kg/day; ages 1 yr and up.			Diarrhea	Begin if H₂ blockers are not effective. Do not use in infants.
Alginates	Simethicone; 20 mg 4 × day for ages 0–2 yr; 40 mg 4 × day for ages 2–12 yr; 40–125 mg 4 × day for ages 12–18 yr.	Reduces gas.	Excessive gas.	Minimal.	Potential for allergic reaction. May be given via dropper or mixed with water or formula.
Prokinetics	Erythromycin; 1.5–12.5 mg/kg q6–8 hr.	Increases gastric motility.	GERD in older children.	Stomach cramping, diarrhea.	Not part of routine GERD treatment. No evidence of effectiveness in infants and younger children.

Surgical Management of GERD

Surgical intervention for GERD in children is controversial, especially in younger children, because symptoms often resolve in 95% of patients by 18 months. While pediatric fundoplication for GERD is decreasing in prevalence, there are certain situations in which surgical anti-reflux management may be indicated (Barnhart, 2016). First, children with neurological impairment are at increased risk for chronic GERD and severe complications. In addition, children with complex feeding regimens for GERD management or other conditions may benefit from surgical intervention. When children require enteral feeding or are unable to maintain a patent airway during eating, they may be considered for surgical intervention (Wakeman et al., 2016).

According to current evidence, *laparoscopic Nissen fundoplication* (LNF) is the operation performed most often for pathological reflux, but open surgery and other types of fundoplication are also treatment options when pharmacological management has failed (Wakeman et al., 2016). LNF has a lower rate of morbidity but a higher rate of failure than open approaches; overall, outcomes of anti-reflux procedures are poorly evaluated (Barnhart, 2016). According to Short et al. (2017), there is wide variation in the utilization of anti-reflux surgery and also in diagnostic testing before surgery. In a large study (n = 5, 299, 943 infants; 149,190 [2.9%] with GERD), less than 4% of infants with GERD underwent diagnostic testing. Current guidelines recommend considering surgery when there are life-threatening complications of GERD, underlying chronic conditions (e.g., neurological conditions, cystic fibrosis) that increase risk of complications, and/or when pharmacotherapy fails (Rosen et al., 2018). There is also a recommendation for larger randomized controlled trials to determine best surgical treatment standards for children with GERD.

Complementary and Alternative Therapies (CAT)

Children with GER/GERD may benefit from *complementary and alternative therapies* (CAT), which reduce the need for pharmacological interventions. Some of these therapies are supported with evidence, whereas others have not been studied thoroughly. Potentially helpful therapies for GER/GERD in children include infant massage, acupuncture, melatonin supplements, relaxation techniques, hypnotherapy, and herbal supplements (chamomile, ginger root, marshmallow root, and slippery elm) (Kiefer, 2015; Salehi, Karegar-Borzi, Karimi, & Rahimi, 2017; Setright, 2017). However, there is disagreement on the efficacy of these therapies, and in the most recent guidelines, the following nonpharmacological approaches were determined to be ineffective despite minimal evidence to support their use: positioning, massage therapy, prebiotics, probiotics, and herbal medications (Rosen et al., 2018).

First, infant massage has been practiced for years to improve infant feeding and has been specifically investigated as a treatment for GERD. Neu and colleagues (2014) completed a randomized, controlled pilot study with 36 mother–baby dyads, using the Nursing Child Assessment of Feeding Scale (NCAFS) as an outcome measure. Initially, the mothers and infants with GERD experienced significantly worse interactions during feeding as compared to those without GERD. After massage twice weekly by a professional resulted in improved interaction during feeding, daily massage by the parent was recommended for infants with GERD (Neu et al., 2014).

While there are no studies to support its efficacy in children, acupuncture has been shown to decrease stomach acid and symptoms of GERD in adults, especially when paired with PPI therapy (Hershcovici & Fass, 2011). Additionally, electroacupuncture, using electrical current along with needles, has also been shown to be effective in adults. Because stress may exacerbate GER, it is reasonable that mind–body therapies, such as meditation and deep breathing, may be effective in older children (age 10 and above) with GERD who are able to practice these interventions. Noninvasive mind–body strategies, such as relaxation and meditation, are a reasonable first choice for a complementary therapy, especially for adolescents, as they have useful transferrable skills with minimal side effects (NIDDKD, 2019). There are limited studies that support hypnotherapy to promote relaxation and decrease GERD symptoms (Hershcovia & Fass, 2011).

Herbs may be used as supplements to aid digestion, specifically the demulcent herbs, such as slippery elm and marshmallow root. These come from plants that contain polysaccharides and form a mucilaginous protectant in the esophagus and stomach against a hyperacidic environment (Kiefer, 2015). Licorice acts as an anti-inflammatory in the GI tract, which can also decrease GERD symptoms; its ability to increase the secretion of mucus by the gastric mucosa has a protective effect (Setright, 2017). When slippery elm and licorice were compared in 58 patients over 6 months, both herbs were associated with significant improvement in GERD symptoms (Setright, 2017). While these limited studies support the use of herbals, there are no studies that support the effectiveness of herbs in treating GER(D) in infants or children (Rosen et al., 2018).

The bean gum of *Ceratonia silique* added to cow's milk has resulted in decreased regurgitation in infants. Similarly, carob bean has been shown to decrease regurgitation and vomiting in infants, and quince has shown similar results along with improved feeding and less fussiness (Salehi et al., 2017). Rikkunshito is a formula that contains several herbs, including jujuba fruit, ginseng root, and tuber; it shows evidence of positive results including decreases in nausea, vomiting, stridor, and esophageal acid clearance time (Salehi et al., 2017). In addition, melatonin, which is produced in the GI tract, can be used as a supplement to decrease abdominal pain and gastric acidity. According to Keifer (2015, p. 59), "Ideally, medications are taken on a regular basis and herbals are used as needed for symptoms relief." The use of herbals varies greatly based on personal preference and also culturally bound health beliefs. In a recent study of young mothers in central Appalachia, women who scored highest in the beliefs about the safety/efficacy of herbal remedies were four times as likely to use herbal remedies (Alwhaibi, Goyat, & Kelly, 2017).

Summary

Nurses who care for children and their families often encounter parents who are concerned about their child's feeding habits, especially infants who regurgitate frequently. It is important to distinguish between the normal infant feeding and the manifestations of GER and GERD. As children age, they are better able to describe their symptoms, but the distinctions between GER and GERD may require diagnostic testing for confirmation. A referral to a pediatric gastroenterologist is recommended in the following situations: if the child's signs/symptoms suggest gastrointestinal disease, poor response to pharmacological treatment after 4 to 8 weeks, or inability to withdraw medications at 6 to 12 months. Therapeutic lifestyle changes are initial interventions for children of all ages for both GER and GERD; surgical therapies are reserved for children with intractable symptoms or who are at risk for life-threatening complications of GERD (Rosen et al., 2018).

Key Points

- Most infants exhibit signs and symptoms of GER, which usually resolve with normal maturation by age 18 months.
- GERD in children can result in feeding problems that may impact growth and development across childhood.

- Lifestyle changes are the first intervention for any age child with suspected GER or GERD and can greatly improve symptoms.
- The histamine H_2 blocker famotidine is usually effective in alleviating GERD symptoms.
- There are several mind-body techniques and herbal remedies with weak supporting evidence of their efficacy in treating GERD in infants and children.

Review Questions

1. The nurse assesses the 8-month-old infant for GER and expects to find which assessment findings? (Select all that apply.)

   a. Frequent spitting up
   b. Projective vomiting
   c. Failure to thrive
   d. Stridor
   e. Mild abdominal distension
   f. Muscle atrophy

2. The nurse teaches the family that medications for GERD may be necessary. Which of the following responses by the parent confirms that the parents have adequate understanding of GERD treatment for a 6-year-old child with medications?

   a. "My child will have to have extensive x-rays and testing before given a diagnosis."
   b. "Lifestyle changes will not be necessary once our child is on medications."
   c. "There are no safe medications for a child this age with GERD."
   d. "If lifestyle changes don't help, a medication will probably be ordered for our child if symptoms persist."

3. The adolescent with GERD wants to add complementary therapies to their GERD treatment regimens. Which of the following would be recommended as a first approach by the nurse?

   a. A mind–body approach, such as deep breathing
   b. Licorice, slippery elm, and/or marshmallow root
   c. Acupuncture
   d. Melatonin

4. In order to effectively assess and manage GERD, the nurse may ask parents to do which of the following?

   a. "Keep a log of your child's daily intake and symptoms."
   b. "Schedule smaller, more frequent feedings."
   c. "Monitor daily weight and report any changes of over 1 pound per week."
   d. "Use thickener for an infant's formula."
   e. "Position your child prone after eating but do not leave them unobserved."

5. When a GERD diagnosis is confirmed in a child, the nurse teaches the parents that appropriate treatment is necessary with which of the following statements?

   a. "Prescribers wait until age 4 to treat with medication because most children outgrow GERD by that age."
   b. "Providers will implement therapeutic lifestyle changes before adding medication."

c. "Providers will determine after 3 months if your child will need surgery for GERD."

d. "Because GERD can have long-term complications, medications will be the first treatment."

6. **The nurse explains that GERD is a complex condition that is influenced by which of the following factors? (Select all that apply.)**

a. Increased lower esophageal sphincter pressure

b. Immature structure and function of GI tract

c. Abdominal obesity

d. Positioning during and after eating

e. Parent and infant interactions

See the appendix for answers to review questions.

References

Alwhaibi, M., Goyat, R., & Kelly, K. (2017). The use of herbal remedies among mothers of young children living in central Appalachian region. *Evidence-Based Complementary and Alternative Medicine, (2017)*, 1–7.

Ambartsumyan, L., & Rodriguez, L. (2014). Gastrointestinal motility disorders in children. *Gastroenterology & Hepatology, 10*(1), 16–26.

Baird, D., Harker, D., & Karmes, A. (2015). Diagnosis and treatment of gastroesophageal reflux in infants and children. *American Family Physician, 92*(8), 705–714.

Barnhart, D. C. (2016). Gastroesophageal reflux disease in children. *Seminars in Pediatric Surgery, 25*(4), 212–218. doi:10.1053/j.sempedsurg.2016.05.009

Capriotti, T. (2020). *Pathophysiology: Introductory concepts and clinical perspectives* (2nd ed.). Philadelphia, PA: F.A. Davis.

Dillon, P. (2017). *Nursing health assessment: A critical thinking, case studies approach* (2nd ed.). Philadelphia, PA: F.A. Davis.

Franciosi, J., Mougey, E., Williams, A., Gomez Suarez, R., Thomas, C., Creech, C., . . . Lima, J. J. (2018). Association between CYP2C19 extensive metabolizer phenotype and childhood anti-reflux surgery following failed proton pump inhibitor medication treatment. *European Journal of Pediatrics, 177*(1), 69–77. doi:10.1007/s00431-017-3051-4

Gold, B., Pilmer, B., Kierkuś, J., Hunt, B., Perez, M., Gremse, D., . . . Perez, M. C. (2017). Dexlansoprazole for heartburn relief in adolescents with symptomatic, nonerosive gastro-esophageal reflux disease. *Digestive Diseases & Sciences, 62*(11), 3059–3068. doi:10.1007/s10620-017-4743-3

Goolsby, M., & Grubbs, L. (2015). *Advanced assessment: Interpreting findings and formulating differential diagnoses*. Philadelphia, PA: F.A. Davis.

Hershcovia, T., & Fass, R. (2011). Gastro-oesophageal reflux disease: Beyond proton pump inhibitor therapy. *Drugs, 71*(18), 2381–2389. doi:10.2165/11597300-000000000-00000

Kiefer, D. S. (2015). Stress-related GERD: Strategies for an integrative treatment approach. *Alternative & Complementary Therapies, 21*(2), 57–60. doi:10.1089/act.2015.21201

Kierkus, J., Oracz, G., Korczowski, B., Szymanska, E., Wiernicka, A., & Woynarowski, M. (2014). Comparative safety and efficacy of proton pump inhibitors in paediatric gastroesophageal reflux disease. *Drug Safety, 37*(5), 309–316. doi:10.1007/s40264-014-0154-y

Kung, Y., Hsu, W., Wu, M., Wang, J., Liu, C., Su, Y., . . . Wang, Y. (2017). Recent advances in the pharmacological management of gastroesophageal reflux disease. *Digestive Diseases & Sciences, 62*(12), 3298–3316. doi:10.1007/s10620-017-4830-5

Leung, A. K., & Hon, K. L. (2019). Gastroesophageal reflux in children: An updated review. *Drugs in Context, 8*, 212591. Retrieved from https://doi.org/10.7573/dic.212591

Li, J. (2019). Is there a connection between asthma and acid reflux? Retrieved from https://www.mayoclinic.org/diseases-conditions/asthma/expert-answers/asthma-and-acid-reflux/faq-20057993

National Institute of Diabetes and Digestive and Kidney Diseases. (2019). Reflux in children. Retrieved from https://medlineplus.gov/refluxinchildren.html

Neu, M., Schmiege, S. J., Pan, Z., Fehringer, K., Workman, R., Marcheggianni-Howard, C., & Furuta, G. T. (2014). Interactions during feeding with mothers and their infants with symptoms of gastroesophageal reflux. *Journal of Alternative & Complementary Medicine, 20*(6), 493–499. doi:10.1089/acm.2013.0223

Quitadamo, P., Miele, E., Alongi, A., Brunese, F. P., Di Cosimo, M. E., Ferrara, D., . . . Staiano, A. (2014). Italian survey on general pediatricians' approach to children with gastroesophageal reflux symptoms. *European Journal of Pediatrics, 174*(1), 91–96. doi:10.1007/s00431-014-2369-4

Rosen, R., Vandenplas, Y., Singendonk, M., Cabana, M., DiLorenzo, C., Gottrand, F., . . . Tabbers, M. (2018). Pediatric gastroesophageal reflux clinical practice guidelines: Joint recommendations of the

North American Society for Pediatric Gastroenterology, Hepatology, and Nutrition and the European Society for Pediatric Gastroenterology, Hepatology, and Nutrition. *Journal of Pediatric Gastroenterology and Nutrition, 66*(3), 516–554. https://doi.org/10.1097/MPG.0000000000001889

Rybak, A., Pesce, M., Thapar, N., & Borrelli, O. (2017). Gastro-esophageal reflux in children. *International Journal of Molecular Sciences, 18*(8), 1671. Retrieved from https://doi.org/10.3390/ijms18081671

Salehi, M., Karegar-Borzi, H., Karimi, M., & Rahimi, R. (2017). Medicinal plants for management of gastro-esophageal reflux disease: A review of animal and human studies. *Journal of Alternative & Complementary Medicine, 23*(2), 82–95. doi:10.1089/acm.2016.0233

Setright, R. (2017). Prevention of symptoms of gastric irritation (GERD) using two herbal formulas: An observational study. *Journal of the Australian Traditional-Medicine Society, 23*(2), 68–71.

Sharma, P. (Ed.). (2018). *The rise of acid reflux in Asia.* New York, NY: Springer.

Short, H. L., Braykov, N. P., Bost, J. E., & Raval, M. V. (2017). Variation in preoperative testing and antireflux surgery in infants. *Pediatrics, 140*(2), 1–9. doi:10.1542/peds.2017-0536

Singendonk, M. J., Brink, A. J., Steutel, N. F., van Etten-Jamaludin, F. S., van Wijk, M. P., Benninga, M. A., & Tabbers, M. M. (2017). Variations in definitions and outcome measures in gastroesophageal reflux disease: A systematic review. *Pediatrics, 140*(1). doi:10.1542/peds.2016-4166

Wakeman, D. S., Wilson, N. A., & Warner, B. W. (2016). Current status of surgical management of gastroesophageal reflux in children. *Current Opinion in Pediatrics, 28*(3), 356–362. doi:10.1097/MOP .0000000000000341

Winter, H. (2020). Long-term issues in pediatric GERD: Identifying children at risk for complications. Retrieved from https://www.medscape.org/viewarticle/517266_30

Winter, H., Gunasekaran, T., Tolia, V., Gottrand, F., Barker, P. N., & Illueca, M. (2015). Esomeprazole for the treatment of GERD in infants ages 1–11 months. *Journal of Pediatric Gastroenterology & Nutrition, 60*(Suppl. 1), S9–S15. doi:10.1097/MPG.0b013e3182496b35

Woo, T., & Robinson, M. (2020). *Pharmacotherapeutics for the advanced practice nurse prescribers* (5th ed.). Philadelphia, PA: FA Davis.

Chapter 17

Traumatic Brain Injury

LEARNING OBJECTIVES

Upon completion of this chapter the student will be able to:

- Integrate knowledge of the physiology, pathophysiology, assessment, and nonpharmacological and pharmacological management for care of a pediatric patient with a traumatic brain injury.
- Appraise current standards of care for pediatric patients with traumatic brain injuries.

Introduction

Unintentional injuries remain the leading cause of death for children (age 1 to 19 years) both in the United States and worldwide (Centers for Disease Control and Prevention [CDC], 2017; World Health Organization [WHO], 2008). According to 2014 CDC data, there were 473,947 emergency department visits in the United States annually as a result of *traumatic brain injury* (TBI) in children age 14 and younger; or approximately 1 in 220 children are seen in *emergency departments* (EDs) related to concussion (American Speech–Language–Hearing Association [ASLHA], 2020; Brain Injury Association of America [BIAA], 2018; CDC, 2017). The estimated annual number for TBI-related emergency room visits, hospitalizations, and deaths combined was 511,257 for this same age range (CDC, 2017). While the high injury incidence affects children and their families across all demographic groups, there are disparately higher injury risks for children from low-income and/or ethnically under-represented groups due to unsafe living conditions and incidence of risky behaviors (Lescano, Koinois-Mitchell, & McQuaid, 2016).

Head injury, or TBI, is the most common type of injury incurred by children. For infants and toddlers (2 years and younger), falls are the leading cause of head injury. For preschool and school-age children (2 to 12 years), falls or being propelled against an object are the most frequent causes of head injury. For adolescents (13 to 17 years), assault, sports, and motor vehicle crashes are responsible for the majority of head injuries. Across all age-groups, incidence rates of TBI are higher in boys than in girls; based on combined data from emergency room visits, hospitalizations, and death, boys ages 0 to 4 years had the highest incidence rates of TBI (BIAA, 2018; CDC, 2017; Quayle, Homes, & Kuppermann, 2014).

The morbidity and mortality rates for TBI among children are notable; TBI is the leading cause of death and disability among U.S. children, across all age-groups. More than 2,600 children, 14 years of age and younger, die annually as a result of TBI; adolescents have the highest mortality rate followed by children less than 5 years of age

(BIAA, 2018; CDC, 2017). Similarly, the rate of hospitalization for TBI is highest among adolescents and then children less than 5 years old. *Abusive head trauma* (AHT), formerly known as *shaken baby syndrome* (SBS), is a specific type of TBI that primarily occurs in children who are younger than 3 years of age and accounts for about one-third of deaths due to child abuse/maltreatment. AHT is the most common traumatic cause of mortality in children less than 1 year of age (Payne, Fernandez, Jenner, & Paul, 2017). Most cases of AHT occur in children less than 6 months of age, although AHT has been reported in children up to 5 years of age.

Globally, the incidence of AHT ranges from 14 to 40 per 100,000 children who are less than 1 year of age, with approximately half of those requiring care in an intensive care unit. In the United States, approximately 1,600 children younger than age 1 are diagnosed and treated for AHT annually (Payne et al., 2017; Schub & Avital, 2018). In an effort to quantify the case burden of TBI globally and possibly explain the higher U.S. incidence, Dewan and colleagues (2018) performed a meta-analysis with the following results: TBI is highest in higher-income countries, possibly due to better data collection, while TBI following traffic collisions is more common in low- and middle-income countries. Additionally, the proportion of TBIs resulting from road traffic collisions was greatest in Africa and southeast Asia (both 56%) and lowest in North America (25%), probably due to safety regulations, including seatbelts and child safety restraint requirements (Dewan et al., 2018).

Physiology

While injuries occur in and across body systems in the pediatric population, this chapter will focus on traumatic brain injuries and the resulting neurological changes that may occur. Therefore, an overview of the normal nervous system, with a focus on the *central nervous system* (CNS), is presented.

First, the CNS works in conjunction with the *peripheral nervous system* (PNS) to receive and interpret transmissions to and from the body in order to maintain and control a myriad of normal functions. While the PNS is composed predominantly of nerves, the CNS includes the brain and spinal column (Quayle et al., 2014). The CNS is protected by tough meningeal membranes and then encased in bones of the skull and spinal vertebrae. The blood–brain barrier also protects the CNS from invasion of foreign substances that may be harmful. Because the CNS acts as an integrative center for the rest of the nervous system, an injury to the CNS often has implications throughout multiple body systems (BIAA, 2018; Bressan & Babl, 2016; CDC, 2017; Quayle et al., 2014).

Basically, the brain collects and interprets information that it receives from the sense organs (via *afferent neurons*) and generates motor responses (via *efferent neurons*). The location of specific functional areas of the brain are shown in Figure 17-1 (Capriotti, 2020). The brain processes input from the current situation and combines it with cognition of past memories (except in the case of a reflexive response) to determine and initiate a response. For example, the interpretation of a sensory perception occurs as the *axons* of the sensory receptor cells enter into the spinal cord or brain (depending on what type of receptor) and transmit their signals to a first-order sensory nucleus that has a specific sensory modality. Then the impulse is sent to a higher-order sensory area with the same modality. As the impulse moves through the CNS, it reaches the thalamus, which sends it to the cerebral cortex where it is interpreted and combined with signals from other sensory systems (BIAA, 2018; Bressan & Babl, 2016; CDC, 2017).

Just as there are areas of the brain that control sensory functions, there are also the areas that initiate movement. Figure 17-2 shows the major areas of the brain

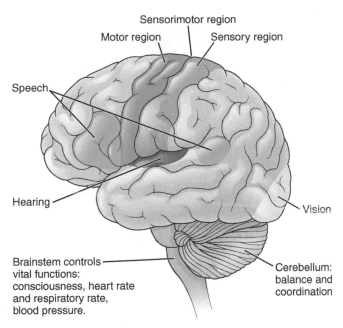

FIGURE 17–1 Functional areas of the brain *(From Capriotti, T. (2020). Pathophysiology: Introductory concepts and clinical perspectives (2nd ed.). Philadelphia, PA: F.A. Davis.)*

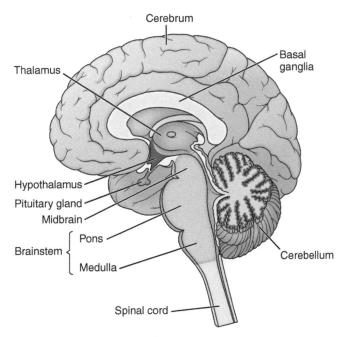

FIGURE 17–2 Major areas of the brain that control movement *(From Capriotti, T. (2020). Pathophysiology: Introductory concepts and clinical perspectives (2nd ed.). Philadelphia, PA: F.A. Davis.)*

that control specific types of movement (Capriotti, 2020). Voluntary muscle movements (except eye movements) are controlled by motor neurons in the spinal cord and hindbrain (cerebellum, pons, and medulla). Spinal motor neurons are controlled by processes both within the spinal cord and from the brain. In the lower brain of the medulla and pons are the motor areas that control automatic movements such as breathing, walking, and swallowing. At higher levels in the brain, such as the red nucleus (in the midbrain), more coordinated movements are controlled. Then at higher levels, such as the primary motor cortex, there is control of fine details of movement. The basal ganglia and cerebellum are particularly important in controlling balance. Therefore, damage to any of these specific areas of the brain results in a certain type of movement or sensory disorder (BIAA, 2018; Bressan & Babl, 2016; CDC, 2017).

 CLINICAL PEARLS

Infants are particularly susceptible to head trauma because their head is large in comparison to their body; neck strength and stability are not fully developed; and nerves are not completely myelinated.

Pathophysiology

Head trauma is a broad category and may include many pathophysiological events/processes. Children with head trauma may experience one or a combination of primary injuries, including trauma to the outer structures of the head (scalp injury, skull fracture) and/or injury to the brain and its structures (concussion or intracranial bleed). There are several types of intracranial bleeds:

• Subarachnoid hemorrhage (bleeding into subarachnoid space, usually from arteries in the circle of Willis)
• Epidural hematoma (bleeding in epidural space frequently caused by skull fracture)
• Subdural hematoma (collection of blood between inner layer of dura mater and arachnoid mater of the meninges)
• Intraventricular hemorrhage (bleeding in any of the ventricles) (Bressan & Babl, 2016; Capriotti, 2020)

TBI is defined as "disruption in the normal function of the brain that can be caused by a bump, blow, or jolt to the head, or by a penetrating head injury" (CDC, 2019, Facts about TBI). The pathological process of brain injury results from either a direct blow to the head (*coup injury*) and/or the acceleration-deceleration movement of the brain within the skull (*contrecoup injury*). In addition to damaging the brain, the movement of the brain may also result in damage to other structures, such as nerves and blood vessels (ASLHA, 2020; BIAA, 2018; Capriotti, 2020).

In a concussion, there is stretching of the brain tissue that causes changes to nerve functioning and metabolic processes, but there are no structural abnormalities with diagnostic imaging. The American Academy of Neurology defines concussion as "a biomechanical alteration of brain function, usually involving the areas of memory and orientation and may or may not include loss of consciousness" (Gillooly, 2016, p. 218). A concussion is a *mild TBI* (mTBI) that occurs after an impact to the head that causes the brain to move in the skull with resulting neurological signs and symptoms (CDC, 2019). Approximately 80% of TBI across the life span, including children, is categorized as mTBI (ASLHA, 2020; BIAA, 2018; CDC, 2017). With a concussion, traumatic biomechanical forces (secondary to force to the head) affect the neurometabolic brain function, while the brain structure remains normal. With head injury, a wave of energy passes through the brain tissue, causing a complex cascade of ionic, metabolic, and physiological changes (i.e., neurometabolic cascade) of concussion. This cascade, as well as microscopic axonal dysfunction, causes concussion symptoms. Specifically, with injury to a neuron, cells release potassium as calcium ions rush into the cell; these shifts in electrolytes result in cellular dysfunction. The neurons also release neurotransmitters inappropriately, which results in additional cell dysfunction due to over- and/or under-stimulation (Choe, 2016). In most cases, this process generally corrects itself and the majority of patients fully recover. However, while the brain is still recovering, reduced cerebral blood flow may result in additional cell dysfunction that increases the vulnerability of the cell to second insult (BIAA, 2018; Capriotti, 2020; CDC, 2019; Choe, 2016).

AHT is a specific type of head trauma and is the most common cause of *non-accidental head injury* (NAHI). In AHT, the brain is injured as a result of a force that causes the brain to hit the skull, resulting in a contusion. Hemorrhage into the extra-dural space may occur due to torn vessels; most commonly there is a subdural hemor-rhage cause by a torn cerebral bridge vein (Payne et al., 2017; Thomas, 2016). Shaking an infant results in a coup-contrecoup injury, which may be followed by secondary brain injury due to decreased cerebral blood flow and cerebral edema. It has been proposed that children's brains possess a plasticity that provides protection from injury and promotes return to normal functioning. Conversely, children's brains may be more vulnerable to the injury; because the infant's head is large compared with body size, the neck muscles are weak, and there is lack of complete myelination of the CNS, they have increased susceptibility to this type of injury. Notably, shaking does not have to be particularly vigorous or last for more than several seconds to cause life-threatening injuries that include subdural hematoma, subarachnoid and/or retinal hemorrhage, spinal cord and/or *diffuse axonal injury* (DAI), and cerebral edema (ASLHA, 2020; Capriotti, 2020; Schub & Avital, 2018; Thomas, 2016).

When the brain is injured, swelling of the tissue begins immediately, which may lead to cerebral edema, ischemia, and *increased intracranial pressure* (ICP). When there is decreased cerebral perfusion, oxygen and nutrient supply to the brain is impaired, which, if prolonged, results in damage and/or death of brain cells. The release of amino acids and an inflam-matory response also decrease the effectiveness of the blood–brain barrier, which permits additional toxins to enter the brain and to cause further damage (Bressan & Babl, 2016; Capriotti, 2020; CDC, 2019; Quayle et al., 2014).

> **HIGH YIELD FACT FOR TESTING**
>
> AHT occurs across cultures; parents, especially first-time parents, benefit from basic education for soothing an infant's crying.

Assessment

The impact of trauma on the neurological system may be immediately evident or may evolve over time, so the nurse must obtain an accurate account of the event in order to treat current alterations and anticipate possible long-term effects. A pediatric patient with head trauma often has additional injuries that affect multiple systems; therefore, a primary assessment survey of the neurological system should be followed by a more in-depth secondary survey that includes a head-to-toe evaluation of structure and function (Dillon, 2017). Because the child may have life-threatening injuries, a focus on airway (often affected by a foreign body, facial laceration, or facial bone fracture), breathing (altered respiratory pattern due to brain injury), and circulation (in particu-lar, Cushing triad: bradycardia, hypertension, altered respirations) is appropriate as an initial assessment (ASLHA, 2020; Dillon, 2017; Goolsby & Grubbs, 2015).

The focused neurological includes assessment of level of consciousness: *alert*, responds to *verbal* stimuli, responds to *pain*ful stimuli, or *unresponsive* (AVPU). The nurse also needs to know the child's previous baseline neurological status (usually from parents' report) and whether there are any sensory and/or developmental conditions that would affect the child's responses. A change in level of consciousness is a cardinal warning of increased intracranial pressure. The secondary survey will usually focus on three systems (musculoskeletal, respiratory, and neurological) but should include all systems. Specifically, the head and/or cervical spine may have malalignment and/or deformity of its normal curvature. On palpation of the skull, a depression and/or bulging of a fontanel may indicate an alteration to the integrity of the skull. In addition, a battle sign (i.e., ecchymoses behind the ear) indicates a basilar skull fracture; similarly, periorbital ecchymoses are indicative of skull trauma. Significant dental injury can indicate severe jarring to the skull. There may also be abnormalities on examination of the ears, such as hemotympanum (blood behind the tympanic membrane) or otorrhea (in particular, cerebrospinal fluid in the ear canal). Because respirations are controlled in the respiratory center in the medulla oblongata and pons, in the brainstem, an injury to that area may result in altered breathing patterns, such as apnea, Cheyne-Stokes, hyperventilation, and/or apneusis (marked sustained inspiratory effort) (ASLHA, 2020; Dillon, 2017; Goolsby & Grubbs, 2015).

Obviously, the neurological assessment is of utmost importance; the nurse should perform a Pediatric *Glasgow Coma Scale* (GCS) assessment, which is outlined in Table 17-1 (Goolsby & Grubbs, 2015). Overall, the GCS is composed of the best responses of the eyes, speaking (verbal), and movement (motor). In addition to the GCS, the neurological examination should concentrate on the following key findings: First, pupillary status and response to light and accommodation should be normal. In addition, any deviation in using the cardinal fields of gaze is considered abnormal. A fundoscopic examination should be completed to rule out retinal hemorrhage. Both motor and sensory function should be assessed bilaterally and using developmentally appropriate techniques for engaging the child to elicit an accurate response, such as "Close your eyes and tell me if you feel the light touch of a feather on your arms" (Bressan & Babl, 2016; Dillon, 2017; Goolsby & Grubbs, 2015).

Brain injury is categorized as mild (i.e., concussion), moderate, or severe with varying manifestations that are presented in Table 17-2. Current data indicate that 1 in 10 high school students who participate in sports experience a concussion, or mild TBI, every 12 months; however, it is estimated that half of all concussions are either not detected or unreported. According to Gillooly (2016), football is the leading cause of concussion in high school athletes, followed by girls' soccer, boys' lacrosse, and boys' soccer. Although data are limited, rugby, ice hockey, volleyball, basketball, and cheerleading are also suspected to contribute to concussion rates due to violent physical contact (BIAA, 2018).

TABLE 17–1 Pediatric Glasgow Coma Scale

Score	Eyes	Verbal	Motor
1	Does not open eyes	No verbal response	No motor response or movement
2	Opens eyes in response to painful stimuli	Inconsolable, agitated	Extends to pain (decerebrate)
3	Opens eyes in response to speech	Inconsistently inconsolable, moaning	Flexes to pain (decorticate)
4	Opens eyes spontaneously	Cries but consolable, inappropriate interactions	Withdraws from pain
5	n/a	Smiles, turns to sounds, interacts	Withdraws from touch
6	n/a	n/a	Moves spontaneously or purposefully

TABLE 17–2 Manifestations of TBI According to Category of Injury

Mild TBI (concussion)	Moderate TBI	Severe TBI
• Normal Glasgow Coma Scale (GCS) score 13–15 • Low-grade persistent headache • Cognitive impairment • Memory loss • Unbalanced abnormal gait • Poor concentration • Fatigue • Hypersensitivity to visual and auditory stimuli • Changes in eating • Nausea • Irritability	• GCS score 9–12 • Loss of consciousness • Post-traumatic amnesia for up to 24 hr	• GCS score 8 or less • Post-traumatic amnesia lasting over 24 hr • Coma • Increased ICP • Seizures

The nurse needs to have knowledge of signs/symptoms that will be present if the child has a concussion. It was previously believed that the child had to lose consciousness in order to incur a concussion, but only 10% of concussions include loss of consciousness. A concussion may result from injury to areas in addition to the head, such as mouth, jaw, neck, face, or anywhere the force is transmitted to the head. There are also established screening tools that may be used in conjunction with physical assessment that guide correct concussion diagnosis. Examples of these tools include CDC's *Acute Concussion Evaluation* (ACE), the *Standardized Assessment of Concussion* (SAC), the *Sport Concussion Assessment Tool 3* (SCAT 3), and child SCAT3 for children under 12 years of age (Gillooly, 2016). SCAT 5 and CHILD SCAT 5 tools are also available (http://dx.doi.org/10.1136/bjsports-2017-097492childscat5).

When assessing a child with a suspected mild TBI, the nurse should ask specifically about headache, which is the most common symptom of concussion and occurs in 90% of mild TBI cases. The next most common symptoms of concussion are sensitivity to light and/or noise, nausea, fatigue, and irritability. Notably, the signs/symptoms of concussion are manifested across physical, cognitive, and emotional areas. (Goolsby & Grubbs, 2015). Based on the "Consensus Statement on Concussion in Sport—the 5th International Conference on Concussion in Sport" (Berlin, October 2016), the suspected diagnosis of concussion can include one or more of the following clinical domains:

1. Symptoms: somatic (e.g., headache), cognitive (e.g., feeling like in a fog), and/or emotional symptoms (e.g., lability)
2. Physical signs (e.g., *loss of consciousness* [LOC], amnesia, neurological deficit)
3. Balance impairment (e.g., gait unsteadiness)
4. Behavioral changes (e.g., irritability)
5. Cognitive impairment (e.g., slowed reaction times)
6. Sleep disturbance (e.g., insomnia), drowsiness (McCrory et al., 2017, p. 840)

Pediatric concussive syndrome is caused by an injury to the brainstem and occurs in children younger than 3 years of age. With this syndrome, the child is stunned at the time of injury but has no loss of consciousness; however, later there may be vomiting and lethargy associated with pale, clammy skin. Children who experience this syndrome should be monitored closely for other changes, including decreased level of consciousness (Bressan & Babl, 2016; Dillon, 2017).

TABLE 17–3   Signs and Symptoms of Increased Intracranial Pressure

Infants	Older Children
• Drowsiness • Separated skull sutures • Bulging fontanels • Vomiting	• Behavioral changes • Decreased alertness • Headache • Lethargy • Nervous system changes: weakness, numbness, double vision, abnormal eye movements • Seizures • Vomiting

There is conflicting evidence about the presence of *post-concussion syndrome* (PCS) in children, a condition in which symptoms of a concussion occur for an extended period of time (at 3 months post-concussion to 1 year post-injury). While the symptoms of PCS in children are similar to those in adults, children often exhibit fewer of them. Currently, the evidence supports that PCS is rare in young children, but nurses who work with children should consider it as a possible diagnosis and be able to identify its presence (Bressan & Babl, 2016; CDC, 2017; Gillooly, 2016)

When assessing a child for concussion, it is important that the child and family plan to prevent another head injury especially in the post-concussive time frame (up to 1 year) when the child's brain is particularly susceptible to incurring long-term harm. For children who are involved in sports, the post-concussion care often includes being restricted from participating in sports for an extended period of time; they should be symptom free at rest and with exertion before resuming normal activities. There may also be restrictions on school attendance, reading, and screen time in order to allow the injured brain tissue to heal (Chaudhary, Pomerantz, Miller, Pan, & Aganwal, 2017; Gillooly, 2016).

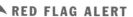 **RED FLAG ALERT**

An early sign of increased ICP is a change in level of consciousness; a parent may be helpful in noticing changes in the hospitalized child, but should not be relied on in place of neurological assessment by a nurse.

The main differences between a mild TBI and one that is considered moderate are loss of consciousness, GCS score, and period of amnesia. With the most severe TBI, the GCS is lower and there is often increased ICP. With preventive measures and/or early identification, increased ICP and its long-term sequelae may be decreased, but it is an ominous occurrence for the child and family (Gillooly, 2016; Goolsby & Grubbs, 2015). The signs and symptoms of increased ICP are based on age and are presented in Table 17-3.

 ASSESSMENT PEARLS

It is important that the baseline concussion assessment is an accurate reflection of the child's condition.

Diagnostic Tests

Diagnostic tests are often critical to the accurate evaluation of a head injury. Laboratory tests that may be performed include the following:

• Serial *complete blood cell counts* (CBCs) (decreased hemoglobin/hematocrit with hemorrhage and/or increased white blood cell count with infection)
• Blood chemistries (elevated amylase and lipase levels with trauma)

- Coagulation studies (establish baseline if anticoagulation is needed and identify abnormalities)
- Arterial blood gas (respiratory acidosis due to altered respiratory patterns)
- Toxicology screening (for drugs and/or heavy metals) (Bressan & Babl, 2016; CDC, 2019)

Diagnostic imaging is critical to the evaluation of pediatric head injuries. First, a *computed tomography* (CT) scan is the most useful imaging study for patients with severe head trauma in order to visualize structures and assess for abnormalities. A *magnetic resonance imaging* (MRI) of the brain may be performed to identify intracranial changes, such as subarachnoid hematoma or intraventricular hemorrhage. In young children with open fontanels, ultrasonography is effective in the identification of skull fractures (Bressan & Babl, 2016; CDC, 2019; Gillooly, 2016).

Interprofessional Team Approach

Because the symptoms of a brain injury of any severity cross multiple systems and components of the child's life, a team approach that includes various disciplines is best suited to managing the child's care. A nurse is often the coordinator/navigator for this team that may include primary care provider, neuropsychologist, neurologist, athletic trainers, school nurses, and teachers (Goolsby & Grubbs, 2015). A team approach has also been used effectively to focus on *non-accidental trauma* (NAT), such as AHT, using detectives and child protectives services workers to provide initial information to be used in the plan of care. Based on input from team members (pediatric trauma surgeon, pediatric hospitalist, pediatric trauma program manager, and other clinicians), clinical practice guidelines have been established and follow-up measures implemented (Draus & Draus, 2017). The complicated care of children with brain injuries is best managed by a team that brings expertise from diverse perspectives to promote the best outcomes (ASLHA, 2020; BIAA, 2018).

Nonpharmacological Management

For children with mild head injuries, the treatment is usually supportive and includes modifications, or accommodations, to their environments that will allow the brain to rest and heal. Proper management of concussion is essential to prevent complications, especially *second impact syndrome* (SIS); this is a life-threatening condition that occurs when a second blow to the head causes rapid brain swelling before the symptoms of the initial concussion have resolved. It is imperative that children who sustain a concussion have complete resolution of symptoms before returning to normal social, school, and sports activities. Recovery times vary greatly, and the plan of care must be individualized according to symptom resolution (CDC, 2017; Gillooly, 2016; McCrory et al., 2017). There are six stages of graduated *return-to-sport* (RTS) that guides the child from symptom-limited activity to full return to sport, with the recommendation that there is an initial period of 24 to 48 hours of both physical and cognitive rest before the RTS is implemented (McCrory et al., 2017). Children often experience symptoms that are very troubling in both the home and school environments, such as migraines, seizures, or aggressive or oppositional behavior; the treatment plan includes any accommodations that are needed in the educational setting along with resources for parents to deal with this stressful situation (BIAA, 2018).

There are many accommodations that can be made at home and school to promote recovery from a TBI. Adequate cognitive rest should be obtained at *subsymptom threshold*, which means that the child does not experience symptoms such as headache

TABLE 17–4   Examples of Accommodations for Students Returning to School After a TBI

Accommodation	Rationale
Allow additional time to complete assignments. May need to postpone standardized testing and limit number of tests per day. May need to reduce amount of homework.	Because there is difficulty focusing, the child may need extended time for any assignment and often for testing.
Allow for additional or frequent breaks during the school day and especially during testing.	The child may experience fatigue or headaches and also have visual changes that increase when tired.
Allow early dismissal if necessary.	Will avoid rushing and collision crowded hallways; reduce noise if noise sensitivity is present; shorten school day if experiencing sleep disturbance.
Seat the student in the front of the class.	This will decrease distractions and promote focus on the teacher.
As needed, reduce computer, smart board, & video use. Wear hat and/or sunglasses. Use audiobooks. Turn off fluorescent lights.	May prevent dizziness and/or visual symptoms.
Allow student to avoid gym, band/music, shop class; use ear plugs; eat lunch in a quiet place.	May have noise sensitivity.
Provide instructions verbally and in written format.	The child may have difficulty focusing, and providing information in two formats will provide an alternate method of processing and promote understanding.
Use assistive technology	There are devices that will assist with note taking and recording class interactions to decrease the need for extended periods of concentration.
Decrease distractions for testing.	With decreased ability to focus and difficulty with problem-solving, a quiet environment will support cognitive function.

or fatigue while engaging in an activity (Gillooly, 2016). Usual activities that require attention and concentration, such as schoolwork and videogames, are prohibited or severely limited, as they often extend recovery time.

A brain injury occurs suddenly and often traumatically, requiring the child and family to adjust to major changes in physical, emotional, intellectual, and social functioning in a short period of time. While parents may be able to achieve a quiet, restful, and supportive environment for the child at home, the child's return to school is often difficult. It is recommended that the parents meet with teachers to discuss the situation and to develop a plan for the child's successful acclimation back into the school setting. This may require documentation of disability and accommodations and may involve a 504 Education Plan. Examples of accommodations with associated rationales for a school-age or adolescent child returning to school after a TBI are listed in Table 17-4 (BIAA, 2018; Bressan & Babl, 2016; CDC, 2019). Because school promotes the child's normal growth and development, it is important to make necessary adaptation so the child can return to school and does not experience significant regression during TBI injury recovery.

Pharmacology

The medical management of a child with head trauma is complicated and is often based on advanced hemodynamic and intracranial monitoring data; the most commonly used medications are addressed briefly in this section. The nurse should expect to administer and monitor the effects of the following medication classifications, shown in Table 17-5 at the end of the Pharmacology section:

- Nondepolarizing neuromuscular blockers (e.g., vecuronium)
- Barbiturate anticonvulsants (e.g., thiopental, pentobarbital, phenobarbital)
- Benzodiazepine anxiolytics (e.g., midazolam, lorazepam)
- Diuretics (e.g., furosemide, mannitol)
- Anesthetics (e.g., fentanyl, propofol)
- Anticonvulsants (e.g., phenytoin, fosphenytoin) (Brennan & Babl, 2016; Woo & Robinson, 2016)

TABLE 17-5   Medications Used to Treat Brain Injury in Children

Class	Example	Action	Dosage	SENC
Nondepolarizing neuromuscular blockers	Vecuronium	Blocks skeletal muscle movement.	Child over 10 yr: 0.04–0.1 mg/kg initially followed by infusion of 0.01–0.05 mg/kg q 12 min then 0.001 mg/kg/min by continuous infusion.	Dosage for children under 10 yr is highly variable and may require higher initial dose. Not recommended for use in children under 1 yr old.
Barbiturate anticonvulsants	Phenobarbital	Inhibits reticular activating system in cerebral cortex.	4–8 mg/kg/day in divided doses.	May be given IV or PO. May affect normal cognitive and developmental functioning if taken long term. Paradoxical reactions (i.e., anger, agitation) are common. Withdrawal may occur if dose is discontinued abruptly.
Benzodiazepine anxiolytics	Midazolam	Increases GABA neurotransmitter that causes muscle relaxation.	For seizures, a loading dose of 0.15 mg/kg in children over 2 mo. An infusion of 1 mcg/kg/min may be titrated.	May be given IV or rectally. Assess for respiratory depression.
Diuretics	Mannitol	Increases plasma osmolality which promotes diffusion of water into plasma and out of cerebrospinal fluid.	0.25–1.5 g/kg IV in a 15%–25% solution infused over 30–60 min.	Do not give if renal function is impaired. ICP may rebound 12 hr after administration. Monitor intake and output.
Anesthetics	Fentanyl	Narcotic analgesia and anesthesia in higher doses.	2–3 mcg/kg IV prn.	Close monitoring of vital signs for effectiveness.
Anticonvulsants	Phenytoin	Reduces and/or prevents seizures by decreasing electrical activity in the brain.	15–20 mg/kg Oral or IV as loading dose, then 5 mg/kg daily divided into 2 doses.	Monitor therapeutic levels of 10–20 mcg/mL. Gingival hyperplasia is common in children so oral hygiene is very important.

Nondepolarizing Neuromuscular Blockers

Always used in combination with a sedative, a nondepolarizing neuromuscular blocker may be part of the intubation process or used to control ICP. Specifically, this type of medication prevents skeletal muscle contraction by blocking acetylcholine in the motor endplate receptors. Frequent monitoring of vital signs and patient response according to established facility protocol must be maintained. Diligent instruction of the family as to the effects on the child is necessary, accompanied by reassurance that the child is sedated and kept comfortable (BIAA, 2018; Traumatic Brain Injury, 2019; Woo & Robinson, 2020).

Barbiturate Anticonvulsants

These medications decrease seizure activity, which is a frequent complication of a head injury. They accomplish this goal by increasing the threshold for stimulation in the motor cortex; they act as a CNS depressant but do not have analgesic effects. Phenobarbital is used effectively to manage different types of seizures in children, including tonic-clonic, partial, and status epilepticus. Initial drowsiness may decrease after the first few weeks, but the child should approach activities requiring alertness and/or balance cautiously and well supervised (BIAA, 2018; Traumatic Brain Injury, 2019; Woo & Robinson, 2020).

Benzodiazepine Anxiolytics

These medications increase the activity of a *gamma-aminobenzoic acid* (GABA), which is an inhibitory neurotransmitter. By inhibiting its reuptake, larger amounts of GABA are in the neural synapse to promote muscle relaxation. Benzodiazepines are often used for conscious sedation in children but are also a valuable adjuvant to preventing and/or treating seizures. The risk of over-sedation with hypotension and depressed respirations must be assessed when multiple agents are used concurrently. Dosing will vary greatly based on the other medications the child receives and their individualized responses (BIAA, 2018; Traumatic Brain Injury, 2019; Woo & Robinson, 2020).

Diuretics

The rate of electrolyte excretion by the kidney is increased by diuretics; as the osmotic pressure of the glomerular filtrate rises, the reabsorption of water and solutes is blocked. This osmotic diuresis decreases intracranial pressure. While the safety of mannitol has not been established in children under 12 years old, it is the preferred diuretic to treat increased ICP in adolescents. Furosemide may be used to decrease fluid volume and associated intracranial pressure in younger children (BIAA, 2018; Traumatic Brain Injury, 2019; Woo & Robinson, 2020).

Anesthetics

Anesthetics may be necessary if the child has a severe TBI and requires sedation for intubation and monitoring. Fentanyl, a potent synthetic narcotic agonist analgesic, may be administered, as it has the advantage of being a short-acting anesthetic, but must be used only when advanced monitoring is in place (BIAA, 2018; Woo & Robinson, 2020).

Anticonvulsants

Nonbarbiturate anticonvulsants may be used to treat the child with a head injury to decrease the risk for seizures; medications that may be used include levetiracetam, phenytoin, and oxcarbazepine. Phenytoin works by decreasing the voltage, frequency, and spread of electric discharges within the motor cortex of the brain, thus reducing the potential for seizure activity. These medications may be used for various types of seizures, including those that occur due to a head injury (BIAA, 2018; Traumatic Brain Injury, 2019; Woo & Robinson, 2020).

There is a wide range of medication regimens that may be used to treat a child, depending on the severity of the TBI and their physiological response. Importantly, when a child is on multiple medications that affect the CNS, there is an increased risk for potentiation of side effects, especially drowsiness. The goal is to control the child's symptoms with the lowest possible doses of only the necessary medications for the shortest period of time. Children should be closely monitored for the medication effectiveness and trial decreased doses as deemed safe (Bressan & Babl, 2016; Traumatic Brain Injury, 2019; Woo & Robinson, 2020).

> **⚑ RED FLAG ALERT**
>
> Children often take multiple medications during recovery from TBI so the potential for drug–drug interactions and potentiated side effects are increased.

Surgical Management

The overall goal of surgical treatment is to prevent secondary injury by helping to maintain blood flow and oxygen to the brain and minimize swelling and pressure. For moderate and/or severe pediatric head injuries, surgical intervention may be necessary to stabilize the child and also to prevent further deterioration. These surgical interventions may include decompression of a hemorrhage, craniotomy with surgical drainage, debridement of an injured tissue, and craniotomy with duraplasty (repair of damaged dura) (BIAA, 2018; Bressan & Babl, 2016; CDC, 2017). Specifically, in closed head injury (skull is intact), surgery does not correct the problem; however, an ICP monitoring device may be placed for advanced assessment. If there is bleeding in the skull cavity, it may be surgically removed or drained; bleeding vessels or tissue may be repaired surgically. With extensive swelling and damaged brain tissue, a portion of tissue may be surgically removed to prevent further damage to healthy tissue. With an open head injury, skull fractures may need to be repaired and damaged tissue removed (Traumatic Brain Injury, 2019).

Complementary and Alternative Therapies (CAT)

There is limited evidence in the area of CAT for TBI in children. While any mind–body techniques that decrease stress are considered potentially helpful to promoting health and healing after a TBI, anticonvulsant medications often cause drowsiness so anxiety may not be a prominent problem. Researchers are investigating natural compounds and vitamins that may have neuroprotective effects that promote brain health. Specifically, curcumin, green tea, essential fatty acids, resveratrol, and vitamin E may have benefits for children recovering from TBI.

Curcumin is an active compound in the spice turmeric and may promote neurological health by increasing brain growth factors, chelating heavy metals, reducing cholesterol, providing antioxidant effects, and protecting mitochondrial function. There are versions of curcumin supplements that include fat-soluble formulations that cross the blood–brain barrier in order to promote brain tissue healing. Similarly, green tea has antioxidant activity, and contains the amino acid L-theanine that may protect from excitotoxic injury that occurs immediately after a concussion. Omega-3 fatty acids are considered essential for brain development and have been added to infant formula. Both *docosahexaenoic acid* (DHA) and *eicosapentaenoic acid* (EPA) are found in nerve membranes and may promote tissue healing. Preliminary animal studies have shown that DHA and omega-3 supplementation improve cognitive function, reduces nerve swelling, stabilizes cellular energy production, and increases nerve repair after TBI. Also, animal studies on vitamin E have found reduced nerve damage and improved cognitive performance after TBI (BIAA, 2018; Epilepsy Society, 2018).

Support Groups

Groups composed of children and families who have experienced TBI may provide effective support during the recovery period. These groups may be based in the rehabilitation setting so the child and family can become involved and obtain valuable information to facilitate the transition back to home. Community-based groups also offer information along with psychosocial support to families who have a child recovering from TBI. Support groups may meet virtually using Zoom or similar technology, so transportation and mobility problems do not prevent participation (BIAA, 2018).

Injury Prevention

A child who has had a head injury is at increased risk for a subsequent injury especially if there are residual impairments that affect gait, balance, and impulse control. Children who participate in physical contact activities are at an increased risk of TBI. It is important to always wear properly fitted head protection during contact sports and recreational activities. Mouth guards are important because they minimize the impact on the jaw. Children should avoid activities that increase the risk of head injuries, such as helmet-to-helmet hits, bike racing, and combat sports. Children who choose to participate in a high-risk sport, such as football, lacrosse, or wrestling, should have a baseline neurological screening so a comparison can be made if a concussion occurs (ASLHA, 2020; BIAA, 2018).

More than 70% of children ages 5 to 14 years ride bicycles, which makes bicycle safety a priority in U.S. pediatric care. Head injuries often occur when a child is involved in a traumatic biking event, which may involve a fall from a bike or being struck by a vehicle (Kaddis, Stockton, & Kimble, 2016). More injuries occur in warmer months when children are playing outside; head injuries are also more prevalent among boys. Many states have laws that require helmet use by all age bike riders, which have made biking much safer. Wearing a helmet also decreases the risk of TBI when there is a traumatic biking event; however, the helmet must be properly fitted in order to provide protection (BIAA, 2018; Elwell, Kulp, & McCue, 2014; Kaddis et al., 2014).

Injuries vary greatly across ages and are associated with developmental stages. For young children, most injuries occur in the home, so interventions should be aimed at enhancing caregiver supervision and providing a safe home environment. Caregiver practices of attention, proximity, and continuity are key determinants of injury to infants (BIAA, 2018; Morrongiello & Schwebel, 2017). As children age and develop, they are away from the home environment for a greater portion of their time and with their peers, rather than a caregiver. While peers often role model and/or encourage risk-taking behaviors in school-age children and adolescents, research has shown that peers can also have a positive effect on decreasing risk behaviors. Adolescents, who may have poor impulse control and may be risk takers, are at increased risk for injury when they are in an altered mood state from drugs (BIAA, 2018; Morrongiello & Schwebel, 2017). Nurses must consider the child's developmental stage along with individual risk factors when planning injury prevention strategies. Some general

SENC BOX 17–1 Safe and Effective Nursing Care for Safety Guidelines to Prevent
Childhood Head Injuries

- Teach children how to safely cross the street, using the crosswalk.
- Advise parents always to use age-appropriate safety restraints in cars.
- Caution children (and parents) to wear a properly fitting helmet anytime riding a vehicle with wheels, even a tricycle.
- Warn parents that children under age 6 should not ride on a snowmobile.
- Advise parents and teenagers that children under the age of 16 should not drive or ride on all-terrain vehicles. Older teens should wear helmets.
- Warn parents of children under age 6 not to let them play in an inflatable bouncer or on trampolines.
- For older children, trampolines should have a safety net wall.
- Teach children to wear helmets and mouth guards when participating in contact sports, even for practice.

guidelines to prevent head injuries so children can be safe in environments both inside and outside their homes are presented in SENC Box 17-1 (CDC, 2019; Ferro et al., 2016; Sciaretta et al., 2016).

Technology is also being used to provide anticipatory guidance in injury prevention. Tse, Nansel, Weaver, Williams, and Botello-Harbaum (2014) evaluated the use of Safe'n'Sound (SNS), a computer-based injury prevention program that provided individualized information to parents via computer while they were in the pediatric waiting room setting. Based on an assessment, a booklet tailored to the child's age and risk factors was printed and reviewed by the provider during the visit. The parental and provider reviews of the program were mixed, but it is an example of how a kiosk-style intervention can be used to deliver health promotion and injury prevention information efficiently.

Legislation exists in all states and the District of Columbia regarding TBI resulting from youth participation in sports. While the laws vary from state to state, this is a starting point for guidelines for removal from play for suspected concussion and providing training in concussion management for coaches and athletic trainers (Gillooly, 2016; Kaddis et al., 2014). Because of the differences in cultures and lifestyles across the globe, it should be investigated whether intervention programs that are developed in high-income countries have applications in lower-income countries (Morrongiello & Schwebel, 2017). Injury prevention programs must be planned with sustainability and cost-effectiveness in mind, too (ASLHA, 2020; BIAA, 2018).

Summary

Children and families bring different cultural backgrounds, medical and developmental histories, learning styles, and experiences to the treatment setting. Each child with TBI has a unique profile of strengths and needs. Nurses must consider age, previous levels of function, developmental status, and pre- and post-injury sensory and motor skills in all phases of care and especially in the development of a treatment plan. Caring for the child with TBI and their family addresses their abilities and challenges in various areas of home, school, work, and community. Across these settings, the focus is on developing and generalizing new skills, remediating lost functions, and/or addressing unwanted behaviors (ASLHA, 2020; BIAA, 2018).

Key Points

- Children who participate in contact sports are at increased risk for concussions.

- Infants and adolescents have the highest rates of head injuries.

- Loss of consciousness is not needed for a diagnosis of concussion, or mild TBI (mTBI).

- A neurological examination should include the Pediatric Glasgow Coma Scale when a child has a suspected head injury.

- Anticonvulsants are often administered after a head injury to prevent and/or treat seizures.

- Mannitol, used to treat increased ICP, should not be administered to children less than 12 years old.

- Resulting motor and sensory deficits relate to the specific area of injury in the CNS.

- Properly fitted helmets reduce head injuries.

Review Questions

1. **The nurse is teaching a 14-year-old adolescent how to prevent head injuries. Select all of the following that the nurse should include in the patient education.**

   a. "Wear a helmet when riding a bike."
   b. "Choose friends who aren't risk-takers."
   c. "Wear a helmet when riding on an ATV."
   d. "Drink green tea for neuro-protection."
   e. "Take concussion testing seriously."
   f. "Don't play football because you can get a concussion."

2. **A family has a 10-year-old child who has been diagnosed with a mild concussion, or mTBI, after falling off their bicycle. Select all of the following the nurse should include in the patient education.**

   a. "Meet with your child's teacher before return to school so changes in the school setting can be planned."
   b. "Once your child has been symptom free for 3 days, they may return to normal activity."
   c. "We will give you guidelines so your child can gradually return to activities."
   d. "Your child is at risk for a second injury if the concussion does not fully heal."
   e. "Plan to distract your child with quiet television shows while they recover."
   f. "You will need to wake your child up every 2 hours for the first week."

3. **A benzodiazepine may be administered as part of the post-concussion treatment to achieve what outcome?**

   a. Decrease anxiety   c. Prevent seizures
   b. Decrease heartrate   d. Decrease intracranial pressure

4. **The Pediatric Glasgow Coma Scale is used to evaluate an infant with a suspected head injury. How does the nurse use this scale appropriately?**

   a. Teach the parents how to use the scale once the child is discharged.
   b. Recognize that a smile is the best verbal response.
   c. Recognize that a lower score is better for an infant.

    d. Assess the infant's response to pain first.

    e. Understand that the score is not as accurate with an infant.

5. After a mild TBI, the parents of a 10-year-old child are told he can return to school after what criteria are met?

    a. Headache free for 3 days

    b. Able to do activities that require concentration without symptoms

    c. Vital signs are within normal limits

    d. When all medication is discontinued

6. The parents want their adolescent child to use complementary therapies to increase the speed of recovery from a head injury. The nurse provides the following guidance. (Select all that apply.)

    a. "We don't have strong evidence that complementary therapies are effective."

    b. "Curcumin is from the herb turmeric and may help."

    c. "DHA and omega-3 fatty acids may be helpful."

    d. "Drinking green tea is a safe option."

    e. "Coping strategies that decrease stress may be helpful."

See the appendix for answers to review questions.

References

American Speech–Language–Hearing Association. (2020). Pediatric traumatic brain injury. Retrieved from https://www.asha.org/PRPSpecificTopic.aspx?folderid=8589942939&section=Incidence_and_Prevalence

Brain Injury Association of America. (2018). *Brain injury in children.* Retrieved from https://www.biausa.org/

Bressan, S., & Babl, F. E. (2016). Diagnosis and management of paediatric concussion. *Journal of Paediatrics & Child Health, 52*(2), 151–157. doi:10.1111/jpc.12967

Capriotti, T. (2020). *Pathophysiology: Introductory concepts and clinical perspectives* (2nd ed.). Philadelphia, PA: F.A. Davis.

Centers for Disease Control and Prevention. (2017). Injury prevention & control: Data & statistics (WISQARS). Retrieved from https://www.cdc.gov/injury/wisqars/

Centers for Disease Control and Prevention. (2019). Facts about TBI. Retrieved from: https://www.cdc.gov/traumaticbraininjury/basics.html

Chaudhary, S., Pomerantz, W. J., Miller, B., Pan, A., & Agarwal, M. (2017). Pediatric injury prevention programs: Identifying markers for success and sustainability. *Journal of Trauma & Acute Care Surgery,* s184–s189. doi:10.1097/TA.0000000000001603

Choe, M. (2016). The pathophysiology of concussion. *Current Pain and Headache Reports, 20*(6), 42. Retrieved from https://doi.org/10.1007/s11916-016-0573-9

Dewan, M. C., Rattani, A., Gupta, S., Baticulon, R. E., Hung, Y. C., Punchak, M., . . . Park, K. B. (2018). Estimating the global incidence of traumatic brain injury. *Journal of Neurosurgery,* 1–18. Advance online publication. https://doi.org/10.3171/2017.10.JNS17352

Dillon, P. (2017). *Nursing health assessment: A critical thinking, case studies approach* (2nd ed.). Philadelphia, PA: F.A. Davis.

Draus, J. M., Jr., & Draus, J. J. (2017). A multidisciplinary child protection team improves the care of nonaccidental trauma patients. *American Surgeon, 83*(5), 477–481.

Elwell, S., Kulp, H., & McCue, J. (2014). Creating a comprehensive bicycle safety program. *Journal of Trauma Nursing, 21*(6), 309–313. doi:10.1097/JTN.0000000000000082

Epilepsy Society. (2018). Complementary therapies. Retrieved from https://www.epilepsysociety.org.uk/complementary-therapies#.Ws6uTC7wbHY

Ferro, V., D'Alfonso, Y., Vanacore, N., Rossi, R., Deidda, A., Giglioni, E., . . . Raucci, U. (2016). Inflatable bouncer-related injuries to children: Increasing phenomenon in pediatric emergency department, 2002–2013. *European Journal of Pediatrics, 175*(4), 499–507. doi:10.1007/s00431-015-2659-5

Gillooly, D. (2016). Current recommendations on management of pediatric concussions. *Pediatric Nursing, 42*(5), 217–222.

Goolsby, M., & Grubbs, L. (2015). *Advanced assessment: Interpreting findings and formulating differential diagnoses.* Philadelphia, PA: F.A. Davis.

Kaddis, M., Stockton, K., & Kimble, R. (2016). Trauma in children due to wheeled recreational devices. *Journal of Paediatrics & Child Health, 52*(1), 30–33. doi:10.1111/jpc.12986

Lescano, C. M., Koinois-Mitchell, D., & McQuaid, E. L. (2016). Introduction to the special issue on diversity and health disparities: Where have we been and where are we going? *Journal of Pediatric Psychology, 41,* 385–390.

McCrory, P., Meeuwisse, W., Dvorak, J., Aubry, M., Bailes, J., Broglio, S., . . . Vos, P. E. (2017). Consensus statement on concussion in sport—the 5th International Conference on Concussion in Sport held in Berlin, October 2016. *British Journal of Sports Medicine, 51*, 838. doi:http://dx.doi.org/10.1136/bjsports-2017-097699

Morrongiello, B. A., & Schwebel, D. C. (2017). Introduction to special section: Pediatric psychology and child unintentional injury prevention: current state and future directions for the field. *Journal of Pediatric Psychology, 42*(7), 721–726. doi:10.1093/jpepsy/jsx072

Payne, F. L., Fernandez, D. N., Jenner, L., & Paul, S. P. (2017). Recognition and nursing management of abusive head trauma in children. *British Journal of Nursing, 26*(17), 974–981.

Quayle, K., Homes, J., & Kuppermann, N. (2014). Epidemiology of blunt head trauma in children in U.S. emergency departments. *New England Journal of Medicine, 371*, 1945–1947.

Schub, T., & Avital, O. (2018). Shaken baby syndrome. *CINAHL nursing guide.*

Sciarretta, J. D., Harris, T., Gibson, S., Wentzel, J. L., Davis, J., & Pepe, A. (2016). Pediatric four-wheel type vehicle injuries: Outcomes and injury patterns. *American Surgeon, 82*(11), 296–297.

Thomas, S. (2016). Soothing crying babies and preventing shaken baby syndrome. *International Journal of Nursing Education, 8*(2), 34–38. doi:10.5958/0974-9357.2016.00043.X

Traumatic Brain Injury. (2019). *Surgical treatment.* Retrieved from https://www.traumaticbraininjury.com/surgical-treatment/

Tse, J., Nansel, T. R., Weaver, N. L., Williams, J., & Botello-Harbaum, M. (2014). Implementation of a tailored kiosk-based injury prevention program in pediatric primary care. *Health Promotion Practice, 15*(2), 243–251. Retrieved from http://ezproxy.queens.edu:2445/10.1177/1524839913504586

Woo, T., & Robinson, M. (2020). *Pharmacotherapeutics for the advanced practice nurse prescribers* (5th ed.). Philadelphia, PA: FA Davis

World Health Organization. (2008). *World report on child injury prevention.* Geneva: Author.

Chapter 18

Otitis Media

Upon completion of this chapter the student will be able to:

- Integrate knowledge of the physiology, pathophysiology, assessment, and pharmacological and complementary management for care of a pediatric patient with otitis media.
- Appraise current standards of care for pediatric patients with otitis media.

Introduction

Otitis media (OM) is a group of inflammatory diseases of the middle ear. The two main types are *acute otitis media* (AOM) and *otitis media with effusion* (OME). AOM, a common childhood illness, is the most frequent reason for health-care visits for U.S. children age 5 and under, affecting 11% of children and their families (709 million cases annually) (American Academy of Otolaryngology–Head and Neck Surgery [AAOHNS], 2017; GBD 2013 Mortality and Causes of Death Collaborators [GBD], 2015; Lieberthal et al., 2013). Globally, it is difficult to track the incidence and prevalence of both AOM and OME due to inconsistencies in reporting; accurately capturing trends, such as overall increase or decrease in incidence, is also difficult (Danishyar & Ashurst, 2020). According to the most recent data, rates of U.S. infant OM have dropped significantly since the 1990s; specifically, rates of OM (includes both AOM and OME) dropped from 18% to 6% in 3-month-old infants, from 39% to 23% in 6-month-olds, and from 62% to 46% in 1-year-olds (The Hearing Review, 2020). From 2014 date, 7.82 million children had primary care visits for the diagnosis of AOM; of these children, 52% were boys, and 48% were younger than 2 years. In 2010, *pneumococcal conjugate vaccine* (PCV13) was implemented; it protects against 13 types of pneumococcal bacteria and is given to children at 2, 4, 6, and 12–15 months of age. Since the implementation of the PCV-13, there has been a downward trend in OM visit rates (Higgins, 2018; Marom et al., 2014). While the rate of OM is decreasing, the rate of *tympanic membrane* (TM) perforation, a complication of OM, has shown a significant increase in children ages 2 to 6 years (2001: 3,721/100,000 to 2011: 4,542/1000); while mastoiditis, a potentially life-threatening complication, has shown a significant decrease (2008: 61/100,000 to 2011: 37/100,000) (Marom et al., 2014).

According to the American Academy of Pediatrics (AAP), AOM is defined as "the rapid onset of signs and symptoms of inflammation in the middle ear" (Hersh, Jackson, Hicks, and the Committee on Infectious Diseases, 2013, p. 1147). While often considered a minor health condition, AOM resulted in 2,400 childhood deaths globally in 2013 due primarily to delay in seeking care or lack of antibiotic therapy and resulting complications (GBD, 2014). Unfortunately, PCV-13 is not available globally; this vaccine is correlated with decreased disease in infants, who are the most vulnerable to life-threatening complications (Marom et al., 2014). In a regional longitudinal 7-year study of otitis media in Boston, Massachusetts, researchers found an annual prevalence rate of at least one AOM in children less than a year of age: 62% had at least one episode of AOM and 17% had three or more episodes of AOM. In this same study, for children younger than 3 years, 83% had at least one episode of acute otitis media, and 46% had three or more episodes (Higgins, 2018). Within the prevalence and incidence rates, AOM has a disproportionate negative impact on the health of children, increases health-care costs, and potentially promotes antibiotic overuse with resulting bacterial resistance. According to qualitative studies on the experience of having a child with AOM, there is often increased family stress, lifestyle disruption, and impaired quality of life for all family members (Chando, Young, Craig, Gunasekera, & Tong, 2016).

Prevalence rates of AOM are 12.8 million episodes annually in U.S. children younger than 5 years (Higgins, 2018). An additional concern is that in children younger than 2 years, 17% had a recurrence of AOM within the year. In addition, in 30% to 45% of cases, OME develops as a complication of AOM; OME may be present for months without resolution. Because AOM has a high recurrence rate, especially in children less than 2 years old and often leads to OME, it is a significant problem for infants/children, their parents, and providers. Additionally, chronic OME has serious side effects, including hearing loss. While AOM usually causes fever and severe pain, OME is more subtle and difficult to identify, especially in younger children. Symptoms of OME are usually hearing loss (detected only with audiogram) or a feeling of aural (ear) fullness that is difficult for children to describe (Higgins, 2018). Because newborn hearing screening is the standard of care in U.S. hospitals nationwide, there should be a record of the child's baseline hearing so that any hearing loss will be detected early. The newborn hearing screen is valuable to identify newborns with medical conditions that involve late-onset hearing loss to guide providers to more aggressive treatment of AOM and OME (American Speech–Language–Hearing Association [ASLHA], 2020).

While most children recover completely from each episode of AOM and do not experience either short-term or long-term complications, the impact of this condition can be very negative on the parents and family. In a systematic review of qualitative studies on caring for a child with AOM, Chando and colleagues (2016) identified the following themes: diminished competence, disrupted schedule, social isolation, potential developmental delays, ownership of situation, valuing support, and appreciating health. In these studies, parents reported that they felt disempowered and that recurrence of AOM often led to doubt about treatment appropriateness and their competence as parents (Chando et al., 2016).

OME is also known as *serous otitis media* (SOM) or *secretory otitis media* (SOM); this condition results from fluid accumulation in the middle ear and may be associated with an infections process (e.g., viral upper respiratory infection or bacterial OM). For normal hearing, the middle ear stays full of air that travels through the eustachian tube; when the tube is blocked, cells lining the middle ear begin to produce fluid that thickens in the middle ear and has been associated with the term *glue ear* for OME (Higgins, 2018). The cause of OME is usually negative pressure produced by dysfunction of the eustachian tube. While 84% to 93% of all U.S. children have at least 1 episode of AOM during childhood, approximately 80% of children are diagnosed with *otitis media with effusion* (OME) by age 10 years (Higgins, 2018). At any given time, 5% of U.S. children age 2 to 4 years have hearing loss due to OME that lasts 3 months or longer; OME prevalence is highest in those age 2 years or younger, as they are also most likely to have AOM. The rates of both AOM and OME decline significantly in children age 6 years and older (Higgins, 2018).

Physiology

Ears are paired organs that are composed of external, middle, and inner compartments. While OM affects the middle ear, as the name implies, abnormalities in other areas of the ear may contribute to the development of this condition. As shown in Figure 18-1, the external ear with its funnel shape conducts sound waves through the ear canal to the *tympanic membrane* (TM) (Capriotti, 2020; Dillon, 2017; Lieberthal et al., 2013). The lining of the external ear is a thin layer of epidermis, covered with fine protective hairs that become more coarse with age, and sebaceous and cerumen glands that have protective secretory functions. Because there is direct communication of the external ear with the TM, any condition (inflammation, blockage, or drainage) in this compartment easily affects functioning of the middle ear (Capriotti, 2020; Woo & Robinson, 2020).

The TM is the division between the external and middle ear. Sound is transmitted via the TM to the cochlea, a small fluid-filled area in the temporal bone within the inner ear. Tiny bones, the auditory ossicles, extend from the roof of the middle ear and are the connector between the TM and the oval window (the opening into the vestibule area of the inner ear). These three tiny ossicles have distinctive shapes and names. First is the *malleus* (hammer); the handle of the malleus connects to the upper portion of the tympanic membrane and can be visualized through the membrane at the umbro. The head of the malleus attaches to the *incus* (anvil), which attaches to the *stapes* (stirrup). The stapes attaches and is sealed into the oval window by the annular ligament.

The middle ear is composed of intricately connected structures that must work together in order to function normally (Capriotti, 2020; Lieberthal et al., 2013; Woo & Robinson, 2020). Sound waves cause the TM to move the ossicles, and in response, the fluid in the oval window vibrates. It is the oval and round windows, two tissue-covered openings that are responsible for transmitting sound from the middle to the inner ear. Vibrations are amplified as they travel from the ossicles in the middle ear to the oval window, which is in the inner ear. The eustachian tube is a structure in the middle ear that connects the nasopharynx to the middle ear; it remains closed unless yawning or swallowing, when equalization between the pressure of the inner ear and

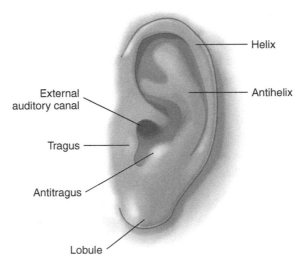

FIGURE 18–1 External and middle ear anatomy *(From Dillon, P. (2017). Nursing health assessment: A critical thinking, case studies approach (2nd ed.). Philadelphia, PA: F.A. Davis.)*

external environment is needed. This is a very important mechanism that maintains normal pressure for the TM and prevents its rupture. Also, optimal sound transmission through the middle ear occurs when air pressure in the ear canal is the same as pressure in the middle ear (Capriotti, 2020). Additionally, the normally functioning eustachian tubes protect the middle ear from nasopharyngeal secretions by providing a mechanism for drainage of these secretions (Ward & Hisley, 2016).

The external and middle ear work in tandem to collect, amplify, transmit and receive sound. Then the inner ear, which consists of sensory and proprioception organs, is responsible for transforming sound waves into neural impulses that are sent to the brain via the auditory nerve. The inner ear is the most complex compartment of the ear as it is responsible for both hearing and balance functions. The *vestibular* system, composed of labyrinths and receptor, regulate movement and balance. The two labyrinths, bony and membranous, make up the semicircular canals. Two separate fluids, *periotic* (perilymph) and *otic* (endolymph), fill the membranous labyrinth and fluctuate during movement, providing a sense of balance and coordinated movement (Capriotti, 2020; Dillon, 2017; Woo & Robinson, 2020). The auditory nerve, cranial nerve VIII, senses the movement of the fluid and contributes to the ability to maintain balance and move with stability. The *cochlea* and the *organ of Corti* in the membranous labyrinth are the special sensory organs that are responsible for hearing. The spiral-shaped organ of Corti is located within the cochlear duct and is composed of supporting cells and many rows of cochlear hair cells. Afferent sensory nerve fibers from the cochlear nerve are wrapped at the base of the cochlear hair cells. The stapes delivers sound waves to the oval window and to the periotic fluid. Sound transmission occurs as cilia of the hair cells in the organ of Corti bend in response to the sound (Capriotti, 2020; Lieberthal et al., 2013; Woo & Robinson, 2020).

HIGH YIELD FACT FOR TESTING

Normal functioning of the ear and subsequent hearing is dependent on the transmission of sound through the three distinct areas of the ear: outer, middle, and inner.

Pathophysiology

It is important to understand the different pathological processes that lead to AOM and to distinguish it from associated ear conditions, such as OME. AOM is an infectious process with an abrupt onset that usually presents with ear pain, causes young children to pull at ears, cry, and have difficulty sleeping, a poor appetite, and fever (Higgins, 2018; Lieberthal et al., 2013; Normandin, 2015). In contrast, OME, defined as an inflammatory condition with the presence of non-infectious fluid in the middle ear for more than three months, is typically not associated with any specific symptoms and is more difficult to identify. The effusion may be serous, mucoid, or purulent. Pain often increases with presence of an effusion because the TM is inflamed, irritated, and bulging. In a related but distinctive condition, *chronic suppurative otitis media* (CSOM) (also known as *chronic otitis media with effusion* (COME), is middle ear inflammation, not infection, that lasts more than 3 months (Outhoff, 2017). Otorrhea, or ear discharge, in a child is usually painless; however, fluid in the middle ear and the resulting impaired mobility of the tympanic membrane may result in hearing loss, balance problems, subsequent poor school performance and/or behavioral problems, ear discomfort, and recurrent AOM (because the fluid is a medium for viral and/or bacterial growth). Overall, there is decreased quality of life for the child and family and the potential for damage to the tympanic membrane that requires surgical repair (Outhoff, 2017; Ward & Hisley, 2016). Children with OME should be re-evaluated at 3- to 6-month intervals with pneumatic otoscopy (to determine tympanic membrane movement), developmental surveillance (for early detection), and hearing testing; if any of these areas shows significant changes, tympanostomy tube placement may be necessary (Outhof, 2017; Ward & Hisley, 2016).

All three of these conditions, AOM, OME, and CSOM (see Table 18-1), may be associated with hearing loss because inflammation and/or infection in the middle ear prevents transmission of sound. Children who have impaired hearing are at a correlated risk for delayed speech development, which may manifest as cognitive or behavioral problems (Capriotti, 2020; Hersh et al., 2013; Woo & Robinson, 2020). Specifically, children with OME are at risk for developing hearing loss in both quiet and noisy settings and have resulting difficulty with both hearing sensitivity and speech perception, which requires interventions (Cai & McPherson, 2017).

TABLE 18–1   Middle Ear Conditions

Condition	Assessment Findings	Treatment	Patient/Family Education
AOM (severe)	Fever >102.2°F Red, bulging TM Otalgia Cholesteatoma Otorrhea Problems sleeping Poor appetite	• If less than 2 yr old, treat with 10 days of antibiotic. • If 2–5 yr, treat with 7 days of antibiotic. • If 6 yr or older, treat with 5 days of antibiotic. • Supportive therapy for pain (alternating acetaminophen and ibuprofen), warm applications locally	• Return to office for TM recheck within 6 weeks. • Promote breastfeeding, especially for infants less than 6 mo. • Decrease exposure to secondhand tobacco smoke. • Decrease day care/similar nursery childcare settings.

AOM (mild)	Afebrile or fever <102.2°F
	    TM non-erythematous or normal
	    Normal TM movement
	    Minimal disruption to everyday activities
		• If this is first occurrence, give a wait and see prescription (WASP).
		• If this is a recurrent AOM, a WASP may still be appropriate, or an antibiotic may be indicated if less than 2 years old.
			• Parents should expect a phone call from the nurse in 48–72 hr to assess for improvement or filling prescription.
			• Parents should demonstrate knowledge of signs/symptoms (s/s) of increasing illness.
			• Parents should demonstrate taking a temperature in an age-appropriate route.

MEE/OME	May be asymptomatic May be associated with AOM	• Reassessment for spontaneous resolution if not association with AOM. • Treat with antibiotic if present with AOM. • Myringotomy (incision in the tympanic membrane) with aspiration may be performed to culture fluid. • Tympanostomy tubes may be necessary for resolution.	• This condition may not resolve for several weeks. • Parents should demonstrate knowledge of s/s of infection. • Keeping return appointment is important for evaluation even if symptoms resolve. • Child's hearing will be monitored.
CSOM/COME	Cloudy TM Otorrhea Decreased hearing	• Tympanostomy tubes may be indicated to promote drainage and decrease inflammation.	• Regular assessment of patency of tubes. • Care of tubes: do not immerse head in water, may swim with ear plugs. • Serial hearing audiometry testing.

(Adapted from: Capriotti, 2020; Hersh et al., 2013; Lieberthal et al., 2013)

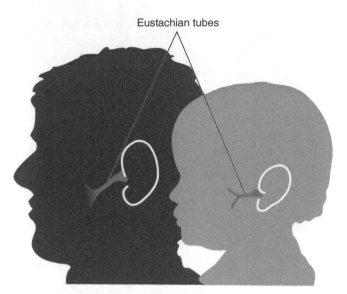

FIGURE 18-2 Position of the eustachian tube as it connects the middle ear space to the back of the nose, or nasopharynx. From: *Rosenfeld, R. M., Shin, J. J., Schwartz, S. R., Coggins, R., Gagnon, L., Hackell, J. M., . . . Corrigan, M. D. (2016). Clinical practice guideline: Otitis media with effusion (update). Otolaryngology–Head and Neck Surgery, 154(Suppl. 1), S1–241. Reprinted by Permission of SAGE Publications, Inc.*

While evidence supports the contribution of various risk factors to the development of AOM, the precise cause of this condition remains unknown but is postulated to be eustachian tube dysfunction. Tubes in infants and children under 5 years old are shorter, wider, and more horizontal in relation to the middle ear (see Figure 18-2), so they do not function as effectively to drain fluid from the middle ear (Ward & Hisley, 2016). Because the cartilage lining of the eustachian tubes is undeveloped, the tubes are more expandable, resulting in pooling of fluid that obstructs the eustachian tube and impairs normal function (Ward & Hisley, 2016). When fluid pools in the middle ear, there is potential for it to become infected from nasopharyngeal bacteria that flows into the area due to the negative pressure (Chonmaitree et al., 2017; Lieberthal et al., 2013). Physiological abnormalities, such as enlarged adenoids and/or obstructed eustachian tubes, may also be responsible for the development of AOM (Capriotti, 2020; Ward & Hisley, 2016; Woo & Robinson, 2020).

When an upper respiratory infection precedes AOM, there is inflammation of the mucous membranes of the eustachian tubes, so they do not work effectively to promote air movement. Air that should flow into the middle ear is reabsorbed into the bloodstream. Then fluid fills the space that is left by the removal of the air, which provides a moist warm environment for rapid growth of pathogens, both viral and bacterial (most commonly *Haemophilus influenzae*, *Streptococcus pneumoniae*, and *Moraxella catarrhalis*) (Hersh et al., 2013; Lieberthal et al., 2013). Infection is often polymicrobial and involves complex interactions between viral and bacterial microorganisms and the child's immune and inflammatory responses. Children's immune systems are still developing so their immature defense mechanisms increase their risk of all types of infections (Chonmaitree et al., 2017; Ward & Hisley, 2016). There is increased blood flow with the inflammatory process that results in injected or red tympanic membrane and fluid accumulation (Capriotti, 2020).

In contrast to the acute infection of AOM, CSOM is a chronic inflammation, not infection, of the middle ear with extension into the mastoid cavity. Children must experience otorrhea through the perforated TM for at least 6 weeks for a confirmatory diagnosis. The child often develops an initial *upper respiratory infection* (URI) that results in AOM, with subsequent CSOM (Lieberthal et al., 2013). When the mucosa is inflamed for an extended period of time, it becomes damaged and may ulcerate. In response to an ulceration, the mucosa proliferates granulation tissue, and polyps often form from the site of an ulceration; this promulgates the cycle of discharge and inflammation. Drainage may be contained to the middle ear (cholesteatoma) or may drain into the ear canal (otorrhea). Globally, CSOM is the most common cause of hearing loss (may be permanent depending on the extent of damage to structure) (Capriotti, 2020; Hersh et al., 2013; Woo & Robinson, 2020).

Risk Factors

Several factors increase a child's risk of developing AOM, including male sex, age between 6 and 24 months, being formula fed as an infant, exposure to secondhand cigarette smoke, day-care attendance (increases the risk of AOM by 100%), presence of allergic rhinitis, and use of a pacifier for several hours each day. Children with cleft lip/palate and Down's syndrome are more likely to develop AOM and CSOM. Alaskan Native children are at higher risk for AOM (Capriotti, 2020; Mayo Clinic, 2020; Woo & Robinson, 2020).

When children suck on a pacifier, they raise the soft palate, which may lessen the effectiveness of the eustachian tube function and allow microorganisms to enter the ear from the oropharynx. Exposure to secondhand tobacco smoke results in irritation of the nasal and throat mucosa and decreases effectiveness of cilia that protect the nasal pharynx and mobilize pathogens away from the ear structures (Capriotti, 2020; Woo & Robinson, 2020). Because URIs are so common in the first year of life, there is associated increased risk for AOM, which often follows these infections.

Children of certain ethnic backgrounds experience OM at a higher rate; these ethnicities are Native American Indian, African American, and Alaskan Native. Researchers are investigating a genetic component to OM, as it is more common in some families. In a Finnish study of 923 children, it was determined that certain genes have a role in the innate immune system and are involved in susceptibility to respiratory infection and AOM; specifically, there was a polymorphism that was tied to increased recurrence of AOM and another one that decreased the risk of infection (Toivonen et al., 2017). Factors related to the health disparity among these ethnicities may also include crowded living conditions, exposure to secondhand tobacco smoke, and lack of breastfeeding (Lieberthal et al., 2013).

The rate of AOM occurrence has decreased over the past 30 years due to pneumococcal vaccination, breastfeeding, and decreased exposure to secondhand smoke. The 7-valent pneumococcal vaccine (PCV7) and the subsequent PCV13 have decreased the overall incidence of AOM and have shifted the primary causative agent from *S. pneumoniae* to *H. influenzae*. Conversely, the *Haemophilus influenzae* type B (Hib) vaccine has not decreased the incidence of AOM caused by *H. influenzae* because the infections are usually caused by non-typeable bacteria (Hersh et al., 2013; Lieberthal et al., 2013).

> **HIGH YIELD FACT FOR TESTING**
>
> As the anatomical ear structures of the child grow and develop, especially the eustachian tubes, the ears function more efficiently, and infection is less likely to occur.

Assessment

The definitive diagnosis of AOM should be based on the presence of either of two assessment findings so accuracy in evaluating patients' signs is critical. First, there should be evidence of *middle ear effusion* (MEE), fluid that is present behind the TM, with moderate to severe bulging of the TM, or otorrhea that is not attributed to an infection of the external ear (otitis externa or *swimmer's ear*). However, AOM may also be diagnosed when the TM is only mildly bulging but is erythematous and the child has recent onset ear pain (otalgia). TM visualization may be difficult with children due to small ear canals, especially when inflamed, presence of drainage, or erythema due to crying and/or fever; an effective examination is dependent on the cooperativeness of the patient (Dillon, 2017; Hersh et al., 2013; Lieberthal et al., 2013; Normandin, 2015).

Assessment begins with obtaining a history from the patient and/or family. For a child, the parent should be asked about risk factors (discussed earlier) that increase the chance of AOM. The nurse should also question the parent/child about any symptoms that may occur with an AOM, understanding that OM may be asymptomatic. Parents may need education about the importance of identifying and treating OM so it does not result in permanent hearing loss, and this part of the assessment provides an opportunity to offer information and answer questions (Dillon, 2017).

While AOM is a condition affecting the middle ear, it is important to thoroughly assess the external ear for any abnormalities that may contribute to AOM development as the structures are connected and interdependent. The auricle, or outer ear, should not be tender with movement and/or palpation. The ear canal should be free of inflammation and discharge. A gross determination of normal hearing can be made, individualized based on the child's age and development. Neonates are screened for hearing abnormalities before discharge from the hospital (Dillon, 2017; Goolsby & Grubbs, 2015). Parents can usually determine and report whether their infant or toddler reacts normally to sounds in the household environment. When the child is old enough to cooperate, they can verify which ear the nurse whispers into with closed eyes. Audiometry is performed routinely with the 4-year-old well-child assessment and for entry into kindergarten, so this may provide a baseline for the child's hearing (Dillon, 2017; Goolsby & Grubbs, 2015).

Assessment focuses on evaluation of the TM by both direct and indirect measures. Direct evaluation requires use of speculum and otoscope. SENC Box 18-1 shows the steps to assure a clear visualization of the ear canal. Note that holding the otoscope with the handle upward allows the examiner to rest that hand against the child's head, so if the child's head moves, the otoscope moves with the child, eliminating potential risk for injury to the ear canal.

The cone of light is a normal finding due to the translucent nature of the TM; it is usually seen at five o'clock (with the TM as the face of a clock) on the right TM, and seven o'clock on the left TM. The TM should be pearly gray, translucent, and nonbulging, with the following structures visible: umbo, pars flaccida, and the cone of

---

SENC BOX 18–1   Safe and Effective Nursing Care for Examining the Ear Canal

- For children <2 years old, *pull the ear lobe down* to straighten the ear canal.
- For children >2 years old, *pull the ear up and back* to straighten the ear canal.
- Insert the speculum about 0.5 in. into the ear canal.
- With the otoscope, visualize and assess the following aspects of the TM:
  - Color
  - Intactness
  - Position of landmarks (bones and cone of light)
  - Mobility

light (Dillon, 2017; Goolsby & Grubbs, 2015). With recurrent AOM, there is scarring of the TM that make take months to resolve or may persist permanently; the presence of tympanostomy tubes may result in visible changes to the TM, and mild scarring that does not interfere with TM function is not unusual (Dillon, 2017; Goolsby & Grubbs, 2015).

The presence of MEE is abnormal and should be described by amount (how far it is visible in proportion to the TM, such as half-way) and color (clear, watery, thick, mucoid, or purulent). When serous OM is present, the TM often appears yellowish with air bubbles noted behind it. With AOM, the TM is often reddened, with absence of the light reflex. It is important to note if the bony landmarks are either more or less visible than what is considered normal; they are more prominent with negative pressure in the middle ear and less prominent with fluid or pus behind the TM. When there is chronic OM, the TM may develop cystic masses of epithelial cells, also known as cholesteatoma. Also, a thin-walled painful bulla forms in the related condition known as *bullous myringitis* (see Table 18-2 for a summary of common signs and symptoms of middle ear conditions) (Dillon, 2017; Goolsby & Grubbs, 2015; Lieberthal et al., 2013).

Evidence that was evaluated to formulate the AAP guidelines concluded that the combination of a bulging *cloudy* (lack of clear landmarks and whitish color) TM that doesn't move normally with pneumatic evaluation was the best predictor of AOM. A TM that is red (including hemorrhagic, very or moderately red) is strongly correlated with AOM. A slightly red TM is not a significant finding in the accurate diagnosis of AOM as it may occur for other reasons (crying, irritation, or inflammation) (Dillon, 2017; Goolsby & Grubbs, 2015; Lieberthal et al., 2013).

The presence of MEE without clinical symptoms is defined as otitis media with effusion (OME); it requires additional monitoring to assure it resolves but does not

TABLE 18–2   Common Signs and Symptoms of Otitis Media

System/Organ	Signs/Symptoms
Ear	Otorrhea (discharge in ear canal) Otalgia (ear pain) TM red, bulging, decreased movement, fluid present behind TM (effusion) Decreased hearing acuity Increased bone conduction (Rinne test) on affected side Lateralization to affected side (Weber test) Tinnitus Decreased hearing Difficultly balancing
Nose	Rhinnorhea (URI may preceded OM) Nasal mucosa: red and boggy Sinus tenderness
Throat	Pharynx: postnasal drainage present Sore throat
Gastrointestinal	Anorexia GI upset (nausea, vomiting, diarrhea)
Immune	Fever (<102.2°F considered not severe) CBC (usually not indicated): leukocytosis and elevate erythrocyte sedimentation rate

(Adapted from: Capriotti, 2020; Goolsby & Grubbs, 2015)

require antibiotic therapy. The TM may rupture when the pressure of the fluid is high, which results in discharge from the ear and decreased pain. When the TM ruptures or perforates, it appears dark; and then as scar tissue forms, there are white, cloud-like, irregularly shaped areas on it (Lieberthal et al., 2013).

Pneumatic otoscopy and/or tympanometry is required for the diagnosis of AOM because physical examination must show both middle ear inflammation and middle ear effusion (Boatright, 2015; Lieberthal et al., 2013). A pneumatic otoscope introduces a small puff of air into the ear canal and tests the mobility of the TM; it is indicated in the following situations: acute or chronic infection, TM perforation or scarring, cholesteatoma, or fluid behind the TM. Tympanometry measures the pressure change in the ear in response to sound at different pressures and plots these pressures as a tympanogram; this diagnostic procedure is minimally invasive and may be valuable when the child has had multiple episodes of AOM and/or the visualization/assessment of the TM provides inconclusive findings (Dillon, 2017; Goolsby & Grubbs, 2015). Alteration in the normal middle ear often results in stiffening of the middle ear, which causes reflection of sound, also known as increased admittance. MEE is also likely when the TM does not move normally.

Two tuning fork tests, the Weber and the Rinne, are part of the assessment of the ear and hearing. Children must be old enough to respond to the associated questions, but these noninvasive, painless tests may provide valuable information about the child's hearing ability. For the Weber test, a vibrating tuning fork is placed on the top of the head and then the child is asked in which ear the sound is heard better or if it is equal; a normal finding is equal hearing or vibratory sense. Lateralization, a sign of conductive or sensorineural hearing loss, is the finding when the sound is heard more clearly on one side and is abnormal. For the Rinne test, the vibrating tuning fork is placed behind the ear on the mastoid bone until the child reports no longer hearing it, and then it is placed in front of the ear where the child should be able to hear it. The child reports at what point it is no longer audible, which should be about twice the time it was heard when on the mastoid bone. Air conduction (in front of the ear) is compared to bone conduction (on the mastoid bone) and should be approximately twice as long with normal hearing (Dillon, 2017; Goolsby & Grubbs, 2015).

While AOM usually resolves without permanent sequelae, two potentially serious complications of AOM are conductive hearing loss and mastoiditis. First, MEE, resulting from AOM, is the most common cause of conductive hearing loss. Fluid accumulates behind the TM and may affect pressure in the eustachian tube; the result is lower pressure in the middle ear as compared to the external ear, causing impaired conduction of sound with decreased motion of ossicles and the TM (Dillon, 2017; Woo & Robinson, 2020). Other conditions associated with AOM may result in conductive hearing loss, such as perforated TM, cholesteatoma, otorrhea, and CSOM.

Mastoiditis occurs when an AOM infection spreads to the air cells of the skull behind the ear and results in inflammation of the mucosal lining of the mastoid process, which is a portion of the temporal bone. Antibiotic therapy has not been shown to decrease the incidence of mastoiditis, a complication of AOM. For every 5,000 children treated appropriately for AOM, only 1 case of mastoiditis is prevented (Hersh et al., 2013). Effective vaccination against some of the bacteria has decreased the incidence of AOM and also may have resulted in decreased mastoiditis rates. Not surprisingly, the same bacteria that are responsible for most AOM infections are also the causative agents for mastoiditis: *Streptococcus pneumoniae, Streptococcus pyogenes, Staphylococcus aureus, Haemophilus influenzae,* and *Moraxella catarrhalis* (Capriotti, 2020; Hersh et al., 2013). Parents should be reassured that mastoiditis is a rare complication and that accurate assessment and treatment of AOM decrease its occurrence. They should also be educated to notify the provider if the child experiences any of the following symptoms: increased otalgia with pain behind the ear, swelling and redness behind an ear, increased fever, headache, and/or brown discharge from the ear canal (Capriotti, 2020; Dillon, 2017; Woo & Robinson, 2020).

ASSESSMENT PEARLS
  Consider the presence of a foreign object in the ear canal as a source of inflammation and subsequent discharge.

Pharmacology

While antibiotics may speed recovery of AOM, they often have associated side effects (vomiting, diarrhea, and skin rash are most common), including the potential for the development of antibiotic resistance. According to the AAP, AOM is typically self limiting, and careful assessment and evaluation minimize the potential for antibiotic overuse (Adler & Lehman, 2016; Hersh et al., 2013). A meta-analyses of randomized controlled trials on the use of antibiotics in children with AOM had the following results:

• More than 50% of children with AOM recover without antibiotic therapy.
• Resolution of AOM is faster with antibiotic therapy compared with placebo.
• Younger children, those with bilateral involvement, and those with more severe disease, are more likely to need antibiotic therapy (Lieberthal et al., 2013; Woo & Robinson, 2020).

For children over 2 years old who have a mild infection (fever under 102.2°F, no purulent drainage, non-bulging TM, eating and sleeping well), it may be appropriate to recommend observing the child for improvement over two or three days. A parent may have a prescription, known as a *watchful waiting* (WW) or *wait and see prescription* (WASP), to fill if the child does not show improvement in signs and symptoms (Boatright, 2015; Lieberthal et al., 2013; Normandin, 2015). This procedure should only be applied to low-risk patients in whom the provider is confident that the parent will follow the protocol and fill/not fill the prescription appropriately. There must also be a process in place for follow-up, so parents communicate with providers if they start the antibiotic administration and how the child responds and recovers. Conversely, parents may expect and often insist on an antibiotic for their child even when they meet criteria for observation; this is an optimal time to discuss the potential risks of early antibiotic therapy compared to the risks for the child and to develop a mutually agreed-upon plan of care. A follow-up phone call at 48 to 72 hours after the office visit may be effective in determining whether the child's symptoms are resolving without antibiotic therapy or whether the prescription was filled and what the child's response was to it (Lieberthal et al., 2013; Woo & Robinson, 2020).

In summary, children with more severe signs and symptoms, including bilateral involvement, and children less than age 2 years are more likely to require and benefit from antibiotics. American Academy of Pediatrics clinical guidelines indicate that OME usually has a viral origin and does not warrant antibiotics, whereas AOM usually has a bacterial origin, but the guidelines recommend WW as an alternative equivalent to antibiotic treatment for nonsevere cases in children 2 years and older (fever less than 102.2°F, pain relieved by analgesics). WW is also recommended for AOM in children age 6 months to 2 years when it is nonsevere and unilateral (single ear) (Boatright, 2015; MacGeorge, Smith, Caldes, & Hackman, 2017). The WW approach involves prescribing an antibiotic (or making a prescription available), but advising parents or caregivers not to administer it unless symptoms worsen or do not improve in a brief period (usually 48 to 72 hours). Following the guidelines,

WW advice should be accompanied by instruction on symptom monitoring and management (especially pain relief) and how to obtain follow-up care if needed (Higgins, 2018; MacGeorge et al., 2017). WW is part of antibiotic stewardship, which is judiciously limiting antibiotic use to appropriate regimens, doses, durations, and administration to prevent the development of resistance and maintain effectiveness of existing antibiotics.

Because AOM is the leading reason that a provider prescribes an antibiotic for children 12 years and younger (ranging from 20% of prescriptions for children age 6 to 12 to 60% of prescriptions for children under 2 years), it is important to evaluate the appropriateness of antibiotic use in each individual situation. Of the prescriptions for antibiotics, over 90% are filled and at least partially administered, despite the WW education. With the goal of antibiotic stewardship, it is proposed that antibiotics are not needed for children unless there is suppurative exudate and in those cases, an antibiotic is necessary in only 10% of cases (MacGeorge et al., 2017).

Determination of the source of infections, bacterial or viral, is based on the child's signs, symptoms, and physical examination. With a moderate to severe bulging TM with otorrhea or a mildly bulging and/or erythematous TM with associated otalgia, the child meets criteria for a bacterial infection that requires an antibiotic (Hersh et al., 2013). According to AAP guidelines, the initial antibiotic of choice is typically amoxicillin for an infection and when the child has not taken an antibiotic in the past 30 days. It is the most commonly dispensed pediatric medication and is generally well tolerated, with most common side effects being diarrhea, nausea, vomiting, and rash (Stitt & Normandin, 2016).

Amoxicillin is effective for gram-positive bacteria that are responsible for the majority of otitis media infections. If the child has received an antibiotic in the past 30 days or has a history of recurrent AOM unresponsive to amoxicillin, then an antibiotic with beta-lactamase coverage should be administered. Augmentin is amoxicillin with clavulanate added; clavulanate neutralizes an enzyme produced by bacteria that inactivates amoxicillin, thereby increasing the effectiveness of amoxicillin. Side effects are similar to those of amoxicillin, with a slightly higher rate of diarrhea, which is usually self-limiting (Stitt & Normandin, 2016). For children who are allergic to penicillin or beta-lactamase, the recommended antibiotics are trimethoprim-sulfamethoxazole or macrolides. There is a 10% to 15% chance of an allergy to cephalosporins in children with a penicillin allergy, so care should be used when prescribing and/or administering these medications, especially via an *intramuscular* (IM) route (Waseem, 2018). When any antibiotic is prescribed, it is best practice to follow up (usually by phone or email) within 48 to 72 hours to make sure the child's symptoms are abating and have not worsened, and there are no adverse reactions to antibiotic therapy (Lieberthal et al., 2013). Prophylactic antibiotic therapy is not recommended to prevent recurrent AOM and is associated with the development of antibiotic-resistant bacteria.

Medications used in the treatment of AOM are presented in Table 18-3 at the end of this section. While once thought to be an effective preventative measure, prophylactic antibiotics do not decrease the occurrence/recurrence of AOM. Evidence does support insertion of tympanostomy tubes in children experiencing a single episode of OME of less than 3 months' duration; even though 3 months is a long period of time for an ongoing infection, most infections of this duration resolve spontaneously with antibiotics. Therefore, WW is recommended for 3 months following the diagnoses of OME unless the child is at risk for developmental delays and hearing is critical for their speech, language, and learning development (Outhoff, 2017). The definition of frequent infection (for the purpose of considering the placement of tympanostomy tubes

TABLE 18–3 Medications for Otitis Media

Class	Example	Action	Dosage	SENC

Antibiotics (penicillin)	Amoxicillin	Bactericidal	80–90 mg/kg/day in 3 divided doses.	First choice for OM if not allergic to penicillin.
				  May be used for subsequent infections but at a higher dose.
				  Instruct parents in importance of completing entire course even when symptoms improve.

Antibiotics Penicillin with beta lactamase inhibitor	Amoxicillin with clavulanic acid	Bactericidal activity is increased because beta-lactamase inhibitors prevent breakdown of antibiotic. If *H. influenzae* or *M. catarrhalis* is suspected.	<3 mo: 30 mg/kg/day of amoxicillin in 2 doses.
			>3 mo:
			  20–45 mg/kg/day of amoxicillin in 2 doses.
				Not used for first episode of AOM.
				  Use for subsequent infections. Do not use with kidney or liver dysfunction.
				  Do not use with penicillin allergy.
				  GI upset is most common side effect.

Antibiotics Cephalosporin	Ceftriaxone	Effective gram-positive and gram-negative coverage.	30 mg/kg in 1 dose IM.	Recurrent and/or severe infection.
				  Resistance to penicillin is suspected.
				  Administer pain medication for injection site.

Analgesic otic preparations	Antipyrine and benzocaine ear drops	Combines pain reliever, numbing agent, and antiseptic.	Fill ear canal with drops every 2–3 hr.	Do not use if TM perforated.
Analgesics/antipyretics	Acetaminophen	Pain and fever relief.	Infant drops: 160 mg/5 mL, follow package instructions. Children: 10–15 mg/kg/dose every 4 hr.	Administer regularly to promote comfort during first 24–48 hr until antibiotic is effective. Then use as needed to promote comfort.
Analgesics/antipyretics	Ibuprofen	Pain and fever relief.	Infant drops: 50 mg/1.25 mL, follow package instructions. Children: 4–10 mg/kg/dose.	Parents may alternate acetaminophen and ibuprofen but do not administer concurrently. Educate parents that other medications may contain analgesics.

(Hersh, et al., 2013; Lieberthal et al., 2013; Woo & Robinson, 2020)

as a treatment and prophylactic measure) is three episodes of AOM within 6 months or four episodes in 1 year with at least one episode in the preceding 6 months (Lieberthal et al., 2013; Woo & Robinson, 2020).

Children who are considered at high risk for complications and the potential for permanent damage due to AOM should be treated with an antibiotic; this includes children less than 2 years of age and those with recurrent AOM. The recommended length of antibiotic therapy has decreased from 10 days to 5 to 7 days because of problems completing the full course of treatment and because evidence supports that shorter regimens are equally effective (Woo & Robinson, 2020). It may require 8 to 12 weeks for the infection and associated MEE to completely resolve; a reevaluation at this point is recommended (Hersh et al., 2013; Lieberthal et al., 2013).

For older children who are afebrile, it is appropriate to monitor and recheck for spontaneous resolution of symptoms in 1 to 5 days; the reassessment may be accomplished by a phone call or by an office visit if deemed necessary. Supportive therapy for pain management and comfort should be given to all children with OM. These measures include antipyretics, analgesics, and application of heat. Medications for fever and pain may include paracetamol (acetaminophen), ibuprofen, or benzocaine ear drops. Antibiotic treatment of AOM does not provide symptomatic relief in the first 24 hours, so analgesics for pain and antipyretics for fever are an important part of the treatment plan (Woo & Robinson, 2020). If a child of any age is not significantly improved at 48 hours after initiation of an antibiotic, it may be that the infection is viral or that antibiotic resistance has developed. A child with previous ear infections and antibiotic administration probably has developed the latter, whereas for a first-time infection, a virus may be the causative agent. Due to the potential for the development of drug-resistant microorganisms, it is preferable to have the child complete a 5-day course of an antibiotic even if it does not seem effective, rather than have a partially treated infection (Hersh et al., 2013; Lieberthal et al., 2013; Normandin, 2015). An additional 5- to 7-day course of a broad-spectrum antibiotic may be required for resolution of a resistant infection due to bacteria. Decongestants and antihistamines are no longer considered effective for promoting resolution of the inflammation and drainage that occur with AOM; these medications may increase the length of infection and expose children to potential side effects (Woo & Robinson, 2020).

Surgical Treatment

Placement of tympanostomy tubes is a surgical intervention for OM that is recommended for children with persistent MEE with or without AOM. Notably it is the presence of the effusion that is related to long-term complications, including hearing loss, rather than the frequency of infections. Tympanostomy tubes are usually placed to achieve one of the following outcomes: improved drainage from behind TM, decreased risk of AOM, improved hearing and/or speech, and normal sleep patterns. Children with tympanostomy tubes may still have ear infections, but usually they are less severe and resolve more quickly. Occasionally, tympanostomy tubes have to be removed surgically but usually they fall out spontaneously at 6 to 9 months and are no longer needed. Rarely, the tubes fall out too soon and replacements are inserted surgically. While evidence is scant to support the use of tympanostomy tubes for recurrent AOM without MEE, this is still widely seen in clinical practice (Hersh et al., 2013; Lieberthal et al., 2013; Woo & Robinson, 2020).

Prevention and Complementary and Alternative Therapies (CAT)

There are several measures that may decrease a child's risk of developing AOM. First, evidence supports that breastfeeding has a dose-related response; any proportion of breastfeeding to bottle feeding has a positive effect, with exclusive breastfeeding for 6 months as the goal (Lieberthal et al., 2013). Breast milk contains *immunoglobulin A* (IgA), which offers protection against viruses and allergies. Positioning with the head elevated, which occurs naturally during breastfeeding, decreases the likelihood of reflux of milk into the ear (Ward & Hisley, 2016). If a child is bottle fed, then they should not be supine when fed or have the bottle propped up with an object (Woo & Robinson, 2020). Day care is associated with higher rates of AOM, but any situation in which the child is exposed to other children, such as a church nursery or indoor play area, poses the same risk due to exposure to respiratory infections. Immunization against *H. pneumoniae* has resulted in decreased AOM caused by this organism (Lieberthal et al., 2013). Xylitol (birch sugar), in lozenge or gum form, is effective in preventing AOM in children older than 2 years, but the highest incidence of AOM is in younger children who cannot use this product (Woo & Robinson, 2020).

A complementary therapy to pharmacological and/or surgical management is the Galbreath technique, an osteopathic technique that was developed in the 1920s. It works by promoting venous and lymphatic drainage in the ear using manipulation of the mandibular area. There is mixed evidence as to its effectiveness, but it may promote eustachian tube functioning and can be taught to parents for use at home. Studies have highlighted a disconnect between parents' expectations and clinical treatment plans, so alternative treatment may be valuable in promoting a sense of competence and confidence in caring for a child with AOM (Chando et al., 2016). Children with impaired hearing often experience social isolation, but less is known about the effect on their parents and it is recommended to connect parents for support and to help them develop resilience (Chando et al., 2016).

Summary

Otitis media occurs when there is an infectious process in the middle ear; normally, this space is filled with air and is critical to the normal functioning of the tiny vibrating bones in the inner ear. The majority of children have at least one infection during childhood, and they are the most common infection among children of all ages, but especially in children less than 2 years of age. Providers are challenged to educate parents that the various forms of otitis media (AOM, OME, and COME) often resolve spontaneously without antibiotic treatment. It is important to manage pain and fever that occur with AOM and to monitor the tympanic membrane in OME and COME so that permanent damage does not occur. Risk factors for OM that are modifiable include group childcare, formula feeding, and exposure to tobacco smoke. Conversely, it is important to identify the following risk factors, but they cannot be modified: age (6 months to 2 years is highest risk), seasonal factors (fall, winter, spring with high pollen counts), poor air quality, Alaskan Native heritage, and cleft palate. While OM may be a common occurrence, there are potential permanent serious complications, including hearing loss, speech and/or developmental delays, spread of infection to the mastoid, and damage to the tympanic membrane (Higgins, 2018; Normandin, 2015; Ward & Hinsley, 2016).

Key Points

- Children under age 2 are at increased risk for the development of middle ear infections due to physiology of the eustachian tube, still developing immune system, and exposure to bacteria in day-care settings.
- Exclusive breastfeeding for the first 6 months is recommended to prevent AOM.
- Assessment of the TM, its color and movement, is critical to the accurate diagnosis and treatment of AOM.

- A child over two years old with mild symptoms (fever less than 102.2°F, non-bulging TM) may be observed for resolution of symptoms with supportive treatment only.
- All children with suspected AOM should be treated for pain and fever.
- Amoxicillin is the first line choice of antibiotic therapy for AOM.

Review Questions

1. **The nurse is teaching the parents of a 15-month-old child who has just been diagnosed with the first AOM. Which of the following is the nurse's best response to the parent's question, "Why does our child have to take an antibiotic when this is their first AOM?"**

   a. "The doctor wants to prevent antibiotic resistance if your child has another infection."
   b. "Based on your child's age, it is appropriate to treat with an antibiotic."
   c. "Even though it was prescribed, you can watch your child for increased symptoms and fill if they do not improve."
   d. "Your child is at high risk for long-term complications with an AOM at this age."

2. **When interviewing the parent of a 1-year-old about risk factors for AOM, which of the following are important red flags for increased risk of developing frequent AOM? (Select all that apply.)**

   a. Male sex
   b. Breastfed until 6 months of age
   c. Grandmother watches child while mother works
   d. Mother had AOM as child
   e. Mother is a smoker

3. **The nurse assesses the TMs of a 6-year-old child who has the following signs/symptoms: slight ear unilateral pain for a week, afebrile, recent history of a URI. When the TM is cloudy with poor mobility, the nurse determines which of the following?**

   a. An AOM is present and the child should be placed on an antibiotic.
   b. There is evidence of MEE and the child should be reassessed in 6 weeks for resolution.
   c. This is a normal finding based on the child's age and history of a URI.
   d. There is damage to the TM and the child should be evaluated for tympanostomy tube.

4. **Parents are stressed by their 1-year-old child's recurrent AOMs because they are having frequent absences from work and are unable to sleep through the night. They ask what they can do to prevent a recurrence. The nurse's best response is:**

   a. "Your child is at increased risk for AOMs due to their age so you can't prevent them."
   b. "As long as the infections are mild, there shouldn't be any long-term effects."
   c. "Your child will be started on an antibiotic to prevent infections until they are 2 years old."
   d. "Day care doubles your child's risk of AOM; are there other childcare options?"

5. **The nurse instructs the parents on how to correctly administer the 5-day course of antibiotic prescribed for AOM for their 7-year-old child. Which of the following statements lets the nurse know that the patient understands instructions?**

   a. "I won't need to give my child Tylenol for pain because the antibiotic will decrease the pain."

   b. "My child needs to take the entire course prescribed even if they are much better in 2 days."

   c. "Because my child is 7, I'll wait to see if they improve before filling the prescription."

   d. "I'll bring my child back to the office in 1 week for an antibiotic injection."

See the appendix for answers to review questions.

References

Adler, C., & Lehman, D. (2016). Upper respiratory infection and acute otitis media common in infancy. *NEJM Journal Watch. Pediatrics & Adolescent Medicine.* doi:http://dx.doi.org/10.1056/nejm-jw.NA40919

American Academy of Otolaryngology–Head and Neck Surgery. (2017). *Clinical practice guidelines: Otitis media with effusion (OME).* Retrieved from https://www.entnet.org/content/clinical-practice-guideline-otitis-media-effusion-ome

American Speech–Language–Hearing Association. (2020). Newborn hearing screening. Retrieved from https://www.asha.org/practice-portal/professional-issues/newborn-hearing-screening/

Boatright, C. (2015). Treatment patterns for pediatric acute otitis media: A gap in evidence-based theory and clinical practice. *Pediatric Nursing, 41*(6), 271–276.

Cai, T., & McPherson, B. (2017). Hearing loss in children with otitis media with effusion: A systematic review. *International Journal of Audiology, 56*(2), 65–76. Retrieved from https://doi.org/10.1080/149920 27.2016.1250960

Capriotti, T. (2020). *Pathophysiology: Introductory concepts and clinical perspectives* (2nd ed.). Philadelphia, PA: F.A. Davis.

Chando, S., Young, C., Craig, J. C., Gunasekera, H., & Tong, A. (2016). Parental views on otitis media: Systematic review of qualitative studies. *European Journal of Pediatrics, 175*(10), 1295–1305. doi:http://dx.doi.org/10.1007/s00431-016-2779-6

Chonmaitree, T., Jennings, K., Golovko, G., Khanipov, K., Pimenova, M., Patel, J. A., . . . Fofanov, Y. (2017). Nasopharyngeal microbiota in infants and changes during viral upper respiratory tract infection and acute otitis media. *PLoS One, 12*(7). doi:http://dx.doi.org/10.1371/journal.pone.0180630

Danishyar, A., & Ashurst J. (2020). *Acute otitis media.* StatPearls [Internet]. Retrieved from https://www.ncbi.nlm.nih.gov/books/NBK470332/

Dillon, P. (2017). *Nursing health assessment: A critical thinking, case studies approach* (2nd ed.). Philadelphia, PA: F.A. Davis.

GBD 2013 Mortality and Causes of Death Collaborators. (2015). Global, regional, and national age-sex specific all-cause and cause-specific mortality for 240 causes of death, 1990–2013: A systematic analysis for the Global Burden of Disease Study 2013. *Lancet, 385*(9963), 117–171. doi:10.1016/S0140-6736(14)61682-2

Goolsby, M., and Grubbs, L. (2015). *Advanced assessment: Interpreting findings and formulating differential diagnoses.* Philadelphia, PA: F.A. Davis.

Hersh, A., Jackson, M., Hicks, L., and the Committee on Infectious Disease. (2013). Principles of judicious antibiotic prescribing for upper respiratory tract infection in pediatrics. *Pediatrics, 132*, 1146–1154.

Higgins, T. (2018). Otitis media with effusion. Retrieved from https://emedicine.medscape.com/article/858990-overview#a5

Lieberthal, A. S., Carroll, A. E., Chonmaitree, T., Ganiats, T. G., Hoberman, A., Jackson, M. A., . . . Tunkel, D. E. (2013). The diagnosis and management of acute otitis media. *Pediatrics, 131*(3), e964–999. doi:10.1542/peds.2012-3488.

MacGeorge, E. L., Smith, R. A., Caldes, E. P., & Hackman, N. M. (2017). Toward reduction in antibiotic use for pediatric otitis media: Predicting parental compliance with "watchful waiting" advice. *Journal of Health Communication, 22*(11), 867–875. Retrieved from https://ezproxy.queens.edu:6464/10.1080/1081 0730.2017.1367337

Marom, T., Tan, A., Wilkinson, G. S., Pierson, K. S., Freeman, J. L., & Chonmaitree, T. (2014). Trends in otitis media-related health care use in the United States, 2001–2011. *JAMA Pediatrics, 168*(1), 68–75. Retrieved from https://doi.org/10.1001/jamapediatrics.2013.3924

Mayo Clinic. (2020). Ear infection (middle ear). Retrieved from https://www.mayoclinic.org/diseases-conditions/ear-infections/symptoms-causes/syc-20351616

Normandin, P. A. (2015). Pediatric infectious diseases. *Journal of Emergency Nursing, 41*(2), 160–161. doi:http://dx.doi.org/10.1016/j.jen.2014.12.008

Outhof, K. (2017). Grommets—an update on common indications for tympanostomy tube placement. *Professional Nursing Today, 21*(2), 12–16.

Rosenfeld, R. M., Shin, J. J., Schwartz, S. R., Coggins, R., Gagnon, L., Hackell, J. M., . . . Corrigan, M. D. (2016). Clinical practice guideline: Otitis media with effusion (update). *Otolaryngology–Head and Neck Surgery, 154*(Suppl. 1), S1–241.

Stitt, G., & Normandin, P. A. (2016). Part 1: Safe administration of oral pediatric medications in the emergency department. *Journal of Emergency Nursing, 42*(3), 276–278. doi:http://dx.doi.org/10.1016/j.jen.2016.03.018

The Hearing Review. (2020). Ear infection rates in US infants have dropped. Retrieved from https://www.hearingreview.com/inside-hearing/research/ear-infection-rates-in-us-infants-have-dropped

Toivonen, L., Vuononvirta, J., Mertsola, J., Waris, M., He, Q., & Peltola, V. (2017). Gene variants relate to risk of respiratory infections and AOM. *Pediatric Infectious Disease Journal, 36*, e114–e122.

Ward, S., & Hisley, S. (2016). *Maternal-child nursing care.* Philadelphia, PA: F.A. Davis.

Waseem, M. (2018). Otitis media treatment and management. *Medscape.* Retrieved from https://emedicine.medscape.com/article/994656-treatment

Woo, T., & Robinson, M. (2020). *Pharmacotherapeutics for the advanced practice nurse prescribers* (5th ed.). Philadelphia, PA: FA Davis.

Case Study 4 (Pediatrics): Acute Lymphoblastic Leukemia

LEARNING OBJECTIVES

Upon completion of this case study the student will be able to integrate knowledge of the pathophysiology, assessment, and pharmacological and nonpharmacological care options for a pediatric patient with *acute lymphoblastic leukemia* (ALL) and their family.

Introduction to Acute Lymphoblastic Leukemia

Leukemia is a hematological neoplasm, affecting the development of all blood cells, especially *white blood cells* (WBCs). The disease forms in precursor stem cells in the bone marrow, from a specific cell line. The abnormal cells are similar to immature cells; however, they do not develop normally, and they proliferate uncontrollably, both of which affect cell functioning (National Cancer Institute [NCI], 2018). There are two types of leukemia: *myelocytic* (affects myeloid cells) and *lymphocytic* (affects lymphoid cells). *Acute lymphoblastic leukemia* (ALL) affects lymphoid cells and is also known as lymphocytic or lymphogenous leukemia (American Cancer Society [ACS], 2019; Leukemia and Lymphoma Society [LLS], 2020; NCI, 2018).

Annually, approximately 3,000 U.S. children are diagnosed with ALL; it is the most common pediatric cancer and the most frequent cause of death from cancer in people younger than 20 years of age (ACS, 2019; NCI, 2018). The incidence of ALL in the United States is about 30 cases per million persons in the younger than 20 age-group, with the peak incidence occurring at 3 to 5 years of age ("About Childhood Acute Lymphoblastic Leukemia [ALL]," 2018; ACS, 2019; Hunger & Mulligan, 2015). Children younger than age 6 comprise 75% of ALL cases across all age-groups. There is a significant disparity across ethnicities: 14.8 cases per million African Americans, 35.6 cases per million Caucasians, and 40.9 cases per million Hispanics. There are disparities across genders, with a higher incidence in males (55% of cases) as compared to females (45%) ("About Childhood," 2018; Hunger & Mulligan, 2015; LLS, 2020; NCI, 2018). ALL survival rates have increased from under 10% in the 1960s to 80% to 90% in 2015; survival rates are lower for babies (50%) and adults (35%). In particular, there is a better prognosis and five-year survival with B cell ALL (84%) as compared to T cell ALL (75%) ("About Childhood," 2018; ACS, 2019; LLS, 2020; NCI, 2018).

Meet JB

JB is a 3-year-old Hispanic male who is brought to the pediatrician's office by his mother. She reports that JB has been well except for the usual childhood illnesses, such as occasional upper respiratory infections *(URIs). However, over the past several weeks, he has had frequent URIs that have not resolved. In addition, last week, he developed multiple bruises that are not explained by injury, and he appears pale and tired. His mother is worried because he is usually an active child, and he has been sleeping more and has recently been asking to take naps after stopping regular napping over a year ago.*

Physiology and Pathophysiology

ALL is a cancer of blood cells characterized by proliferation of the immature lymphocytes (Capriotti, 2020). Refer to Chapter 16 for a review of the specific functions of lymphocytes. Briefly, lymphocytes are subtypes of white blood cells that provide immunity through two mechanisms: natural killer cells and T cells (cell-mediated immunity) and B cells (humoral, antibody-driven immunity) ("About Childhood," 2018; Hunger & Mullighan, 2015; NCI, 2018). In the bone marrow, the stem cell precursors for these T and/or B lymphocytes do not function, which results in cells that do not mature past the lymphoblast phase (NCI, 2018). With the abnormal proliferation of these immature cells, there is no room for normal blood cells, including white blood cells, red blood cells, and platelets (ACS, 2019; Capriotti, 2020). Shifts in blood cell components result in multiple conditions, such as anemia, compromised immunity, and impaired clotting. These abnormal cells enter the circulation and also grow outside the bone marrow in the *central nervous system* (CNS), kidneys, liver, and testicles. With T-cell ALL, there is 85% chance of meningeal infiltration ("About Childhood," 2018; Capriotti, 2020; LLS, 2020)

The cause of ALL is not known, however there are risk factors for its development, including gene mutations (e.g., *ARID5B, CDKN2A/2B, CEBPE, IKZF1, GATA3, PIP4K2A*) and genetic syndromes such as Down's syndrome, Fanconi's anemia, X-linked agammaglobulinemia, severe combined immunodeficiency, and neurofibromatosis type 1 (ACS, 2019; Hunger & Mullighan, 2015; NCI, 2018). Specifically, Philadelphia Chromosome (PhC) is an abnormality due to the translocation of a gene between chromosomes 9 and 22 that is also referred to as the Breakpoint Cluster Region-Abelson proto-oncogene (BCR-ABL). These resulting abnormal genes form a protein, tyrosine kinase, that causes leukemic changes in the hematopoietic cells (ACS, 2019; Capriotti, 2020; NCI, 2018). Also, a large for gestational age birth weight (over 8.8 pounds for a full-term birth) is associated with increased risk of developing ALL.

In ALL, lymphocytes do not develop normally, and there is defective control over the number of lymphoid cells that are produced. When a lymphoblast, an immature lymphocyte, gains mutations to genes that affect blood cell maturation, ALL may develop. These inherited gene mutations interact with certain environmental risk factors to ultimately determine whether ALL occurs (ACS, 2019; LLS, 2020). There is lack of consistent evidence about the factors that are responsible for ALL. Evidence exists to support that having a common infection, such as influenza, may indirectly contribute to ALL. The *delayed-infection hypothesis* proposes that ALL is due to an abnormal immune response to infection; a child with genetic risk factors who has limited exposure to diseases may have excessive lymphocyte production during an illness. Prenatal exposure to radiation may be a controllable environmental risk factor for the development of ALL (Capriotti, 2020; NCI, 2018).

Gathering Information

When taking the health history, Nurse NN learns that JB's birth was a normal vaginal delivery, weighing 9 pounds. JB's mom says, "We have big babies in our family." JB has two older sisters, who are healthy except that one sister had influenza this year. JB's mom worked in a doctor's office as a radiology technician before and during her pregnancy with JB but is now home with her three children; JB's father works at a bank. JB is currently taking acetaminophen as needed for a low-grade fever and generalized aches/pain. JB says his chest hurts and "my legs don't feel like running." While he has had normal growth and development to this point, his mom reports that he hasn't been eating well recently. He has no known medication or environmental allergies.

Assessment and Diagnosis

Diagnosis of ALL may be difficult based on history and physical examination alone. The clinical signs and symptoms present are related to the replacement of normal cells with the proliferating abnormal cells in the bone marrow and potentially other sites (ACS, 2019). With compromised immune functioning, there may be a history of frequent infections, including URIs, canker sores, and/or diarrhea. With advanced disease, the child may present with pneumonia (Capriotti, 2020; Dillon, 2017; NCI, 2018). The child is often pale, fatigues easily, and is dyspneic (due to anemia). There may be vague symptoms due to compromised immunity, such as fever, chills, night sweats, and body aches. Lymph nodes and spleen may be enlarged as the initial signs ("About Childhood," 2018; ACS, 2019; LLS, 2020; NCI, 2018). Within the child's abdominal cavity, splenic and/or liver enlargement may lead to nausea/vomiting and unintentional weight loss. The child may have bone pain, which is often most intense in the sternum, tibia, and femur. Impaired platelet functioning may cause nosebleeds (epistaxis), gingival bleeding, and unexplained bruising (Capriotti, 2020; Dillon, 2017; Goolsby & Grubbs, 2019). A *complete blood count* (CBC) shows an abnormally increased WBC count with ALL; the lymphoblast component of the CBC is increased while the other components are decreased (see Table CS4–1). Normally, the higher the WBC on initial diagnosis is, the poorer the prognosis is ("About Childhood," 2018; Capriotti, 2020; NCI, 2018).

TABLE CS4–1 Normal CBC Values and Changes with ALL/Treatment

CBC Component Normal Value*	Initial Change With ALL	With Desired Response to Treatment
Hematocrit (31.7%–39.9%)	Decreased	Increase to normal
Hemoglobin (10.2–13.4 g/dL)	Decreased	Increase to normal
Red blood cells (3.89–5.03)	Decreased	Increase to normal
Platelets (150–400)	Decreased	Increase to normal
White blood cells (4.86–11.4)	Increased	Decrease to normal
• Neutrophils (22.4%–74.7%)	Decreased	Increase to normal
• Eosinophils (0%–4.7%)	Decreased or unchanged	Increase to normal
• Basophils (0.1%–0.8%)	Decreased or unchanged	Increase to normal
• Lymphocytes (18.1%–68.7%)	Decreased	Increase to normal
• Atypical lymphocytes (2%–4%)	Increased	Decrease to normal
• Monocytes (4.1%–12.3%)	Decreased	Increase to normal

(Goolsby & Grubbs, 2019; NCI, 2018)
*All blood components decrease during chemotherapy.

Diagnosis

During JB's examination, Nurse NN obtains a height and weight, and notes that there has been a 0.5 pound weight loss since his last appointment 3 months ago for a URI. His skin is light brown, and his nailbeds are pale pink. His gums are pale pink, and there's slight bleeding noted at the gum line. There are bruises on JB's thighs and abdomen, along with petechiae on his chest. JB guards his chest and abdomen, saying, "My chest hurts." He has not complained of headaches. Nurse NN auscultates the heart and lungs and defers the abdominal assessment until the end of the examination. JB sits on his mom's lap while the nurse observes a normal abdominal contour without visible pulsations or retractions. Auscultation reveals normal bowel sounds. As the nurse lightly palpates JB's abdomen, he starts to cry and resists; deep palpation is contraindicated in this situation. While JB stays on his mom's lap, a CBC is obtained and reveals marked WBC elevation (25 g/dL). Based on the initial CBC, JB is referred to a pediatric oncologist. A bone marrow aspiration is performed to confirm the ALL diagnosis, based on a lymphoblast count of over 20% of total WBCs (ACS, 2019; Capriotti, 2020). Leukemic cells are classified by the World Health Organization (WHO); ALL is categorized as B-lymphoblastic leukemia/lymphoma or T-lymphoblastic leukemia (Seiter, 2019). A DNA analysis is also done to establish the treatment protocol (ACS, 2019).

Treatment Options

There are several aims of the ALL treatment plan. First, the abnormal cells must be destroyed, and normal bone marrow function must be restored. Prophylactic treatment of sanctuary sites (especially CNS) is aimed at killing cells in those areas. Maintenance treatment may be administered over a period of years to achieve and maintain remission. This additional chemotherapy may be administered via the intrathecal route, especially if brain metastasis has occurred ("About Childhood," 2018; LLS, 2020). Radiation therapy may also be implemented in this situation. The child's response to treatment is monitored via laboratory values; a rapid response is a sign of a better prognosis for all types of ALL (ACS, 2019; NCI, 2018). Chemotherapy (presented in Table CS4–2) is usually a multidrug approach, lasts for approximately 36 months, and is delivered in the following phases: induction, consolidation, delated intensification, and maintenance. The plan, or *protocol*, is based on the particular cell type and cancer staging for ALL ("About Childhood," 2018; LLS, 2020; Woo & Robinson, 2020).

A specific chemotherapeutic agent, Kymriah (tisagenlecleucel), was U.S. Food and Drug Administration approved in August 2017 for treatment of B-cell precursor ALL that is refractory or in second or later relapse. Chemotherapy given intravenously or orally does not penetrate the blood–brain barrier sufficiently to destroy leukemic cells in the brain; prophylaxis of CNS recurrence is a priority because the brain and spine are often first sites for relapsing leukemia (called *sanctuary disease sites*) ("Acute Lymphocytic Leukemia," 2020; NCI, 2018). The child usually has a port placed for intravenous therapy, and it is important that the family understands how to care for the access port at home. While receiving chemotherapy, the child is immunocompromised and may be treated prophylactically with both antibiotics and antifungals to prevent infection (NCI, 2018; Woo & Robinson, 2020). Additionally, *granulocyte colony-stimulating factors*, or G-CSF (lenograstim, filgrastim), may be given with chemotherapy to stimulate the normal white blood cell growth.

Parents should be taught that certain side effects commonly occur and usually can be anticipated and ameliorated with both pharmacological and nonpharmacological measures. These include, within the gastrointestinal system, appetite changes, constipation and/or diarrhea, and pain and/or sores in the mouth/tongue/throat; in the integument, dry skin and color changes; and within the neurological system, numbness, tingling,

TABLE CS4–2 Drugs Commonly Used to Treat ALL in Children

Class	Example	Action	Dosage	SENC
Antineoplastic	Vincristine	Used in induction phase. Arrests mitosis at metaphase by inhibition of mitotic spindle function.	If child is over 10 kg, 1–2 mg/m^2 IV weekly.	Monitor for musculoskeletal adverse effects, especially muscle weakness in hands, paresthesias, and decreased Achilles tendon reflex. Hepatotoxicity. Prevent constipation.
Antineoplastic	Doxorubicin	Used in consolidation phase. Blocks DNA and RNA transcription.	30 mg/m^2 weekly × 4 weeks.	Irreversible myocardial toxicity with congestive heart failure and arrhythmias.
Antineoplastic, alkylating agent	Cyclophosphamide	Used in delayed intensification phase. Blocks synthesis of DNA, RNA, and protein as an alkylating agent.	2–8 mg/kg IV or PO.	Give on empty stomach. Risk for anaphylaxis. Interstitial pulmonary fibrosis. Report hematuria as sign of hemorrhagic cystitis. Administer IV fluids to attain specific gravity of 1.01 before administration.
Antimetabolite and antineoplastic	Methotrexate	Used in maintenance phase. Blocks mitosis by inhibiting folic acid.	Intrathecal 10–15 mg/m^2.	Hepatotoxicity. Sudden death. Pulmonary fibrosis.
Colony-stimulating factor	Filgrastim	Increases bone marrow production of lymphocytes.	5 mcg/kg/day IV.	Discontinue when neutrophil count is 10,000. Monitor for fever. Report bone pain.
Colony-stimulating factor	Epoetin	Stimulates bone marrow to produce red blood cells.	50 U/kg 3 × weekly subcutaneously based on hematocrit.	Headache is common. Monitor for thrombotic events.

("About Childhood," 2018; ACS, 2019; NCI, 2018; Woo & Robinson, 2020)

and pain. Conversely, the following side effects constitute potential emergencies and should be reported immediately to the provider: fever 100.5°F or greater/chills, bleeding/bruising, rash, shortness of breath, allergic reaction (swelling of mouth/throat, itching, dysphagia), intense headache, bloody stool or urine, and long-lasting (over 48 hours) diarrhea or vomiting (ACS, 2019; LLS, 2020).

The child receiving chemotherapy should be monitored for liver and kidney damage; increased uric acid levels may result in kidney damage (NCI, 2018; Woo & Robinson, 2020). Hypercalcemia may affect normal heart function by precipitating arrhythmias. High-dose steroids (prednisolone) are often given with chemotherapy and may result in adrenal gland suppression, even with short-term treatment ("Acute Lymphocytic Leukemia," 2020; Woo & Robinson, 2020).

Note that administration of chemotherapeutic agents often requires additional education with demonstration of competency and/or certification, depending on the facility policies. Chemotherapy doses are based on *body surface area* (BSA), which may be calculated using one of several formulas based on height/weight ratios (preferred) or a quick reference age-based chart. BSA reflects metabolic mass rather than body weight, as it is less affected by abnormal fatty tissue and results in more specific dosing. In addition to medications, platelets and/or packed red blood cells may be necessary due to the disease process and/or the child's response to chemotherapy (NCI, 2018; Woo & Robinson, 2016).

Radiation may be used to cause breaks in the DNA molecules, which destroys abnormal cells; it is indicated when ALL has entered the CNS. Bone marrow transplantation from a tissue match, often a sibling, may also be used in conjunction with chemotherapy. If the child does not respond to this standard regimen or there is recurrence of the disease, stem cell transplantation may be used. Immunotherapy is also being investigated and implemented as a treatment option for ALL, usually after initial therapy does not result in remission or there is recurrence of disease ("About Childhood," 2018; ACS, 2019; NCI, 2018). For example, in *chimeric antigen receptor* (CAR) T-cell therapy, the child's T cells are genetically altered to include the CARs that attach to proteins on leukemia cells. These genetically altered cells are then infused into the child to attach to and kill leukemic cells. Another example is tisagenlecleucel, which targets the CD19 protein on leukemic cells; the child's T cells are removed using leukapheresis. Cells are frozen, genetically altered into CAR T cells, multiplied, and then infused into the child; this process occurs over several weeks and usually involves adjuvant chemotherapy (ACS, 2019).

Generally, a child may have to be hospitalized during the initial phase of diagnosis and initiation of treatment, but then can be treated effectively on an outpatient basis. For the time of hospitalization, the care priorities include pain management, maintaining adequate nutrition and hydration, risk for infection, and coping with a life-threatening situation. Once the child is discharged to home, the priorities may shift to compliance with oral chemotherapeutic regimen, risk for delayed development (physical, emotional, and cognitive), and management of fatigue (ACS, 2019; LLS, 2020; NCI, 2018; Woo & Robinson, 2020). Meeting the physical and emotional needs of the child and family during and after treatment is also a care priority. These priorities are outlined in Table CS4–3.

TABLE CS4–3 Care Priorities for Child Who Is Receiving Chemotherapy

Physical	Emotional
• Take frequent rest breaks during the day. • Avoid crowds. • Remain hydrated. • Take antiemetic regularly. • Assess skin daily for bruises, cuts, reddened pressure areas. • Eat small, healthy meals. • Assess for signs/symptoms of infection: fever, cough, fatigue, diarrhea. • Use soft toothbrush or irrigation system for frequent mouth care. • Take oral, axillary, or temporal (not rectal) temperature routinely.	• Prepare for hair loss with hats, scarves, wigs. • Keep in touch with friends via phone, Internet. • Learn and practice relaxation and stress reduction techniques. • Seek support from established (e.g., pastor, family, friends) and new (e.g., providers, counselors, other children/families with cancer) sources of support.

("About Childhood," 2018; ACS, 2019; NCI, 2018)

Despite having a life-threatening condition, children with ALL should be treated based on their developmental level. A preschool child, such as JB, may need help understanding that he did not do something wrong and is not being punished by being sick. An older school-age child will most likely need help coping with the barriers that ALL presents in meeting the developmental task of industry. And teenagers are often most concerned with changes due to ALL that make them different from and/or separate them from their peers ("About Childhood," 2018; ACS, 2019; LLS, 2020). Nurses are integral in promoting coping for the patient and their family and also providing education to understand the disease process and importance of adherence to treatment plan and preventing complications, both short term and long term.

Treatment Follow-Up

Survivors of childhood leukemia are at risk for certain health problems once they reach adulthood. The risks are dependent on several factors, including type of leukemia, treatment type and dosage, and age at time of treatment. One of the most serious long-term side effects of ALL for childhood survivors is the 5% risk of developing *acute myelogenous leukemia* (AML). This risk is linked to receiving the chemotherapeutic agents, epipodophyllotoxins, or alkylating agents ("About Childhood," 2018; ACS, 2019; Woo & Robinson, 2020). Heart disease risk, including hypertension and stroke, are also increased, along with the potential for learning problems (especially after brain radiation), delayed growth and development (especially with stem cell transplant), and infertility for both genders (ACS, 2019).

While the physical care of the child and family is complex, the Institute of Medicine also recommends services to address functional and psychosocial consequences of cancer in their report, *From Cancer Patient to Cancer Survivor: Lost in Transition*. In a study based on this need, Cartmell and colleagues (2018) developed a mechanism to collect data and document service availability in South Carolina and recommended implementation of this process in other states to identify available services and/or gaps.

A long-term support option that may be offered to children and their families is a weekend retreat with other cancer survivors. There is evidence that overnight and day camps are effective in promoting quality of life and a sense of well-being in school-age children and teens with cancer, while also providing much-needed respite for families (ACS, 2019; NCI, 2018). In a related study by Bashore and Bender (2017), participants focused on the positive aspects of surviving cancer and gained support from sharing their experiences with other families. In another study, Terp and Sjöström-Strand (2017) interviewed parents 2 years after their child was admitted to the intensive care unit and found parents had vivid memories and feelings of powerlessness. Spousal relationships were often strengthened by the experience, and parents reported that they had different life values as a result. These studies indicate that the care of the child and family does not end with successful treatment of the cancer and may need to extend years into the future to promote healthy coping (ACS, 2019; NCI, 2018).

Treatment and Follow-Up

Following his diagnosis of ALL, JB was prescribed a multidrug chemotherapeutic regimen that lasted 36 months. To promote continuity of care, JB and his family were assigned a pediatric oncology nurse navigator, CA, who coordinated his appointments with his primary care pediatrician and the oncology specialists. It was necessary to administer chemotherapy for the usual 36-month regiment to ensure remission. During this prolonged treatment regimen, there were several priorities for JB's care, both physical and emotional, which Nurse CA explained to JB's parents. Nurse CA also urged JB's parents to encourage him to select activities he wanted to participate in, so he could remain active while having adequate opportunities for rest during the day. Because the treatment regimen can be very restrictive, JB's parents were also told to give him choices whenever possible so he could retain a sense of control and agency. JB responded quickly to the medications, with a decrease in the lymphoblasts and a normal lymphocyte count and components. Red blood cells and platelets are also now within normal range.

Summary

A child's cancer diagnosis creates an immediate crisis and many feelings (e.g., anxiety, panic, uncertainty) for the child, their parents, and other family members. The nurse provides family-centered care throughout the process, which includes initial diagnosis, treatment planning and implementation decisions (which often change based on the child's response to treatment), and long-term care. With access to information and coordination of care, the child and family can continue to have quality of life during the treatment process, which often spans 2 to 3 years, and afterward.

Key Points

- The child with ALL is at risk for infection; the child and family should be taught how to prevent infection and recognize its signs/symptoms early.
- ALL develops as a result of genetic and environmental factors.
- Assessment of the child with ALL may reveal any of the following signs/symptoms: generalized weakness, anemia, fever, frequent infections, weight loss, bruising, bone pain, dyspnea, enlarged lymph nodes, petechiae, testicular enlargement, and/or mediastinal mass.
- If there is CNS involvement, the child may experience headache, vomiting, lethargy, nuchal rigidity, or neuropathies.
- ALL requires a chemotherapeutic regiment that may span three years and be supplemented with radiation therapy. Immunotherapy is also a promising option.

Review Questions

1. **The nurse is reviewing the health history of JB, a 3-year-old Hispanic American male. The nurse understands that which of the following increases the patient's risk for ALL? (Select all that apply.)**

   a. Age

   b. Male sex

   c. Mother's advanced maternal age

   d. His birth weight of 9 lb

   e. Prenatal exposure to radiation

2. **When explaining chemotherapy to JB's family, which of the following statements made by the nurse is correct?**

   a. "Your child will probably need chemotherapy over the next 3 years."

   b. "Your child will have to be hospitalized while receiving all chemotherapy."

   c. "All chemotherapy will be delivered intravenously."

   d. "Chemotherapy will ensure that your child's cancer does not recur."

3. **Which of the following statements made by JB's mother indicates accurate understanding of care for JB while taking chemotherapy at home?**

   a. "I will take his temperature rectally every day to check for fever."
   b. "I will limit his fluid intake, so he doesn't develop swelling."
   c. "I will keep him away from crowds, especially during flu season."
   d. "I will insist he takes a 1-hour nap in the morning and the afternoon."

4. **The nurse is providing education about the potential for spread of ALL to the CNS. Which of the following statements made by JB's mother indicates a need for further education?**

   a. "It's rare that ALL spreads to the brain, so I won't worry."
   b. "If JB's cancer spreads to his brain, he won't recover."
   c. "It's important that I report any headache to the provider."
   d. "Because we caught JB's cancer early, it probably won't spread."

5. **The nurse understands that JB has which of the following presenting sign/symptoms of ALL? (Select all that apply.)**

   a. Chest pain
   b. Fatigue
   c. Weight loss
   d. Constipation
   e. Bruising

See the appendix for answers to review questions.

References

About childhood acute lymphoblastic leukemia (ALL). (2018). Dana-Farber Cancer Institute. Retrieved from http://www.danafarberbostonchildrens.org/conditions/leukemia-and-lymphoma/acute-lymphoblastic-leukemia.aspx

Acute lymphocytic leukemia (2020). Johns Creek: Ebix Inc. Retrieved from https://ezproxy.queens.edu:2048/login?url=https://ezproxy.queens.edu:2078/other-sources/acute-lymphocytic-leukemia/docview/2087732234/se-2?accountid=38688

American Cancer Society. (2019). Leukemia in children. Retrieved from https://www.cancer.org/cancer/leukemia-in-children.html

Bashore, L., & Bender, J. (2017). Benefits of attending a weekend childhood cancer survivor family retreat. *Journal of Nursing Scholarship, 49*(5), 521–528. doi:10.1111/jnu.12320

Capriotti, T. (2020). *Pathophysiology: Introductory concepts and clinical perspectives.* Philadelphia, PA: F.A. Davis.

Cartmell, K. B., Sterba, K. R., Pickett, K., Zapka, J., Alberg, A. J., Sood, A. J., & Esnaola, N. F. (2018). Availability of patient-centered cancer support services: A statewide survey of cancer centers. *PLoS One, 13*(3). doi:10.1371/journal.pone.0194649

Dillon, P. (2017). *Nursing health assessment: A critical thinking, case studies approach* (2nd ed.). Philadelphia, PA: F.A. Davis.

Goolsby, M., & Grubbs, L. (2019). *Advanced assessment: Interpreting findings and formulating differential diagnoses* (4th ed.). Philadelphia, PA: F.A. Davis.

Hunger, S., & Mullighan, C. (2015). Acute lymphoblastic leukemia in children. *New England Journal of Medicine, 373,* 1541–1552. doi:10.1056/NEJMra1400972

Leukemia and Lymphoma Society. (2020). Childhood ALL. Retrieved from https://www.lls.org/leukemia/acute-lymphoblastic-leukemia/childhood-all

National Cancer Institute. (2018). Childhood acute lymphoblastic leukemia treatment (PDQ®)–health professional version. Retrieved from https://www.cancer.gov/types/leukemia/patient/child-all-treatment-pdq

Seiter, K. (2019). Acute lymphoblastic leukemia staging. Retrieved from https://emedicine.medscape.com/article/2006661-overview

Terp, K., & Sjöström-Strand, A. (2017). Parents' experiences and the effect on the family two years after their child was admitted to a PICU—An interview study. *Intensive & Critical Care Nursing, 43,* 143–148. doi:10.1016/j.iccn.2017.06.003

Woo, T., & Robinson, M. (2020). *Pharmacotherapeutics for the advanced practice nurse prescribers* (5th ed.). Philadelphia, PA: FA Davis.

Geriatric

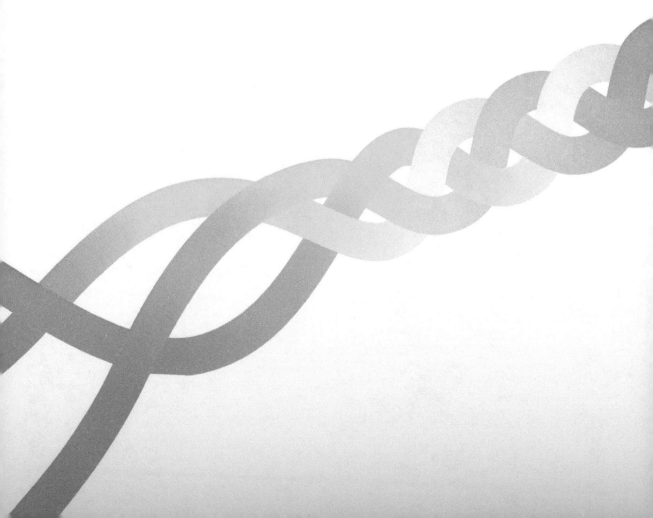

Chapter 19

Healthy Aging

LEARNING OBJECTIVES

Upon completion of this chapter the student will be able to:

• Integrate knowledge of the normal physiological changes of aging and assess how these changes impact quality of life for the older adult.

• Appraise current recommendations regarding health promotion and injury prevention for the older adult.

• Understand and discuss issues that place the older adult at risk for poverty and marginalization.

Introduction

The older population is expected to reach 74 million and will represent 21% of the total population by the year 2030 (Federal Interagency Forum on Aging-Related Statistics [FIFARS], 2016) and 98 million (23.5% of the population) by the year 2060 (Office of Disease Prevention and Health Promotion [ODPHP], 2018). The main factors in this growth are the aging of the baby-boom generation and longer life spans (Centers for Disease Control and Prevention [CDC], 2013b). Older adults are categorized by their age-groups: *young old* (65 to 74 years); *middle old* (75 to 84 years), *old old* (85 to 99 years) and *elite old* (100 years or older), with the old old being the fastest growing segment of the elderly population (Ignativicius, 2018b).

Quality of life is an issue for the older adult since independence, productivity, security, and socialization are directly related to health status (Ignativicius, 2018b; National Council on Aging [NCOA], 2018b). Older adults have a high incidence of chronic illness with 80% reporting one chronic illness and 70% reporting two or more chronic illnesses (NCOA, 2018b), making health promotion and chronic disease management key initiatives to improve the overall health of our aging population (Blair, 2012). Additionally, less than half of the estimated 1 in 3 older adults who falls report their falls, yet falls lead the causes of injury in this population (ODPHP, 2018). *Healthy People 2020* goals for older adults include initiatives that seek to address common chronic conditions and to increase the number of older adults who take advantage of cancer screenings and who receive recommended immunizations (ODPHP, 2018).

Estimates indicate that as many as 5 million older adults experience elder abuse each year, including between 47% and 50% of older adults with some form of dementia. The financial impact on the health-care system from injuries incurred because of elder abuse exceeds $5.3 billion, with more than $2.8 billion in Medicare payments attributed to preventable harm (understaffing, inadequate care and treatment) events that occurred in long-term care facilities (National Center on Elder Abuse [NCEA], n.d.).

The health-care economic burden is higher for marginalized individuals (Kim & Belza, 2017) and exponentially higher for Medicare households (65+ years old), accounting for 14% of their 2012 budget compared to only 5% of the household budgets of younger adults, with nearly two-thirds of these costs spent on health insurance. In general, health-care spending costs typically increase with age, with 11.7% (65 to 69 years), 13.3% (70 to 74 years), 16.1% (75 to 79 years), and 15.4% (80 years or older) of the household budget spent on health care in 2012 (Cubanski, Swoope, Damico, & Neuman, 2014). Currently, the yearly direct costs for treatment of falls in the elderly are $50 billion and are projected to approach $101 billion by 2030 (NCOA, 2018b), with payments for nonfatal falls being distributed between Medicare ($29 billion), Medicaid ($9 billion), and private insurance or other payers ($12 billion) (CDC, 2019). In addition to direct costs of falls, there are indirect costs in terms of loss of independence, lost productivity (at work or home), disability, and overall quality of life (CDC, 2016). Additionally, the estimated overall Medicare costs to manage chronic disease in older adults is 93% (NCOA, 2018b), making health promotion and injury prevention initiatives an important part of holistic care of this population.

This chapter reviews the normal physiological changes of aging, which may impact independence and quality of life, and discusses health issues and health promotion strategies that reduce risk factors and improve health status and overall quality of life for the older adult. Physiological changes discussed in this chapter include sensory perception (vision and hearing loss), nutrition (including oral health), and mobility (falls). Common pathological conditions related to these normal physiological changes and health promotion strategies to address these changes are outlined. Additional information on the impact of polypharmacy and a discussion of elder abuse are included.

The Physiology of Aging

The normal changes of aging impact all body systems (see Table 19-1); however, some changes are more likely to impact the individual's ability to remain independent and maintain a satisfactory quality of life (Ignatavicius, 2018b). These include vision, hearing, nutrition and oral health, and musculoskeletal changes, and are described in more detail in the sections that follow. Older adults who report no limitations with their *activities of daily living* (ADLs) are more likely to report well-being and to feel they are successfully aging (Mejía, Ryan, Gonzalez, & Smith, 2017).

Vision

Light reaches the retina by entering the eyeball through the cornea, is refracted or focuses as it travels through the pupil (center of the iris) and then through the vitreous humor (gel-like substance that makes up the body of the eye), and finally focuses on the retina at the back of the eyeball. Vision extends to 6 cardinal fields of vision through a symmetrical movement of the oblique and rectus muscles that are controlled by cranial nerves III, IV, and VI. Visual acuity requires a normal cornea shape for pupils to constrict and dilate as they adapt to light levels and for the lens to accurately focus light rays onto the retina. Additionally, normal eye pressure is controlled by parasympathetic innervation of the eye's ciliary muscle,

TABLE 19–1 Physiological Changes of Aging by Body System

Body System	Change	Clinical Importance

Cardiovascular	Heart muscle and heart valves become stiffer due to fibrosis and calcification of tissue
	   ↓ heart rate and AV conduction
	   ↓ elasticity of blood vessels
	   Arterial baroreceptors respond slower to blood pressure changes
	   Beta-adrenergic response ↓
		↓ heart rate
		↑ murmurs
		↑ dysrhythmias
		hypertension
		orthostatic hypotension

Endocrine	↓ secretion of aldosterone, insulin, thyroid-stimulating hormone (TSH) and T_4, and other hormones ↑ insulin resistance	↑ risk for diabetes ↑ risk of hypothyroidism ↓ basal metabolism rate ↓ stress response
Gastrointestinal tract (GI)	↓ taste buds ↓ salivation ↓ GI motility Atrophy of stomach lining (↓ HCl and intrinsic factor secretion) GI flora changes ↓ Liver size and function	↓ absorption, particularly of vitamin B_{12} Constipation / diarrhea ↑ risk of *Clostridium difficile* Lactose intolerance ↓ drug metabolism
Immune system	↓ B cell and T cell function	↑ risk of cancer ↑ risk of infection ↓ effectiveness of immunization
Integumentary	Dermal thinning and ↓ collagen Adipose fat redistributed ↓ function of sweat glands Fewer melanocytes	↑ risk for skin tears Temperature regulation impaired Skin pigment becomes irregular

Neurological (CNS)	↓ number of neurons
	   Neurotransmitters including b-endorphins, dopamine, *gamma-aminobutyric acid* (GABA), norepinephrine, serotonin change in their balance and function in various areas of the CNS
	↑ loss of myelin
		Changes in sleep patterns
		May have higher pain thresholds
		   ↑ risk of neurological disorders like Parkinson's and memory loss

Pulmonary	↓ number of cilia
	↓ cough reflex
	↑ residual volume
	↓ lung capacity
	   Calcification of costal cartilage and changes in shape of thorax
	↓ respiratory muscle strength
		↓ vital capacity
		   Shortness of breath (SOB) and fatigue with exertion
		   Secretions tend to pool, ↑ risk of pneumonia or other respiratory infections

Renal	↓ number of nephrons ↓ renal tubule function ↓ blood flow	↓ creatinine clearance and filtration ↑ fluid retention ↓ response to fluid overload ↑ nocturnal urine formation ↓ drug excretion
Sensory	Ears: high-frequency hearing loss Eyes: lenses become less flexible	↓ ability to distinguish speech Cataracts Presbyopia ↓ acuity and accommodation
General body composition	Bone and muscle mass decline and adipose tissue % increases ↓ % of water	↑ risk of balance and gait issues ↑ fracture risk ↓ muscle strength

(Besdine, 2016; Blair, 2012; Capriotti, 2020; Goolsby, 2019; Huether, 2012)

which is responsible for adjusting aqueous fluid flow, thus controlling eye pressure (Capriotti, 2020).

Hearing

An estimated 33% of all older adults experience some degree of hearing loss. As one ages, the ear's pinna elongates due to decreased elasticity and loss of subcutaneous tissues; however, this normal change does not impact hearing (Belden, DeFriez, & Huether, 2012). Age-related changes that impact hearing include increasing coarseness and length of ear hair that leads to clumping of cerumen which blocks the ear canal and leads to decreased hearing acuity. The tympanic membrane begins to lose elasticity as one ages, and the resultant dull and retracted appearance of the membrane, in the absence of other symptoms, does not indicate otitis media (Borchers & Borchers, 2018b).

Nutrition/Oral Health

Nutritional health in the elderly begins with oral health, which, while important throughout the life span, becomes particularly important for the older adult, with both external factors and physical changes contributing to oral health status. For example, the financial situation after job retirement often reduces access to dental care as a result of loss of dental insurance and inability to pay for routine dental care. While Medicaid provides some minimal benefits for dental care, the Medicare program does not cover dental care (Bassim, 2018; CDC, 2013a). The number of older adults who visit the dentist declines as one ages, with 2014 data showing that in the 65-to-74 years age-group, 66% reported a dental visit in the last year, while in those over 85 years, only 56% reported a similar visit (FIFARS, 2016). Reduced income also contributes to poor nutrition as healthy foods typically cost more than less-healthy options, while the inability to drive because of physical or cognitive limitations also reduces access to dental care and grocery stores (Bassim, 2018; CDC, 2013a).

Normal physiological changes of aging also contribute to oral health status. As one ages, tooth enamel deteriorates, increasing risk for cavities. Another contributor to the high rates of dental cavities in older adults is the reduction in the production of saliva (*xerostomia*), which develops as a part of normal aging, as a side effect of some medications, or as the result of cognitive decline, diabetes, or neurological diseases (American Dental Association [ADA], 2018). Finally, individuals with cognitive impairment, those who lack coordination or fine motor skills, and those who have arthritis in the fingers, hands, or upper extremities are limited in their ability to perform adequate oral hygiene (ADA, 2018).

Sensory changes impact appetite and food preparation, with the loss of taste sensation (salty, bitter, sweet) and reduction in the sense of smell, leading to excessive use of salt and sugar to improve flavor (Ignatavicius, 2018b; Johnston & Chernoff, 2012). A decline in thirst sensitivity occurs as one ages and, coupled with a reduced total body water content, places the older adult at increased risk of dehydration and complications of dry mouth, including cavities, cracked lips, mucositis, and development of tongue fissures (ADA, 2018; Johnston & Chernoff, 2012).

Finally, caloric and nutritional needs change as the body ages. The decline in body muscle mass, coupled with lower physical activity levels, requires a reduction in daily caloric intake to maintain normal weight. However, protein needs increase with age because retention of nitrogen declines with a decrease in caloric intake, making it important to increase protein intake to maintain a positive nitrogen balance (Johnston & Chernoff, 2012).

Musculoskeletal Function

Bone remodeling is a constant process that occurs across the life span, with bone-building (osteoblastic) activity occurring first at a more rapid rate, as bone resorption (osteoclastic) activity. Around age 25 to 30 years, *bone mineral density* (BMD) is strongest; a gradual decline in bone density occurs as one ages, and bone resorption occurs at a more rapid rate than bone is built (Ignatavicius, 2018a). Additionally, muscle mass loss occurs at a rate of about 5% every 10 years as one ages, contributing to the predisposition of the older adult to musculoskeletal injury (Capriotti, 2020).

Pathophysiology

Many changes due to aging are gradual and easily manageable at first, but eventually move into the area of pathology, creating more serious problems and requiring more intervention. This section discusses pathologies that can develop in the areas of vision, hearing, oral health, and musculoskeletal function.

Vision Changes

Visual acuity decreases as a result of *structural changes* within the eye and its supporting structures. The ability to focus on a particular object becomes diminished as eye muscles lose tone, and *dry eye* occurs as the lower eyelid relaxes away from the eye and tear production decreases. Individuals with dry eye symptoms are at increased risk for infections and corneal damage. As the cornea loses its regular shape and contour, the eye loses its ability to focus light rays on the retina, and vision blurs (*astigmatism*). Another structural change that limits the older adult's ability to see in lower light is the result of structural changes in the iris, limiting dilation and accommodation to environmental changes in light. A normal change within the eye that does not inhibit vision is the accumulation of fat deposits along the outer edge of the cornea, which is seen as a bluish-white, opaque ring (*arcus senilis*) (Borchers & Borchers, 2018a).

Functional changes that limit visual acuity occur in the lens, which loses its elasticity and hardens, resulting in the formation of a cataract. These lens changes contribute to limiting accommodation to light, which, along with the lens's tendency to yellow with age, diminishes its ability to convey light to and focus light on the retina. As a result of these changes, older adults develop *presbyopia*, or the inability to see close objects clearly (Borchers & Borchers, 2018a).

Two of the most common visual disorders are cataracts and age-related macular degeneration. While *cataracts* can develop at any stage in life, they are a major cause of visual impairment in the elderly. Risk factors include age, diabetes, kidney disease, eye trauma, and the use of certain medications (steroids, alfuzosin, and tamsulosin). Other risk factors include eye trauma, ultraviolet light exposure, and cigarette smoking (Capriotti, 2020; Goolsby, 2019).

Age-related macular degeneration (AMD) is subdivided into *dry* or *wet* AMD based on the underlying pathological changes within the eye. *Dry* AMD results from blockages in the retinal capillaries, which lead to ischemia and necrosis of the retinal cells, while *wet* AMD develops from growth of new, thin-walled blood vessels that leak fluid and blood into the eye.

CLINICAL PEARLS
Risk factors for developing AMD include smoking, gender (female > males), hypertension, family history, short stature, and long-standing dietary deficiencies of carotene and vitamin E (Borchers & Borchers, 2018c).

Hearing Loss

Pathological changes in the structure and function of the ear lead to three types of hearing loss. The loss of auditory neurons in the organ of Corti leads to loss of the ability to hear high-frequency sounds (*sensorineural loss* or *presbycusis*), the primary cause of hearing loss in older adults. Common causes of sensorineural hearing loss include damage to cranial nerve VIII or prolonged exposure to loud music or noise (Belden et al., 2012). Conditions that impair sound conduction (*conductive hearing loss*) from the external and middle ear to the inner ear include tumors (benign or malignant), impacted cerumen, foreign bodies, eustachian tube dysfunction, and viruses. The third type of hearing loss is *mixed and functional hearing loss*, which results from a combination of sensorineural and conductive changes (Belden et al., 2012; Borchers & Borchers, 2018b).

Nutrition/Oral Health Decline

Periodontal disease contributes to dental cavities and tooth loss as gingival recession exposes roots that often become brittle with age and tend to break (ADA, 2018; Huether, 2012). In fact, an estimated 23% of older adults (ages 65 to 74 years) have been diagnosed with severe periodontal disease, with the highest incidence among men and low-income groups (CDC, 2013b). Tooth loss contributes to inadequate nutrition by impacting the ability to chew and necessitating choosing mechanically soft foods and eliminating fresh vegetables and fruits from the diet. A softer diet is also frequently chosen by denture wearers because they may not fit well and are less efficient than natural teeth in chewing food (CDC, 2013a).

Obesity and malnutrition can also be attributed to choosing fast foods as low-cost, quick, and easy food choices. Vitamin deficiencies can result from poor nutritional intake or from decreased absorption related to normal aging or pathological changes in the *gastrointestinal* (GI) tract, creating the need to consciously include vitamin-rich foods in the diet (Ignatavicius, 2018b).

Musculoskeletal Changes/Falls

Physiological changes in the musculoskeletal system, including a decrease in bone density (*osteopenia*) and in muscle mass and strength, place the older adult at increased risk for falls. Bone loss begins in the inner bone (*trabecular*) layers, first in the vertebrae and then in the ends (*cancellous*) of long bones. By the mid-40s to around 50 years of age, bone loss extends to the outer (*cortical*) bone layers, creating softer bones that are more prone to fracture (Blair, 2012; Ignatavicius, 2018a). Vertebral collapse occurs as the intervertebral bodies lose their sponginess and become thin, leading to kyphosis and loss of height.

Just as bones change with aging, joint cartilage and connective tissue become stiffer (less elastic) and deteriorate, leading to joint deformities and impaired joint function. This is particularly the case in weight-bearing joints and the joints of the cervical and lumbar spine, which may affect the hands and fingers, causing difficulty eating and performing ADLs (Blair, 2012; Ignatavicius, 2018a). Skeletal muscles and ligaments also change with aging, decreasing in mass and strength, and contributing to increased flexion in weight-bearing joints such as the knees and hips. This contributes to decreased *range of motion* (ROM) and changes in gait, and predisposes the older adult to falls (Palmer, 2013).

Individuals who experience a fall are twice as likely to fall again as their peers who have not experienced a fall. Injuries sustained in a fall cause more than 2.8 million older adults to seek treatment in the *emergency department* (ED), with more than

300,000 of these visits culminating in a hospital admission to treat a fractured hip (CDC, 2016). Additionally, most traumatic brain injuries in older adults occur as the direct result of a fall, with more than 46% of these injuries being fatal (NCA, 2018b).

Geriatric Functional Assessment

Functional assessment measures "the degree to which an individual can perform those activities that enable him or her to live independently" (Byrd & Pierson, 2019, p. 641) and has the goal of maximizing and maintaining older adults' ability to remain independent in their ADLs. Additionally, functional assessment

becomes important in early recognition of illness, since in the older adult a sudden change in baseline cognition, decline in ADLs, changes in appetite, or urinary incontinence are often the first signs that they are ill (Byrd & Pierson, 2019).

Functional abilities are evaluated using two assessment tools that evaluate physical self-maintenance (ADLs) and *instrumental activities of daily living* (IADLs). Categories in the ADLs tool are scored on a 1 to 5 scale based on their independence in performing each activity: toileting, feeding, dressing, grooming, physical ambulation, and bathing. Categories in the IADLs tool are scored on a 1 to 10 scale giving credit for ability to perform the specific items within each category: use of a telephone, shopping, preparing food, performing housekeeping chores, doing laundry, assuming responsibility for their own medications, handling their own finances, and relying on their mode of transportation. Administered at different points over time, these tests provide an overall picture of the older adult's ability to live independently and indicate when assistance is needed or living independently is no longer safe (Byrd & Pierson, 2019).

Vision Assessment

The eye assessment includes a general assessment of the individual's past medical history including eye conditions or concerns with vision. Habits such as the use of contact lens (inquire about the type, how often they are changed, and how they are cleaned/stored), or occupational and recreational risk for eye injury should be included in this assessment (Goolsby, 2019). Inspection of the outer eye including accessary structures (eyebrows, lashes, and lids) accompanies the assessments for visual acuity. Next, peripheral vision, eye movement, and pupillary response are assessed. Cranial nerves III, IV, and VI are assessed both as part of the eye examination and as part of a comprehensive neurological examination (Capriotti, 2020; Goolsby, 2015).

Pathological changes of the eye that lead to cataract development are part of the aging process, and the result of loss of water and increased density within the lens (Capriotti, 2015). Individuals with cataracts describe diminished visual acuity (blurred, dimmed, and hazy vision) along with difficulty adjusting to bright lights, seeing a halo or glare, especially when driving at night. Cataracts are diagnosed based on signs and symptoms and visualization of the dilated eye (Goolsby, 2019).

Patients with AMD describe variations in their visual acuity and have difficulty reading and seeing faces, because central vision is impaired while peripheral vision remains intact (Capriotti, 2020). Diagnosis is based on symptoms and the presence of hemorrhage, exudates (hard and soft), and altered retinal pigmentation visualized during the fundoscopic eye exam. Additionally, central vision is measured by using an Amsler grid (Capriotti, 2020; Goolsby, 2019).

Hearing Assessment

Accurate assessment of hearing loss begins with the health history, including past history of infection ear surgery, history of chronic diseases (atherosclerosis, kidney disease, or diabetes), and any long-term exposure to loud noises. Assessment of the individual's medication history, including use of ototoxic medications (high-dose aspirin products, aminoglycoside antibiotics, cisplatin chemotherapy, or loop diuretics), may give clues to the origin of hearing loss. Current history including progression of loss (sudden or gradual), bilateral or unilateral hearing loss, and presence of tinnitus or vertigo helps present an accurate picture of the individual's condition (Phan, McKenzie, Huang, Whitfield, & Chang, 2016). An additional component of the patient's history focuses on the presence or absence of behaviors that indicate hearing loss, such as turning the head or leaning forward to hear others speak, asking others to repeat what they have said, and the appropriateness of responses to the conversation or question (Borchers & Borchers, 2018b).

Basic physical assessment hearing tests include the whisper test and use of a tuning fork to distinguish laterality of hearing loss and between conductive or sensorineural hearing loss. The *Rinne test* measures air and bone conduction of sound. Normally, air conduction time is twice the time as bone conduction and should be similar for both ears. The *Weber test* measures how well the individual hears sound bilaterally. Lateralization of sound to be louder in one ear than the other indicates conductive or sensorineural loss and again results should be similar bilaterally (Borchers & Borchers, 2018b; Goolsby, 2019). The most accurate diagnostic test for hearing loss is an *audiometry*, where frequency (high or low tones), intensity (measured in decibels), and threshold (lowest intensity heard) are measured. *Pure-tone audiometry* assesses tones, while a *speech audiometry* measures speech discrimination (the ability to hear words clearly) (Borchers & Borchers, 2018b; Phan et al., 2016).

 ASSESSMENT PEARLS

To achieve an accurate hearing assessment, excess cerumen must be removed, and the individual must be assessed for allergies, current upper respiratory infection, and excessive fluid in the middle ear, all of which can result in an inaccurate test result (Goolsby, 2019; Phan et al., 2016).

Oral Health and Nutrition Assessment

Careful assessment of oral health, including any conditions that limit the ability to perform oral care, is an essential component of nutritional assessment. Normal oral cavity changes of aging include thinning of the epithelium and loss of taste buds, atrophy of soft tissues, and a decrease in saliva. Other age-related changes in the oral cavity include a recession of the gums and accompanying erosion of the teeth at the gum line. If these changes result in tooth loss, malocclusion of the teeth and difficulty with chewing follows. In addition to inspection of the oral cavity, assessment questions should focus on dry mouth (xerostomia), tooth loss (or presence of dentures), the client's ability to chew, or changes in smell or taste (Jarvis & Eckhardt, 2020).

Nutritional assessment is important for all older adults, as being undernourished increases risk for malnutrition, which increases risk for dependence, frailty, and death. Components of a nutritional assessment include accurate height and weight measurements, which may be challenging if the older adult has kyphosis or is unable to stand. Weight should be always measured in the same type of clothes, and on the same scale if possible. Significant weight loss or weight gains are quality indicators of functional decline. Nutritional assessment includes asking about foods and fluid intake, as dehydration is also a common condition in the older adult.

The Nutritional Screening Tool is a 10-question tool that gives points for a yes answer, with the nutritional score indicating risk for poor nutritional health. Below-normal serum albumin levels (3.1 to 4.3 g/dL) and total cholesterol levels (less than160 mg/dL) are useful in identifying protein-energy malnutrition, while above-normal blood urea nitrogen/creatinine ratio levels (greater than a 20:1 ratio) are useful in identifying dehydration (Byrd & Pierson, 2019; Corbett & Banks, 2013). Finally, questions about bowel movements are important, as constipation is a common compliant as GI motility slows with aging, and constipation has serious implications for mortality if fecal impaction or bowel obstruction occurs (Byrd & Pierson, 2019; Ignatavicius, 2018b).

Musculoskeletal Assessment

A baseline *dual-energy x-ray absorptiometry* (DEXA) scan to screen for osteoporosis should be ordered for all adults beginning at age 65 and should be repeated per recommendations based on the degree of bone loss (Palmer, 2013).

Gait and mobility assessments are critical in identifying older adults at risk for falls. Specific performance tests include the *timed get-up-and-go test*, which measures the individual's ability to rise up from sitting, walk 20 feet across the floor, turn around, and walk back to the chair. The process should take less than 15 seconds. The *Tinetti Performance-Oriented Mobility Assessment* (POMA) specifically tests balance (sitting, arising, standing, turning, and sitting down, and balance with eyes closed) and gait mobility (hesitancy, step length and height, symmetry of steps, continuity or stop/start pattern, path, swaying, and use of walking aid) (Byrd & Pierson, 2019).

Nonpharmacological Treatments and Prevention

The only treatment for cataracts is surgical removal of the hardened lens, which is replaced with an artificial intraocular lens (Capriotti, 2020). There is currently no cure for AMD, but it is thought that progression of dry AMD can be slowed by including adequate amounts of antioxidants, carotenoids, and vitamin B_{12} in one's diet. Additionally, patients with wet AMD may experience improved vision following laser therapy (to prevent further blood vessel leakage) or ocular injections using bevacizumab or ranibizumab (*vascular endothelial growth factor inhibitors* [VEGFIs]) (Capriotti, 2020). The role of the nurse in caring for patients with visual impairment is to provide education on the disease process and treatment options, encourage follow-up care, and suggest interventions that promote safety and improve quality of life.

Age-related physiological changes in the ear (dryer cerumen and a stiffening of the cilia, which impedes movement of cerumen) lead to cerumen buildup, a common case of conductive hearing loss. Use of a wax-softening medication and regular wax removal by the health-care provider can improve hearing (Jarvis & Eckhardt, 2020). For many older patients with hearing loss, it should be noted that not all benefit from hearing aids. Individuals with frequency hearing loss may benefit from hearing aids, while those with deficits in speech discrimination may not benefit. Some patients may be appropriate for a cochlear implants (Phan et al., 2016). Preventive interventions that are appropriate at any age include avoiding cleaning the ear with a cotton-tipped applicator and pushing cerumen further into the ear canal. A major cause of hearing loss is noise, and avoiding exposure to loud sounds and wearing either headphones or ear plugs if exposure can't be avoided is important health promotion activity at any age (Jarvis & Eckhardt, 2020).

Oral hygiene interventions include regular tooth brushing using a toothbrush with oscillating or rotating brushes, daily flossing and use of mouth rinse, and application of fluoride varnish. The use of water flossing is effective, particularly when gums are sensitive (ADA, 2018). Additionally, use of fluoride toothpaste protects against cavities, as does drinking fluoridated water. For older adults who cannot perform their own oral care, caregivers should be encouraged to assist with brushing or brush the teeth, and all older adults should see the dentist regularly, including those with dentures (CDC, 2013b).

Fall prevention measures are important for all older adults but are critical for those who have been identified as "at risk" for falls. The older adult's medication regimen should be evaluated to identify any that increase fall risk, including antihypertensives and tricyclic antidepressants, and to evaluate the effectiveness of medications for diseases like Parkinson's, where the prescribed medications are aimed at improving mobility (Nelson, 2016). Exercises in the form of tai chi or yoga can be helpful in improving balance (Ignatavicius, 2018a), while home safety measures such as removing scatter rugs, using grab bars in the shower or tub, adding higher-wattage lightbulbs or using a night light, and adding or using rails on both sides of stairs are important fall prevention strategies (CDC, 2017).

CLINICAL PEARLS

Encouraging water intake, use of sugarless gum, and avoidance of alcohol and tobacco help with symptoms of dry mouth. Adequate water intake also helps prevent constipation (ADA, 2018; CDC, 2013a).

Pharmacology: Pharmacokinetics, Pharmacodynamics, and Polypharmacy

Age-related changes in the GI tract, including the liver and kidneys, impact how drugs are absorbed, distributed, metabolized, and excreted (*pharmacokinetics*). Drug *absorption* in the GI tract is not usually a problem in aging; however, this normal change of aging in combination with a proton pump inhibitor can impair bioavailability of some drugs (Nelson, 2015). *Distribution* of some drugs is impacted as the aging process changes the total body fat (increases up to 30%) and water (decreases of up to 10% to 15%), and lean muscle mass ratios (up to 20% reduction in lean muscle mass), elevating the concentration circulating at peak times. For example, drugs that are water soluble (e.g., digoxin or lithium), along with drugs with narrow therapeutic ranges, may have higher blood concentrations with a "normal" dose (Nelson, 2015), and drugs that tend to concentrate in body fat (e.g., benzodiazepines) take longer to be excreted, prolonging duration of action (Nelson, 2015; Shea & Townsend, 2012). Finally, serum albumin levels decrease up to 20% as one ages, limiting the how much drug can bind to protein in the blood, increasing the risk for drug toxicity in normal amounts (Nelson, 2015).

Metabolism of drugs changes as the aging liver becomes smaller and has decreased blood flow. Despite these changes, most liver enzyme activity remains unchanged in older adults; however, some drugs have altered clearance due to decline in the function of the *cytochrome P450* (CYP450) system, while other drugs, such as propranolol, are more bioavailable because of a decline in effectiveness of first-pass metabolism (Nelson, 2015). *Excretion* of drugs is directly related to kidney function, which declines by about 50% by the mid-70s. Along with a slow decline in renal blood flow (about 10% every 10 years), impaired excretion of drugs can lead to high serum levels and adverse drug reactions (Shea & Townsend, 2012).

Changes of aging also impact the body's ability to effectively respond to a drug (*pharmacodynamics*). Changes in the permeability of the blood–brain barrier in the *central nervous system* (CNS) make the older adult particularly sensitive to drugs (e.g., antidepressants, antipsychotics, or sedatives) and create a more extreme response than needed with a normal dose. Additionally, drugs with anticholinergic effects (particularly if combined with other anticholinergic drugs) and those with narrow therapeutic ranges can cause adverse drug reactions (Shea & Townsend, 2012). In contrast to sensitivity to certain drugs, older adults have an insensitivity to other drugs (e.g., beta agonists or beta blockers) and may require higher doses to obtain a therapeutic response (Nelson, 2015).

Thus *polypharmacy* (use of 5 to 10 medications that are prescribed, over the counter [OTC], or herbals), along with the normal changes of aging, puts the older adult at increased risk of adverse effects (Nelson, 2015). While the number of drugs itself does not create a problem, it is the concurrent use of several medications that may have similar therapeutic effects that puts the older adult at risk. Adverse drug reactions are common due to drug–drug interactions. Older adults may not take their prescribed medications regularly due to costs, drug–drug interactions, or other side effects. Additional factors that contribute to polypharmacy can be attributed to (1) multiple providers treating different comorbid conditions; (2) the use of different clinical practice guidelines for several comorbid conditions, each with medications that may interact with medications on another guideline (Nelson, 2015; Shea & Townsend, 2012); and (3) borrowing or sharing medications rather than seeking medical attention for symptoms (Shea & Townsend, 2012).

The Beers Criteria, originally developed by the American Geriatrics Society to evaluate the risks/benefits of certain medications commonly prescribed to nursing home residents and updated in 2015 to address the broader older adult population, provides guidance to prescribers based on strength of evidence. Drug categories included in the 2015 updated Beers Criteria include antidepressants, anticholinergics, barbiturates, and proton pump inhibitors, and include recommendations for dose adjustment based on renal function (Simonson, 2016). In addition to the Beers Criteria, mnemonics have been found useful in prevention or reduction of polypharmacy: The SAIL (1998) (*simple, adverse reactions, indication, list*); ARMOR (2009) (*assess, review, minimize, optimize, reassess*); TIDE (2012) (*time, individualize, drug interactions, educate*); and MASTER (2011) (*minimize, alternatives, start low and go slow, titrate, educate, review*) all have the common goal of guiding the prescriber to thoughtfully assess medications for their benefits and risks at each visit (Skinner, 2015). Actions the health-care provider can take to avoid issues with polypharmacy are outlined in SENC Box 19-1.

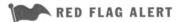 **RED FLAG ALERT**

Patient education regarding prescribed anticholinergic drugs should include a caution about simultaneous use of OTC drugs that also have anticholinergic effects.

SENC BOX 19-1 Safe and Effect Nursing Care for Interventions to Prevent or Reduce Polypharmacy

Several interventions are useful in preventing or reducing polypharmacy in the older adult.

1. At each visit, carefully review all of the older adult's prescribed, OTC, and herbal medications with attention to any interactions and to the benefit of continued use of the medication (Nelson, 2015).
2. Inquire about any recent hospitalizations or medications that have been prescribed by another provider (Skinner, 2016).

Continued

> **SENC BOX 19-1** Safe and Effect Nursing Care for Interventions to Prevent or Reduce Polypharmacy—cont'd
>
> 3. Discontinue drugs no longer needed and avoid a combination of medications that cause adverse reactions or increase fall risk.
> 4. Listen for clues that the patient may not be taking the medication as prescribed to help prevent additional conditions or progression of current medical conditions.
> 5. Provide patient/family education on normal aging and lifestyle alternatives to medications; these have the potential to decrease both the number of medications taken and to improve quality of life for older adults (Nelson, 2012; Shea & Townsend, 2012).

Elder Abuse and Marginalization

Elder abuse may present in one or more of the following ways: *abandonment* (caregiver deserts the older adult at a health-care facility or leaves them alone in a public place), *confinement* (isolation or restraining for reasons that are not medically required), *emotional abuse* (verbal threats, intimidation, or harassment), *financial exploitation* (older adult's resources are withheld or misused by another person), *passive or willful neglect* (caregiver fails in their obligation to provide necessities or to pay for those services if they have financial responsibility for the older adult), *physical abuse* (injury or physical pain), or *sexual abuse* (nonconsensual forced sexual activity) (NCEA, n.d.; NCOA, 2018a). Nearly 60% of all abuse incidents are instigated by a family member.

Another troubling type of neglect is *self-neglect*, which occurs when the older adult is mentally competent to make their own financial and health-care decisions but chooses to behave in a way that is detrimental to their own health and safety. The individual may appear dehydrated or malnourished and may refuse medical care or to take prescribed medications. They may be ungroomed and dirty and live in an unsanitary home or choose to be homeless (NCEA, n.d.).

Risk factors for elder abuse include gender (older women experience more elder abuse than men), dementia, history of prior domestic violence or other traumatic events, impaired functional abilities and physical health, living in poverty, and having a minimal social support system. Additionally, African Americans, those without a spouse or partner, younger older adults, those who do not use social services, those who need assistance with ADLs, and those who self-rate their health status as poor have an increased risk of financial exploitation (NCEA, n.d.). Several screening tools are available for use in detecting elder abuse, and states have mandatory reporting laws for suspected cases of elder abuse (Ignatavicius, 2018b). Unfortunately, while 1 in 10 older adults are estimated to be affected by elder abuse, only 1 in 14 of these incidents are reported to authorities (NCOA, 2018a). Statistics on elder abuse are impacted by failure to recognize signs of abuse and by failure to report by cognitively impaired older adults. Signs of elder abuse are outlined in Table 19-2.

Marginalization and Isolation

Marginalized older adults endure health inequities that impact health status. As older adults' health-care expenditures increase, their ability to afford housing decreases, making affordable housing for low-income older adults a priority. Even for those who own their own home, the costs of maintaining the residence often exceed their monthly income. An estimated 93,000 older adults will be homeless by 2050 (Goldberg, Lang, & Barrington, 2016). Low socioeconomic status limits access to resources and

TABLE 19–2   Signs of Elder Abuse by Type

Abuse	Warning Signs
Abandonment	Desertion of the older adult in a public place or at an institution (hospital, care facility, etc.)
Emotional	Frequent arguments with caregiver Strained relationships Sudden changes in alertness or depression Verbal belittling or threats by caregiver Withdraws from their normal activities
Financial exploitation	Perpetrator: Charges excessive amounts for either necessary or unnecessary services rendered Forges check signatures, misuses money or the elder's personal property Pressures the older adult to change a will or initiate a property transfer Funds or valuables suddenly disappear without explanation
Passive or willful neglect	Health problems that have not been addressed with provider Inadequate clothing Poor nutrition: dehydration and/or malnutrition Presence of dirt / fleas / lice / or smells like urine or feces Unsafe or hazardous living conditions
Physical	Broken bones Broken eyeglasses Caregiver refuses to allow others to be alone with the abused adult Laboratory results that indicate under- or overutilization of prescribed medications Presence of abrasions, burns, bruises, or pressure marks
Sexual	Anal or vaginal bleeding that cannot be explained Bruising: genital or breast areas Underclothing is found to be bloody, stained, or torn Sexually transmitted infections that cannot be explained Self-report of sexual assault

(NCEA, n.d.; NCOA, 2018a; Toole, 2012)

healthy foods and may limit the individual's physical activity if they live in a community where they feel "unsafe" to get out and walk. Lower educational levels have also been linked to Alzheimer's disease (Kim & Belza, 2017).

Older adults who are marginalized for many reasons (race, income, sexual identity, and physical or intellectual impairment) or who are homeless or incarcerated often have multiple chronic health conditions that impact their quality of life (Ignativicius, 2018b). As older adults, they may face increased discrimination and social isolation and are at higher risk for dementia (Kim & Belza, 2017). Health promotion initiatives aimed at marginalized older adults are important to improving quality of life for these vulnerable populations.

In an effort to help older adults remain independently in their own homes for as long as possible (commonly called "aging in place"), avoid social isolation, and reduce overall costs of living, programs like Livable Communities (AARP non-profit program) engage communities in purposeful planning and location of healthcare and supportive services, housing, and transportation, to make access to these services easier for the older adult who no longer drives (Wick, 2017). The decision to stop driving is difficult and is known to lead to social isolation and loneliness, which are tied to the development of depression and dementia and increased health-care costs (Kim & Belza, 2017). Additionally, weekend transportation with access to health-care services and social events are important needs for older adults who desire to age in place (Wick, 2017).

Summary

The older adult's sense of healthy aging and overall sense of well-being is influenced by the individual's social embeddedness; their degree of cognitive function, physical health and independence in ADLs; and their socioeconomic situation (Megía et al., 2017). Normal physiological changes, compounded by comorbid conditions and polypharmacy, put the older adult at risk for falls and injury. Older adults are at increased risk for marginalization due to lifestyle choices or socioeconomic status, and elder abuse often goes unreported by vulnerable older adults. This chapter has highlighted some of the most common physiological changes of aging and their impact on healthy aging. Understanding the challenges of aging is key to health prevention and health promotion interventions and to providing resources to support older adults in their quest for independence and well-being in their final years of life.

Key Points

- Changes in functional ability, cognitive level, appetite, or continence, particularly urinary, may be the first signs of illness in the older adult.
- All body systems are impacted by the aging process, and while some changes are insignificant, others increase risk factors for injury and serious medical conditions.
- Medications used to treat older adults should be started at low dosages and then slowly titrated to an effective level to avoid adverse drug reactions.

Review Questions

1. **Which of the following does the nurse recognize as important to decreasing polypharmacy? (Select all that apply.)**
   a. Asking the older adult to bring all their medication bottles to each visit.
   b. Inquiring about other health-care providers that are prescribing medications for health-related conditions.
   c. Telling the patient to take all the prescribed antibiotic even if they feel better.
   d. Understanding that they may not comply with taking the medication if they have financial difficulties.

2. **When taking the health history, which of the following suggests to the nurse that the older adult might be a victim of elder abuse or passive neglect?**
   a. The caregiver brings the client to the office only when they have a health concern.
   b. The caregiver fails to pay medical bills when they are due.
   c. The older adult exhibits signs of dehydration and undernutrition.
   d. The caregiver refuses to allow the nurse to interview the patient in private.

3. **Normal aging of the central nervous system can cause which of the following symptoms?**
   a. Decreased pain thresholds
   b. Decreased stress response
   c. Increased basal metabolism rate
   d. Sleep pattern changes

4. **Which of the following laboratory findings indicates that the older adult may be malnourished?**

   a. Blood urea nitrogen 40 mg/dL

   b. Serum albumin level 2.8 g/dL

   c. Serum cholesterol 210 mg/dL

   d. Urine specific gravity 1.005

5. **When educating a caregiver about the oral health needs of an aged parent with cognitive impairment, the nurse includes which of the following statements?**

   a. "Eating soft foods is not necessary because teeth remain strong throughout the life span."

   b. "Encourage fluids to prevent dental cavities because older adults have less saliva."

   c. "Mouth care is not as important when the older adult has upper and lower dentures."

   d. "Visiting the dentist will not be necessary if the older adult becomes afraid of going out."

See the appendix for answers to review questions.

References

American Dental Association. (2018). Aging and dental health. Retrieved from https://www.ada.org/en/member-center/oral-health-topics/aging-and-dental-health

Bassim, C. W. (2018). Editorial: Oral health in healthy aging. *Journal of the American Geriatrics Society, 66*(3), 439–440. https://doi.org/10.1111/jgs.15253

Belden, J., DeFriez, C., & Huether, S. E. (2012). Pain, temperature, sleep and sensory function. In S. E. Huether & K. L. McCance (Eds.), *Understanding pathophysiology* (5th ed.). St. Louis, MO: Elsevier Mosby.

Besdine, R. W. (2016, Sept). Physical changes with aging. *Merck manual: Professional version*. Retrieved from https://www.merckmanuals.com/professional/geriatrics/approach-to-the-geriatric-patient/physical-changes-with-aging

Blair, K. A. (2012). Health priorities for the older adult. In J. W. Lange (Ed.), *The nurse's role in promoting optimal health of older adults: Thriving in the wisdom years*. Philadelphia, PA: F.A. Davis.

Borchers, S. A., & Borchers, A. A. (2018a). Assessment of the eye and vision. In D. D. Ignatavicius, L. Workman, & C. R. Rebar (Eds.), *Medical-surgical nursing: Concepts for interprofessional collaborative care* (9th ed.). St. Louis, MO: Elsevier.

Borchers, S.A., & Borchers, A.A. (2018b). Care of patients with ear and hearing problems. In D. D. Ignatavicius, L. Workman, & C. R. Rebar (Eds.), *Medical-surgical nursing: Concepts for interprofessional collaborative care* (9th ed.). St. Louis, MO: Elsevier.

Borchers, S. A., & Borchers, A. A. (2018c). Care of patients with eye and vision problems. In D. D. Ignatavicius, L. Workman, & C. R. Rebar (Eds.), *Medical-surgical nursing: Concepts for interprofessional collaborative care* (9th ed.). St. Louis, MO: Elsevier.

Byrd, L., & Pierson, C. (2019). Older patients. In M. J. Goolsby & L. Grubbs (Eds.), *Advanced assessment: Interpreting findings and formulating differential diagnoses* (4th ed.). Philadelphia, PA: F.A. Davis.

Capriotti, T. (2020). *Pathophysiology: Introductory concepts and clinical perspectives* (2nd ed.). Philadelphia, PA: F.A. Davis.

Caswell, W. (2018, January 17). Income levels for aging Americans are increasing, but not as quickly as aging costs. *Modern Health Talk*. Retrieved from www.mhealthtalk.com/aging-cost/

Centers for Disease Control and Prevention. (2013a). *Oral health for older Americans* [Fact sheet]. Retrieved from https://www.cdc.gov/oralhealth/publications/factsheets/adult_oral_health/adult_older.htm

Centers for Disease Control and Prevention. (2013b). The state of aging and health in America 2013. Retrieved from https://www.cdc.gov/aging/pdf/State-Aging-Health-in-America-2013.pdf

Centers for Disease Control and Prevention. (2016). Costs of falls among older adults. Retrieved from https://www.cdc.gov/homeandrecreationalsafety/falls/fallcost.html

Centers for Disease Control and Prevention. (2017). Important facts about falls. Retrieved from https://www.cdc.gov/homeandrecreationalsafety/falls/adultfalls.html

Centers for Disease Control and Prevention. (2019). Falls data: Cost of older adult falls. Retrieved from https://www.cdc.gov/homeandrecreationalsafety/falls/fallcost.html

Corbett, J. V., & Banks, A. D. (2013). *Laboratory tests and diagnostic procedures with nursing diagnoses* (8th ed.). Upper Saddle River, NJ: Pearson Education.

Cubanski, J., Swoope, C., Damico, A., & Neuman, T. (2014, January 9). *Health care on a budget: The financial burden of health spending by Medicare households*. Kaiser Family Foundation. Retrieved from

https://www.kff.org/medicare/issue-brief/health-care-on-a-budget-the-financial-burden-of-health
-spending-by-medicare-households/

Federal Interagency Forum on Aging-Related Statistics. (2016). *Older Americans 2016: Key indicators of well-being*. Washington, DC: U.S. Government Printing Office. Retrieved from https://agingstats.gov/docs
/LatestReport/OA2016.pdf

Goldberg, J., Lang, K., & Barrington, V. (2016, April). How to prevent and end homelessness among older adults. *Justice in Aging*. Retrieved from www.justiceinaging.org

Goolsby, M. J. (2019). The eye. In M. J. Goolsby & L. Grubbs (Eds.), *Advanced assessment: Interpreting findings and formulating differential diagnoses* (4th ed). Philadelphia, PA: F.A. Davis.

Huether, S. E. (2012). Structure and function of the digestive system. In S. E. Huether & K. L. McCance (Eds.), *Understanding pathophysiology* (5th ed.). St. Louis, MO: Elsevier Mosby.

Ignatavicius, D. D. (2018a). Assessment of the musculoskeletal system. In D. D. Ignatavicius, L. Workman, & C. R. Rebar (Eds.), *Medical-surgical nursing: Concepts for interprofessional collaborative care* (9th ed.). St. Louis, MO: Elsevier.

Ignatavicius, D. D. (2018b). Common health problems of older adults. In D. D. Ignatavicius, L. Workman, & C. R. Rebar (Eds.), *Medical-surgical nursing: Concepts for interprofessional collaborative care* (9th ed.). St. Louis, MO: Elsevier.

Jarvis, C., & Eckhardt, A. (2020). *Physical examination and health assessment* (8th ed.). St. Louis, MO: Elsevier.

Johnston, R. E., & Chernoff, R. (2012). Healthy eating. In J. W. Lange (Ed.), *The nurse's role in promoting optimal health of older adults: Thriving in the wisdom years*. Philadelphia, PA: F.A. Davis.

Kim, B., & Belza, B. (2017). Toward an equitable society for every generation. *Journal of Gerontological Nursing, 43*(11), 2–4. doi:10.3928/00989134-20171012-01

Mejía, S. T., Ryan, L. H., Gonzalez, R., & Smith, J. (2017). Successful aging as the intersection of individual resources, age, environment, and experience of well-being in daily activities. *The Journals of Gerontology, Series B: Psychological Sciences and Social Sciences, 72*(2), 279–298. Doi: 10.1093/geronb/gbw148

National Center on Elder Abuse. (n.d.). *What we do: Research statistics/data*. Retrieved from https://ncea.acl
.gov/whatwedo/research/statistics.html

National Council on Aging. (2018a). *Elder abuse facts*. Retrieved from https://www.ncoa.org/public-policy
-action/elder-justice/elder-abuse-facts/

National Council on Aging. (2018b). *Healthy aging fact sheet*. Retrieved from https://d2mkcg26uvg1cz
.cloudfront.net/wp-content/uploads/2018-Healthy-Aging-Fact-Sheet-7.10.18-1.pdf

Nelson, J. M. (2016). Geriatric patients. In T. M. Woo & M. V. Robinson (Eds.), *Pharmacotherapeutics for advanced practice nurse prescribers* (4th ed.). Philadelphia, PA: F.A. Davis.

Office of Disease Prevention and Health Promotion. (2018). *Healthy People 2020: Older adults*. Retrieved from https://www.healthypeople.gov/2020/topics-objectives/topic/older-adults

Palmer, D. M. (2013). Musculoskeletal assessment. In L. Schoenly (Ed.), *Core curriculum for orthopaedic nursin* (7th ed.). Chicago, IL: National Association of Orthopaedic Nurses.

Phan, N. T., McKenzie, J., Huang, L., Whitfield, B., & Chang, A. (2016). Diagnosis and management of hearing loss in elderly patients. *Australian Family Physicians, 45*(6), 366–369. Retrieved from https://www
.racgp.org.au/afp/2016/june/diagnosis-and-management-of-hearing-loss-in-elderly-patients/

Shea, C., & Townsend, H. (2012). Using medications safety and effectively. In J. W. Lange (Ed.), *The nurse's role in promoting optimal health of older adults: Thriving in the wisdom years*. Philadelphia, PA: F.A. Davis.

Simonson, W. (2016). The 2015 updated Beers Criteria: The evolution continues. *Geriatric Nursing, 35*, 61–62. Retrieved from http://dx.doi.org/10.1016/j.gerinurse.2015.12.006

Skinner, M. (2015). A literature review: Polypharmacy for primary care. *Geriatric Nursing, 36*, 367–371. Retrieved from http://dx.doi.org/10.1016/j.gerinurse.2015.05.003

Toole, M. (2012). Legal considerations. In J. W. Lange (Ed.), *The nurse's role in promoting optimal health of older adults: Thriving in the wisdom years*. Philadelphia, PA: F.A. Davis.

Wick, J. (2017). Aging in place: Our house is a very, very, very, fine house. *The Consultant Pharmacist, 32*(10), 566–575.

Chapter 20

Heart Failure

Upon completion of this chapter the student will be able to:

- Integrate knowledge of the physiology, pathophysiology, assessment, and nonpharmacological and pharmacological management for care of an older patient with heart failure.

- Appraise current standards of care for older patients with heart failure.

Introduction

Congestive heart failure (CHF), or *heart failure*, occurs when the heart's pumping ability is not adequate to support the body organs' needs for blood and oxygen. Heart failure is included in the broad category of *cardiovascular disease* (CVD) (with cerebrovascular disease, peripheral vascular disease, hypertension, valvular heart disease, and coronary artery disease) (Capriotti, 2020). While CVD is more prevalent in men before age 50, after that age, the incidence of heart disease is equally high across sexes (Goolsby & Grubbs, 2015). Heart failure is both a national and global health problem. Approximately 5.7 million U.S. adults have heart failure, and this number is expected to rise to over 8 million by 2030 (Centers for Disease Control and Prevention [CDC], 2017). Heart failure affects about 40 million people globally; it is estimated that 2% of adults overall and 6% to 10% of adults over the age of 65 have heart failure. Patients with heart failure account for about 1 million hospital admissions each year, with an additional 2 million hospitalized with heart failure as a secondary diagnosis (Hoffman & Sullivan, 2020).

The World Health Organization (WHO, 2017) reports that 17.7 million people died from cardiovascular disease in 2015, more than any other cause. Half of people diagnosed with heart failure die within 5 years of their diagnosis. Many patients die from progressive pump failure and resulting congestion, although one-half die from sudden cardiac death. Death can also be due to end-organ failure due to inadequate systemic circulation, particularly to the kidneys (American Heart Association [AHA], 2017a; CDC, 2017; Hoffman & Sullivan, 2020).

Paradoxically, people are surviving acute conditions due to improved medical and surgical treatments, but many of these *survivors* of acute coronary syndrome, cancer, hypertension, and diabetes develop heart failure as older adults (Agnetti, Piepoli, Siniscalchi, & Nicolini, 2015). Heart failure is also a very expensive disease, costing an estimated $39.2 billion annually in the United States, including cost of provider services and hospitalization, medications, and lost workdays (Hoffman & Sullivan, 2020). According to the Centers for Medicare & Medicaid Services (CMS), patients with heart failure are readmitted to the hospital at a rate of 22%, and at an average cost 18% greater than the initial stay; heart failure is the most common indication for readmission among Medicare patients (Harmon, 2016). The incidence and prevalence of heart failure is expected to continue rising. Specifically, heart failure is more common in people who are 65 years old or older, African Americans, overweight, and/or have had a myocardial infarction (Hoffman & Sullivan, 2020; National Heart, Lung, and Blood Institute [NHLBI], 2018).

This disease is especially impactful in geriatric patients, who have an increased risk for developing this condition due to an aging and weakened heart muscle. These patients often also have decreased resources for treatment. Because many nurses are in daily contact with patients with heart failure, the majority of whom are older, it is important to understand the management of this condition in this patient population.

Physiology

Normal heart physiology has been addressed in previous chapters (Chapters 1 and 5); however, when the patient has heart failure, there are sequelae for multiple organs. For example, a weakened myocardium cannot provide adequate blood to the kidneys, which leads to impaired functioning and fluid overload. The lungs and liver are often the end points for this additional fluid volume accumulation, leading to left-sided (systolic or diastolic) and right-sided heart failure. Additionally, the intestines are affected by impaired circulation and are less efficient in absorbing nutrients (AHA, 2017b; Capriotti, 2020; Hoffman & Sullivan, 2020). The heart and the primarily affected organs—kidneys and liver—often incur end-organ damage; therefore, the normal physiology and resulting pathophysiology of all these organs are presented in this chapter. If left untreated, however, worsening heart failure affects virtually every organ in the body (Capriotti, 2020).

It is the heart's pumping ability that circulates oxygen-rich blood from the lungs to the left atrium, then to the left ventricle, which pumps it to the body. Because the left ventricle is the heart's primary pumping chamber, it is larger than the other chambers and has a thicker muscle wall. With left-sided or *left ventricular* (LV) heart failure, the left ventricle must compensate and work harder to pump the same amount of blood. The heart's pumping action moves blood that returns to the heart through pulmonary veins through the right atrium into the right ventricle. Because the right ventricle pumps blood back into the lungs to be oxygenated, it does not normally have a thickened myocardial wall. The pumping capability of both ventricles is necessary for normal heart function and supplying oxygenated blood to all organs (AHA, 2017b; Capriotti, 2020; Dillon, 2017).

Basic kidney function is affected by the pumping ability of the heart and also by the body's fluid volume, both intravascular and interstitial. Each kidney contains up to a million functioning units, nephrons, which are filtering units of tiny blood vessels called a glomerulus attached to a tubule. Within the nephron, blood enters the glomerulus and is filtered, and the remaining fluid then passes along the tubule. In the tubule, chemicals and water are either added to or removed from the filtrate in order to maintain homeostasis. The final filtrate product is urine and is excreted as waste (AHA, 2017b; Capriotti, 2020; CDC, 2017).

Similarly, the liver has many necessary functions, including phagocytosis of damaged red blood cells and bacteria; production and management of glucose and cholesterol; synthesis of plasma proteins (albumin, globulin, protein C, insulin-like growth factor, clotting factors); biotransformation of toxins, hormones, and drugs; and storage of vitamins and minerals (Capriotti, 2020).

Reticuloendothelial cells in the liver (also in spleen and bone marrow) are primarily responsible for clearing pathogens and *red blood cells* (RBCs). Kupffer cells are reticuloendothelial cells in the liver that scavenge damaged and nonfunctioning RBCs and bacteria as they pass through the hepatic circulation. Hundreds of millions of RBCs are removed by this system each minute. Kupffer cells lyse RBCs into heme and globin; the globin is further catabolized into components for reuse, and heme is broken into biliverdin and iron. The liver receives a variety of lipid molecules from the circulating blood, including chylomicrons remnants, *very low-density lipoproteins* (VLDL), *low-density lipoproteins* (LDL), *high-density lipoproteins* (HDL), and fatty acids. Large lipoprotein molecules are broken into smaller units by the liver enzymes. The liver also performs three metabolic processes to maintain normal blood glucose: glycogenesis, glycogenolysis, and gluconeogenesis. The liver uses dietary amino acids and those released during normal tissue catabolism to synthesize its own proteins and enzymes (AHA, 2017b; Capriotti, 2020; Harrison, Evans, Shaffer, & Romero, 2016).

Pathophysiology

In general, heart failure occurs because the pumping ability of the heart is not adequate to meet the body's demands. Heart failure can occur in the left side, ride side, or both pumping chambers (biventricular). Heart failure may result from many different causes that decrease the heart muscle's pumping efficiency, such as cardiovascular disease (specifically myocardial infarction), hypertension, diabetes, and lifestyle factors (Hoffman & Sullivan, 2020; NHLBI, 2018). With heart failure, there is decreased contractile ability, rather than a normal increased contractile force, due to overloading of the ventricle. This condition results from inability of actin and myosin filaments to cross-link in the heart muscle (Capriotti, 2020; CDC, 2017). Reduced stroke volume may occur in heart failure with an associated increased end systolic volume from decreased contractility. With increased cardiac workload and loss of reserve, it is an initial challenge to meet oxygenation demands with exertion. Eventually the heart is challenged to meet the basal metabolic demands at rest (Capriotti, 2020; Hoffman & Sullivan, 2020).

There are two types of left-sided heart failure, and drug treatments are different for the two types because the pathophysiological processes are distinctive. First, left-sided *heart failure with reduced ejection fraction* (HFrEF), is also known as systolic heart failure. In this condition, the left ventricle cannot contract normally and does not pump with enough force to push adequate amounts of blood into circulation. In systolic heart failure, the body activates neurohormonal pathways that result in increased circulating blood volume (CDC, 2017). Also, the sympathetic nervous system stimulation causes increased heart rate and myocardial contractility, arteriolar vasoconstriction in nonessential vascular beds, and renin secretion in the kidney. Catecholamines may have negative effects, such as ischemia, arrhythmias, cardiac remodeling, and myocyte toxicity. The renin-angiotensin system activation results in further arteriolar vasoconstriction, sodium and water retention, and release of aldosterone. Increased aldosterone level also results in sodium and water retention, along with endothelial dysfunction and organ fibrosis (Capriotti, 2020; Hoffman & Sullivan, 2020).

In the other type of left-sided heart failure, there is *preserved* (above 40%) *ejection fraction* (HFpEF). This condition is also called diastolic heart failure. In contrast to systolic heart failure, the left ventricle may still have pumping ability but loses its ability to relax because the muscle has become stiff. In diastolic heart failure, the heart does not fill properly with blood during the resting period between each beat. Therefore, the primary symptoms of left-sided heart failure are dyspnea and peripheral edema

(Capriotti, 2020; Hoffman & Sullivan, 2010). Dyspnea in heart failure is multifactorial; pulmonary congestion may be a primary cause, along with impaired renal function that occurs with fluid retention. Kidney failure may be both causative and a result of heart failure (Goolsby & Grubbs, 2015; Hoffman & Sullivan, 2020). Also, the dyspnea that occurs with heart failure is often more pronounced with physical exertion but may occur primarily when lying down (orthopnea), or it may occur suddenly during sleep (*paroxysmal nocturnal dyspnea* [PND]). In recent years, doctors have recognized a "new" symptom of CHF called *bendopnea*, or dyspnea when bending over due to an increase in already elevated ventricular filling pressures (Hoffman & Sullivan, 2020).

As a result of left-sided failure, there is a backup of blood into the right side of the heart, which stresses the right ventricle and causes difficulty propelling blood into the lungs. Once the blood gets to the lungs, there is already increased pressure in the pulmonary vasculature, and the right-side of the heart has to work harder. Eventually, the right-side of the heart is not able to compensate and right-sided heart failure ensues. While dyspnea and edema are the most prominent symptoms of heart failure, in right-sided failure there may be additional symptoms from the peripheral circulation congestions, such as jugular venous distension, ascites, and hepatic enlargement (AHA, 2017; NHLBI, 2018). Right-sided heart failure can also occur in isolation, without concurrent left-sided failure; this is known as *cor pulmonale* and is usually caused by respiratory disease, particularly *chronic obstructive pulmonary disease* (COPD), and/or living at a high altitude for many years (Hoffman & Sullivan, 2020; NHLBI, 2018).

After heart failure is diagnosed, it can be classified for better specificity and treatment based on symptom severity The *New York Heart Association* (NYHA) Functional Classification (Table 20-1) is the most commonly used system and places patients in a category based on limitation of their physical activity (AHA, 2017). Low output heart failure is advanced heart failure in which the heart is no longer able to pump enough blood to sustain normal organ function. The most prominent symptoms are dangerously low blood pressure, which causes extreme weakness, severe fatigue, lightheadedness, and/or syncope (AHA, 2017a; NHBLI, 2018).

Risk Factors

According to the CDC (2017), three diseases present risk factors for the development of heart failure: coronary heart disease, hypertension, and diabetes. Lifestyle factors also increase a person's risk factors for heart failure, especially if they have one these three diseases. Contributing lifestyle behaviors include smoking tobacco, eating a high-fat and high-sodium diet, physical inactivity, and obesity. Finally, age can be a

TABLE 20–1 NYHA Heart Failure Classification Categories

Class	Patient Symptoms
I	No limitation of physical activity. Ordinary physical activity does not cause heart failure symptoms.
II	Slight limitation of physical activity. Comfortable at rest. Ordinary physical activity results in fatigue, palpitation, and/or dyspnea.
III	Marked limitation of physical activity. Comfortable at rest. Minimal activity causes fatigue, palpitation, and/or dyspnea.
IV	Unable to engage in physical activity without discomfort. Symptoms of heart failure at rest. Discomfort increases with physical activity.

(AHA, 2017a)

contributing factor in the development of heart failure (Hoffman & Sullivan, 2020; NHLBI, 2018).

Coronary Heart Disease

When the heart muscle is damaged by impaired circulation within the coronary arteries, there is a subsequent risk for heart failure. Specifically, myocardial damage to the left ventricle, the primary pumping chamber of the heart, will decrease the heart's ability to adequately pump the body's circulating blood volume. While the heart may compensate for this increased workload with a concomitant increased heart rate, this mechanism may not be adequate to maintain normal fluid volume balance (CDC, 2017; Hoffman & Sullivan, 2020). Arrhythmias, especially atrial fibrillation, may occur with coronary heart disease; these abnormal heart rhythms decrease the pumping effectiveness of the heart (AHA, 2017b; Hoffman & Sullivan, 2020; NHLBI, 2018).

Hypertension

Elevated blood pressure increases cardiac workload, as narrowed arteries that are less elastic decrease blood flow. Over time, the heart may enlarge, thickening and increasing in size, to meet increased demands. This resulting cardiomegaly decreases the heart's ability to pump effectively. Studies report a positive association between hypertension and insulin resistance (AHA, 2017). For patients with comorbidities, such as hypertension and diabetes, there is a 100% increase in risk for developing cardiovascular disease (AHA, 2017b; Hoffman & Sullivan, 2020).

Diabetes

The risk of developing cardiovascular disease increases for adults with type 1 or type 2 diabetes. According to the AHA (2017), at least 68% of people age 65 or older with diabetes die of some form of heart disease, including heart failure. Adults with diabetes are two to four times more likely to die of heart disease than adults without diabetes. Patients with diabetes often have abnormal lipid levels including high LDL cholesterol, low HDL cholesterol, and elevated triglycerides. This triad of abnormal lipids is correlated with coronary heart disease (Hoffman & Sullivan, 2020).

Lifestyle Factors

There are several modifiable lifestyle behaviors that increase the risk of developing heart failure. First, tobacco smoking contributes to the risk of cardiovascular disease, in addition to the risk for impaired lung function and decreased peripheral circulation. Smoking also decreases cardiac output, especially in patients with a history of myocardial infarction. Increased heart rate and systemic blood pressure with smoking result in higher levels of the following: pulmonary artery pressure, ventricular filling pressures, and total systemic and pulmonary vascular resistance (CDC, 2017; Hoffman & Sullivan, 2020). By causing vasoconstriction, smoking increases oxygen demand and also decreases myocardial oxygen supply with reduced diastolic filling time. The effects of smoking are especially pronounced in older patients who have comorbidities and changes due to normal aging (AHA, 2017b; Hoffman & Sullivan, 2020).

Alcohol, a myocardial depressant, should be restricted to moderate levels (one drink/day for women; two drinks/day for men). High alcohol intake increases the risk of arrhythmias (especially atrial fibrillation). Hypertension is also associated with alcohol intake and may cause impaired cardiac function and fluid retention. With diagnosed alcohol-induced cardiomyopathy, abstinence is necessary and can result in improved cardiac function (AHA, 2017b; NHLBI, 2018).

Obesity is another major risk factor for cardiovascular disease; a diet high in cholesterol and fat often leads to this condition. A diet high in sodium is also associated with the development and/or worsening of heart failure due to resultant fluid retention. Physical inactivity is another modifiable major risk factor for cardiovascular disease; the combination of exercising and losing weight can prevent or delay the onset of type 2 diabetes, reduce blood pressure, and help reduce the risk for heart disease (AHA, 2017b; Hoffman & Sullivan, 2020; NHLBI, 2018).

Age

Certain physiological changes that occur with normal aging predispose an elderly person to heart failure (Capriotti, 2020; Mohammadi, Khoshab, & Kazemnejad, 2016). Fibrous tissue and fat deposits in the heart's conduction system, especially the *sinoatrial* (SA) node, may result in a slightly slower heart rate. Heart failure may occur if the heart rate cannot increase to compensate for another normal change with aging, decreased cardiac output. A slight atrophy in heart size due to loss of muscle, especially the left ventricle, may occur with aging. The heart wall thickens with aging, so capacity decreases and pumping capability is also decreased despite the increased overall heart size (AHA, 2017b; Hoffman & Sullivan, 2020; NHLBI, 2018).

Myocardial contractility decreases with normal aging but is also affected by cardiovascular disease, especially myocardial infarction, and some medications such as chemotherapeutic agents (Dillon, 2017; Goolsby & Grubbs, 2015). Heart chamber filling time may increase, which decreases the ability to increase cardiac output in response to increased demand. Preload and afterload changes also may lead to heart failure; pump failure can result from increased preload as the heart muscle fails from overload. Elevated afterload, usually from hypertension or aortic stenosis, may also lead to heart failure as the heart cannot pump against the high resistance (Goolsby & Grubbs, 2015; Hoffman & Sullivan, 2020). Arrhythmias, often due to cardiovascular disease, are more common in older people; they also affect cardiac efficiency and output. Another normal change in the aging heart is lipofuscin deposits, which are lipid-containing pigment granules that are correlated with muscle cell degeneration. Heart valves thicken and stiffen with age, which affects blood flow and may result in audible murmurs (Dillon, 2017; Hoffman & Sullivan, 2020).

> **HIGH YIELD FACT FOR TESTING**
>
> Because heart failure can quickly progress, it's important to correctly classify its severity and maximize treatment.

> **CLINICAL PEARLS**
>
> If systolic heart failure has early diagnosis and treatment, diastolic heart failure may be prevented.

Assessment

There are assessment classes developed by the NYHA that correlate with assessment findings (see Table 20-2). The patient qualifies for one of the classes (I–IV) based on their subjective symptoms related to physical activity and also an associated class (A–D) based on objective findings and physical activity. For example, a patient with shortness of breath at rest but normal coronary arteries on an angiogram is classified: Functional Capacity IV, Objective Assessment A (AHA, 2017a). With this system, both the patient's experience in daily life (subjective) and physical/diagnostic findings (objective) are included in the assessment. As shown in the example, the categories are not necessarily aligned; the subjective patient experience is not always accurately reflected in or correlated to the objective findings.

TABLE 20–2 NYHA Heart Failure Class Assessment

Class	Objective Assessment
A	No observed evidence of heart failure. No symptoms and no limitation in ordinary physical activity.
B	Objective evidence of minimal cardiovascular disease. Mild symptoms and slight limitation during ordinary activity. Comfortable at rest.
C	Objective evidence of moderate cardiovascular disease. Marked limited physical activity due to symptoms, even during light activity. Comfortable only at rest.
D	Objective evidence of severe cardiovascular disease. Severe limitation. Symptomatic at rest.

(AHA, 2017a)

Obtaining an Accurate Daily Weight

1. Weigh at the same time every day, preferably in the morning after voiding and before ingesting food or liquids.
2. Have someone in attendance for weighing, to verify the measurement if there is visual impairment and also to provide support when getting on and off scales to prevent a fall. If the older patient lives alone, the risk of injury from a daily weighing may be greater than benefits; other measures of fluid balance can be used.
3. Wear the same clothing in terms of heaviness and/or layering when weighing.
4. Use the same scales for weighing. Keep the scale in a location where the temperature stays nearly constant and on a flat, hard, level surface (hardwood, concrete, or very hard linoleum).
5. Inform provider of any weight changes, especially an increase of more than 2 lb.

Signs and Symptoms of Left-Sided Failure

One of the most accurate assessments of heart failure is provided by measuring a daily weight. This measurement can be monitored by the patient at home and any changes reported to the provider so that changes in medications can be made (Almkuist, 2017; Dillon, 2017; Hoffman & Sullivan, 2020). In order for data obtained by the patient to be accurate and appropriate for making changes in treatment, the patient should follow the guidelines for daily weight measurement given in the accompanying box.

Because left-sided failure results in congestion in the lungs, the primary symptoms are respiratory, as well as fatigue due to insufficient circulating oxygenated blood. The respiratory signs are usually tachypnea and dyspnea. The patient often complains of dyspnea with exertion and a nonproductive cough. On auscultation, rales or crackles are heard initially in the lung bases. As the heart failure advances, the adventitious sounds spread throughout the lung fields and may progress to pulmonary edema. With insufficient oxygenation, cyanosis may occur peripherally (nailbeds in fingers and toes) and centrally (circumoral) as the disease advances (Dillon, 2017; Hoffman & Sullivan, 2020). When performing cardiac auscultation, the *point of maximal impulse* (PMI) may be laterally displaced from the fifth intracostal space midclavicular line (due to cardio-megaly). A gallop rhythm due to a third heart sound (S3) may occur due to increased blood flow or increased intra-cardiac pressure with heart failure. Heart murmurs may indicate valvular heart disease, which may either be a cause of (e.g., aortic stenosis) or result from (e.g., mitral regurgitation) heart failure. In older patients, confusion may be a sign of worsening heart failure, especially if there are electrolyte imbalances (particularly hyponatremia) as side effects of pharmacological management (Dillon, 2017; Goolsby & Grubbs, 2015; Hoffman & Sullivan, 2020).

Signs and Symptoms of Right-Sided Failure

The patient with right-sided heart failure will often have the respiratory signs of tachypnea and dyspnea because this condition often results from and follows left-sided heart failure. In addition to the respiratory signs, the patient may experience pitting peripheral edema, ascites, and liver enlargement because there is backup into the peripheral and hepatic circulation. Jugular venous pressure is often elevated and may be further accentuated by eliciting hepatojugular reflux (Dillon, 2017; Goolsby & Grubbs, 2015). If right ventricular pressure is increased, a parasternal heave may be observed, due to increased contraction strength. Right-sided failure leads to congestion in the systemic capillaries, which results in edema. Dependent areas are usually affected first; feet swell in people who are standing up, and sacral edema develops in people who are immobile. Nocturia may occur when excess peripheral fluid is reabsorbed into the circulation from being in a recumbent position. As right-sided heart failure progresses, ascites and liver enlargement may develop from congestion in the hepatic circulation. Impaired liver function and jaundice with coagulopathy also may occur (Hoffman & Sullivan, 2020; NHLBI, 2018).

Accurate assessment of peripheral edema may be achieved by using a scale. There are numerous types available, but the primary measurements of most scales combine the amount of indentation present and the time required for the induration to resolve. Indentation should be assessed over a bony prominence, preferably the tibia or medial malleolus. If there are disparate measures in indentation and duration to rebound, the more severe assessment finding is used to assign the level of edema. In other words, if the pitting is 6 mm but resolves quickly, the higher rating of 3+ is applied (see Table 20-3) (Dillon, 2017; Hoffman & Sullivan, 2020).

A scale developed by UNICEF (2018) is more easily applied and uses a 1 to 3 grading scale as follows:

1+ Mild swelling in hands and ankles/feet
2+ Swelling in feet, hands, lower arms, and lower legs
3+ Generalized bilateral pitting edema, in extremities and face

Nurses may find it helpful to share the UNICEF scale with patients to use as a home monitoring strategy, while the more specific scale is more appropriate for the nurse's assessment of edema in patients with heart failure.

Jugular venous distension (JVD) is a cardinal sign that right-sided heart failure is present. This finding alerts the nurse that there is progression of existing left-sided heart failure and potential for decreased respiratory effectiveness and for ensuing end

TABLE 20–3 Peripheral Edema Scale: Indention Depth and Rebound Time

Grade	Definition
+1	Barely detectable 2 mm indentation; immediate rebound
+2	4 mm indention; 10–15 sec to rebound
+3	6 mm indention; more than 60 sec to rebound
+4	8 mm indentation; 2–3 min to rebound

(Dillon, 2017)

organ damage. Therefore, accurate assessment of *jugular venous pressure* (JVP), and potentially JVD, may be essential to identifying underlying physiological changes that require changes in the plan of care. It is optimal to position the patient with the head of the bed elevated 30 to 45 degrees; the patent's position should be noted in the finding documentation. The highest level of jugular pulsation should be noted; if unable to see the pulsation, due to neck size and/or adipose tissue, then note the level of distention. Measurement is obtained by applying a flat edge (usually a ruler, but any flat edge) along the chest at the angle of Louis and then making a right angle with another flat edge to measure the pulsation/distension (see Figure 20-1). Normally, the JVP is visible at 3 cm along the jugular vein; if either is visible above this point, JVD is present.

Because heart failure has implications for all body systems, many diagnostic tests could be performed to assess the presence and/or impact of heart failure. The focus here is on the initial testing for purposes of diagnosing acute heart failure. According to the NHLBI (2018), the following tests are essential:

- *Brain-type natriuretic peptide* (BNP) level
- Complete blood count
- Creatinine
- Thyroid-stimulating hormone levels

BNP was initially identified in the brain but is released primarily from the heart, particularly the ventricles. BNP is increased in heart failure due to high ventricular filling pressures and is representative of myocardial function. *Atrial-type natriuretic peptide* (ANP) is also a measure of heart failure. Myocardial muscle stretching results in increased NP levels and suggests worsening heart failure. BNP assessment is deemed simple and reliable; serial BNP assessment at home is used to identify decompensation in high-risk patients (Harrison et al., 2016; Hoffman & Sullivan, 2020; NHLBI; 2018).

A complete blood count reveals low hemoglobin and hematocrit levels that indicate anemia. This results in a compensatory increase in cardiac output to compensate for lower oxygen carrying capacity. When the increased cardiac output is not enough to meet the body's needs, heart failure results (Hoffman & Sullivan, 2020).

Normal renal function maintains fluid volume balance and especially prevents hypervolemia. By diagnosing impaired renal function with elevated creatinine and *blood urea nitrogen* (BUN), a contributing factor to heart failure development can be addressed (Hoffman & Sullivan, 2020).

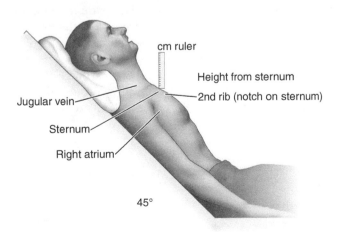

FIGURE 20–1 Measuring jugular venous pressure *(Capriotti, T. (2020). Pathophysiology: Introductory concepts and clinical perspectives (2nd ed.). Philadelphia, PA: F.A. Davis.)*

Thyroid abnormalities, specifically hypothyroidism, lead to heart failure by decreasing myocardial pumping, which eventually leads to weakening of the myocardium. Appropriate treatment of these conditions, specifically anemia and/or hypothyroidism, may result in significant improvement of HF, especially for older patients who are more sensitive to these alterations (AHA, 2017; Harrison et al., 2016).

Overall, indicators of poor outcomes of CHF include the following:

- Impaired renal function
- Cachexia
- Valve regurgitation
- Ventricular arrhythmias
- Higher NYHA heart failure class
- Decreased *left ventricular ejection fraction*
- High catecholamine and BNP levels
- Low serum sodium level
- Hypocholesterolemia
- Left ventricular dilation (Hoffman & Sullivan, 2020)

 ASSESSMENT PEARLS

When determining the type of heart failure, consider the patients' most prominent symptoms and particularly the site and extent of edema.

Nonpharmacological Management of Heart Failure

While heart failure often requires medical management, nonpharmacological measures may be effective adjuvants. Comprehensive home management programs, including education on these interventions along with medication regimens and regular primary care appointments, have been shown to improve patients' outcomes, decrease hospital readmissions, and increase patients' confidence in self-management (Liou et al., 2015; Mohammadi et al., 2016). If family members of older patients with heart failure are involved in the home management, then the patient is more likely to have higher quality of life along with decreased risk of re-hospitalization (Hasanpour-Dehkordi, Khaledi-Far, Khaledi-Far, & Salehi-Tali, 2016).

While the effectiveness of a sodium-restricted diet (1.5 to 2 g daily intake) remains part of the guidelines, it is not supported by current evidence. In patients with acute HF, there is little effect; in chronic HF, patients on a diet with normal sodium levels have better outcomes when they are on a high dose of a loop diuretic. When heart failure is identified in its early stage and is categorized as HFpEF, patients are instructed not to overeat, as this is often associated with increased blood flow to the intestines and away from the myocardium. A low-sodium diet is recommended for short-term management and preventing fluid retention, but has not been effective in preventing disease progression. Current recommendations are to limit sodium in the diet, but excessive dietary sodium restriction does not significantly promote better outcomes (AHA, 2017; Harrison et al., 2016; Hoffman & Sullivan, 2020).

Daily weight measurement is an accurate way to self-monitor fluid status and provides early identification of hypervolemia. When impaired renal function is a contributing factor in a patient's heart failure diagnosis, they may be placed on fluid restriction. A restriction of 2 liters/day is the guideline, but a more individualized fluid restriction is based on the patient's 24-hour urine output plus 500 mL for insensible losses. Although fluid restriction is an intervention mentioned by current guidelines for patients with HF, a recent meta-analysis of five studies suggests this therapy has no benefit, compared with liberal fluid intake, on the following: mortality, hospital admission, or thirst in patients with HF (Agnetti et al., 2015). Because fluid imbalances can occur quickly in older patients, especially dehydration, fluid restriction for management of HF should be medically supervised (Hoffman & Sullivan, 2020; NHLBI, 2018). Home blood pressure monitoring may also be an accurate reflection of fluid status but does not show changes as quickly as daily weights. Smoking cessation is vital to improved myocardial function, in addition to improving respiratory system effectiveness (AHA, 2017b).

Nonstrenuous and gradual aerobic exercise will improve both cardiac and respiratory system functioning. Patients should be directly supervised in their initial exercise efforts or have detailed instruction in what symptoms signal the need to stop activity and call for emergency assistance (chest pain, palpitations, shortness of breath) (AHA, 2017; Hoffman & Sullivan, 2020; NHLBI, 2018). While exercise may increase cardiac demand, at very moderate and controlled levels it has a beneficial effect for patients with HF. It's important that HF is well controlled by medication before any type of exercise is initiated. The patient also should not exercise in conditions that increase cardiac workload, such as cold weather. When approached with moderation and by following guidelines, exercise may result in improved cardiac, lung, and circulatory system functioning and decrease signs and symptoms of HF (AHA, 2017b; Hoffman & Sullivan, 2020).

As nurses focus specifically on older patients with HF, they should take into consideration certain factors related to aging that may affect patients' ability to exercise, including arthritis and resulting limited mobility, decreased vision and hearing, and risk for falls. Walking in a safe area, using an assistive device if necessary, is deemed the most efficacious exercise for older patients. Involving the spouse and/or other family members in the lifestyle changes, particularly exercise, provides support to the patient's continued participation (Hasanpopur-Dehkordi et al., 2016; Hoffman & Sullivan, 2020; Mohammedi et al., 2016).

Heart failure care coordination may help to prevent acute exacerbations of HF and, in particular, pulmonary edema, a life-threatening complication. Nurses may work as navigators to coordinate care among the primary care provider and specialist and to support the patient in self-monitoring their condition (Harmon, 2016; Liou et al., 2015; Mohammadi et al., 2016). It's important that partnerships are formed among the interprofessional team members and the patient and their family to promote better outcomes and improve the patient's ability to perform activities of daily living safely (Hoffman & Sullivan, 2020; Mohammadi et al., 2016).

If changes are identified early, they may be managed safely at home; supportive home monitoring of HF may include daily weights, blood pressure monitoring, serial BNP, and peripheral edema assessment (Almkuist, 2017). When family members are involved in monitoring the older patient's health status at home, the patient may experience increased quality of life along with the decreased risk and cost of hospital readmissions (Hasanpopur-Dehkordi et al., 2016; "Health and Wellbeing," 2013; Liou et al., 2015; Mohammadi et al., 2015). Monitoring compliance with medication regimen and follow-up health-care provider appointments can also be supported by an HF care coordinator.

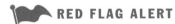
RED FLAG ALERT
Older patients can be empowered to effectively manage heart failure at home with the requisite care coordination, support, and resources.

CLINICAL **PEARLS**
With home self-monitoring, early signs and symptoms of HF can be identified and treated.

Pharmacology

Many of the medications that are used to treat HF are also used to treat other cardiovascular conditions, such as hypertension and *ST-elevation myocardial infarction* (STEMI). Information is focused on their use for HF in this chapter but references to information in other chapters are also noted. Patients with HF often have complicated medication regimens that require frequent changes based on their condition and/or response to their effectiveness (Mohammadi et al., 2015). Medications that follow the current guidelines and are appropriate for older patients with HF are presented, which are based on the NYHA heart failure classes. For classes I through III, an angiotensin-converting enzyme and a beta blocker in combination are generally recommended (Hoffman & Sullivan, 2020; Woo & Robinson, 2020). An example of a medication from each of the primary classifications that may be used to manage heart failure is presented in Table 20-4 at the end of this section, with Safe and Effective Nursing Care (SENC) that is focused on the older patient.

Angiotensin-Converting Enzyme (ACE) Inhibitors

Angiotensin-converting enzyme (ACE) inhibitors are first line medications in treating HF because they prevent weakening of the myocardium and thus may prolong life for patients. Specifically, ACE inhibitors treat HF caused by systolic dysfunction (e.g., dilated cardiomyopathy). ACE inhibitors prevent the formation of angiotensin II, which is a potent vasoconstrictor (Hoffman & Sullivan, 2020; Woo & Robinson, 2020). The benefits of medication with ACE inhibitors in heart failure are presented in the accompanying box.

ACE inhibitors have a relatively low incidence of side effects and are well tolerated in patients, especially in older patients. Approximately 10% of patients experience a dry, hacking cough as a side effect, which may be related to elevated bradykinin. Hypotension, a common side effect, is especially problematic in older people who are at increased risk of orthostatic hypotension and resulting fall (Hoffman & Sullivan, 2020; Woo & Robinson, 2020). Nurses must teach older patients to change positions slowly, especially when rising from bed during the night for toileting and/or in the morning. Angioedema, a life-threatening airway swelling and obstruction, occurs in 0.1% to 0.2% of patients and is two to four times more likely to occur in African Americans as compared to European Americans. Because hyperkalemia is a potential side effect, renal function should be assessed before initiating therapy with an ACE inhibitor and should be monitored frequently (usually every 3 months) in older patients who often have age-related decreased renal function (Hoffman & Sullivan, 2020; Woo & Robinson, 2020; Yancey et al., 2017).

Angiotensin II Receptor Blockers (ARBs, or Inhibitors)

By preventing angiotensin II from binding to angiotensin II receptors on the muscles surrounding blood vessels, *angiotensin II receptor blockers* (ARBs) result in decreased

---

Benefits of ACE Inhibitors for Older Patients With HF

- Reduced afterload, which enhances ventricular stroke volume and improves ejection fraction.
- Reduced preload, which decreases pulmonary and systemic congestion and edema.
- Reduced sympathetic activation, preventing increases in preload and afterload.
- Improved oxygen supply/demand ratio by decreasing afterload and preload.
- Prevents angiotensin II from triggering cardiac remodeling.

TABLE 20–4 Primary Medications for Treating Heart Failure

Class	Example	Action	Indication	Adverse Effects	SENC
ACE inhibitors	Captopril Dosage for HF is higher than for HTN: 6.25–12.5 mg tid up to 75 mg tid for elderly	Decreases blood pressure by blocking angiotensin-converting enzyme.	Used with diuretics to improve dyspnea and activity tolerance.	Hypotension, angioedema.	It must be taken tid and q 8h is preferable. Taste may be affected. Orthostatic hypotension and fall prevention.
Angiotensin-Receptor Neprilysin Inhibitors (ARNIs)	Sacubitril/valsartan 50–200 mg bid	Lowers blood pressure and promotes diuresis.	Decreases extracellular fluid and cardiac workload.	Angioedema, hypotension, impaired renal function.	This is a combination medication. Monitor blood pressure and urine output.
If(f) current inhibitors	Ivabradine 5 mg bid Increase dose to keep pulse <50–60 and maintain basal blood pressure.	Decreases conduction through SA node.	Decreases cardiac workload by slowing pulse. Doesn't affect myocardial contractility.	Bradycardia, dizziness, visual changes, and halos.	Teach patients to take pulse. Caution with driving especially at night.
Combined alpha-beta blockers	Carvedilol 3.25 mg bid; may increase to 5.5 mg bid based on weight.	Adrenergic alpha and non-selective beta blocker.	Decreases myocardial oxygen demand and workload.	Hypotension, syncope, bradycardia.	Take with food. When increasing dose, give larger dose at bedtime to decrease risk of orthostatic hypotension.
Aldosterone receptor antagonists	Spirolactone 25–100 mg/day	Promotes sodium and water excretion from distal tubule.	Diuresis without potassium loss.	Electrolyte imbalances.	Daily weights.
Cardiac glycoside	Digoxin 0.1–0.375 mg/day	Positive inotropic and negative chronotropic effects.	Increases myocardial contractility.	GI symptoms: nausea, vomiting, anorexia.	Assess for bradycardia and/or AV block that may progress.
Loop diuretics	Hydrochlorothiazide	Reduces sodium chloride (NaCl) and water re-absorption in the ascending g limb of the loop of Henle. Initial therapy for volume overload.	25–50 mg daily. One a.m. dose. Use lower dose with elderly (6.25–12.5 mg daily).	Hypokalemia, hyponatremia, headache, dizzy-ness, thirst, postural hypotension, and syncope.	Closely monitor blood pressure, urine output, and serum potassium levels. May be used in patient with impaired kidney function with careful monitoring of renal laboratory test results.

(Hoffman & Sullivan, 2020; NHLBI, 2018; Woo & Robinson, 2020)

afterload by dilating blood vessels and decreasing cardiac workload. With decreased afterload, the heart is able to pump against less resistance, which improves its effectiveness and decreases deleterious effects of HF. ARBs have also been shown to have a protective effect on renal function and to slow the progression of HF (Hoffman & Sullivan, 2020; Woo & Robinson, 2020). Common side effects of ARBs include cough (though not as common as with an ACE), hyperkalemia, hypotension (especially orthostatic in older patients), dizziness, headache, drowsiness, diarrhea, abnormal metallic taste sensation, rash, indigestion, and upper respiratory tract infection. An ARB may be preferred to an ACE in patients with diabetes and paired with a beta blocker for heart failure management (Hoffman & Sullivan, 2020; Woo & Robinson, 2020; Yancy et al., 2017).

Angiotensin-Receptor Neprilysin Inhibitors (ARNIs)

This new class of medication, the *angiotensin-receptor neprilysin inhibitors* (ARNIs), combines a neprilysin inhibitor and an ARB. These two medications exert a synergistic effect, thereby improving heart failure through several mechanisms (Hoffman & Sullivan, 2020; Woo & Robinson, 2020). The neprilysin inhibitors sacubitril/valsartan work by inhibiting sustained stimulation of neurohormonal systems. These systems often cause hypertension to progress to heart failure by inhibiting *neutral endopeptidase* (NEP) and suppressing the *renin-angiotensin-aldosterone system* (RAAS) via blockade of the *angiotensin II type 1* (AT1) receptors. The neprilysin inhibitor portion inhibits the enzyme neprilysin, thus increasing levels of vasoactive peptides, including natriuretic peptides, bradykinin, and adrenomedullin. Thus, sacubitril increases the levels of these peptides, causing blood vessel dilation and reduction of *extracellular fluid* (ECF) volume via sodium excretion (Hoffman & Sullivan, 2020; Woo & Robinson, 2020; Yancey et al., 2017).

These medications decrease blood pressure, especially the systolic, with decreased remodeling and improved prognosis. They reduce the risk of death from a cardiovascular event and hospitalization for heart failure in patients with chronic heart failure (NYHA classes II through IV); they also reduce ejection fraction. An ARNI is contraindicated for a patient who is on an ACE inhibitor or has been on one in the past 36 hours (Hoffman & Sullivan, 2020; Woo & Robinson, 2020). The major side effects are similar to those of an ACE inhibitor and/or ARB and include angioedema, hypotension, impaired renal function, and hyperkalemia (Cook et al., 2016; Yancey et al., 2017).

I$_{(f)}$ Current Inhibitor

Ivabradine (Corlanor) is the first in a new class of medications: I$_{(f)}$ current inhibitors used in the management of heart failure. This medication blocks the *hyperpolarization-activated cyclic nucleotide-gated* (HCN) channel, or $I_{(f)}$, in the SA node and inhibits the heart's primary pacemaker. Because calcium channel blockers decrease the strength of contraction (negative inotropic effect), they are contraindicated in heart failure. Ivabradine blocks inflow of sodium and potassium into the I$_{(f)}$ channels, thereby preventing depolarization and decreasing SA node activity. By decreasing the heart rate, there is more time for efficient filling of the chambers and flow to the myocardium itself. There is no concomitant decrease in cardiac contractility, as in beta blockers and calcium channel blockers (Hoffman & Sullivan, 2020; Woo & Robinson, 2020).

Based on these properties, this medication is especially effective in treating heart failure with reduced ejection fraction when used in combination with a beta blocker. Adding ivabradine to a beta blocker has been shown to result in decreased hospitalization for patients with NYHA classes II through IV HF (Cook et al., 2016). The side effects of this medication include bradycardia, headache, first degree atrioventricular block, dizziness, and blurred vision. A unique side effect experienced by over 10% of patients on ivabradine is known as luminous phenomena, in which there is enhanced brightness of images probably due to blockage of $I_{(f)}$ ion channels in the retina. This side effect is usually mild and resolves after a month of therapy. However, for the older patient who may have diminished visual acuity, it is important to warn them that they may have this sensation and to follow safety recommendations to prevent falls (Cook et al., 2016; Woo & Robinson, 2020; Yancy et al., 2017).

Beta Blockers (or Beta-Adrenergic Blocking Agents)

For patients with decreased left ventricular function, the inclusion of a beta blocker in the medication regimen has been shown to improve life expectancy. Beta blockers block the beta receptors on heart muscle, resulting in negative chronotropic and ino-tropic effects. Non-selective beta blockers, such as carvedilol, also block alpha recep-tors, which are found on blood vessels, and relax the blood vessels, dilating them, which lowers blood pressure and vascular resistance. While not a first line medication in the treatment of heart failure, a beta blocker is used in combination with diuret-ics and ACE inhibitors to reduce mortality and hospitalization (Hoffman & Sullivan, 2020; Woo & Robinson, 2020). The three beta blockers that are recommended for heart failure management are bisoprolol, carvedilol, and sustained-release metopro-lol (Woo & Robinson, 2020). In particular, carvedilol is indicated for patients in the NYHA classes II and III but is not part of the AHA guidelines (Woo & Robinson, 2020). It is proposed that beta blockers prevent cardiac remodeling and its complica-tions (Woo & Robinson, 2020; Yancy et al., 2017).

Aldosterone Receptor Antagonists

This class of medications blocks the effect of aldosterone, which is reabsorption of sodium and fluid from the collecting ducts in the kidneys' nephrons. By acting as a diuretic, it decreases blood pressure and edema, which reduces the cardiac work-load and mitigates heart failure. Aldosterone receptor antagonists are not a first line medication but are particularly effective in advanced heart failure and as an adjuvant to other medications (Hoffman & Sullivan, 2020; Woo & Robinson, 2020). This is another medication that has been shown to decrease mortality and hospitalization for patients with heart failure. Because aldosterone receptor antagonists are dependent on normal kidney function, the dose may need to be decreased for older patients who have age-related decreased renal function. Because patients with heart failure are often on a combination of medications that affect renal function, it is important to closely monitor serum BUN, creatinine, and potassium levels (Hoffman & Sullivan, 2020; Woo & Robinson, 2020).

Older medications in this class were often responsible for gynecomastia; however, this side effect does not occur with newer ones. Common side effects of this class of medications include frequent urination, dehydration, hyponatremia, hypotension, ataxia, drowsiness, dizziness, dry skin, and rashes. Older patients, who have the poten-tial for fluid imbalances should be monitored closely for dehydration, which can occur quickly. The potential for falls also increases if patients have problems with their gait due to ataxia and dizziness (Hoffman & Sullivan, 2020; Woo & Robinson, 2020). When skin dryness associated with aging is increased due to the medication, the patient may experience uncomfortable itching and increased risk for skin irritation and breakdown. It is usually 2 to 3 days before any diuretic effect from these medications occurs, and the maximal therapeutic effect may take 2 to 3 weeks, so they are not appropriate when immediate diuresis is the goal. Aldosterone receptor antagonists are potassium sparing because of their site of action in the kidney, which is mostly impenetrable to potassium (Woo & Robinson, 2020; Yancy et al., 2017).

Loop Diuretics

Loop diuretics are an important part of the pharmacological management of heart failure in older patients (see Chapter 1 for basic information about their action and side effects). While loop diuretics can promote safe and prompt fluid loss in treating heart failure in the older patient, there are also precautions that should be followed. Dry mouth, which may occur as a side effect, may impact older patients as they already have age-related decreased secretions and decreased taste. When older patients live alone, they are often tempted to skip meals, leading to poor nutrition, when foods do not have their usual appealing taste. Next, dehydration can occur very quickly in older patients, so doses of a loop diuretic may need to be decreased to prevent this complication. A related complication, which may be life threatening, is hyponatremia; this electrolyte imbalance may result in severe neurological (confusion, lethargy, seizures) and cardiac (arrhythmias) sequelae (Hoffman & Sullivan, 2020; Woo & Robinson, 2020).

Digoxin

This medication has been one of the mainstays of pharmacological treatment of heart failure, but is no longer the first choice because it may increase the risk of death. Use of digoxin may be indicated when the use of diuretics and ACE inhibitors has been maximized and heart failure continues to worsen. It is also indicated when a beta blocker is ineffective or the patients do not tolerate a beta blocker (Hoffman & Sullivan, 2020; Woo & Robinson, 2020). When atrial fibrillation is present, digoxin is often used to convert the heart rhythm and/or control the rate. Digoxin results in improved cardiac functioning during heart failure by its positive inotropic (increased myocardial contractility) and negative chronotropic (decreased heart rate that allows for more effective ventricular filling) effects. The combination of decreased heart rate and increased blood pressure leads to improved cardiac output (Hoffman & Sullivan, 2020; Woo & Robinson, 2020).

The most common side effects are fatigue, nausea and vomiting, anorexia, and bradycardia, which are quite vague and often attributed to other conditions and/or medications in older patients. For these patients, who often have decreased renal function, it is necessary to monitor serum digoxin levels in order to maintain a therapeutic level. A smaller dose of digoxin is often indicated in older patients. Taking a pulse before administering digoxin is a long-standing practice in acute care settings; however, older patients at home who are not able to palpate a pulse can use the pulse value from a digital blood pressure machine. The definition of bradycardia may be individualized, based on the older patient's baseline heart rate and their tolerance of a decreased heart rate while on digoxin. Note that digoxin toxicity can occur quickly in older patients due to dehydration and electrolyte imbalances, especially hypokalemia. The symptoms of digoxin toxicity are also vague, including fatigue, malaise, and visual disturbances. The cardiac manifestations are life-threatening arrhythmias, such as ventricular tachycardia/fibrillation, and SA and *atrioventricular* (AV) blocks (Hoffman & Sullivan, 2020; Woo & Robinson, 2020).

It is important to address pharmacological management of heart failure in older patients from the current guidelines, while also taking into account age-related changes that may be present and individualizing care. Medications should be adjusted to help the patient achieve and maintain their best possible quality of life, while taking the fewest medications in the lowest doses possible to decrease the potential for side effects. Few studies of HF have samples exclusively composed of older adults.

There is no consensus as to the over/underutilization of HF medications in older adults; nor is there consensus that intensive medication therapy is associated with additional benefits. Older patients are especially vulnerable to HF medications' hypotensive effects or cause nocturia, which may increase fall risk. Careful risk-benefit analysis should be conducted for all medication adjustments. With age-related decreased renal function, poor nutritional status, and greater risk for dehydration, older patients are at risk for both side and adverse effects.

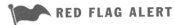

RED FLAG ALERT

Nurses should evaluate dosing of prescribed medications and assess if lower doses can be used in older patients to compensate for impaired renal function and decrease the potential for side effects.

Telehealth may be used to monitor medication effectiveness and side effects (AHA, 2017b; Hoffman & Sullivan, 2020; NHLBI, 2018; Woo & Robinson, 2020).

Complementary and Alternative Therapies (CAT)

Older patients with heart failure may benefit from complementary therapies, but there is limited evidence that these therapies are effective. While the older patient may not be familiar with some of these approaches, they often embrace them as they are a source of relaxation from the stress of managing a chronic illness. First, tai chi is a mind–body practice that includes postures and gentle movements combined with focused breathing and relaxation; movements can be performed while walking, standing, or sitting, so patients with arthritis and/or other musculoskeletal disorders can participate. Based on evidence, tai chi may promote quality of life and mood in older patients with heart failure by providing psychological benefits, such as reducing anxiety ("Health and Wellbeing," 2013).

While there are multiple supplements that are purported to improve heart disease, there are not many that are specifically targeted at heart failure. Hawthorn extract is recommended for heart, kidney, and digestive diseases in addition to decreasing anxiety. Because of its effects in multiple organ systems, it may improve the widespread complications that occur with heart failure. However, the side effects are similar to those of digoxin, including dizziness, nausea, and digestive symptoms. Hawthorn also has many potential interactions with prescribed medications (AHA, 2017b; "Health and Wellbeing," 2013). Another supplement, *coenzyme Q10* (CoQ10) may provide benefits for some patients with cardiovascular disorders, including heart failure but research is not conclusive. CoQ10, an antioxidant, is found in large amounts in the heart, and because its levels decrease with age, it is reasonable to infer that supplemental CoQ10 in older patients is helpful. Generally, CoQ10 has minimal side effects and is tolerated by older adults (AHA, 2017b; Woo & Robinson, 2020). It is important to ask patients if they are taking supplements, as these may have interactions with prescribed medications.

Summary

Heart failure is a complex illness that is difficult to manage, especially when it is diagnosed in older adults who have age-related system changes and comorbidities. As nurses perform focused assessments on older patients with heart failure, they are particularly attentive to the cardiovascular, respiratory, and peripheral circulatory systems. With education, support, and coordination of care, older patients are able to safely monitor and manage heart failure at home, maintaining quality of life and decreasing hospitalizations (Almkuist, 2017; Harmon, 2016; "Health and Wellbeing," 2013). While there are no accepted guidelines for a target blood pressure for patients with heart failure, it is generally accepted that lower blood pressures are preferred, especially systolic. However, in older patients, nurses must be alert to increased risk of falling due to orthostatic hypotension when blood pressures are maintained at such low levels (Hoffman & Sullivan, 2020; Woo & Robinson, 2020).

Key Points

• Older patients are at increased risk for heart failure due to normal aging along with comorbidities.

• Healthy lifestyle changes can greatly improve signs and symptoms of heart failure in older patients.

• Heart failure classification guides the pharmacological management.

• Older patients can successfully monitor and manage heart failure at home.

• Effective pharmacological management of heart failure often requires multiple medications, which increases the risk for side effects and interactions.

Review Questions

1. **The nurse assesses a patient with left-sided heart failure NYHA class III and expects to find which assessment findings? (Select all that apply.)**

   a. Fatigue
   b. Sleep disorders
   c. Orthopnea
   d. Hepatomegaly
   e. Jugular venous distension
   f. Tissue wasting

2. **The family asks you, the nurse, why so many medications are necessary to manage heart failure. The nurse's best response is:**

   a. "If the patient stops smoking, they probably could decrease the number of medications."
   b. "When an older person has a disease, they usually require more medication and in higher doses."
   c. "This is a complex disease that affects many body systems; lifestyle changes may decrease the need for some medications."
   d. "Taking medications regularly is the only intervention to prevent rehospitalization."

3. **The 85-year-old patient with heart failure asks what they can do so they don't feel so fatigued. What interventions may promote their abilities to perform activities of daily living? The nurse tells them to do which of the following? (Select all that apply.)**

   a. "Keep a log of your activity and when you are most tired during the day."
   b. "Schedule frequent rests during the day for recovery from activity."
   c. "Monitor daily weight and report any changes of over 1 lb in a day."
   d. "Include light aerobic activity in your day when you feel best."
   e. "Elevate your legs when you are sitting down to decrease swelling."

4. **When initiating pharmacological management of NYHA class II heart failure for a 77-year-old patient, the nurse anticipates what treatment plan?**

   a. A loop diuretic and an angiotensin converting enzyme inhibitor (ACE inhibitor)
   b. Digoxin and a beta blocker
   c. An ACE inhibitor and an angiotensin receptor blocker (ARB)
   d. An angiotensin receptor neprilysin inhibitor (ARNI) and beta blocker
   e. An aldosterone receptor antagonist and a loop diuretic

5. The patient with heart failure asks when to seek emergent care. The nurse provides education that includes which of the following signs and symptoms? (Select all that apply.)

a. Chest pain

b. Shortness of breath with activity

c. Abdominal swelling

d. Pitting edema

e. Dry, hacking cough

See the appendix for answers to review questions.

References

Agnetti, G., Piepoli, M. F., Siniscalchi, G., & Nicolini, F. (2015). New insights in the diagnosis and treatment of heart failure. *Biomed Research International, 30*, 151 116. doi:10.1155/2015/265260

Almkuist, K. D. (2017). Using teach-back method to prevent 30-day readmissions in patients with heart failure: A systematic review. *MEDSURG Nursing, 26*(5), 309–351.

American Heart Association. (2017a). Classes of heart failure. Retrieved from https://www.heart.org/en/health-topics/heart-failure/what-is-heart-failure/classes-of-heart-failure

American Heart Association. (2017b). Congestive heart failure. Retrieved from http://www.heart.org/HEARTORG/Conditions/HeartFailure/AboutHeartFailure/Classes-of-Heart-Failure_UCM_306328_Article.jsp#.WkWG2FWnGpo

Capriotti, T. (2020). *Pathophysiology: Introductory concepts and clinical perspectives* (2nd ed.). Philadelphia, PA: F.A. Davis.

Centers for Disease Control and Prevention. (2017). Heart failure fact sheet. Retrieved from https://www.cdc.gov/dhdsp/data_statistics/fact_sheets/fs_heart_failure.htm

Cook, J. C., Tran, R. H., Patterson, J. H., & Rodgers, J. E. (2016). Evolving therapies for the management of chronic and acute decompensated heart failure. *American Journal of Health-System Pharmacy, 73*(21), 1745–1754. doi:10.2146/ajhp150635

Dillon, P. (2017). *Nursing health assessment: A critical thinking, case studies approach* (2nd ed.). Philadelphia, PA: F.A. Davis.

Goolsby, M., & Grubbs, L. (2015). *Advanced assessment: Interpreting findings and formulating differential diagnoses*. Philadelphia, PA: F.A. Davis.

Harmon, D. (2016). Preparing for certification. The problem with heart failure. *MEDSURG Nursing, 25*(3), 192–193.

Harrison, G., Evans, M. M., Shaffer, A., & Romero, L. (2016). Treating a patient experiencing an acute exacerbation of chronic heart failure. *Med-Surg Matters, 25*(4), 8–10.

Hasanpour-Dehkordi, A., Khaledi-Far, A., Khaledi-Far, B., & Salehi-Tali, S. (2016). The effect of family training and support on the quality of life and cost of hospital readmissions in congestive heart failure patients in Iran. *Applied Nursing Research, 31*, 165–169. doi:10.1016/j.apnr.2016.03.005

Health and wellbeing for people living with heart failure. (2016). *Foundation of Nursing Studies: Improvement Insights, 11*(3), 1.

Hoffman, J., & Sullivan, N. (2020). *Medical-surgical nursing: Making connections to practice* (2nd ed.). Philadelphia, PA: F.A. Davis.

Liou, H., Chen, H., Hsu, S., Lee, S., Chang, C., & Wu, M. (2015). The effects of a self-care program on patients with heart failure. *Journal of the Chinese Medical Association, 78*, 648–656.

Mohammadi, E., Khoshab, H., & Kazemnejad, A. (2016). Activities of daily living for patients with chronic heart failure: A partnership care model evaluation. *Applied Nursing Research, 30*, 261–267. doi:10.1016/j.apnr.2015.01.008

National Heart, Lung, and Blood Institute. (2018). Heart failure. Retrieved from https://www.nhlbi.nih.gov/health-topics/heart-failure

UNICEF. (2018). Measuring edema. Retrieved from https://www.unicef.org/nutrition/training/3.1/20.html

World Health Organization. (2017). Cardiovascular diseases. Retrieved from http://www.who.int/mediacentre/factsheets/fs317/en/

Woo, T., & Robinson, M. (2020). *Pharmacotherapeutics for the advanced practice nurse prescribers* (5th ed.). Philadelphia, PA: F.A. Davis.

Yancy, C., Jessup, M., Bozkurt, B., Butler, J, Casey, D. E. Jr., Colvin, M. M., . . . Westlake, C. (2017). 2017 ACC/AHA/HFSA focused update of the 2013 ACCF/AHA Guideline for the Management of Heart Failure: A report of the American College of Cardiology/American Heart Association Task Force on Clinical Practice Guidelines and the Heart Failure Society of America. *Circulation 136*(6), e137–e161.

Chapter 21

Pneumonia

LEARNING OBJECTIVES

Upon completion of this chapter the student will be able to:

- Integrate knowledge of the physiology, pathophysiology, assessment, and pharmacological management for care of a geriatric patient with pneumonia.
- Appraise current standards of care for older adult patients with pneumonia.

Introduction

Each year between 2 and 5 million people are diagnosed with pneumonia, an accumulation of fluid in the lungs that results from an inflammatory or infectious process. Pneumonia is differentiated based on the location where the individual acquired the infection (Blair, 2018):

- *Community-acquired, CAP* (living in the community outside of a hospital or a long-term care facility)
- *Health-care-associated, HCAP* (less than 48 hours after hospital admission or while living in an assisted or long-term care facility)
- *Hospital-acquired, HAP* (more than 48 hours after hospital admission)
- *Ventilator-assisted, VAP* (within 48 to 72 hours after being intubated)

Community-acquired pneumonia (CAP) and *health-care-associated pneumonia* (HCAP) are more common in older adults and increase mortality in this population (Blair, 2018); 157,500 cases of HCAP were reported in 2011 (Centers for Disease Control and Prevention [CDC], 2018). CAP statistics are difficult to capture but an estimated 900,000 or more older adults contract CAP each year (Lawrence & Karakashian, 2018), and incidence rates increase with age, with approximately 18.2:1000 individuals in the 65-to-69-year age range as compared to 52.3:1000 individuals over 85 years contracting CAP each year (Blair, 2018). Advanced age is associated with the severity of CAP, the need for hospital care, and increased mortality from the disease (Blair, 2018; Jain et al., 2015).

In 2015, approximately 1.3 million older adults (65 and older) were diagnosed with CAP, with around 40% of these individuals requiring an average hospital stay of 5.6 days to treat their pneumonia (Brown, Harnett, Chambers, & Sato, 2018). Almost 52,000 deaths each year are related to a pneumonia diagnosis, and despite the availability of pneumococcal vaccines, only 66.9% of all older adults have ever received the vaccine (CDC, 2017). Finally, estimated total costs of treating CAP among Medicare patients reaches nearly $13 billion annually (Brown et al., 2018). Despite the availability of vaccines that reduce the risk for developing CAP, the disease remains costly in terms of economic burden and mortality. This chapter reviews the effects of aging on lung physiology, pathophysiology related to older adult respiratory assessment, and pneumonia. Risk factors and treatment options for community-acquired, health-care-associated pneumonias, hospital-acquired, ventilator-assisted, and aspiration pneumonia are discussed.

Physiology

Responsible for gas exchange, the respiratory system is composed of the upper and lower airways, the blood vessels that innervate them, and the supporting structures of the thoracic cage (Brashers, 2012b), as shown in Figure 21-1. Protection of the airway begins with the nasal hairs and turbinates, which filter and trap foreign particles (Brashers, 2012b; Capriotti, 2020). As air moves from the nose through the airway, the larynx with the glottis and epiglottis serve as the next line of defense for the respiratory system. The epiglottis opens during inspiration and closes over the glottis during swallowing to prevent aspiration of liquids and food into the trachea (Franco, 2017). As one ages, laryngeal muscles atrophy and lose some of their elasticity as airways lose cartilage, increasing the risk for aspiration. The voice also becomes softer, increasing difficulty in hearing and understanding the older adult's words (Rees, 2018).

Mucus and cilia continue the filtering process as air moves downward toward the lungs. The upper airway (nose, mouth, throat) has a normal flora of bacteria, while the lower airway's mucociliary system, when functioning properly, maintains a bacteria-free environment in the bronchial tree and lungs by transferring filtered, humidified, and warmed air to the lungs (Brashers, 2012b; Capriotti, 2020). Aging changes the effectiveness of the protective function of cilia and alveolar macrophages, placing the older adult at risk for infection (Rees, 2018).

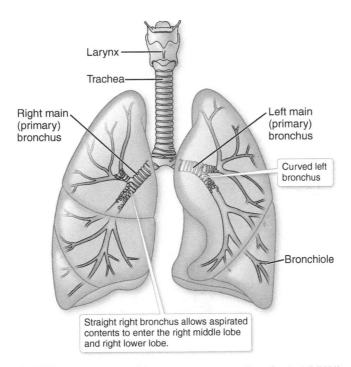

FIGURE 21–1 Anatomy of the respiratory system *(From Capriotti, T. (2020). Pathophysiology: Introductory concepts and clinical perspectives. 2nd ed. Philadelphia, PA: F.A. Davis Company.)*

Anatomically, the lower respiratory tract consists of the trachea, bronchi, bronchioles, and alveolar ducts. Of particular importance to lung function are the lungs themselves, shown in Figure 21-2. The left lung is composed of two lobes, while the right lung has three lobes and performs approximately 60% to 65% of the lungs' work (Rees, 2018). The right mainstem bronchi is shorter and straighter than the left and is more prone to aspiration, penetration by foreign objects, or accidental intubation (Capriotti, 2020; Rees, 2018). The bronchioles branch from the mainstem bronchi, become smaller as they advance deep into the lung tissue, and are dependent on the lung's elastic recoil to remain open. The alveolar ducts and sacs are found at the terminal ends of the bronchioles and are the location of gas exchange. Their ability to remain open and available for gas exchange is dependent on the presence of surfactant (Rees, 2018). Epithelial cells in the alveoli secrete surfactant, which lowers surface tension during expiration and prevents the lungs from collapsing. The alveoli also contain macrophages that help protect the lungs by ingesting any foreign matter that may reach the lower lungs (Brashers, 2012b). As one ages, there is a decrease in alveolar surface accompanied by dilation of the alveolar ducts and bronchioles that place the older adult at increased risk for development of atelectasis and infection (Rees, 2018).

There is a distinct difference in *ventilation*, the process by which air is mechanically moved in and out of the lungs, and *respiration*, the cellular process of oxygen and carbon dioxide exchange (Brashers, 2012b). Oxygen from the air is transported across membranes of the alveoli and enters the *red blood cells* (RBCs), where the oxygen attaches to heme and forms oxyhemoglobin. Simultaneously, carbon dioxide (created as a by-product of cell metabolism) moves out of the RBCs and is removed from the lungs through exhalation (Capriotti, 2020).

Normally the process of ventilation and *perfusion* (the transfer and movement of oxygen and carbon dioxide in the blood) creates an equilibrium. However, when there is a discrepancy in the amount of oxygen and blood reaching the alveoli, the pulmonary arteries compensate by vasoconstricting to redistribute blood flow from well-ventilated areas to less-ventilated areas of the lung (Capriotti, 2020). However, the ventilation perfusion rates are not equal in all areas of the lungs. In fact, in the lung bases perfusion surpasses ventilation, while in the apices ventilation surpasses

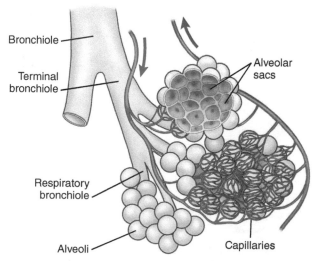

FIGURE 21–2 Close-up of the lung *(From Hoffman, J. J., & Sullivan, N. J. (2020). Medical-surgical nursing: Making connections to practice (2nd ed.). Philadelphia, PA: F.A. Davis.)*

perfusion (Brashers, 2012b). As one ages, there is an increase in vascular resistance in the pulmonary vasculature with a concurrent decrease in the volume of capillary blood flow, and less heme to transfer oxygen for cellular metabolism. This leads to hypoxia, and explains why the first signs of respiratory disease, particularly infection, include confusion (Rees, 2018).

Effective inspiration depends on lung and chest wall elasticity, major muscles (diaphragm and intercostal), accessory muscles (sternocleidomastoid, scalene), and normal airway resistance. Expiration is normally a passive process, not requiring muscle effort (Brashers, 2012b). As one ages, the diaphragm and intercostal muscles lose their strength, and respiratory effort increases. A combination of changes in the chest wall further increase respiratory effort as chest wall elasticity decreases, kyphosis progresses, and the *anteroposterior* (AP) diameter ratio changes, creating a more barrel chest appearance in the older adult (Rees, 2018).

Pathophysiology

Lower respiratory tract infections are the result of an impairment of the body's natural defense mechanisms, including impaired immunity and the inability to clear foreign materials from the respiratory tract (Brashers, 2012a). Macrophages found in the alveolar spaces protect against infection from pathogens that reach the lower lungs. Pneumonia develops when an infectious organism or inhaled irritant enters the respiratory system and migrates to the alveoli. The alveolar macrophages activate the inflammatory response by releasing interleukin-1 and tumor necrosis factor alpha, B cells, and T cells, initiating the inflammatory response to the pathogen (Brashers, 2012a). Neutrophils are drawn to the inflamed area, and the accumulation of neutrophils triggers capillary leakage of red blood cells, edema, and the accumulation of exudate in the alveoli (Blair, 2018; Capriotti, 2020; Franco, 2017). Compounding the situation, alveolar goblet cells become overstimulated and produce excessive mucus, which, along with exudate, makes normal alveolar opening and closing difficult, creating the *crackles* sounds commonly heard in pneumonia (Capriotti, 2020).

In this first stage of pneumonia, congestion occurs as alveolar walls thicken and diffusion of oxygen and carbon dioxide in the alveoli is compromised, leading to hypoxemias. In the second stage of pneumonia, a solid mass forms as fibrin, neutrophils, and red blood cells consolidate (Franco, 2017). Dyspnea results, vital capacity is diminished, and *atelectasis* occurs, as damaged alveoli collapse and gas exchange is further impaired (Blair, 2018; Brashers, 2012a). Capillary leakage and formation of fibrin allow the infection to spread into other areas of the lungs and, if left untreated, into the bloodstream (*septicemia*) and/or the pleural cavity (*empyema*) (Blair, 2018).

Described based on location and causative pathogen, pneumonia may be confined to one area (*lobar*) of a lung or diffusely spread throughout the lungs (*bronchial*). Causative pathogens (*bacterial* or *viral*) vary based on whether the pneumonia is CAP, HCAP, HAP, or VAP, and may be difficult to identify, particularly in CAP, where about 20% to 30% of the causes are unknown (Franco, 2017). Additionally, aspiration pneumonia is common among those who are comatose, who have difficulty swallowing (*dysphagia*), who have gastric reflux, or who are impaired from drug or alcohol intoxication (Capriotti, 2020). Table 21-1 highlights the common pathogens of pneumonia.

Viral infections increase risk of developing a secondary bacterial pneumonia by altering the lungs' immune response (Hoffman & Sullivan, 2020). During the recent 2019 novel coronavirus (COVID-19) pandemic, many individuals, particularly those with existing comorbidities, developed severe viral pneumonia symptoms. In response to a virus, the body produces cytokines (inflammatory mediators) to prevent replication and kill the virus. In COVID-19, the lungs' immune response overreacts to the

TABLE 21-1 Common Pathogens in Pneumonia

Community-Acquired	Health-Care-Associated	Hospital-Acquired	Immunocompromised
Most common: *Streptococcus pneumoniae* *Haemophilus influenzae* Other: *Chlamydia pneumoniae* *Mycoplasma* *Legionella* *Staphylococcus aureus*	Methicillin-resistant *Staphylococcus aureus* (MRSA) *Pseudomonas*	MRSA Vancomycin-resistant *Enterococcus* (VRE) *Acinetobacter* *Klebsiella* *Pseudomonas*	*Pneumocystis* pneumonia (PCP)

(Brashers, 2012a; Capriotti, 2020; Franco, 2017)

virus, cytokines overproduce, and large amounts of inflammatory exudate are deposited in the alveoli. As the pneumonia progresses, *acute respiratory distress syndrome* (ARDS) develops, which may lead to respiratory failure and death (Casey, 2020).

 CLINICAL PEARLS

Influenza and other respiratory viruses can also lead to pneumonia, especially in the older adult and other individuals whose immune systems may be compromised.

Assessment

Assessment of the respiratory system begins with a thorough health history. Because cough and dyspnea can be attributed to a wide variety of respiratory conditions, careful questioning regarding the onset, duration, quality of symptoms, and anything that contributes to the symptoms must be considered. The patient's family and medical history as well as their habits, including exposure to first- or secondhand smoke, respiratory toxins, or inhaled allergens, are helpful in making the diagnosis (Goolsby & Jones, 2019). At increased risk of developing pneumonia are individuals who are over age 65; have a history of allergies, asthma, *chronic obstructive pulmonary disease* (COPD), or other chronic respiratory conditions; and who smoke, are immunocompromised, or who have been diagnosed with recent influenza (Capriotti, 2020; Franco, 2017). Risk factors for community-acquired and hospital-acquired pneumonia are highlighted in Table 21-2.

As with other systems (except for the *gastrointestinal* [GI] tract), physical assessment begins with inspection of the chest, including the rate and rhythm of respirations, the amount of effort, and depth of inspirations. Next, any deformities should be palpated, followed by posterior percussion of the lung fields. In pneumonia, a dull tone is heard when percussing the consolidated area. Finally, with the patient breathing through their mouth, a complete respiratory cycle should be auscultated over the bronchial and peripheral lung fields. Timing and quality of any abnormal (*adventitious*) sounds during the respiratory cycle should be noted (Goolsby & Jones, 2018).

Symptoms of pneumonia vary with the individual, but include cough, dyspnea, chest discomfort, fever with shaking chills, hypoxemia, and malaise (Blair, 2018; Franco, 2017; Goolsby & Jones, 2019). Sputum from a productive cough may be blood

TABLE 21–2   Risk Factors for Pneumonia in Older Adults

Community-Acquired	Health-Care-Associated/Hospital-Acquired
Alcoholism	Administration of alkaline pH tube feedings
Aspiration (recent)	Altered level of consciousness
Chronic obstructive pulmonary disease (COPD)	Aspiration (recent)
Exposure to environmental irritants	Chronic respiratory disease
Immunocompromised due to chronic illness	Gram-negative bacteria colonization in mouth, nose, or stomach
Recent exposure to influenza or respiratory virus	Immunocompromised
Smoke (smoker or secondhand)	Mechanical ventilation
Has not been vaccinated for.	Poor nutritional status
Pneumococcal pneumonia (within the past 5 years)	Use of histamine blockers or antacids
Influenza (the current year)	

(Blair, 2018; Brown et al., 2018; Kaysin & Viera, 2016)

tinged, purulent, or rust colored. Auscultation may reveal diminished breath sounds, crackles related to fluid accumulation, or wheezing as airways become narrow. Finally, in pneumonia, *tactile fremitus* (vibrating sound made when the patient speaks either "1, 2, 3" or "99") is increased (*bronchophony*) over consolidated areas, and consolidation is also confirmed when the patient is actually repeating "E-E-E." The sound is nasal and is heard as "A-A-A" (*egophony*) (Blair, 2018; Goolsby & Jones, 2018). In older adults, impaired oxygenation may present as changes in mental status (confusion), and older adults (as well as some younger adults) may be afebrile or have a subnormal temperature (Capriotti, 2020; Franco, 2017).

Diagnostic studies useful in diagnosing pneumonia include a *complete blood count* (CBC) and collection of a sputum for culture and sensitivity, and a Gram stain to differentiate between bacterial and viral pathogens (Brashers, 2012a; Capriotti, 2020; Goolsby & Jones, 2019). Arterial blood gases (for critically ill patients) and pulse oximetry assess oxygenation. The chest x-ray is a key component of early pneumonia diagnosis. Chest x-rays show a dense, white area of consolidation, but this density may not appear on x-ray until about 12 to 48 hours after the first symptoms of pneumonia, and typically clears on x-ray earlier in viral than in bacterial pneumonias (Blair, 2018; Franco, 2017). *Computer tomography* (CT) is another standard radiological test used to diagnose pneumonia and is useful in visualizing any abnormalities too small to see on regular x-ray (Franco, 2017).

There are a couple of tools that help determine whether the patient with community-acquired pneumonia requires hospitalization for treatment of their disease. The *Pneumonia Severity Index* (PSI) uses age, sex, comorbidities, residence (assisted or long-term care), physical examination, laboratory findings, and findings from radiological studies to assign points that assess mortality risks (Franco, 2017; Kaysin & Viera, 2016). PSI scores range as follows (Capriotti, 2020):

0–90   Low risk
91–130   Moderate risk
>130   High mortality risk (requires hospitalization for treatment)

The *CURB-65* tool awards one point for each of the following:

New onset of **C**onfusion
Elevated B**U**N (blood urea nitrogen) (>20 mg/dL)

Rapid **R**espiratory rate (≥30/min)
Low **B**lood pressure (<90 mm Hg systolic or ≤60 mm Hg diastolic)
Age ≥**65** years.

A score ≥3 indicates that hospitalization is needed to provide appropriate treatment, while a lower score (0–1) indicates that home management of pneumonia symptoms is safe (Goolsby & Jones, 2019; Kaysin & Viera, 2016).

 ASSESSMENT PEARLS

While the process of inhalation and exhalation makes one respiratory cycle, observing respiratory effect, patterns, and rates is not adequate to determine the effectiveness of ventilation, which can only be measured by $Paco_2$ levels of the arterial blood gas (Brashers, 2012b).

Pharmacology

While pharmacological treatment of pneumonia is ideally focused on treating a particular organism, identification is often delayed until culture reports are finalized, and for approximately 30% to 40% of patients with CAP, the causative organism is not identified (Franco, 2017; Kaysin & Viera, 2016). Therefore, empirical treatment with antibiotics is initiated at the time of diagnosis and will vary based on whether the infection was acquired while in a community or health-care setting (Blair, 2018; Kaysin & Viera, 2016). Choice of anti-infective is also based on the hospital-specific antibiogram (Kalil et al., 2016). Any ordered culture/sensitivity specimens should be obtained *prior* to the first dose of antibiotic (Vallerand & Sanoski, 2021).

Identification of the causative bacteria and use of sensitivity tests to confirm the most effective antibiotic to treat the infection are key to the treatment plan, with a goal of reducing the bacterial load so that the body's immune system can respond to eliminate the infection. Other important considerations include limiting antibiotic use to the recommended course of therapy and avoiding use of antibiotics to treat viral infections, which, along with not finishing the course of treatment, have contributed to the rising numbers of resistant organisms. Finally, some classes of antibiotics may be contraindicated in individuals who are debilitated, have severe GI conditions, or who are immunocompromised (Karch & Tucker, 2020). Figure 21-3 provides an algorithm for pharmacological treatment of community-acquired pneumonia in adults.

Duration of anti-infective treatment varies based on the severity of the pneumonia and ranges from 5 to 7 days to as long as 21 days (Blair, 2018). Current treatment guidelines for patients admitted to the hospital with pneumonia indicate that anti-infective therapy should start within 4 to 8 hours of arrival at the hospital (Kaysin & Viera, 2016). For patients with CAP, the first line of anti-infective therapy is the macrolides. Antibiotics commonly prescribed to treat pneumonia are highlighted in Table 21-3.

RED FLAG ALERT

It is important to note that many antibiotics interact with other drugs and may be IV incompatible with other drugs, so a careful drug history is important (Jordan, Turner, & Woo, 2016).

The use of methylprednisolone as an adjunct to anti-infective therapy has been shown to decrease *intensive care unit* (ICU) and hospital length of stay and the risk for development of ARDS for patients with aspiration pneumonia (Kaysin & Viera, 2016). Based on symptoms, administration of oxygen, antipyretics, and bronchodilators may also be indicated. Guaifenesin, or another expectorant, may also be indicated (Blair, 2018; Capriotti, 2020).

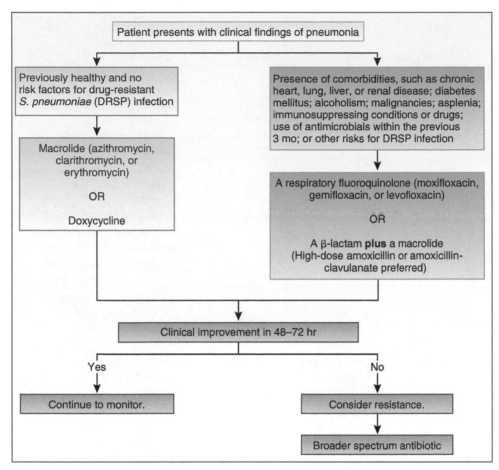

FIGURE 21–3 Treatment algorithm: outpatient treatment of adults with community-acquired pneumonia
(From Woo, T. (2020). Pharmacotherapeutics for advanced practice nurse prescribers *(5th ed.). Philadelphia, PA: F.A. Davis.)*

Complementary and Alternative Therapies and Prevention

Providing sufficient oxygenation is one of the first interventions used to treat pneumonia and can be implemented in the hospital or outpatient setting. Oxygen may be delivered via mask or nasal cannula, and effectiveness is measured by improvement in oxygen saturation levels and decrease in dyspnea. Incentive spirometry is another method of improving oxygenation by helping alveoli expand and improve oxygenation. As with oxygen therapy, incentive spirometry can be initiated in either the hospital or outpatient setting. In either setting, patients need to be taught how to use the incentive spirometer and encouraged to use it hourly when awake. Encouraging fluid intake of up to 2 liters a day (if appropriate for any comorbid conditions) helps thin secretions and prevents dehydration associated with fever and malaise (Blair, 2018).

Prevention of pneumonia is an important part of patient education, and all adults should be encouraged to get an annual influenza vaccination (many cases of pneumonia are the direct result of influenza). Prevention with pneumococcal vaccine is encouraged for all older adults (≥65 years). The pneumococcal conjugate (Prevnar 13® or PVC13) or vaccine and the pneumococcal polysaccharide (Pneumovax 23® or PPSV23) vaccines are both currently available. Timing of vaccine administration

TABLE 21–3 Antibiotics Commonly Used to Treat Pneumonia

Class	Example	Action	Dosage	SENC
Aminoglycosides	Amikacin Gentamicin	Inhibits protein synthesis.	5 mg/kg q 8 hr Or 7.5 mg/kg q 12 hr 1–2 mg/kg q 8 hr 　Max: 6 mg/kg/day in 3 doses	Used for gram-negative infection; *Klebsiella pneumoniae.* Adverse reactions: ataxia, ototoxicity; nephrotoxicity.
Aminopenicillin/beta-lactamase inhibitors	Ampicillin/sulbactam (Unasyn)	Cell death by binding to bacterial cell wall.	1–2 g IV q 6–8 hr max dose: 12 g/day	Caution with renal impairment; hepatotoxic; diarrhea.
Anti-pseudomonal penicillins (extended spectrum)	Piperacillin-tazobactam	Cell death by binding to bacterial cell wall.	4.5 g IV q 6 hr	Stevens-Johnson syndrome; *Clostridium difficile*–associated diarrhea (CDAD). 　Caution with renal impairment or sodium restrictions.
Carbapenems	Imipenem	Cell death by binding to bacterial cell wall.	500 mg IV q 6 hr	CDAD; Caution with renal impairment; infuse slowly; rapid infusion causes nausea / vomiting.
Cephalosporins	Ceftazidime	Cell death by binding to bacterial cell wall.	2 g IV q 8hr	Caution with renal impairment; CDAD; Stevens-Johnson syndrome.
Fluoroquinolones	Ciprofloxacin Levofloxacin	Inhibit DNA synthesis by inhibiting the DNA enzyme gyrase.	400 mg IV q 8 hr 750 mg IV q 24 hr	Caution with CNS disease (may increase ICP), renal impairment; Stevens-Johnson syndrome; warning for tendon rupture. particularly in older patients and those on concurrent steroids.
Glycopeptides	Vancomycin	Cell death by binding to bacterial cell wall.	15 mg/kg IV q 8–12 hr	Ototoxicity; nephrotoxicity; local phlebitis; "red man" syndrome when given rapidly.
Macrolides	Azithromycin	Inhibit protein synthesis.	IV 500 mg IV q 24 hr × 2 days or PO: 　500 mg PO day 1; then 250 mg/day for 4 days.	Stevens-Johnson syndrome; increases liver function tests, prothrombin time, blood glucose, BSN, and serum creatinine.
Oxazolidinones	Linezolid (Zyvox)	Inhibits protein synthesis.	600 mg IV or PO q 12 hr × 10–14 days	CDAD; serotonin syndrome if on serotonergic meds; oral can be given with or without food.
Tetracyclines	Doxycycline	Inhibits protein synthesis.	PO: 100 mg q 12 hr day 1; 100–200 mg daily or 50–100 mg q 12 hr	Dizziness; CDAD; hepatotoxicity; Stevens-Johnson syndrome; used when patient is allergic to penicillin.

(Jordan, Turner & Woo, 2016; Kalil et al., 2016; Kaysin & Viera, 2016; Vallerand & Sanoski, 2021)

SENC BOX 21–1   Safe and Effective Nursing Care for Drug Administration Education for Patients With Pneumonia

- Instruct patient on time of day to take medication.
- Inform patient of possible drug/food interactions.
- Advise patient whether to take with or without food.
- Caution patient about possible adverse reactions and common side effects.

should be determined by the patient and provider through shared decision making, with one dose of PCV13 recommended for those 19 and older who are at higher risk due to medical conditions and for those over 65 who have not already had the vaccine. All persons over age 65 should receive the PPSV23 vaccine even if they have already received the PCV13 vaccine. Additional doses of vaccine can be administered according to a timing of vaccine algorithm (CDC, 2020). Persons at high risk for pneumonia should be taught additional prevention strategies, including careful hand washing, monitoring of high-risk patients for aspiration, and avoiding crowds and those with known upper respiratory infections, particularly during peak infectious seasons. Prevention of HAP and VAP, with their high mortality rates, requires strict adherence to hospital-based protocols (Blair, 2018).

Once pneumonia is diagnosed, patient education needs to take a different approach, as shown in SENC Box 21-1.

Cautioning the patient on the importance of taking the full course of a prescribed antibiotic is another essential component of patient education (Jordan, Turner, & Woo, 2016; Lawrence & Karakashian, 2018). Patients should be encouraged to increase fluid intake, stop smoking, get extra rest, and call their provider if symptoms get worse or do not improve within 48 to 72 hours after starting their antibiotics (Lawrence & Karakashian; Richardson, 2020).

Summary

Pneumonia directly impacts quality of life and health-care costs and has a high rate of morbidity and mortality, particularly in older patients or in those with dysphagia, an impaired immune system, or chronic diseases (Lawrence & Karakashian, 2018). Preventive strategies start with annual influenza immunization and pneumococcal pneumonia vaccination and the use of protocols to reduce the incidence of HAP and VAP. Treatment with antibiotics and other supportive therapies is based on the type of pneumonia acquired and the prevailing effective antibiotics of the region. Understanding the changes in the aging respiratory system and how these increase pneumonia risks, along with key preventive strategies and accurate assessment and early diagnosis, is key to reducing the death rates from this common respiratory disease.

Key Points

- Pneumonia care is dependent on the location where the infection was acquired (community-acquired, health-care-associated, hospital-acquired, ventilator-assisted, or aspiration).
- The upper airway structures are the first lines of defense against lower respiratory infections. With the normal changes of aging, this defense system becomes less effective.

- Alveolar function in pneumonia is impaired due to accumulation of excessive goblet cell mucus, exudate, and edema that results from the inflammatory response to foreign materials in the lungs.
- Antibiotics are prescribed based on empirical treatments for the particular pneumonia and hospital-specific antibiograms.

Review Questions

1. **The nurse is assessing breath sounds of the older patient with newly diagnosed community-acquired pneumonia and hears wheezes. The nurse understands that the patient is experiencing which of the following?**

   a. Bronchophony
   b. Fluid accumulation in the main bronchi

   c. Hypoxemia
   d. Narrowed airways

2. **When conducting a physical assessment of the respiratory system, which of the following is correct?**

   a. Auscultating breath sounds prior to percussion ensures an accurate assessment.
   b. Auscultate breath sounds while asking the patient to breathe through their open mouth.
   c. Percussion of the chest is the last component of the respiratory assessment.
   d. In pneumonia, percussion over the area of infection yields a sharp tone.

3. **To assess for consolidation of the lungs, the nurse should expect consolidation, if which of the following is true?**

   a. A productive cough is followed by wheezing upon auscultation.
   b. Consolidation cannot be heard during auscultation.
   c. The sounds "E-E-E" are heard as a nasal-sounding "A-A-A."
   d. While listening with the stethoscope as the patient states "E-E-E," the sound is muffled.

4. **When assessing the severity of a patient's newly diagnosed community-acquired pneumonia, which of the following criteria are used in the Pneumonia Severity Index? (Select all that apply.)**

   a. Age
   b. Comorbidities

   c. New-onset confusion
   d. Residence

5. **When educating the patient with newly diagnosed pneumonia, the nurse suggests that the patient increase fluid intake. Which of the following statements lets the nurse know that the patient understands instructions?**

   a. "Careful hand washing will be more effective than fluids to help me recover from pneumonia."
   b. "Increasing fluids will help me get rid of any infection."
   c. "It is not necessary to drink more than one large glass of water a day to help with secretions."
   d. "To help my expectorate work better, I should drink at least 2 liters of water a day."

See the appendix for answers to review questions.

References

Blair, M. (2018). Care of patients with infectious respiratory problems. In D. D. Ignatavicius, L. Workman, & C. R. Rebar (Eds.), *Medical-surgical nursing: Concepts for interprofessional collaborative care* (9th ed.). St. Louis, MO: Elsevier.

Brashers, V. L. (2012a). Alterations of pulmonary function. In S. E. Huether & K. L. McCance (Eds.), *Understanding pathophysiology* (5th ed.). St. Louis, MO: Elsevier Mosby.

Brashers, V. L. (2012b). Structure and function of the pulmonary system. In S. E. Huether & K. L. McCance (Eds.), *Understanding pathophysiology* (5th ed.). St. Louis, MO: Elsevier Mosby.

Brown, J. D., Harnett, J., Chambers, R., & Sato, R. (2018). The relative burden of community-acquired pneumonia hospitalizations in older adults: A retrospective observational study in the United States. *BMC Geriatrics, 18*(92). Retrieved from https://doi.org/10.1186/s12877-018-0787-2

Capriotti, T. (2020). *Pathophysiology: Introductory concepts and clinical perspectives.* 2nd ed. Philadelphia, PA: F.A. Davis Company.

Casey, G. (2020). A pandemic in action. *Kai Tiaki Nursing New Zealand, 26*(3), 17.

Centers for Disease Control and Prevention. (2018). HAI data and statistics. Retrieved from https://www.cdc.gov/hai/surveillance/index.html

Centers for Disease Control and Prevention. (2020). Pneumococcal vaccine timing for adults. Retrieved from https://www.cdc.gov/vaccines/vpd/pneumo/downloads/pneumo-vaccine-timing.pdf

Franco, J. (2017). Community-acquired pneumonia. *Radiologic Technology, 88*(6), 621–638.

Goolsby, M. J., & Jones, C. S. (2019). Respiratory system. In M. J. Goolsby & L. Grubbs (Eds.), *Advanced assessment: Interpreting findings and formulating differential diagnoses* (4th ed.). Philadelphia, PA: F.A. Davis.

Hoffman, J. J., & Sullivan, N. J. (2020). *Medical-surgical nursing: Making connections to practice* (2nd ed.). Philadelphia, PA: F.A. Davis.

Jain, S., Self, W. H., Wunderink, R., Fakhran, S., Balk, R., Bramley, A. M., . . . Qi, C. (2015). Community-acquired pneumonia requiring hospitalization among U.S. adults. *New England Journal of Medicine, 373*(5), 415–427. doi:10.1056/NDJMoa1500245

Jordan, J., Turner, R. B., & Woo, T. M. (2016). Drugs used in treating infectious diseases. In T. M. Woo & M. V. Robinson (Eds.), *Pharmacotherapeutics for advance practice nurse prescribers* (4th ed.). Philadelphia, PA: F.A. Davis.

Kalil, A. C., Metersky, M. L., Klompas, M., Muscedere, J., Sweeney, D. A., . . . Brozek, J. L. (2016). Management of adults with hospital-acquired pneumonia: 2016 clinical practice guidelines by the Infectious Diseases Society of America and the American Thoracic Society. *Clinical Infectious Diseases, 63*(5), e61–e111. Retrieved from https://doi.org/10.1093cidciw353

Karch, A. M., & Tucker, R. G. (2020). *Focus on nursing pharmacology* (8th ed). Philadelphia, PA: Wolters luwer

Kaysin, A., & Viera, A. J. (2016). Community-acquired pneumonia in adults: Diagnosis and management. *American Family Physician, 94*(9), 698–706. Retrieved from www.aafp.org/afp.

Lawrence, P., & Karakashian, A. L. (2018). *Pneumonia in older adults.* CINAHL Information Systems.

Rees, H. (2018). Assessment of the respiratory system. In D. D. Ignatavicius, L. Workman, & C. R. Rebar (Eds.), *Medical-surgical nursing: Concepts for interprofessional collaborative care* (9th ed.). St. Louis, MO: Elsevier.

Richardson, K. (2020). Pneumonia. In T. M. Woo & M. V. Robinson (Eds.), *Pharmacotherapeutics for advanced practice nurse prescribers* (5th ed.). Philadelphia, PA: F.A. Davis.

Vallerand, A. H., & Sanoski, C. A. (Eds.). (2021). *Davis's drug guide for nurses* (17th ed.). Philadelphia, PA: F.A. Davis.

Woo, T., & Robinson, M. V. (Eds.). (2020). *Pharmacotherapeutics for advanced practice nurse prescribers* (5th ed.). Philadelphia, PA: F.A. Davis.

Chapter 22

Osteoarthritis and Rheumatoid Arthritis

LEARNING OBJECTIVES

Upon completion of this chapter the student will be able to:

- Integrate knowledge of the physiology, pathophysiology, assessment, and nonpharmacological and pharmacological management for care of a geriatric patient with osteoarthritis or rheumatoid arthritis.

- Appraise current standards of care for patients with joint disorders.

Introduction

Arthritis is a common term used to describe chronic and painful joint conditions. There are more than 100 forms of this disabling condition (Arthritis Foundation, 2018; Centers for Disease Control [CDC], 2017a). This chapter will focus on the chronic joint disorders of osteoarthritis and rheumatoid arthritis. Approximately 54 million American adults have been diagnosed with arthritis by a health-care provider, with 23.7 million reporting arthritis-associated activity limitations (Arthritis Foundation, 2018; CDC, 2018b). Risk for development of some form of arthritis increases with age and is projected to include approximately 25.9% (78.4 million) of U.S. adults by the year 2040; of these adults, more than 43.2% (34.6 million) will report limitations in their activities (CDC, 2017b).

Age-adjusted data from the 2013–2015 National Health Interview Survey indicated that non-Hispanic American adults (European American, 22.6%, African American, 22.2%, and Asian American, 11.8%) and a lower number of Hispanic/Latino American adults (15.4%) reported they had received a diagnosis of arthritis from their health-care provider (CDC, 2017c), indicating that ethnicity is a risk factor for arthritis. Comorbidities also increase the risk for arthritis. Additional age-adjusted data from the survey estimated that individuals were more likely to have arthritis if they also had other chronic conditions, including obesity (1.5 times), diabetes (1.7 times), and heart disease (1.9 times) (CDC, 2018b).

With a total yearly economic burden of over $303.5 billion in 2013, arthritis treatment is a significant contributor to rising health-care costs. Breaking down the costs, estimated annual medical costs (including prescriptions) for U.S. adults were $140 billion, with an additional $164 billion attributed to lost wages. Individuals with arthritis incurred pay losses of approximately $4,040 more than their counterparts without an arthritis diagnosis. Notably, osteoarthritis, the most common form of arthritis, accounted for hospital costs of over $6.2 billion in 2013 (CDC, 2020).

This chapter discusses joint physiology, pathophysiology and the treatment options for two of the most common types of arthritis: *osteoarthritis* (OA) and *rheumatoid arthritis* (RA). While the pathophysiological processes are different, both conditions cause pain due to compromised joint mobility; workplace absence and disability; and loss of income and independence in activities of daily living (Arthritis Foundation, 2018). The chronic pain of arthritis, along with a decline in physical functioning, contributes to anxiety and depression (Arthritis Foundation, 2018). Appropriate assessment and management of arthritis hinge on understanding the differences in these chronic orthopedic joint conditions.

Physiology

Joints are formed where two bones meet and are defined by the degree of joint movement: *synarthrosis* (immovable) joint, *amphiarthrosis* (slightly moveable) joint, or *diarthrosis* (freely moveable) joint. Skull bones are an example of a synarthrosis joint, which occurs where bones touch each other and are attached by a fibrous connective tissue. The rib to sternum joints and vertebral joints are examples of an amphiarthrosis joint, which is created when fibrocartilage connects two bones. A diarthrosis or *synovial* joint is created when the bones are connected by a fibrous capsule which contains articular cartilage, synovial fluid, and membranes. Synovial joints are the most common joints and are subdivided into six additional categories described in Table 22–1 (Altizer, 2013; Capriotti, 2020).

TABLE 22–1   Types of Diarthrosis Joints

Type	Description	Movement Allowed	Examples
Ball-and-socket	One bone end is rounded and ball shaped and fits into the cup-like end of the adjoining bone; allows movement in several directions including rotation.	Flexion, extension, abduction, adduction, external and internal rotation. Circumduction (shoulder).	Hip Shoulder
Condyloid	The end of one bone is oval shaped and fits into the elliptical-shaped cavity of the adjoining bone; motion is angular without rotation.	Flexion, extension	Metacarpals, phalanges; metatarsals, phalanges
Gliding	Bone ends are mostly flat and allow bones to slide or twist but allow no circular motion.	Flexion, extension	Carpals Tarsals
Hinge	Connecting bones fit convex to concave ends, allowing flexion and extension motions.	Flexion, extension Supination/pronation (elbow) Medial and lateral rotation (knee)	Elbow Knee
Pivot	Ends of one bone have a conical or rounded shape and fit into the adjoining bone's opening ring, permitting rotation.	Flexion, extension, lateral flexion, rotation	Axis and atlas
Saddle	Bone ends are both concave and convex.	Movement in most directions	Thumb

(Capriotti, 2020)

Articular cartilage, a form of connective tissue without dedicated nerve innervation or blood supply, arises from chondroblasts found in the bone lacunae, and consists of a firm matrix of *proteoglycans* (primarily glycoproteins, chondroitin, and keratin sulfate), *chondrocytes*, and an elastic substance called *collagen*. Chondrocytes are responsible for cartilage synthesis and matrix remodeling, and cartilage tissue can store more sodium than plasma can store, leading to increased water storage in the cartilage tissues. Normally, there is an equilibrium in the cartilage remodeling process; degeneration occurs at the same slow rate as formation of new cartilage. (BJC Health, 2018; Goff & Vanderbeck, 2018; Roberts, 2013; Sovani & Grogan, 2013; Vernes, 2017). Collagen provides cartilage a smooth, elastic, and strong joint surface, while synovial fluid lubricates the joint space. Together, they create a shock-absorbing cushion for bone surfaces that supports smooth joint movement with minimal friction (Roberts, 2013; Sovani & Grogan, 2013).

 CLINICAL PEARLS

Keeping joints healthy impacts an individual's independence, productivity, and overall quality of life. Arthritis is a common comorbidity among individuals who have other chronic conditions.

Pathophysiology

While joint pain and edema are common in all arthritis conditions, the underlying pathophysiological changes, symptom presentations, and treatment approaches are different. Understanding the underlying pathophysiology that contributes to joint damage and disease progression is key to successful diagnosis and treatment of arthritis. The distinguishing changes found in osteoarthritis and rheumatoid arthritis are presented in this section.

Osteoarthritis

Osteoarthritis is commonly referred to as *degenerative joint disease* (DJD) or "wear-and-tear" arthritis, and the etiology is based on the cause of joint deterioration (Arthritis Foundation, 2018; Goff & Vanderbeck, 2018; Ogle, 2020). *Primary* OA is attributed to aging and mechanical stress, while *secondary* OA is attributed to joint injury, metabolic disease, or obesity (Goff & Vanderbeck, 2018). Several changes in joint structure contribute to the development of OA. First, chondroblasts, the precursor cells of cartilage, cannot travel beyond the lacunae, and therefore are not available for effective remodeling of cartilage damage that occurs as a result of repetitive injury to the joint over time. Second, articular cartilage has no dedicated blood supply and, as the cartilage matrix blocks access of immune cells to damaged areas, there is a limited availability of immunoglobulins and lymphocytes and repair of damaged cells is reduced (BJC Health, 2018; Sovani & Grogan, 2013). Cartilage destruction can also be attributed to synovial inflammation. As inflammation increases, there is a decreased production of lubricin, the bone lubricant, and an increased production of enzymes that lead to further cartilage destruction (Capriotti, 2020; Ogle, 2020).

When cartilage is exposed to repeated and excessive force, the resulting damage triggers a disequilibrium in the remodeling process, leading to cartilage destruction and the formation of clusters of new cells that lead to uneven remodeling, degradation of the articular surface, and calcification of the cartilage matrix. Figure 22–1 illustrates the effects of OA. As a direct result of this calcification, the inflammatory process is activated, leading to further cartilage destruction. Joint effusions and edema are a direct result of the inflammatory process (BJC Health, 2018; Capriotti, 2020). Additionally, changes in subchondral bone surfaces lead to the formation of *osteophytes*, which over time increase in size and may break off within the joint space with repeated injury, leading to nerve impingement and pain (Capriotti, 2020; Ogle, 2020).

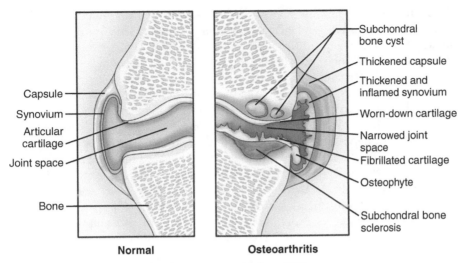

FIGURE 22–1 Osteoarthritis of the knee *(Hoffman & Sullivan, 2020)*

Three different biological processes have been identified as potential sources of the joint destruction common to OA: estrogen deficiency, genetic predisposition, and age-related changes. When *estrogen* levels decline, musculoskeletal menopause occurs, a condition characterized by alterations to the structure of extracellular matrix and chondrocytes, increased bone turnover, decreased bone and muscle mass, and increased joint laxity and fat mass. Joint instability and injury result (BJC Health, 2018). Some individuals are *genetically predisposed* to OA due to alterations in bone mineral density, chondrocyte and matrix mutations, and their genetic skeletal shape. In these individuals, cell regeneration is altered, leading to early development of osteoarthritis (Bruyère et al., 2015). Studies have identified genetic association in the development of OA of the hand, hip, and knee (Sovani & Grogan, 2013).

Age-related joint changes include cell changes that lead to thinner and less dense chondrocyte and matrix cells. Synovial fluid production decreases with age due to reduction in body fluids and hyaluronic acid synthesis, decreasing the cushioning effect during joint stress and increasing cartilage fragility and fissure formation. As more and more fissures are formed, displaced cartilage floats in the joint space; small pieces of bone dislodge as bones move directly against each other and the joint space narrows, producing *crepitus* (the grating sound heard with joint movement) (BJC Health, 2018; Goff & Vanderbeck, 2018). As cell regeneration decreases with age, tendons become less elastic, leading to joint laxity. Additionally, aging leads to changes in balance and proprioception, putting the individual at risk for musculoskeletal injury (Bruyère et al., 2015).

Rheumatoid Arthritis

While genetics, hormones, infection, and environmental triggers are thought to influence the abnormal immune response, the underlying mechanisms that lead to the joint and systemic inflammation of RA are not clearly understood. Genetic predisposition to RA has been identified in about 50% of all RA patients, and female hormone levels have shown disease regression during pregnancy with exacerbations recurring after delivery. When synovial fluid is analyzed, the presence of anaerobic bacteria in high levels suggests that bacterial infection can lead to RA development. Other infectious causes are attributed to Epstein-Barr and rubella viruses and mycoplasma organisms. Regardless of the trigger, synovial tissues are assaulted by the body's own immune system, leading to chronic exacerbations and remissions of the disease and progressive joint damage, as shown in Figure 22–2 (Capriotti, 2020; Roberts, 2013).

There are four recognizable stages of RA. In stage 1, synovial fluid within the joint becomes inflamed (*synovitis*) and increases in volume (*joint effusion*). Antibodies, including rheumatoid factor (*RF*) and anti-cyclic citrullinated peptide (*anti-CCP*), are produced by plasma cells; as the synovial cells become more inflamed, macrophages arrive to ingest the inflamed tissues. In addition, lymphocytes, particularly tumor necrosis factor (*TNF*), work with macrophages to produce a variety of pro-inflammatory mediators that contribute to further destruction of cartilage and bone. Radiological studies in early RA reveal edema of the soft tissues, but no joint destruction (Kontzias, 2017; Roberts, 2013).

In stage 2 RA, hypertrophy of synovial fluid occurs, and very vascular and fibrous scar tissue (*pannus*), develops. Once this process begins, the inflammatory mediators contribute to further joint destruction, and the disease transitions to stage 3 RA. As the cartilage continues to erode, bone cysts, spurs, and erosions of the subchondral bone develop. Tendons and ligaments are damaged from the growing pannus formations, contributing to contractures, laxity of the tendons and ligaments, and the development of contractures. End-stage RA (stage 4) occurs as the joints become non-functional and inflammation subsides. Rheumatoid nodules are associated with this stage of the disease (Capriotti, 2020; Kontzias, 2017; Roberts, 2013).

Prostaglandins contribute to the pain of arthritis and are formed after tissue damage as arachidonic acid, produced by cell membrane breakdown, is broken down by *cyclooxygenase* (COX) enzymes. COX-1 enzymes are found in the endothelium and contribute to platelet aggregation, regulate the production of mucus and acid in the stomach, and aid in the regulation of water excretion by the kidneys. COX-2 enzymes are produced due to the inflammatory process. As inflammation increases, COX-2 enzymes lead to increased prostaglandin levels, the pain threshold is lowered, and the individual experiences an increase in pain (Hudspeth, 2020).

Risk Factors

Risk factors for arthritis are classified as non-modifiable (age, sex, genetics) and modifiable (infection, joint injury, excess weight, and occupation). Osteoarthritis risk factors include age, genetics, ethnicity, a history of participating in a sport or other athletic

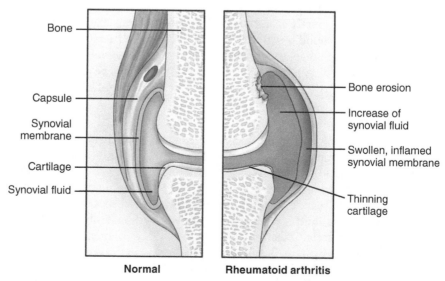

Normal   **Rheumatoid arthritis**

FIGURE 22–2 Rheumatoid arthritis of the hand   *(From Hoffman, J. J., & Sullivan, N. J. (2020). Davis advantage for medical-surgical nursing: Making connections to practice (2nd ed.). Philadelphia, PA: F.A. Davis.)*

activities, prior joint or bone injury, occupational risk for musculoskeletal injury (i.e., heavy lifting), medication use (including over-the-counter medications), and other medical conditions (estrogen deficiency, hypercalcemia, low bone density, obesity, and vitamin D deficiency).

Rheumatoid arthritis is defined as an autoimmune disease; as such, its etiology is thought to be a combination of genetic and environmental abnormal immune responses that lead to joint inflammation and cartilage damage. Thus, the risk factors are less clearly identified (Arthritis Foundation, n.d.; Bryuère et al., 2015; Goff & Vanderbeck, 2018; Roberts, 2013).

Assessment

Understanding the differences in pathophysiology and symptomatic presentation is the first step to accurate assessment of the client with arthritis. Diagnosis is based on an accurate and complete health history (personal and family), including identification of risk factors, and a focused motor-musculoskeletal assessment that includes pain assessment, muscle strength/weakness, stiffness, balance, and coordination assessment. Diagnostic laboratory and radiological findings, including plain x-ray and *magnetic resonance imaging* (MRI), help complete the profile. Additionally, close attention to the client's description of symptom management strategies (pharmacological and nonpharmacological and response to those interventions), along with the impact of symptoms on activities of daily living and quality of life subjective symptoms are essential to an accurate arthritis diagnosis (Bruyère et al., 2015; Dillon, 2007; Roberts, 2013; Sovani & Grogan, 2013). Characteristics and presentation of OA and RA are compared in Table 22–2.

Physical Assessment

Along with the health history, a musculoskeletal assessment is a key component of the diagnostic process. Assess balance, gait, and coordination by observing the patient's stance and gait for any difficulties with posture, weight-bearing, and the swing. The patient's ability to walk heel-to-toe and stand or hop on one foot while in place, perform deep knee bends (if the patient is able), and the Romberg test are the most common assessment tests. The health-care provider should look at the patient's shoes for

TABLE 22–2 Comparison of Characteristics and Presentation of Osteoarthritis and Rheumatoid Arthritis

Characteristic	OA	RA
Onset	Age >50 years	Mid-life (35–45 years)
Sex	Female > male after age 60	Female > male in younger population
Etiology	Degenerative or age related	Inflammatory autoimmune
Progression	Localized	Systemic
Joint involvement	Localized, typically unilateral, most commonly found in weight-bearing joints (hips and knees); also hands, shoulders, spine (cervical and/or lumbar)	Bilateral and symmetrical, typically beginning in small joints (PIP, metacarpophalangeal [MCP]) of the hands, wrists, and progressing to lower extremities (knees and hips)
Nodules	Bouchard's (proximal interphalangeal [PIP]) Heberden's (distal interphalangeal [DIP])	Rheumatic nodules Swan-neck deformity: wrist Boutonniere deformity: fingers

Continued

TABLE 22–2 Comparison of Characteristics and Presentation of Osteoarthritis and Rheumatoid Arthritis—cont'd

Characteristic	OA	RA

Pain	"Aching"; insidious onset
	    Increased following prolonged inactivity (i.e., sitting), which is relieved by movement
	    Increased with activity and at the end of the day and relieved by rest
		Pain with joint palpation
		Pain increased with passive motion

Motion	Stiffness is relieved with movement Crepitus during movement Decreased range of motion (ROM)	Morning stiffness that is relieved with activity Decreased ROM related to edema and/or joint deformity

(Goff & Vanderbeck, 2018; Roberts, 2013)

uneven wear, which often occurs when the patient is unable to bear full body weight equally during ambulation (Dillon, 2007; Palmer, 2013).

Focused joint assessment is directed by the patient's symptoms and includes a comparison of symmetrical joints, beginning with the unaffected side. Inspect joints for color, shape, and size and observe for any deformities. Note any joint tenderness, pain, or any differences in skin temperature on palpation. Warmth may indicate infection, while ecchymosis occurs following trauma, and skin pallor or redness may indicate disruption of blood flow to the extremity. Determining the onset of edema, in addition to describing the extent (localized or diffuse), is important to accurate diagnosis (Palmer, 2013).

Joint movement depends on the type of joint (see Table 22-1). *Range of motion* (ROM) assessment includes active and passive movement, along with ROM against resistance to test muscle strength. ROM testing should be performed with caution, because a joint should never be forced beyond its ease of movement. Note any crepitus that may be heard with joint movement (Dillon, 2007; Palmer, 2013). Localized edema is common when the joint contains blood (hemarthrosis), infection (pyarthrosis), or excessive synovial fluid (effusion), while diffuse edema is found with circulatory dysfunction (lymphatic or venous), infection, tumor, or following a traumatic injury (Palmer, 2013).

Diagnostic Tests

Laboratory findings in OA include a normal or slightly *elevated sedimentation rate* (ESR) and *C-reactive protein* (CRP) levels along with a negative RF level. In comparison, the CRP, RF, ESR, and antinuclear factor levels are typically elevated in RA. Approximately 70% of RA patients also have elevated *anti-citrullinated protein antibodies* (ACPAs), serological markers that indicate the amount of synovial membrane erosion (Capriotti, 2020).

Joint pathology also presents differently in OA and RA. Synovial fluid in the OA shows normal viscosity and few cells, while the synovial fluid in RA reveals a decreased viscosity and elevated WBCs. Similarly, there are specific differences in radiological findings. Radiological findings in OA include the presence of osteophytes, cysts, and an asymmetrical narrowing of the joint space. In RA, while plain x-ray films show joint narrowing and subluxation of the joint bones, these changes are found earlier in the disease process using MRI (Roberts, 2013).

HIGH YIELD FACT FOR TESTING

Osteoarthritis and rheumatoid arthritis have different pathophysiological origins, requiring accurate assessment, diagnosis, and early intervention to maintain functional ability and QOL.

Nonpharmacological Management

Both OA and RA are chronic illnesses and require an individualized treatment plan that helps the patient develop coping strategies and a self-care plan that enables them to maintain as much independence as possible. While a healthy diet is important for everyone, the arthritis patient who is overweight or obese will benefit from weight reduction interventions (Roberts, 2013). There is not a specific diet that the arthritis patient should follow, but current evidence indicates a Mediterranean diet is beneficial to all patients with arthritis because it includes anti-inflammatory foods such as those high in omega-3 fatty acids. Other beneficial dietary choices include green tea (anti-inflammatory effects) and foods high in fiber (reduces CRP levels) (Arthritis Foundation, 2015).

Exercise is another important part of an arthritis treatment plan and should be individualized to prevent further injury to inflamed joints. Because muscle and ligament weakness lead to further joint damage, exercise programs should include a combination of strengthening exercises and low-impact aerobic exercises, which work together to improve joint stability, muscle strength, and joint mobility. A physical therapist can guide the patient to develop an individualized exercise plan that can be followed at home after the patient meets their therapy goals.

Pharmacology

Pharmacological management is based on diagnosis and should be selected with consideration of the patient's other medications. However, because OA is not the result of an altered immune response, these patients do not require treatment with the immunosuppressant drugs required to treat RA. Pain medications are an essential part of all arthritis treatment plans (Capriotti, 2020; Roberts, 2013). Addressing pain as the individual's personal experience and understanding the impact of pain on the patient's quality of life are essential to successful pain management. Table 22-3 at the end of the Pharmacology section details medications used in the treatment of OA and RA.

Pain Management

Initial pain management includes local analgesics and non-opioid medications such as *acetaminophen* or *NSAIDs*. While acetaminophen is a safe choice for most patients with mild or moderate pain, those with hepatic disease must be carefully monitored for toxicity. It is also important to monitor the total daily dose of acetaminophen as the drug is often found in other medications (Hudspeth, 2020).

NSAIDs and *salicylate* drugs reduce mild or moderate pain by inhibiting the action of COX enzymes. While some NSAIDs are nonselective, celecoxib acts specifically to inhibit COX-2 enzymes; while the drug does not reduce the protective actions of COX-1 enzymes in the *gastrointestinal* (GI) track, it does increase the individual's cardiovascular risks. Both non-specific NSAIDs and salicylates affect platelet function, increase bleeding risk, and increase the patient's risk for ulcers. *Tramadol* is a non-narcotic that acts on the *central nervous system* (CNS) to inhibit mild to moderate pain. Opioids are classified based on their duration of action and are reserved for use in severe pain (Hudspeth, 2020).

Corticosteroids

Because of their anti-inflammatory actions, *corticosteroids* are often used as a short-term therapy to manage acute exacerbations of RA. Glucocorticoids (cortisol) have a major impact on the body's metabolic processes including the CNS (altered sleep and memory recall in high doses), blood glucose levels (elevate), protein synthesis (inhibit), and gastric acid secretion (elevate); and, because of their impact on sex hormones, they impact bone mineral density (decrease). Mineralocorticoids (aldosterone) have a major role in balancing sodium and water retention and excretion of potassium. Steroids are selected for use based on the amount of cortisol or aldosterone activity, and the drugs with more cortisol activity are typically chosen for use in treating the inflammatory processes at work in RA. Cortisone (natural and primarily cortisol), prednisolone (synthetic with mixed cortisol and aldosterone), dexamethasone, and methylprednisolone (synthetic with primarily cortisol) are often prescribed to treat inflammatory processes. Because corticosteroids are immunosuppressive and have the potential to mask signs and symptoms of infection, patients on these drugs should avoid exposure to contagious diseases and should not receive live vaccinations during treatment (Vallerand & Sanoski, 2017; Woo, 2020). Adverse effects of long-term or high-dose corticosteroid use include development of cataracts and glaucoma, cardiovascular events (MI and heart failure), diabetes, and decreased bone mineral density (Soubrier, Tatar, Couderc, Mathieu, & Dubost, 2013). Oral corticosteroids are not appropriate for use in treatment of OA (Capriotti, 2020; Roberts, 2013).

Interarticular injections are often used to treat OA and RA and can be effective in decreasing pain and inflammation for a period of weeks to several months. The choice of corticosteroid used for injections is based on the desired duration of effects because corticosteroids vary in their pharmacokinetics and are absorbed at a much slower rate when injected into a joint (Capriotti, 2020; Roberts, 2013; Woo, 2016). Injection of a hyaluronic acid (viscosupplement) is another alternative to corticosteroid injections or to NSAIDs (when not well tolerated or no longer effective) and may improve symptoms for up to a year, although their action and benefits are not clearly understood (Gower, n.d.; Roberts, 2013).

Antirheumatic Drugs (DMARDs)

Disease-modifying antirheumatic drugs (DMARDs) have immunosuppressive actions that slow the progression of a disease. Methotrexate is the most commonly prescribed DMARD used to slow the progression of RA. The weekly oral dose for RA patients is 7.5 mg and can be titrated up to a maximum of 20 mg/week. Once titrated to effective response, a subcutaneous version can be used (Vallerand & Sanoski, 2017). It takes about 6 to 8 weeks to see a decrease in the patient's symptoms and a slowing in joint damage on x-ray. (Roberts, 2013). As with many other drugs, older patients are at higher risk for adverse reactions; therefore, methotrexate should be used with caution in this population. Additionally, there are many drug–drug interactions with both prescription and natural herbs including melatonin and echinacea. Patients on DMARD therapy should be taught to report fever, chills, rash, and other signs of infection (cough, sore throat), bleeding, or exposure to contagious disease. They should also be instructed to avoid alcohol, aspirin, and NSAIDs due to the risk of GI bleeding (Roberts, 2013; Vallerand & Sanoski, 2017).

Monoclonal Antibodies

Monoclonal antibodies are proteins that act to suppress the immune response by their ability to block T lymphocyte cell function. Adalimumab and infliximab specifically deactivate tumor necrosis factor and thereby reduce the inflammatory response. They are only available for subcutaneous, IV, or IM administration because, as proteins, if they are introduced to the GI tract, the drugs are broken down and not utilized by the body. Erlotinib is the only oral monoclonal antibody drug. These drugs also decrease the patient's symptoms and slow joint deterioration on x-rays. Major adverse effects include acute pulmonary edema, cytokine release syndrome, and increased risk of infection due to immunosuppression. Patients may also report feelings of malaise, GI symptoms, and tremors. While these drugs provide an important component of RA treatment, it is also important to teach patients that it may take time to see the effects of these medications (Karch, 2020; Roberts, 2013). Table 22–3 further describes medications used to treat arthritis.

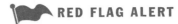 **RED FLAG ALERT**

Education for patients receiving corticosteroids must address potential weight gain, need for vitamin D and calcium to decrease osteoporosis risk, and appropriate treatment for elevated blood glucose levels, particularly in the diabetic patient.

Surgical Intervention: Total Joint Arthroplasty

Surgical intervention is an appropriate therapy when joint damage is so severe that conservative treatments no longer control symptoms and the person's quality of life is significantly impaired. If joint space is not compromised, an arthroscopy performed to remove torn cartilage or loose bodies may relieve pain. However, once joint space is significantly reduced and bone rests on bone or when the joint becomes deformed and unstable, total joint arthroplasty is another surgical option and is commonly performed for severe arthritic changes of hips, knees or shoulder joints (Capriotti, 2020; Roberts, 2013). Preoperative education includes what to expect during the hospital stay, postoperative recovery, changes to the home environment that promote safety, wound care, pain management, exercises, ambulation, and assistive device needs and is key to a successful recovery from the procedure (Goff & Vanderbeck, 2018).

Complementary and Alternative Therapies

Chondroitin sulphate and glucosamine are found in cartilage and have been developed to be used as adjunctive therapy to reduce arthritic pain. However, while some studies have indicated that pain reduction, along with a decrease in cartilage destruction and joint space narrowing, occurs with use of these supplements, other studies have not shown functional improvement or reduction in pain (National Center for Complementary and Integrative Health [NIH], 2017; Sovani & Grogan, 2013). While studies have not revealed significant side effects of these supplements, they do have interactions when used with warfarin and, if used by diabetic patients, may lead to insulin resistance. Based on laboratory rat studies, glucosamine has the potential to cause kidney damage (NIH, 2017). Therefore, patients should begin these supplements with caution and should be aware that results may not be seen for up to 6 weeks, and that if improvement is not seen, the supplements should be discontinued (Roberts, 2013).

Summary

Estimates indicate that more than 54 million adults have been diagnosed with a form of arthritis. Living with joint pain leads to decreased physical function, lost time at work, increased health-care costs, and often anxiety and depression (Arthritis Foundation, 2018). Understanding the complexities of OA and RA is essential to providing an accurate diagnosis, appropriate treatment options, and support for the patient with a chronic, painful condition. With a wide variety of pharmacological, nonpharmacological, and complementary therapies available, the patient may become confused about which options will be most effective in managing their condition. One of the most important roles of the nurse is to assess the patient's learning needs and to provide evidence-based education that helps them make the best decisions for their situation and condition.

TABLE 22–3 Medications Used to Treat Osteoarthritis and Rheumatoid Arthritis

Class	Example	Action	Dosage	SENC
Non-opioids	Acetaminophen	In CNS, inhibits prostaglandin synthesis; used for pain and fever	Oral, rectal, IV Max 24 hr dose is 3,000 mg; in hepatic disease 2,000 mg/24 hr.	Caution with hepatic or renal disease; alcoholism; malnutrition or hypovolemia; drug–drug interactions.
	NSAIDs Celecoxib Ibuprofen Ketorolac	In CNS, inhibits prostaglandin synthesis; used for pain and fever	Celecoxib (PO): 200 mg/day (or 100 mg bid. Ibuprofen (PO, IV): max dose: 3,200 mg/day. Ketorolac (PO, IV, IM): initial dose 30 mg IV q 6 hr, then 10–20 mg PO for no more than 5 days total.	Contraindication: aspirin allergy; caution with aspirin, warfarin, and other thrombolytic drugs (↑ bleeding and GI irritation). Decrease dose of Ketorolac based on age ≥65.
	Tramadol	Norepinephrine and serotonin reuptake inhibitor; analgesic (moderate/severe pain)	Immediate and extended release. Titrate to 300 mg/day maximum dose.	Seizures are a major adverse reaction; caution for serotonin syndrome or physical dependence/tolerance; drug–drug interactions with other CNS depressants.
Opioids	Oxycodone Hydrocodone Fentanyl	Alter pain perception and response: act as CNS agonists by binding to CNS opiate receptors; used for severe pain	Oxycodone (PO, immediate and extended release): 5–10 mg tid/qid. Hydrocodone (PO, immediate and extended release): 2.5–10 mg q 3–6 hr. Fentanyl (IV, transdermal patch, transmucosal): dose based on route.	Use opioids with caution if taking any other CNS depressants. Avoid with MAOIs due to unpredictability of reactions. Transdermal patches for use in long-term pain management. Change sites and disposal follows narcotic policy.
Local analgesics	Capsaicin Lidocaine	Minor pain	Topical Transdermal patch: apply up to 3 patches/24 hr. May cut to smaller size.	Avoid application of any patch or cream to irritated or broken skin. Avoid use near eyes. Avoid in hot pepper hypersensitivity.

Corticosteroids	Prednisone Hydrocortisone	Reduce inflammation	Prednisone: 5–60 mg/day. Hydrocortisone: 20–240 mg/day (can also be used for interarticular injections).	Taper to avoid adrenal insufficiency symptoms (life threatening). Report signs/symptoms of GI bleeding. May mask infection symptoms.
DMARDs	Methotrexate	Immunosuppression (RA only)	7.5 mg weekly (max 20 mg/week).	Immunosuppression reduced with echinacea or melatonin; caffeine. Caution with renal impairment; contraindicated with hepatic disease.
Monoclonal antibodies	Adalimumab Infliximab	Immunosuppression (RA only)	Adalimumab: 40 mg every other week; or 40 mg weekly (if not receiving methotrexate). Infliximab: initial: 3 mg/kg, repeating in 2 and 6 weeks; then every 8 weeks.	With all monoclonal antibodies: Assess for history of or exposure to TB prior to starting therapy.
Hyaluronic acid	Hyalgan® Orthovisc® Synvisc®	Arthritis joint pain	1 injection every 3–5 weeks (depends on drug).	Full benefits may not be seen for about 5 weeks and response is individual.

(Hudspeth, 2020; Vallerand & Sanoski, 2017)

Key Points

- Osteoarthritis and rheumatoid arthritis have different pathological beginnings but both result in joint destruction, pain, and, as the disease progresses, lead to impaired physical functioning.

- While corticosteroids are effective in treating RA, the only use for this drug class in OA is as an interarticular joint injection.

- Education for the patient with arthritis includes the importance of a well-balanced diet, weight management strategies, appropriate physical exercise, and nonpharmacological and pharmacological interventions.

Review Questions

1. **Which of the following statements by the patient would indicate a need for further education on the risk factors for osteoarthritis?**

   a. "My old football knee injury contributed to my arthritis."
   b. "The fact that I'm older has increased my risk for arthritis."
   c. "My arthritis was caused by my body's immune response."
   d. "I need to lose weight because obesity contributes to my arthritis."

2. **When performing a range of motion assessment, the nurse understands that it is important to do which of the following?**

   a. Avoid assessing any edematous joints.
   b. Include both active and passive movements.
   c. Move the joint forcefully to reach maximum extension.
   d. Only assess the involved joints.

3. **The nurse understands that when evaluating laboratory findings, the patient with osteoarthritis may have which of the following?**

   a. Elevated antinuclear factor
   b. Elevated anti-citrullinated protein antibiotics
   c. Normal or slightly elevated C-reactive protein
   d. Normal erythrocyte sedimentation rate

4. **One of the most important nonpharmacological interventions for arthritis includes which of the following?**

   a. Appropriate use of pain medications
   b. Developing effective coping strategies
   c. Ice and heat application daily
   d. Maintaining muscle strength and agility

5. **Patient education for the patient taking a disease-modifying antirheumatic drug (DMARD) includes which of the following? (Select all that apply.)**

   a. Avoid crowds and exposure to contagious diseases.
   b. Effects may not be seen for up to 8 weeks.
   c. Take on an empty stomach before meals.
   d. Use of echinacea is allowed during DMARD therapy.

See the appendix for answers to review questions.

References

Altizer, L. (2013). Anatomy and physiology. In L. Schoenly (Ed.), *Core curriculum for orthopaedic nursing* (7th ed.). Chicago, IL: National Association of Orthopaedic Nurses.

Arthritis Foundation (2015). *The ultimate arthritis diet*. Atlanta, GA: Author. Retrieved from https://www.arthritis.org/living-with-arthritis/arthritis-diet/anti-inflammatory/the-arthritis-diet.php

Arthritis Foundation. (2018). *Arthritis by the numbers: Book of trusted facts & figures* (2nd annual ed.). Atlanta, GA: Author. Retrieved from https://www.arthritis.org/Documents/Sections/About-Arthritis/arthritis-facts-stats-figures.pdf

BJC Health. (2018). Pathophysiology of osteoarthritis. Retrieved from http://www.bjchealth.com.au/what-is-the-pathophysiology-of-osteoarthritis-and-what-are-the-risk-factors-towards-its-development

Bruyère, O., Cooper, C., Arden, N., Branco, J., Brandi, M. L, Herrero-Beaumont, G., . . . Reginster, J.-Y. (2015). Can we identify patients with high risk of osteoarthritis progression who will respond to treatment? A focus on epidemiology and phenotype of osteoarthritis. *Drugs & Aging, 32*(3), 179–187. doi:10.1007/s40266-015-0243-3

Capriotti, T.. (2020). *Pathophysiology: Introductory concepts and clinical perspectives*. Philadelphia, PA: F.A. Davis.

Centers for Disease Control and Prevention. (2017a). Arthritis basics: Frequently asked questions. Retrieved from https://www.cdc.gov/arthritis/basics/faqs.htm

Centers for Disease Control and Prevention. (2017b). Arthritis: National facts. Retrieved from https://www.cdc.gov/arthritis/data_statistics/national-statistics.html

Centers for Disease Control and Prevention. (2017c). Health disparity statistics. Retrieved from Retrieved from https://www.cdc.gov/arthritis/data_statistics/disparities.htm

Centers for Disease Control and Prevention. (2018b). Comorbidities. https://www.cdc.gov/arthritis/data_statistics/comorbidities.htm

Centers for Disease Control and Prevention. (2020). Arthritis: Cost statistics. Retrieved from Retrieved from https://www.cdc.gov/arthritis/data_statistics/cost.htm

Dillon, P. M. (2007). *Nursing health assessment: A critical thinking, case studies approach* (2nd ed.). Philadelphia, PA: F.A. Davis.

Goff, R., & Vanderbeck, K. (2018). Care of patients with arthritis and other connective tissue diseases. In D. D. Ignatavicius, M. L. Workman, & C. R. Rebar (Eds.), *Medical-surgical nursing: Concepts for interprofessional collaborative care* (9th ed.). St. Louis, MO: Elsevier.

Gower, T. (n.d.). *Hyaluronic acid injections for osteoarthritis*. Atlanta, GA: Arthritis Foundation. Retrieved from https://www.arthritis.org/living-with-arthritis/treatments/medication/drug-types/other/hyaluronic-acid-injections.php

Hoffman, J. J., & Sullivan, N. J. (2020). *Davis advantage for medical-surgical nursing: Making connections to practice* (2nd ed.). Philadelphia, PA: F.A. Davis.

Hudspeth, R. S. (2020). Pain management: Acute and chronic pain. In T. M. Woo & M. V. Robinson (Eds.), *Pharmacotherapeutics for advance practice nurse prescribers* (5th ed.). Philadelphia, PA: F.A. Davis.

Karch, A. M. (2020). *Focus on nursing pharmacology* (8th ed.). Philadelphia, PA: Wolters Kluwer / Lippincott Williams & Wilkins.

Kontzias, A. (2017, February). Rheumatoid arthritis. In *Merck manual: Professional version* [Online]. Retrieved from https://www.merckmanuals.com/professional/musculoskeletal-and-connective-tissue-disorders/joint-disorders/rheumatoid-arthritis-ra

National Center for Complementary and Integrative Health. (2017). Glucosamine and chondroitin for osteoarthritis. Retrieved from https://nccih.nih.gov/health/glucosaminechondroitin

Ogle, K. (2020). Coordinating care for patients with connective tissue disorder. In J. J. Hoffman & N. J. Sullivan (Eds.), *Medical-surgical nursing: Making connections to practice*. Philadelphia, PA: F.A. Davis.

Palmer, D. M. (2013). Musculoskeletal assessment. In L. Schoenly (Ed.), *Core curriculum for orthopaedic nursing* (7th ed.). Chicago, IL: National Association of Orthopaedic Nurses.

Roberts, D. (2013). Arthritis & connective tissue disorders. In L. Schoenly (Ed.), *Core curriculum for orthopaedic nursing* (7th ed.). Chicago, IL: National Association of Orthopaedic Nurses.

Soubrier, M., Tatar, Z., Couderc, M., Mathieu, S., & Dubost, J. (2013). Rheumatoid arthritis in the elderly in the era of tight control. *Drugs & Aging, 30*(11), 863–869. doi:10.1007/s40266-013-0122-8

Sovani, S., & Grogan, S. P. (2013). Osteoarthritis: Detection, pathophysiology, and current/future treatment strategies. *Orthopaedic Nursing, 32*(1), 25–36.

Vallerand, A. H., & Sanoski, C. A. (Eds.). (2017). *Davis's drug guide for nurses* (15th ed.). Philadelphia, PA: F.A. Davis.

Vernes, D. (Ed.). (2021). *Taber's cyclopedic medical dictionary* (24th ed.). Philadelphia, PA: F.A. Davis.

Woo, T. M. (2020). Drugs used in treating inflammatory processes. In T. M. Woo & M. V. Robinson (Eds.), *Pharmacotherapeutics for advanced practice nurse prescribers* (5th ed.). Philadelphia, PA: F.A. Davis.

Chapter 23

Chronic Kidney Disease

LEARNING OBJECTIVES

Upon completion of this chapter the student will be able to:

- Integrate knowledge of the physiology, pathophysiology, assessment, and nonpharmacological and pharmacological management for care of a geriatric patient with chronic kidney disease.

- Appraise current standards of care for older adult patients with chronic kidney disease.

Introduction

A disease of impaired filtering, *chronic kidney disease* (CKD) is reported to be the ninth leading cause of death, impacting more than 37 million of the U.S. adult population (Centers for Disease Control and Prevention [CDC], 2019, 2020a). Age impacts kidney filtration rates, with a normal decrease of 1% each year after age 40 (World Kidney Day, 2019) with a worldwide estimated incidence of CKD among men (1 in 5) and women (1 in 4) age 65 to 74 years old (National Kidney Foundation, 2015). Additionally, older individuals are at high risk for CKD due to age and comorbidities common to the older population including cardiovascular disease, diabetes, and hypertension (Mallappallil, Friedman, Delano, McFarlane, & Salifu, 2014).

Unfortunately, about 96% of adults with mild kidney function impairment and 48% of those who are not on dialysis but have severe renal impairment remain unaware of their disease (CDC, 2019). Prevalence of CKD in the United States is higher in non-Hispanic blacks (18%) than non-Hispanic whites (13%), and an estimated 15% of Hispanic individuals have CKD. However, while women (15%) are more likely than men (12%) to develop CKD, progression of the disease to *end-stage renal disease* (ESRD) is more likely to occur in men (3 men for each 2 women) (CDC, 2019). Additionally, the cost of treating CKD in the United States for Medicare recipients was estimated to be $84 billion in 2017, with cost of ESRD treatment adding $36 billion to that total (CDC, 2020a). This disease places a large financial and quality of life burden on the individual with CKD as well as on the community.

CKD often remains a "silent" disease in its early stages and often accompanies other chronic diseases, (McManus & Wynter-Minott, 2017; Norton et al., 2017a), making recognition of the disease key to slowing the disease process. The purpose of this chapter is to describe the normal physiology of the aging kidney, the pathophysiology of CKD, and appropriate pharmacological and nonpharmacological interventions for the disease. Understanding these concepts is essential to providing appropriate care with the goals of managing symptoms, slowing disease progression, and improving quality of life for this patient population (McManus & Wynter-Minott, 2017).

Physiology

The major role of the kidneys includes endocrine and metabolic functions that sustain homeostasis. Normal renal function contributes to overall health by maintaining acid–base balance and fluid and electrolyte balance, and by filtering metabolic waste products (including drugs) from the blood to be excreted via urine. Kidneys also secrete hormones that influence metabolism and *red blood cell* (RBC) levels. (Norton et al., 2017a; Winkelman, 2018a).

Most individuals have two functioning kidneys, each about 10 to 13 cm in length, 5 to 7 cm across, with a thickness of approximately 2.5 to 3 cm (Winkelman, 2018a), located adjacent to and on each side of the vertebral column in the retroperitoneal area of the abdomen (Huether, 2012b). The kidneys are not identical in size; the right kidney is slightly smaller and lower than the left because of the location of the liver (Huether, 2012b; Winkelman, 2018a). However, it is not abnormal for some individuals to have only one large kidney or to have more than two kidneys without evidence of renal disease (Winkelman, 2018a).

The kidney, as shown in Figure 23–1, is made up of several layers. The outer *cortex* consists of the Bowman's capsule (glomeruli), proximal tubules, loop of Henle, and some parts of the distal tubules. This layer covers all of the kidney except the indented *hilum* region, the location of blood and lymphatic vessels and nerve intervention and the point at which the ureter leaves the kidney (Huether, 2012b). The *medulla*, or inner layer of the kidney. is divided into fan-shaped *pyramids* interspersed with columns of *renal cortex* that extend downward between the pyramids. This layer contains the *loop of Henle*, the *distal tubules*, and *collecting ducts*. Most inward, the *renal pelvis* consists of chambers called *calyces* that transport urine from the collecting ducts to the upper regions of the ureter (Huether, 2012b; Winkelman, 2018a).

Each section of nephrons within the glomerulus has a different role in blood filtration. Beginning in the proximal tubule, the reabsorption of amino acids, glucose, potassium, sodium, urea, and water begins, while hydrogen ions and foreign substances are secreted into the urine. The loop of Henle is responsible for concentrating the urine with water reabsorption (descending loop) and sodium reabsorption by diffusion (descending loop) and active transport (ascending loop). As urine moves through the

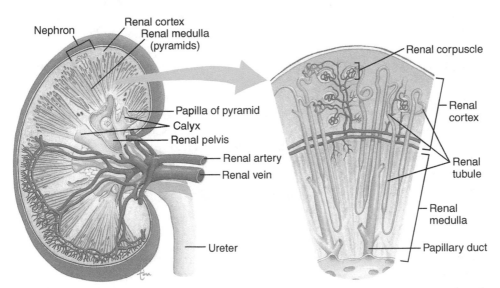

FIGURE 23–1 Layers and components of the adult kidney *(Scanlon, V. C., & Sanders, T. (2019). Essentials of anatomy and physiology (8th ed.). Philadelphia, PA: F.A. Davis.)*

distal tubules, reabsorption of sodium, water, and bicarbonate continues, while ammonium, hydrogen ions, potassium, and some drugs are secreted into the urine. Finally, in the collecting tubules, continued reabsorption of water, sodium potassium, hydrogen ions, and ammonium occurs. Of note is the need for *antidiuretic hormone* (ADH) to facilitate water reabsorption in the distal and collecting tubules (Huether, 2012b).

Blood flow through the kidney is autoregulated using hydrostatic pressure to force blood through the kidney at a normal *glomerular filtration rate* (GFR) between 90 and 120 mL/minute. The end result of normal filtration is the production of concentrated urine that removes waste products, while maintaining normal electrolyte and acid–base balance (Capriotti, 2020). Each of the approximately 1 million nephrons found in each kidney work independently as the afferent arterioles of the renal artery deliver blood to the Bowman's capsule to begin the filtration process. As blood is filtered here, large protein molecules are blocked from entering the tubules and, in the healthy kidney, remain in the bloodstream (Karch, 2020). Next, blood flows to the *efferent* arterioles and on to the peritubular and *vasa recta* capillaries found in the *juxtamedullary* nephrons. *Cortical* nephrons make up about 80% of all nephrons, are located in the renal cortex, and contain the loop of Henle, are short and mostly located within the medulla. In contrast, the *juxtamedullary* nephrons extend into the medulla layer and have an important role in concentrating urine, particularly during periods of low fluid volume when they are responsible for reabsorption of more water while still concentrating urine (Huether, 2012b; Winkelman, 2018a).

The kidney produces *erythropoietin*, a hormone influential in RBC production in bone marrow. Glucose levels are influenced by kidney function in two ways. First, glucose is reabsorbed in the glomeruli up to blood levels 180 mg/dL (the renal threshold), at which point excessive glucose remains in the glomerular filtrate to be excreted. Second, the kidney is also capable of producing glucose (*gluconeogenesis*) and of breaking down insulin. However, in the diseased kidney, insulin clearance declines (Capriotti, 2020). Finally, prostaglandins and bradykinins found in the kidney tissues influence renal blood flow, glomerular filtration rates, excretion of sodium and water, and production of renin (Winkelman, 2018a).

Homeostasis is supported through the *renin-angiotensin-aldosterone system* (RAAS). In response to low sodium levels, *renin* is produced by kidney cells found in the distal convoluted tubule. In response to low blood pressure, decreased perfusion through the nephron, or an increase in activity of the sympathetic nervous system, *renin* is produced in the distal convoluted tubules. Renin stimulates angiotensinogen conversion to angiotensin I, causing an increased secretion of *aldosterone*, and resulting in an increased reabsorption of sodium and water, excretion of potassium, and vasoconstriction (Capriotti, 2020; Winkelman, 2018a).

HIGH YIELD FACT FOR TESTING

The kidney has more than twice the nephrons needed to adequately filter the blood, making identification of nephron damage difficult in the early stages (Capriotti, 2020).

A part of a complex metabolic process that begins in the liver, low blood calcium levels stimulate the production of parathyroid hormone, which in turn stimulates the conversion of inactive vitamin D to the active form (*1,25-dihydroxyvitamin D_3*). Serum phosphorus levels also have a role in this process. Low serum phosphorus levels stimulate the conversion, while high serum phosphorus levels inhibit the process (Huether, 2012b).

Pathophysiology

Chronic kidney disease is a progressive disease characterized by "abnormalities of kidney structure or function, present for > 3 months, with implications for health" (KDIGO, 2013). Disease progression is divided into five stages based on GFR and is also classed into three stages based on albuminuria levels (KDIGO, 2013; Winkelman, 2018b). Other criteria that are used to classify the stage of CKD include abnormalities in serum electrolyte levels; structural changes in the kidneys; the presence of albumin, blood, and/or sedimentation in the urine; and a progressive decrease in the GFR (McManus & Wynter-Minott, 2017; Norton et al., 2017a). During normal aging, the kidney is less efficient in conserving water and maintaining fluid balance, causing a decrease in GFR and increasing the older adult's risk for dehydration, which further inhibits renal blood flow and increases risk for nephrotoxicity (Winkelman, 2018a). Interestingly, because individuals with a history of renal transplantation remain at risk for kidney failure and early death, they are considered to have CKD (McManus & Wynter-Minott, 2017).

Underlying causes of CKD include both systemic and local processes that cause kidney damage in one of three processes. *Systemically*, cardiovascular diseases (hypertension), diabetes mellitus, systemic infections, and some drugs are known to damage nephron function. *Locally*, the presence of renal stones, obstruction of renal blood flow, urinary tract infections, and dysplasia are known to damage the renal filtration system (McManus & Wynter-Minott, 2017). Additionally, *genetic* conditions such as hypoplastic kidneys, polycystic kidney disease, and connective tissue disorders including systemic lupus erythematosus and polyarthritis are known causes of CKD (Winkelman, 2018b).

Damage can also be classed based on the origin of kidney damage. In *prerenal* damage, blood flow and kidney perfusion are decreased, typically from hypovolemia, shock, or decreased cardiac output that decreases the hydrostatic pressure required to force blood through the glomeruli. *Intrarenal* damage occurs as a result of nephron exposure to nephrotoxic drugs, renal infections, or diseases such as poststreptococcal glomerulonephritis. *Postrenal* disease is typically caused by urinary obstruction that prevents urine from moving through the kidney to the bladder. Urine collects in the ureter, backs up into the kidney, and fills the kidney with toxic waste products that damage renal cells (Capriotti, 2020; Quallich & Lajiness, 2015).

Regardless of the underlying cause, as nephrons become damaged, healthy nephrons adapt by hypertrophying and are able to maintain normal filtering functions until about 75% of the nephrons are lost. At this point, sodium and water balance is impaired, creatinine, potassium and urea levels increase, and symptoms appear (Huether, 2012a; Winkelman, 2018b). The initial renal injury results in nephron loss, increased levels of angiotensin II, inflammation and fibrosis of the renal tubules, and glomerular capillary hypertension. This leads to an increase in glomerular permeability and filtration, along with increased protein reabsorption in the renal tubules. Inflammation and fibrosis lead to renal scarring, which contributes to further nephron loss, creating a cycle of impaired glomerular filtration and nephron destruction (Huether, 2012a).

The effects of CKD are related to kidney damage, and the metabolic changes that occur as a result of declining glomerular filtration are evidenced systemically. Creatinine and urea blood levels rise as the kidney is unable to excrete the by-products of protein metabolism. In early CKD, sodium levels drop as the kidney is not able to reabsorb sodium and, along with polyurea, predisposes the individual to hyponatremia. In contrast, in advanced CKD, as urine production declines, serum sodium levels rise, predisposing the individual to peripheral edema and hypertension. As potassium levels rise in the later stages of CKD and are coupled with inadequate restriction of potassium from other sources (diet, transfusions, medications), the individual is at increased risk for lethal dysrhythmias. Acid–base imbalance occurs as kidney function declines, because bicarbonate is not reabsorbed and ammonia is not produced in sufficient amounts to facilitate cellular transfer of hydrogen ions into the urine. These changes lead to acidosis, which is manifested by Kussmaul breathing as the lungs attempt to accommodate for the decreased blood pH (Capriotti, 2020; Norton et al., 2017b; Winkelman, 2018b).

Changes in lipid concentrations result from uremia. Levels of hepatic triglyceride lipase decline, leading to elevated triglycerides. *Low-density lipoprotein* (LDL) levels increase as *high-density lipoprotein* (HDL) levels decrease, predisposing the individual to atherosclerosis. After the GFR falls to around 25%, hypocalcemia develops, as the kidney is no longer able to synthesize 1,25-dihydroxyvitamin D$_3$. As serum calcium levels fall, the parathyroid glands are stimulated to secrete parathyroid hormone, leading to osteoporosis as calcium is reabsorbed from bone into the blood. Additionally, glucose intolerance as insulin action is impaired due to hyperparathyroidism along with adipokine and proinflammatory cytokine alterations (Huether, 2012a).

Assessment

Urinary system assessment that leads to a diagnosis of chronic kidney disease begins with a health history that includes personal and family history of renal disease, percussion of the *costovertebral angle* (CVA) for renal tenderness, and palpation of the kidneys during the abdominal examination for presence of kidney masses, which when associated with abdominal or flank pain and hematuria, trigger a prompt referral to a urologist. Palpation of the kidney can be accomplished by placing one hand over the area of the 10th to 12th ribs, while placing the other hand over the CVA. Following a deep breath as the patient exhales, the kidney's lower pole can be felt by the hand placed over the ribs (Quallich & Lajiness, 2015). In addition to abnormal urinalysis findings, the effects of inadequate filtration of waste products are seen in many body systems. Severity of symptoms increase, as fewer healthy nephrons are available and as CKD progresses. Common symptoms of CKD are highlighted in Table 23–1.

Diagnostic studies are performed to identify the cause of any red flags identified in the renal assessment, including reports of hematuria, pain, oliguria, anuria, or urinary retention. Typical laboratory studies include CBC, urinalysis, GFR, serum creatinine, *blood urea nitrogen* (BUN), and serum and urine electrolyte studies. Presence of albumin, blood, or protein in the urine is an indication of abnormal kidney function (Quallich & Lajiness, 2015). Additional tests, including *urine albumin-to-creatinine ratio* (UACR), are performed based on the initial laboratory findings (Norton et al., 2017a).

Several laboratory tests are used to evaluate kidney function by measuring the kidney's ability to filter substances from the blood within a given period of time (Huether, 2012b). The GFR is a measurement of kidney function and is dependent on perfusion pressure within the glomerular capillaries (Winkelman, 2018a). Normally, 20% to 25% of cardiac output, or between 90 and 120 mL of blood, flows through the kidneys each minute (Capriotti, 2020). Of this volume, between 600 mL to 700 mL is plasma (Huether, 2012b). Glomerular filtration rate is used to determine the effectiveness of nephron function (Norton et al., 2017a).

Elevated urine albumin levels indicate kidney damage (Winkelman, 2018b). Healthy nephron tubules reabsorb almost all protein from the glomerular filtrate. The UACR is a spot urine test (as opposed to a timed test over a period of hours) used to evaluate glomerular permeability by measuring the amount of albumin in the urine. While urine albumin levels fluctuate, creatinine excretion is about 1 g/24 hours, making the test a good reflection of 24-hour urine albumin levels. A urine dipstick will turn positive when urine albumin levels reach 300 mg/g, and persistent albuminuria is often the first sign of declining kidney function (Norton et al., 2017a).

Muscle metabolism produces creatinine that moves into circulation to be excreted by the kidneys, and rising *serum creatinine* levels are indicative of reduced kidney

TABLE 23–1   Common Systemic Symptoms of Chronic Kidney Disease

System	Symptoms
Cardiovascular	Heart failure Hypertension Lethal dysthymias Peripheral edema
Gastrointestinal	Anorexia GI upset (nausea, vomiting, diarrhea) Metallic taste
Hematological	Anemia Thrombocytopenia
Integumentary	Bruising Pruritus Sallow skin color
Immune	Increased risk of infection
Metabolic	Dyslipidemia Elevated creatinine and BUN Hyperkalemia Hypoalbuminemia Metabolic acidosis (when GFR falls to 30%–40%)
Musculoskeletal	Decreased bone density (fractures) Muscle cramps Muscle weakness
Neurological	Confusion, disorientation *Later stages*: Stupor, coma, peripheral neuropathy
Respiratory	Kussmaul breathing Pulmonary edema Shortness of breath Tachypnea
Reproductive	Disruption of menstrual cycle Infertility Sexual dysfunction
Urinary	Hematuria Proteinuria Presence of white blood cells *Early stages*: Polyuria, diluted urine *Later stages*: Oliguria, concentrated urine

(Adapted from Capriotti, 2020; Huether, 2012a; Norton et al., 2017b; Winkelman, 2018b)

function. Because serum creatinine levels are influenced by age, muscle mass, race, and sex, creatinine clearance results must be used in conjunction with other tests to determine kidney function (Norton et al., 2017a). The *creatinine clearance* test is also used to measure decline in nephron filtering function and is a more sensitive test than the serum creatinine, which often remains within normal limits until creatinine clearance levels fall to less than one-half normal levels. This timed urine test compares urine creatinine levels with serum creatinine levels during the timed study and may be repeated at intervals to evaluate the progression of kidney disease (Corbett & Banks, 2013).

Protein metabolism results in the creation of *urea* in the liver, which moves through circulation to be excreted by the kidneys. Although extremes in hydration levels along with liver disease influence serum urea levels, the BUN test is often used as a method of assessing the kidney's ability to filter and concentrate urine (Corbett & Banks, 2013; Huether, 2012b). Normal reference values for estimated GFR (eGFR), BUN, and creatinine clearance are highlighted in Table 23-2.

Monitoring kidney function over a 3-month period allows time to distinguish between an acute kidney injury that resolves and a chronic condition that requires a different treatment approach (McManus & Wynter-Minott, 2017). Unfortunately, patients with CKD are often asymptomatic in the early stages, leading to delays in diagnosis, failure of individuals to recognize the importance of interventions, and further progression of the disease (Norton et al., 2017a). A kidney biopsy is typically used to determine the underlying cause of CKD; however, individuals with diabetes are diagnosed without a biopsy based on a UACR greater than 30 mg/g or a diagnosis of type 1 diabetes for at least 10 years and diabetic retinopathy in conjunction with a UACR greater than 30 mg/g (Norton et al., 2017).

The five stages of CKD are based on a classification system that assesses GFR and degree of albuminuria, which has been associated with cardiovascular disease, increased mortality, and development of renal failure (KDIGO, 2013; McManus & Wynter-Minott, 2017; Winkelman, 2018b). In *stage 1*, GFR ranges from normal to levels above 90 mL/minute. The disease is usually asymptomatic at this stage, but some individuals may exhibit signs of hypertension. *Stage 2* disease signs are often subtle with only mild degrees of kidney damage, a slightly decreased GFR of 60 to 89 mL/minute, slightly increased creatinine and BUN levels, and hypertension. Moderate kidney damage with decreased GRF between 30 to 59 mL/minute describes *stage 3* disease. Signs and symptoms continue to be subtle and mild. However, as the disease progresses to *stage 4*, there is severe kidney damage and GFR is decreased to 15 to 29 mL/min. In this stage, patients experience edema from sodium and water retention; hypertension; anemia related to erythropoietin deficiency; and increased serum phosphorus, potassium, and triglyceride levels; and management of symptoms becomes a priority to prevent further kidney damage. Progression of CKD to *stage 5* is known as

TABLE 23–2 Normal Values for Common Kidney Function Tests

Test	Normal	Abnormal Results
BUN	10–20 mg/dL	(Will be higher in older adults)
Serum creatinine	Men: 0.6–1.5 mg/dL Women: 0.6–1.1 mg/dL	Increased in kidney disease
Creatinine clearance	Men: 95–135 mL/min Women: 85–125 mL/min	Decreased with decreased glomerular function; may be lower in the older adult without kidney disease
BUN/creatinine ratio	6:1 to 20:1	
estimated GFR	>60 mL/min for both African Americans and non–African Americans	Used to stage (3, 4, or 5) chronic kidney disease May be elevated in the older adult without kidney disease
UACR	<30 mg/g	Elevated in chronic kidney disease

(Corbett & Banks, 2013; Norton et al., 2017a; Winkelman, 2018b)

end-stage kidney disease (ESKD) and is diagnosed based on a GFR of less than 15 mL/minute with more severe exacerbation of the signs and symptoms of stage 4 disease (Huether, 2012a; Winkelman, 2018a).

As mentioned above, CKD classification now includes albuminuria staging. In stage A1 (microalbuminuria), UACR ratios are negative or only slightly increased to less than 30 mg/g with creatinine levels less than 30 mg/mmol. In stage A2, UACR levels rise to between 30 and 300 mg/g with creatinine of 3 to 30 mg/mmol. As the disease progresses to stage A3, UACR levels exceed 300 mg/g with a creatinine of greater than 30 mg/mmol (KDIGO, 2013; Winkelman, 2018b). As the urine albumin levels rise, the individual is at increased risk of progression to ESKD and death (Winkelman, 2018b). A comprehensive plan of care considers the stage of renal disease as defined by laboratory findings, symptoms, and comorbidities and is aimed to slow or stop disease progression (Mallappallil et al., 2014).

ASSESSMENT PEARLS

The least invasive and inexpensive method of assessing kidney function is the urinalysis, which evaluates urine for color, clarity, specific gravity, pH, and presence of bacteria, blood, casts, glucose, and protein (Huether, 2012b). The presence of protein in the urine is a classic sign of kidney disease (Capriotti, 2020).

Risk Factors for CKD

As with most diseases, there are modifiable and nonmodifiable risk factors for CKD. Nonmodifiable risk factors include age, ethnicity/race, gender, family history, and low birth weight. Behaviors that increase risk (modifiable) include smoking and use of NSAIDs and antibiotics known to be nephrotoxic. Cessation of smoking and discriminate use of medications known to be nephrotoxic are ways to mitigate risks of CKD. Conditions that increase risk of CKD include cardiovascular disease, diabetes, high-protein diets, hypertension, obesity, and hyperlipidemia. Careful management of these conditions decreases risk of developing CKD (Mallappallil et al., 2014).

Patient education focused on kidney health includes tips on maintaining normal blood pressure, achieving blood glucose target levels, smoking cessation (if applicable), weight control, and physical activity (CDC, 2020a). Dietary recommendations are essential to the teaching plan. Nutritional considerations for the patient with kidney disease include regulation of protein and sodium intake and inclusion of complex carbohydrates, fruits, and vegetables in the diet (Kalantar-Zadeh & Fouque, 2017).

Nonpharmacological Management

One of the first steps to managing chronic kidney disease is completion of a risk assessment with the goal of early identification and slowing of progression of kidney damage (Mallappallil et al., 2014). Acute care treatment is often focused on the acute disease, while primary care treatment focuses on controlling disease progression. Treatment algorithms can be useful in guiding primary care providers in determining whether the patient at risk for CKD has evidence of the disease or requires a referral to a nephrologist for further evaluation. Patients assessed with hyperkalemia, heart failure, uremia, or unexplained kidney function decline meet the requirements for urgent/emergent care in an acute care setting (Chronic Kidney Disease Working Group, 2014).

Successful management of CKD requires an interdisciplinary team approach to monitoring comorbid conditions and a collaborative effort to engage the patient in self-management of this chronic disease. Self-management strategies include behavior

---

SENC BOX 23–1 Safe and Effective Nursing Care for Support and Self-Management for CKD Patients

Encouraging self-care, use of coping strategies, and family involvement and support are keys to decreasing the anxiety and depression commonly associated with CKD (Winkelman, 2018b). Key to self-management is education on the disease process and the importance of lifestyle changes that slow progression of nephron damage (Rivera, 2017).

---

modifications related to diet, exercise, and weight management with a goal of improving overall health (Chronic Kidney Disease Working Group, 2014). The goals of nutritional disease management are to slow progression of CKD while providing a healthy diet that avoids malnutrition and complications directly related to diet (Kalantar-Zadeh & Fouque, 2017; Norton et al., 2017a). See SENC Box 23–1.

Dietary restrictions are essential to controlling the effects of excessive protein and sodium on damaged nephrons. Limiting protein consumption reduces albuminuria and has been shown to slow progression of CKD and reduce risk for metabolic acidosis. Therefore, protein consumption for non-diabetics with CKD should be limited to 0.8 g/kg/day, and for diabetic patients, limited to 0.8 to 1.0 g/kg/day (Norton et al., 2017a).

To effectively support blood pressure control, it is recommended that sodium consumption be limited to no more than 1,500 mg each day (USDHHS, 2015). Patients should be educated that sea salt has the same amount of sodium as regular table salt. Additionally, potassium intake should be limited once the serum potassium levels rise above 5.0 mEq /L, and patients should be cautioned to avoid salt substitutes that contain potassium (Norton et al., 2017a). Avoidance of foods high in potassium content, including certain juices (grapefruit, orange, or prune), is important, particularly if the patient is also taking an *angiotensin-converting enzyme* (ACE) or *angiotensin receptor blocker* (ARB), as this combination increases risk for hyperkalemia. Substitution of cranberry juice, which has less potassium, is appropriate for those who want a juice drink. Light colas that are typically lower in phosphates are better choices than dark colas, which are typically higher in phosphates (Norton et al., 2017a). An important part of dietary education is to teach patients how to read food labels and, because the source of a majority (75%) of daily sodium intake is consumed from processed foods or when eating out, to encourage purchase of fresh foods that can be prepared at home (Norton et al., 2017a).

It is important to note that dietary and fluid volume management requirements change as kidney disease progresses and that patients will need dietary guidance from a registered dietitian to customize the diet to meet their economic situation, and personal and ethnic preferences. Patients with renal disease will also need support from those living with them to successfully follow a restricted diet (Winkelman, 2018b). Fluid volume management is important to managing blood pressure and controlling edema. To avoid hyponatremia in stage 3 CKD, fluid restriction to 1.5 L/day is suggested, but adjusted for fever or other conditions where insensible fluid loss is increased or in hot environmental conditions (Kalantar-Zadeh & Fouque, 2017).

RED FLAG ALERT

Because patients with CKD are at significant risk for infection and death related to infections, it is important for these patients to receive a yearly influenza vaccination and initial and follow-up pneumococcal pneumonia vaccinations, and for those in stage 4 and 5 CKD to receive a hepatitis B vaccination (McManus & Wynter-Minott, 2017). Administration of live vaccines is contraindicated for most CKD patients, particularly those on immunosuppressive drugs (Chronic Kidney Disease Working Group, 2014).

Accurate daily weights are needed to monitor fluid gain. These are best obtained by weighing on the same scales at the same time of day while wearing approximately the same weight of clothing. Additionally, the daily weight should be obtained after the patient has voided. When tracking weight trends, remember that 1 L of fluid weighs 1 kg. When fluid restrictions are ordered, fluids from all sources are counted in the daily total, which should be divided throughout the 24 hours (Winkelman, 2018b).

Pharmacology

Because CKD affects all body systems, a wide variety of drugs may be used to treat symptoms. The goals of pharmacological management of CKD are to manage symptoms while slowing or preventing progression of kidney damage. In particular, doses for older patients or for those with advanced CKD may need to be adjusted to avoid accumulation of toxic blood levels (Mallappallil et al., 2014). Plasma protein is lost as large protein molecules are allowed into the urine filtrate (albuminuria), leading to *hypertension* (HTN) and edema. Pharmacological options to treat HTN and edema include drugs that block the RAAS, including ACEs used to block angiotensin I conversion to angiotensin II, and ARBs, which are angiotensin II blockers. These drug classes work to decrease glomerular pressure with a goal of prolonging exposure of blood to the filtration process (McManus & Wynter-Minott, 2017; Norton et al., 2017a). However, due to the risks of hyperkalemia and hypotension, it is not recommended to combine these drug classes when treating CKD (Prasad-Reddy, Isaacs, & Kantorovich, 2017). See Chapter 20 for a more detailed discussion of ACEs and ARBs.

Loop diuretics are used to treat peripheral edema that results from failure of damaged nephrons to prevent albumin excretion and water reabsorption. Anemia can be treated with *erythropoiesis-stimulating agents* (ESA), and accompanying iron deficiency can be treated with oral or intravenous iron drugs. Vitamin D deficiency is addressed by supplemental replacement (Atkinson & Warady, 2018; McManus & Wynter-Minott, 2017; Norton et al., 2017a; Prasad-Reddy et al., 2017). However, when nephron damage is extensive, serum levels of diuretics rise, causing further injury; thus, diuretics are discontinued when the patient begins dialysis (Winkelman, 2018b). Drugs in these classes used to treat CKD are highlighted in Table 23-3.

Some drugs should be avoided in the presence of CKD, including most *over-the-counter* (OTC) drugs. Most drugs are excreted by the kidneys and may need to be avoided or to have their dosage and timing adjusted based on the kidney's declining ability to filter and excrete drugs. Once identified as being in stage 3 CKD, patients are cautioned to avoid NSAIDs, but they can use low-dose aspirin therapy (Garcin, 2015). Additionally, magnesium-containing antacids should be avoided, because the kidney cannot excrete magnesium. In later stages of CKD, when drugs are known to accumulate in the blood, dose adjustments must be made for analgesics including opioids, antibiotics, digoxin, lipid-lowering statins, insulin, or other antidiabetic drugs to avoid toxic levels and adverse reactions (McManus & Wynter-Minott, 2017; Winkelman, 2018b).

Dialysis and Surgical Treatment

As kidney disease progresses to stages 4 and 5, additional filtration methods may be required to maintain fluid and electrolyte balance. *Hemodialysis* requires a permanent vascular access but has the advantage of a shortened time for each (3 to 4 hours) treatment. It is more efficient in filtering wastes, but has higher hemodynamic complications including hypotension, dysrhythmias, and cell lysis. Hemodialysis must be

TABLE 23–3   Drugs Used to Treat Chronic Kidney Disease

Class	Example	Action	Dosage	SENC
Loop diuretics	Furosemide	Diuresis and hypokalemic effects.	20–80 mg day to a max of 600 mg/day. Renal impairment: 2–2.5 g/day.	Give at 8 a.m. and 2 p.m; many drug–drug interactions including some effects that may be ↑ in CKD (e.g., digoxin–dig toxicity), ↑ anticoagulant effects.
Erythropoietin-stimulating agents (exogenous erythropoietin)	Epoetin-alpha	Stimulates the bone marrow to produce RBCs.	50–100 units/kg subcutaneous (or IV) 3 × / week.	If given to patients with normal renal function, ↑ risk of endogenous erythropoietin production leading to ↑ severity of anemia. May cause arthralgias, fatigue, and weakness (asthenia).
Iron preparations	Ferrous sulfate Iron dextran	Increases serum iron concentration, converted to hemoglobin (Hgb) or is stored in the liver, spleen, bone marrow.	100–200 mg/day PO Test dose of 0.5 mL (25 mg) 1 hr prior to regular dose. Dose calculated based on lean body weight and desired Hgb. Max dose 100 mg/day over 4–5 hr.	Take 2 hours before or after antacids, cimetidine; ciprofloxacin or ofloxacin; levodopa; tetracyclines. Also avoid taking with eggs, coffee, tea, or milk. Keep patient recumbent for 30 min after administration to avoid orthostatic hypotension.
Parathyroid hormone modulators Antihypocalcemics	Cinacalcet (Sensipar®) Calcitriol	Hypocalcemic used to ↓ parathyroid hormone production to reduce serum calcium levels. Vitamin D compound; regulates calcium and phosphate absorption in the small intestine, reabsorption of calcium in the bone and phosphate in the renal tubules.	300 mg daily; ↑ every 2–4 weeks with a range of 30–180 mg/ daily. 0.5–2 mcg/day PO in the a.m.	Avoid use if serum calcium is <8.0 mg/dL. Monitor for hypocalcemia (cramping, myalgias, paresthesias, seizures). May cause metallic taste, dry mouth, nausea/vomiting, and weakness.
Vitamins/minerals	**Vitamin D** Calcitriol (1,25-dihydroxycholecalciferol)	Active form of vitamin D used in CKD dialysis to treat vitamin D deficiency.	0.25 mcg/day with average dose 0.5–1 mcg/day	Caution with digoxin; side effects related to hypercalcemia.
	Phosphate binders Calcium carbonate	Inhibits GI absorption of phosphates by binding to dietary phosphate; the resulting calcium phosphate complex is then excreted in feces.	1–2 g/day	Take with meals; has many drug–drug interactions. Avoid with digoxin and hypocalcemia or with use of other calcium supplements (calcium citrate) due to increased aluminum absorption

(Karch, 2020; McManus & Wynter-Minott, 2017; Robinson, 2020a, 2020b; Vallerand & Sanoski, 2015; Winkelman, 2018b)

SENC BOX 23–2   Safe and Effective Nursing Care for Support and Self-Management for Dialysis Patients

Nurses can help patients and their families adjust to dialysis by providing resources that help them with informed decision making and active participation in their care. Start with individualized education that includes basic information on dialysis (hemodialysis or peritonea), infection prevention, and patient education sheets. Patient resources include links to the National Kidney Foundation and End Stage Renal Disease (ESRD) networks. These websites include information on infection prevention, preparing for natural disasters (flood, hurricane, power outages), support networks, and insurance and Medicare (CDC, 2019).

performed at least three times a week; if traveling, the patient must arrange for treatment at a different location.

If the individual needs a flexible schedule and has no history of abdominal surgery that would prevent catheter placement, *peritoneal dialysis* may be a better option. Although less stringent dietary restrictions are required and fewer hemodynamic complications are reported, there is a high risk for infection, hyperglycemia, and peritonitis. Patients must restrict potassium and are at risk of weight gain from the additional dextrose that is absorbed from the dialysate. Additionally, peritoneal dialysis must be performed daily and length of dwell time (time dialysate is kept in the abdominal cavity) is individualized. Equipment must be stored and carefully maintained (Norton et al., 2017b; Winkelman, 2018b). Regardless of the type of dialysis, the older patient is at higher risk for HTN related to the procedure (Winkelman, 2018b). See SENC Box 23–2 for guidelines on support and self-management for dialysis patients.

Kidney transplantation is a treatment, not a cure, for end-stage kidney disease, and with the short supply of donor organs, careful consideration of likelihood of successful transplant is essential when evaluating the CKD patient for surgery. In 2016, approximately 100,000 people were on the kidney transplant list, with about 3,000 being added each month. While wait times are dependent on the patient's health status and the availability and compatibility of available organs, a typical median time between listing and first transplant is 3.6 years (NKF, 2017). While eligibility requirements vary among transplant centers, the recipient of a live or deceased donor kidney must be healthy enough to survive the lengthy surgical procedure and must be willing to adhere to the strict regimen of antirejection drugs and careful follow-up following the surgery (Norton et al., 2017b; Winkelman, 2018b). The average transplant candidate is under 70 years of age, but older adults are considered on an individual basis (Winkelman, 2018b). Individuals with a recent cancer diagnosis, chronic infections, chronic pulmonary disease, or substance abuse issues are at high risk for complications. Those with a recent cancer diagnosis or who have coronary artery disease are not considered appropriate candidates for transplant. Those with significant gastrointestinal (GI) conditions including diverticulitis or peptic ulcers must have their conditions treated prior to transplant to avoid worsening of the condition as a result of high steroid doses in the post-transplant period (Norton et al., 2017b; Winkelman, 2018b).

Summary

An estimated 10% of the worldwide population has CKD, and of individuals 65 to 74 years old the disease affects approximately "one in five men and one in four women"

(NKF, 2015). Understanding the aging kidney, risk factors for kidney disease, and treatment options is important to preventing disease progression and maintaining quality of life of patients with kidney disease. Finally, regardless of the stage of renal disease or treatment options under consideration, the patient with CKD requires access to a wide variety of resources to achieve optimal outcomes. Key members of an interdisciplinary team include primary and specialist providers, nurses who understand the complex needs of the CKD patient, dietitians to guide food and fluid choices, physical therapists to maintain activities of daily living and functional abilities, pastoral care for spiritual needs and/ or psychiatric support for depression, pharmacists to answer questions about medication regimens, and social workers to help obtain needed resources.

Key Points

- The kidney has twice the number of nephrons needed to adequately filter blood waste products and compensate as nephrons are damaged, delaying identification of CKD until about 75% of nephrons are damaged.
- Glomerular filtration rate and urine albumin-to-creatinine ratio findings are used to stage the degree of kidney damage from CKD.
- Pharmacological treatment of CKD includes a combination of ACE inhibitors, ARBs, loop diuretics, and vitamin and minerals supplements aimed at managing symptoms of inadequate glomerular filtration.
- Regardless of the stage of CKD, the individual requires a coordinated interdisciplinary approach to care planning.

Review Questions

1. **The nurse is teaching a 70-year-old patient who has just been diagnosed with chronic kidney disease (CKD). Which of the following is the nurse's best response to the patient's question, "Why did the doctor not 'catch' this before I had so much kidney damage?"**

   a. "The doctor did the best that he could to monitor your kidney function."
   b. "The body has more nephrons than it needs and compensates until most nephrons are damaged."
   c. "Kidney disease is rare in older adults, so the doctor did not anticipate you would get CKD."
   d. "You should have come in for your 6-month checkup and he would have found it."

2. **When conducting a history assessment of the renal system, which of the following are important red flags for CKD? (Select all that apply.)**

   a. Hematuria
   b. Orthostatic hypotension
   c. Sodium intake 1,200 mg/day
   d. Urine protein +1
   e. Urine albumin level 330 mg/day

3. **The nurse is caring for a patient CKD and understands that the patient with a history of which of the following would not be a candidate for diagnostic kidney biopsy?**

   a. Coronary artery disease
   b. Diabetes mellitus
   c. Hematuria
   d. Pulmonary fibrosis

4. **According to the KDIGO classification system, a glomerular filtration rate (GFR) of 58 mL/minute indicates that the nurse should include which of the following in patient education?**

    a. "This is a normal rate, and you only need to adjust your diet to restrict protein and sodium."
    b. "You only have mild kidney damage, and the doctor will order more tests in 2 months."
    c. "You will need to start hemodialysis to treat your severe kidney disease."
    d. "Your elevated blood pressure and laboratory values indicate that you have moderate kidney damage."

5. **The nurse is providing education to the patient with newly diagnosed CKD on how to take a loop diuretic. Which of the following statements lets the nurse know that the patient understands instructions?**

    a. "I can take Tylenol to help with my joint pain while on this medication."
    b. "I will take this medication at 8 a.m. and 2 p.m. to be effective and help me sleep at night."
    c. "I will take this medication with at least one 8-ounce glass of water three times a day."
    d. "To help my diuretic work better, I should drink cranberry juice instead of orange juice."

See the appendix for answers to review questions.

References

Atkinson, M. A., & Warady, B. A. (2018). Anemia in chronic kidney disease. *Pediatric Nephrology, 33*, 227–238. doi:10.1007/s00467-017-3663-y

Capriotti, T. (2020). *Pathophysiology: Introductory concepts and clinical perspectives* (2nd ed.). Philadelphia, PA: F.A. Davis.

Centers for Disease Control and Prevention. (2020a). *Dialysis safety:*. Retrieved from https://www.cdc.gov/dialysis/patient/index.html

Centers for Disease Control and Prevention. (2020b). *Chronic kidney disease basics*. Retrieved from https://www.cdc.gov/kidneydisease/basics.html

Chronic Kidney Disease Working Group. (2014). *VA/DoD clinical practice guideline for the management of chronic kidney disease in primary care: Guideline summary*. Department of Veterans Affairs/Department of Defense. Retrieved from https://www.healthquality.va.gov/guidelines/CD/ckd/CKDSUM5fIA542017.pdf

Corbett, J. V., & Banks, A. D. (2013). *Laboratory tests and diagnostic procedures with nursing diagnose*. (8th ed.). Upper Saddle River, NJ: Pearson Education.

Garcin, A. (2015). Care of the patient with chronic kidney disease. *Med-Surg Matters, 24*(5), 4–7.

Huether. S. E. (2012a). Alterations of renal and urinary tract function. In S. E. Huether & K. L. McCance (Eds.), *Understanding pathophysiology* (5th ed.). St. Louis, MO: Elsevier Mosby.

Huether. S. E. (2012b). Structure and function of the renal and urologic systems. In S. E. Huether & K. L. McCance (Eds.), *Understanding pathophysiology* (5th ed.). St. Louis, MO: Elsevier Mosby.

Kalantar-Zadeh, K., & Fouque, D. (2017). Nutritional management of chronic kidney disease. *New England Journal of Medicine, 377*(18), 1765–1776.

Karch, A. M. (2020). *Focus on nursing pharmacology* (8th ed.). Philadelphia, PA: Wolters Kluwer / Lippincott Williams & Wilkins.

KDIGO. (2013). Kidney disease improving global outcomes. In *KDIGO 2012. Clinical practice guideline for the evaluation and management of chronic kidney disease*. https://kdigo.org/wp-content/uploads/2017/02/KDIGO_2012_CKD_GL.pdf

Mallappallil, M., Friedman, E. A., Delano, B. G., McFarlane, S. I., & Salifu, M. O. (2014). Chronic kidney disease in the elderly: Evaluation and management. *Clinical Practice, 11*(5), 525–535.

McManus, M. S., & Wynter-Minott, S. (2017). Guidelines for chronic kidney disease: Defining, staging, and managing in primary care. *The Journal for Nurse Practitioners, 13*(6), 400–410.

National Kidney Foundation. (2015). Global facts: About kidney disease. Retrieved from https://www.kidney.org/kidneydisease/global-facts-about-kidney-disease

National Kidney Foundation. (2017). *Organ donation and transplantation statistics*. Retrieved from https://www.kidney.org/news/newsroom/factsheets/Organ-Donation-and-Transplantation-Stats

Norton, J. M., Newman, E. P., Romancito, G., Mahooty, S., Kuracina, T., & Narva, A. S. (2017a). Improving outcomes for patients with chronic kidney disease: Part 1. *American Journal of Nursing, 117*(2), 22–32.

Norton, J. M., Newman, E. P., Romancito, G., Mahooty, S., Kuracina, T., & Narva, A. S. (2017b). Improving outcomes for patients with chronic kidney disease: Part 2. *American Journal of Nursing, 117*(3), 26–35.

Prasad-Reddy, L., Isaacs, D., & Kantorovich, A. (2017). Considerations and controversies in managing chronic kidney disease: An update. *American Journal of Health-Systems Pharmacists, 74*(11), 795–810.

Quallich, S. A., & Lajiness, M. (2015). Genitourinary system. In M. J. Goolsby & L. Grubbs (Eds.), *Advanced assessment: Interpreting findings and formulating differential diagnoses.* Philadelphia, PA: F.A. Davis.

Rivera, S. (2017). Identifying and eliminating the barriers to patient education for patients in the early stages of chronic kidney disease. *Nephrology Nursing Journal, 44*(3), 211–216.

Robinson, M. V. (2020a). Drugs affecting the cardiovascular and renal systems. In T. M. Woo & M. V. Robinson (Eds.), *Pharmacotherapeutics for advance practice nurse prescribers* (5th ed.). Philadelphia, PA: F.A. Davis.

Robinson, M. V. (2020b). Hyperlipidemia. In T. M. Woo & M. V. Robinson (Eds.), *Pharmacotherapeutics for advance practice nurse prescribers* (5th ed.). Philadelphia, PA: F.A. Davis.

Scanlon, V. C., & Sanders, T. (2019). *Essentials of anatomy and physiology* (8th ed.). Philadelphia, PA: F.A. Davis.

Vallerand, A. H., & Sanoski, C. A. (Eds.). (2017). *Davis's drug guide for nurses* (15th ed.). Philadelphia, PA: F.A. Davis.

Winkelman, C. (2018a). Assessment of the renal/urinary system. In D. D. Ignatavicius, L. Workman, & C. R. Rebar (Eds.), *Medical-surgical nursing: Concepts for interprofessional collaborative care* (9th ed.). St. Louis, MO: Elsevier.

Winkelman, C. (2018b). Care of patients with acute kidney injury and chronic kidney disease In D. D. Ignatavicius, L. Workman, & C. R. Rebar (Eds.), *Medical-surgical nursing: Concepts for interprofessional collaborative care* (9th ed.). St. Louis, MO: Elsevier.

World Kidney Day. (2019). CKD in elderly people. Retrieved from https://www.worldkidneyday.org/faqs/chronic-kidney-disease/

Case Study 5 (Geriatrics): Osteoporosis

LEARNING OBJECTIVES

Upon completion of this case study the student will be able to integrate knowledge of the pathophysiology, assessment/diagnosis, and treatment options for care of a patient with osteoporosis.

Introduction to Osteoporosis

Osteoporosis, a metabolic disease of decreased *bone mineral density* (BMD), is a worldwide major health concern, with more than 8.9 million fractures attributed to the disease each year (International Osteoporosis Foundation [IOF], 2017). It is a "silent disease," with symptoms typically not presenting until the individual experiences their first fracture (Ignatavicius, 2018). In the United States, more than 55% of adults over 50 years old are estimated to have either decreased bone mass (*osteopenia*) or diagnosed osteoporosis. Worldwide, for this same population, at least 1 in 3 women and 1 in 5 men are anticipated to experience one fracture related to osteoporosis (IOF, 2017). The disease increases mortality and negatively impacts quality of life in terms of disability, pain, and increased health-care costs related to fracture care, hospitalization, nursing home placement, and pharmacological management of the disease (IOF, 2017; Jeremiah, Unwin, & Greenawald, 2015). Early identification of risk factors, appropriate screening, and health promotion intervention, along with appropriate treatment of the disease, are key to reducing the overall impact of osteoporosis. This case study focuses on the pathophysiology, assessment and diagnosis, and treatment options for management of osteoporosis.

Meet Mrs. JS

Mrs. JS is a 70-year-old Asian woman who lives with her son and his family. She has presented to the emergency room (ER) following a fall at home and is accompanied by her son. The ER nurse (Nurse MA) discovers that English is her second language and is able to answer questions about her history and current conditions. She has been in the United States for 30 years but was not employed outside the home. Mrs. JS complains of severe pain (10 on a scale of 0 to 10) in her right wrist. Her vital signs are normal; however, when measuring weight (100 pounds) and height, Nurse MA finds that Mrs. JS's measured height is one-half inch shorter than her reported height.

Physiology and Pathophysiology

Cortical bone (85% of all bone) is made up of the Haversian system, a complex system of canals surrounded by layers of *osteocytes*, minerals and proteins that form a dense matrix. Cancellous bone (15% of all bone) is porous bone that forms an irregular network containing bone marrow. Bone remodeling is facilitated by the interactions of *osteoblasts* (bone-forming cells) and *osteoclasts* (bone-resorption cells), while osteocytes make up the majority (90% to 95%) of the bone's matrix and mediate the remodeling process (Abel, 2013; Curtis, Moon, Dennison, Harvey, & Cooper, 2016).

Bone remodeling occurs over a period of months as osteoblasts and osteoclasts work to together to create new bone and reabsorb old bone. Normally, new bone growth occurs faster than resorption of old bone until around age 30, the point at which bone density is at its peak. After this, bone density remains stable during mid-life, then changes as one ages, so that over time, bone resorption occurs at a faster rate than new bone is formed (Abel, 2013; Curtis et al., 2016; Hallock, 2017). If the process accelerates and bone loss significantly exceeds bone formation, cortical bone becomes thin, porous, and fragile, predisposing the individual to fracture. Despite the normal shift in the remodeling process, osteoporosis is not a normal part of the aging process (Crowther-Radulewicz & McCance, 2012).

The etiology of *primary* osteoporosis can be related to genetics, environment, and certain lifestyle choices. These include inadequate calcium intake; lack of sunlight exposure and low vitamin D levels inhibiting calcium absorption; and sedentary lifestyle with limited weight-bearing exercise. *Secondary* osteoporosis has its origins in hormonal disorders, bowel conditions, or as the result of prolonged use of certain medications (Capriotti, 2020; Ignatavicius, 2018). Table CS5–1 highlights risk factors for osteoporosis.

TABLE CS5–1   Risk Factors for Primary and Secondary Osteoporosis

Primary	Secondary
Genetic • Age • Body frame (thin, small bones) • Ethnicity (Asian, Caucasian) • Family history of osteoporosis or hip fracture • Gender (Female > Male) • History of falls	**Hormonal** • Early menopause (natural or after surgery) without hormone replacement therapy (HRT) • Late menarche • Nulliparity

Nutrition
• ↓ calcium and vitamin D intake
• Protein intake in excess or low levels
• Lactose intolerance
	Metabolic Conditions
	• Chronic diseases:
	  ○ Diabetes mellitus
	  ○ Chronic obstructive pulmonary disease (COPD)
	  ○ Liver disease
	  ○ Renal disease
	• Cushing's disease
	• Hyperthyroidism
	• Hyperparathyroidism
	• Hypogonadism
	• Prolonged immobility
	• Malabsorption conditions

TABLE CS5–1   Risk Factors for Primary and Secondary Osteoporosis—cont'd

Primary	Secondary
Behavior • Excessive alcohol intake • Excessive caffeine or carbonated soda intake • Sedentary (↓ weight-bearing exercise) • Smokes	**Medications** • Aluminum-based antacids • Anticonvulsants (carbamazepine, phenobarbital, or phenytoin) • Corticosteroids (prolonged use >3 months) • Cytotoxic agents • Immunosuppressants • Loop diuretics • Methotrexate • Proton pump inhibitors (used >1 year) • Thyroid medications

(Abel, 2013; Capriotti, 2020; Crowther-Radulewicz & McCance, 2012; Curtis et al., 2016; Hallock, 2017; Ignatavicius, 2018; Robinson, 2020)

Gathering Information

While Mrs. JS is in the emergency room, Nurse MA takes Mrs. JS's medical history, which includes a history of hypothyroidism, gastroesophageal reflux disease (GERD), *a total abdominal hysterectomy at the age of 29, and menopause at age 55 with no hormone replacement therapy. Current medications include levothyroxine 88 mcg daily, esomeprazole 40 mg bid, and low-dose aspirin 88 mg daily. Nurse MA follows up with lifestyle questions that reveal a sedentary lifestyle since retirement 4 years ago. Additionally, Mrs. JS reports that she drinks three cups of coffee a day and, based on her description of nutritional habits, has a low intake of calcium-rich foods. She denies allergies to medications, foods, or environmental triggers or use of herbals or vitamin supplements. She receives Medicare Parts A and B but has no prescription drug plan.*

Assessment and Diagnosis

Diagnosis of osteoporosis depends on a careful assessment of risk factors, physical examination, and laboratory testing. The nurse should be alert to skeletal changes that may indicate the patient has osteoporosis, starting with a decrease in height as vertebrae lose their density and collapse. Kyphosis (commonly known as a Dowager's hump) also becomes more prominent as the thoracic spine curves, and individuals with osteoporotic changes in their vertebrae may lose up to 6 inches in height over time (Crowther-Radulewicz & McCance, 2012; Ignatavicius, 2018; Palmer, 2013). Often kyphosis or a fragility fracture (osteoporotic fracture) of the distal radius (Colles' fracture), hip, or vertebrae is the first sign of osteoporosis (Capriotti, 2020; National Association of Orthopaedic Nurses [NAON], 2014; Palmer, 2013). Women age 65 and older, men age 70 and older, individuals with history of fracture after age 50, and individuals with known risk factors should be screened for osteoporosis (NOF, 2018).

While laboratory findings may be normal in osteoporosis, serum phosphate, alkaline phosphatase, and protein electrophoresis results, in addition to serum calcium levels, may be helpful in determining the extent of the metabolic process. Notably, the *dual-energy x-ray absorptiometry* (DEXA) scan is the gold standard test for diagnosing and monitoring the progression of osteoporosis. During this test, the hip and lumbar spine are exposed to radiation to measure BMD and density, and the size and thickness of bone is calculated to estimate the bone's ability to withstand mechanical stress. The test uses a T-score to compare the individual's BMD with the mean score

TABLE CS5–2   DEXA T-Scores, BMD and Osteoporosis

Category	T-Score
Normal	≥ –1.0
Osteopenia	Between –1.0 to –2.5
Osteoporosis	≤ –2.5
Severe osteoporosis	≤ –2.5 with a fracture

Note: Measurements are based on hip or spine BMD and mean score of healthy 30-year-old female.

(Capriotti, 2020; Jeremiah et al., 2015; National Osteoporosis Foundation [NOF], 2018)

of a healthy 30-year-old female (Brown, 2013; Crowther-Radulewicz & McCance, 2012; Jeremiah et al., 2015; U.S. Preventive Services Task Force [USPSTF], 2018). The test is noninvasive, but the nurse must caution the patient to avoid taking calcium supplements prior to the procedure, to remove any jewelry, to wear clothes without zippers or buttons, and to remove any braces or prosthetics prior to the procedure. The nurse should also inquire whether the patient has a metal implant in the area to be scanned, because the procedure may be contraindicated in this event (Brown, 2013). Table CS5–2 describes osteoporosis categories based on T-score findings.

Similarly, *peripheral dual-energy x-ray absorptiometry* (pDXA) can be used to evaluate BMD in the radius when hip and spine DEXA scan is not possible. Screening with a *quantitative ultrasound* (QUS) evaluation of the calcaneus does not involve radiation and may be helpful as an initial screening tool in rural areas where access to DEXA scanning technology is not available or to identify individuals who are appropriate for DEXA scan; however, the test should be used with caution, as the results do not correlate well with the DEXA scan and cannot be used as a diagnostic tool (Jeremiah et al., 2015; USPSTF, 2018). An additional screening tool is the *Fracture Risk Assessment Tool* (FRAX). This tool uses age, height, weight, and history information to calculate the individual's absolute fracture risk and scores measure the risk of fracture within the next 10 years. Results can be used to plan preventive and treatment interventions (Jeremiah et al.; NOF, 2018).

Diagnosis

ER laboratory findings for Mrs. JS are normal except for a slightly low serum calcium of 8.0 mg/dL (normal 8.5 to 10.2 mg/dL). Following an x-ray, Mrs. JS is diagnosed with a Colles' fracture of the right distal radius and suspected osteoporosis. She is treated with a cast application and is prescribed tramadol 50 mg PO every 4 to 6 hours as needed for severe pain. Nurse MA notes that Mrs. JS has no prescription drug plan, and she inquiries about Mrs. JS's ability to purchase her medication. Her son responds that he will be able to help his mom with any costs for medications and medical care not covered by Medicare. Nurse MA provides medication education and cast care instructions to the patient and her son. Using the "teach-back" format, the nurse presents the information and asks the patient and her son to repeat back the instructions to ensure that the instructions are understood. Mrs. JS is then discharged with referrals to her primary health-care provider for osteoporosis screening and to an orthopedic provider for follow-up fracture care.

Mrs. JS sees her primary provider the following week. The primary provider nurse practitioner (Nurse EM) reviews Mrs. JS's history and ER laboratory results. When asked about her current pain level, Mrs. JS reports a pain level of 2 on a 0 to 10 scale, and that she no longer requires the prescription pain medication. Nurse EM records this information and performs a brief, focused physical assessment. She then informs Mrs. JS that further laboratory and other testing will be needed, provides education on the needed laboratory tests, and gives Mrs. JS instructions on DEXA scan procedures. Laboratory results reveal a low serum vitamin D level of 10 ng/mL (normal 20 to 100 ng/mL), and the DEXA scan reveals her BMD T-score is –2.5. Mrs. JS is diagnosed with osteoporosis.

Treatment Options

Treatment of osteoporosis includes a combination of lifestyle and pharmacological changes designed to slow bone and calcium loss and to prevent fractures (Crowther-Radulewicz & McCance, 2012; Ignatavicius, 2018). Lifestyle changes in diet and activity (regular exercise and exposure to sunlight) are important features of self-care interventions and may be used independently or in conjunction with medication. Common medications include calcium and vitamin D dietary supplements, as well as bisphosphonates or other drugs prescribed to help slow bone reabsorption or to increase bone production (Abel, 2013; Capriotti, 2020; Jeremiah et al., 2015; IOF, 2017). Medications used to treat osteoporosis are highlighted in Table CS5–3.

TABLE CS5–3 Drugs Commonly Used to Treat Osteoporosis

Class	Example	Action	Dosage	SENC
Bisphosphonates	Alendronate	Slows bone resorption but does not inhibit bone formation or mineralization.	Prevention: 35 mg/ weekly. Treatment: 70 mg / weekly.	Drink plenty of fluids to prevent renal complications. Take on empty stomach before breakfast and remain upright for at least 30 min to avoid esophageal irritation; used for men to ↓ vertebral fractures.
Monoclonal antibodies	Denosumab	Inhibits osteoclast formation and inhibits bone resorption.	Subcutaneous injection: 120 mg every 4 weeks; additional doses on days 8 and 15 during the first month of treatment.	Do not shake prefilled syringe; may cause pancreatitis or anaphylaxis; patients need to consume 1,000 mg calcium and 400 IU of vitamin D each day.
Selective estrogen receptor modulators	Raloxifene	Selectively activates estrogen pathways to reduce bone resorption actions of parathyroid hormone. Has antiestrogen effects on breast and uterus.	60 mg/day.	Take with or without food; ↑risk of CVA or thromboembolic event; leg cramps or hot flashes are common side effects.

Continued

TABLE CS5–3 Drugs Commonly Used to Treat Osteoporosis—cont'd

Class	Example	Action	Dosage	SENC
Hormones	Calcitonin	A hypocalcemic that slows progression of postmenopausal bone loss.	Nasal spray most commonly prescribed. Can also be prescribed intravenous and subcutaneous.	Alternate nostrils to avoid irritating nasal mucosa; do not double up on missed doses and discard after 30 days.
	Forteo	Synthetic parathyroid hormone that regulates calcium function.	Subcutaneous injection: 20 mcg daily.	Used if patient has experienced fragility fracture; not recommended for use longer than 2 yr; must be refrigerated. Side effects include arthralgias and orthostatic hypotension.
Calcium	Calcium carbonate	Supplement		Cheapest; highest in elemental calcium/dose; take with food because acid is required for absorption.

Note: Many of these drugs are known to increase serum cholesterol levels. Due to increased risk of osteonecrosis (jaw) and atypical fractures, bisphosphonates are often discontinued after 5 years of therapy.

(Curtis et al., 2016; Jeremiah et al., 2015; Karch, 2020; Robinson, 2020; Vallerand & Sanoski, 2017)

As many as 40% of patients are not compliant with taking their medications after 1 year, however, and this number drops to less than 20% after 2 years (IOF, 2017). Patient education by the nurse is therefore a key component of self-management of osteoporosis and is outlined in SENC Box CS1–1.

Finally, kyphoplasty and vertebroplasty are outpatient surgical procedures that may be indicated to relieve the pain and immobility caused by vertebral compression fractures (Capriotti, 2020).

Treatment and Follow-Up

Following her diagnosis of osteoporosis, Mrs. JS is prescribed Os-Cal with vitamin D and alendronate, a bisphosphonate. Nurse EM encourages Mrs. JS to begin walking as a weight-bearing exercise. She also advises Mrs. JS to decrease her coffee intake, increase her dietary calcium intake, and follow a healthy diet of fruits, vegetables, and proteins. Nurse EM discusses fall prevention strategies and provides information on the disease process and mediation options. She stresses the importance of taking medications as ordered and educates Mrs. JS on how and when to take alendronate. Finally, Nurse EM informs Mrs. JS that she will be scheduled for a repeat DEXA scan in 1 to 2 years after beginning alendronate and encourages her to contact her provider with any questions or concerns. Mrs. JS leaves the provider visit with a clear sense of the scope of her condition and information on what she must do to manage it for optimal quality of life going forward. When repeating the DEXA scan to evaluate medication effectiveness and disease progression, it is recommended to use the same DEXA machine in the same facility to obtain the most accurate comparison of bone density. The nurse includes this information in the patient instructions (Finkelstein & Yu, 2019).

SENC BOX CS5–1   Safe and Effective Nursing Care for Patient Education for Individuals With Osteoporosis

1. Teach the patient about the disease process and treatment plan, symptom management, and when to call the provider. (This is key to successful management of osteoporosis.)
2. Advise patient to combine weight-bearing exercise such as walking for 30 minutes at least three times a week with balance and strengthening exercises. Avoid high-impact exercises that raise the risk of vertebral compression fractures (e.g., running or horseback riding).
3. Teach the patient how to read food labels and to eat a healthy diet that is high in calcium, proteins, and vitamins (including fruits and dark-green, leafy vegetables).
4. Inform patient that pain is best managed by including rest periods and application of ice or heat as adjuncts to prescribed pain medications.
5. Instruct the patient to take prescribed bisphosphonates in the early morning before breakfast with a full glass of water and to remain upright for at least 30 minutes after taking the medication to avoid side effects.
6. Teach the patient strategies for smoking cessation or weight loss if applicable.

(Abel, 2013; Ignatavicius, 2018; Robinson, 2020)

Summary

Nurses have an integral role in improving the quality of life for individuals at risk for or who have been diagnosed with osteopenia or osteoporosis. Early identification of the factors that increase risk of osteoporosis and fragility fractures is key to developing a treatment plan that slows development or progression of bone loss. Patient education on the disease process, helpful lifestyle modifications, and the importance of diet and exercise are key to adherence and successful management of the disease.

Key Points

• Osteoporosis is a "silent disease," and decreasing modifiable risk factors through lifestyle modifications is key to preventing or slowing bone loss.

• Fragility fractures and skeletal changes such as kyphosis are often the first sign of osteoporosis.

• Low impact, weight-bearing exercise, such as walking three times a week, and a calcium-rich diet have been shown to improve bone health.

• The nurse is key to educating patients on when and how to take bisphosphonates to avoid side effects and achieve the best absorption of the drugs.

• The DEXA scan is a noninvasive test that is considered the best resource for diagnosis and monitoring of osteoporosis.

Review Questions

1. **The nurse is reviewing the health history of a 70-year-old Asian female. The nurse understands that which of the following increases the patient's risk for osteoporosis? (Select all that apply.)**

    a. Drinks three cups of coffee every day
    b. History of total abdominal hysterectomy at age 29
    c. Walks 5 miles at least 3 days a week
    d. Takes a proton pump inhibitor for GERD

2. **When explaining DEXA results to a patient, which of the following statements made by the nurse is correct?**
   a. "A score in the negative numbers indicates you are not at risk for developing osteoporosis."
   b. "A score of –1.0 indicates you have some bone loss."
   c. "The DEXA scan is only a screening tool and does not show osteoporosis."
   d. "The DEXA score compares your bone density to others your age."

3. **Which of the following choices would the nurse be expected to include when teaching a patient about calcium-rich foods?**
   a. Apple juice
   b. Green beans
   c. Spinach
   d. Walnuts

4. **The nurse is providing education about bisphosphonates to the patient newly diagnosed with osteoporosis. Which of the following statements made by the patient indicates a need for further education?**
   a. "I can take this medication with my lunch to avoid an upset stomach."
   b. "I will drink plenty of water with my medication to prevent kidney damage."
   c. "The medication will help me grow back the bone I've lost."
   d. "This medication can be taken with or without food."

5. **The nurse is educating the patient with osteoporosis on how to take their newly prescribed denosumab. Which of the following statements lets the nurse know that the patient understands instructions?**
   a. "Careful handwashing is important to prevent infection."
   b. "Increasing my water intake will help the medication absorb better."
   c. "It is important to switch nostrils each day to avoid irritation."
   d. "It is important not to shake the syringe as I'm preparing the injection."

See the appendix for answers to review questions.

References

Abel, L. E. (2013). Metabolic bone conditions. In L. Schoenly (Ed.), *Core curriculum for orthopaedic nursing* (7th ed.). Chicago, IL: National Association of Orthopaedic Nurses.

Brown, D. A. (2013). Diagnostic studies in orthopaedics. In L. Schoenly (Ed.), *Core curriculum for orthopaedic nursing* (7th ed.). Chicago, IL: National Association of Orthopaedic Nurses.

Capriotti, T. (2020). *Pathophysiology: Introductory concepts and clinical perspectives* (2nd ed.). Philadelphia, PA: F.A. Davis.

Crowther-Radulewicz, C. L., & McCance, K. L. (2012). Alterations of musculoskeletal function. In S. E. Huether & K. L. McCance (Eds.), *Understanding pathophysiology* (5th ed.). St. Louis, MO: Elsevier Mosby.

Curtis, E. M., Moon, R. J., Dennison, E. M., Harvey, N. C., & Cooper, C. (2016). Recent advances in the pathogenesis and treatment of osteoporosis. *Clinical Medicine, 16*(4), 360–364.

Finkelstein, J. S., & Yu, E. W. (2019). Patient education: Bone density testing. In J. E. Mulder (Ed.), *UpToDate*. Retrieved Feb. 27, 2021 from https://www.uptodate.com/contents/bone-density-testing -beyond-the-basics

Hallock, A. (2017). Osteoporosis in patients with CKD: A diagnostic dilemma. *Nephrology Nursing Journal, 44*(1), 13–18.

Ignatavicius, D. D. (2018). Care of patients with musculoskeletal problems. In D. D. Ignatavicius, M. L. Workman, & C. R. Rebar (Eds.), *Medical-surgical nursing: Concepts for interprofessional collaborative care* (9th ed.). St. Louis, MO: Elsevier.

International Osteoporosis Foundation. (2017). Facts and statistics. Retrieved from https://www.iofbonehealth .org/facts-statistics#category-14

Jeremiah, M. P., Unwin, B. K., & Greenawald, M. H. (2015). Diagnosis and management of osteoporosis. *American Family Physician, 92*(4), 261–268.

Karch, A. M. (2020). *Focus on nursing pharmacology* (8th ed.). Philadelphia, PA: Wolters Kluwer / Lippincott Williams & Wilkins.

National Association of Orthopaedic Nurses. (2014). NAON position statement: Bone health and osteoporosis screening.

National Osteoporosis Foundation. (2018). Bone density exam / testing. Retrieved from https://www.nof .org/patients/diagnosis-information/bone-density-examtesting/

Palmer, D. M. (2013). Musculoskeletal assessment. In L. Schoenly (Ed.), *Core curriculum for orthopaedic nursing* (7th ed.). Chicago, IL: National Association of Orthopaedic Nurses.

Robinson, M. V. (2020). Hormone replacement therapy. In T. M. Woo & M. V. Robinson (Eds.), *Pharmacotherapeutics for advanced practice nurse prescribers* (5th ed.). Philadelphia, PA: F.A. Davis.

U.S. Preventive Services Task Force. (2018). Screening for osteoporosis to prevent fractures. *JAMA, 319*(24), 2521–2531. doi:10.1001/jama.2018.7498

Vallerand, A. H., & Sanoski, C. A. (Eds.). (2021). *Davis's drug guide for nurses* (17th ed.). Philadelphia, PA: F.A. Davis.

Mental Health Disorders Across the Life Span

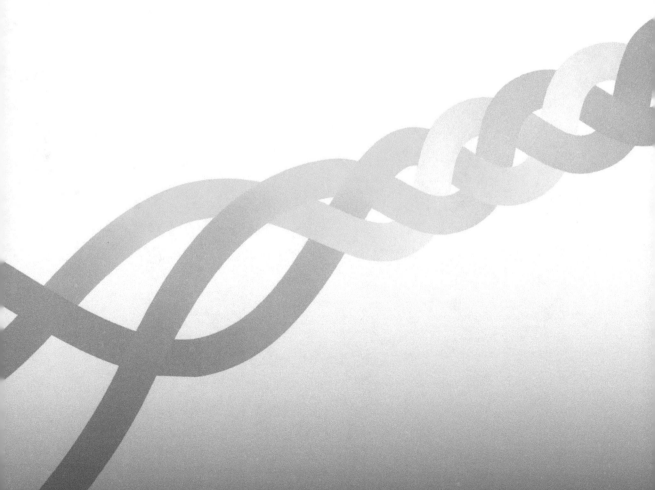

Chapter 24

Altered Cognitive Function

LEARNING OBJECTIVES

Upon completion of this chapter the student will be able to:

- Integrate knowledge of the physiology, pathophysiology, assessment, and pharmacological management for care of an adult with altered cognitive function.
- Compare and contrast dementia and delirium.
- Appraise current standards of care for older adult patients with altered cognitive function.

Introduction

The normal aging process includes changes in neurological processing, as the brain processes information at a slower rate while maintaining stability in intelligence (Alzheimer's Association, n.d.). However, altered cognitive function is not a sign or a consequence of normal aging (Capriotti, 2020). Cognitive changes that result in memory loss range in severity from mild cognitive impairment (small changes in thinking and memory only noticed by family and friends) to significant loss of ability to perform activities of daily living such as bathing, feeding, and grooming, and instrumental activities of daily living that support independent living including housekeeping, meal preparation, and one's ability to manage personal finances (Jarvis, 2020). *Dementia* is a general term often used to describe the symptoms of mental decline common in a variety of diseases; according to the Alzheimer's Association (n.d.), approximately 60% to 80% of all dementias are attributed to Alzheimer's disease, the most common form of dementia. Other forms of dementia include vascular (or multi-infarct) dementia (15% to 20%), Lewy body disease (26%), and other forms of dementia (7%). Lewy bodies are associated with Parkinson's disease and Alzheimer's dementias (Alzheimer's Association, 2020). Approximately 45% of individuals with Alzheimer's disease also have brain changes common in vascular dementia; this combination of dementia forms is referred to as *mixed dementia* (Alzheimer's Association, 2018b).

Approximately 10%, or 5.5 million, of Americans age 65 or older have Alzheimer's dementia, and as age increases, the incidence rises from 3% (ages 65 to 74), to 17% (ages 75 to 84), to 32% (ages 85 and older). As the population continues to age, the total number of individuals with dementia will rise. Estimates indicate that by 2025 there will be approximately 7.1 million Americans (29% increase from 2018) diagnosed with Alzheimer's dementia. As the baby boomer segment of the population ages and lives longer, by 2050 about 7 million Americans (51%) age 85 and older will have an Alzheimer's diagnosis. Finally, an Alzheimer's diagnosis by age 70 lowers life expectancy, with 61% of individuals with Alzheimer's, as compared to 30% without the disease, being expected to die before age 80 (Alzheimer's Association, 2018b).

Traumatic brain injury (TBI) is another condition that results in memory or thinking impairments. The Centers for Disease Control and Prevention (CDC) reported (most recent statistics from 2014) that more than 2.87 million injuries, hospitalizations, and deaths were related to a traumatic brain injury, with more than 837,000 of these injuries occurring in children 17 years or younger. Older adults (81%) and children (49%) are most likely to receive emergency department (ED) care related to a TBI following a fall, highlighting the need to be vigilant with safety for these vulnerable populations (CDC, 2019). Effects of a mild TBI may be resolved in a few weeks to 6 months. while a more serious TBI may lead to lifelong neurological effects (Capriotti, 2020).

The burden of Alzheimer's and other dementias is significant in terms of financial cost and in caregiver burden. In 2018, the total cost of dementia care is estimated at $277 billion, spread across several payer sources: Medicare (50%, $140 billion); Medicaid (17%, $47 billion), out of pocket (22%, $60 billion), and other sources (11%, $30 billion). Of Medicare recipients with a dementia diagnosis, approximately 11% also have Medicaid insurance to aid with assisted living and long-term care expenses, greatly increasing the overall costs of the Medicaid program. Usage of financial resources from both programs is 23% greater by those with dementia diagnosis. Additionally, unpaid caregiver (family and/or friends) costs must be considered, based on the number of hours spent and on the length of time these services were provided to the dementia patient. Approximately 18.4 billion hours of care were provided in 2017 by unpaid caregivers; using an estimated $12.63/hour as a basis for calculation, these hours equal approximately $232.1 billion in caregiving costs (Alzheimer's Association, 2018b).

Individuals with dementia are at high risk of developing delirium during an illness or hospital stay. As the number of individuals over age 65 with a dementia diagnosis rises, the number of older adults who develop delirium is also predicted to increase (Brooke, 2018; Brooks, Spillane, Dick, & Stuart-Shor, 2014). According to the American Delirium Society (2015), approximately 7 million hospital patients experience an episode of delirium each year. The overall economic burden is seen in terms of complications and increased length of stay and is estimated to exceed $100 billion each year (Brooks et al., 2014).

Altered cognitive function negatively impacts an individual's ability to remain independent, their overall health status, and their quality of life. The nurse must understand the normal changes of the aging brain and recognize the various forms of dementia and delirium in order to make appropriate care decisions. The purpose of this chapter is to describe normal brain physiology as it relates to aging and cognitive function and to highlight the effects of TBI on cognitive function. Alzheimer's, vascular, and Parkinson's dementias will be described and contrasted to the symptoms of delirium, and treatment options will be highlighted.

Physiology

The brain is the center of cognitive functioning and the body's interaction with the external and internal environment. Approximately 15% to 20% of the total cardiac output is transported to the brain to support its functions. Blood flow in the brain is regulated by *carbon dioxide* (CO_2) levels. As CO_2 levels rise, vasodilation is triggered and blood flow to the brain increases. *Neuroplasticity* is a complex process by which the brain is able to adapt to changing conditions, reorganize neural pathways, and create new synapses. The degree to which this adaptation occurs impacts learning, memory, and development. Changes in neurotransmission, genetics, and the environment contribute to this complex process and the development of cognitive impairment or other neurological diseases (Sugerman & Huether, 2012).

The brain is divided into the *cerebral cortex* (frontal lobe, parietal lob, temporal lobe, and occipital lobe), the *cerebellum*, and the *diencephalon*, which is responsible for neurotransmission of sensory impulses to various regions of the brain as well as autonomic regulation within the peripheral nervous system. The *brainstem* is the area of the brain that controls vital body functions (blood pressure, heart rate, and respirations). Functions of the cerebral cortex are outlined in Figure 17–1 in Chapter 17. Neurological symptoms and disease presentation vary based on the portion of brain impacted by pathological changes (Capriotti, 2020).

The *central nervous system* (CNS) and *peripheral nervous system* (PNS) make up the nervous system. Normal function of the human nervous system requires complex interactions between the CNS (brain and spinal cord) and the PNS (cranial and spinal nerves). The PNS can be further divided into the *autonomic nervous system* (ANS), which regulates involuntary functions of the body, and the *somatic nervous system* (SNS), which regulates voluntary skeletal motor muscle activity (Sugerman & Huether, 2012).

Within the central nervous system, *neurons* are responsible for transmission of impulses across electrical synapses and for processing information, thus maintaining homeostasis. As shown in Figure 24–1, each neuron is composed of a central body, many dendrites (which receive incoming signals and carry them to the cell body), one axon (which sends out signals from the cell body), and an axon terminal (which contains various neurotransmitters).

Neurotransmitters are secreted from axon terminals and allow impulse transmission across the synapse from one neuron to the next (Capriotti, 2020). *Neuroglial* cells are found in the CNS where they serve as the neuron scaffold while providing neurons with nutrition and removal of cellular waste and foreign material (Ignatavicius, 2018a; Sugerman & Huether, 2012). As part of this structure, the microtubules allow the flow of nutrients along a pathway between the neuron's cell body and axon. *Tau proteins* help stabilize these microtubules (Capriotti, 2020). Neuroglial cells are also involved in the blood–brain barrier and *cerebrospinal fluid* (CSF) regulation. *Schwann* cells provide this same function to neurons in the PNS (Ignatavicius, 2018a; Sugerman & Huether, 2012). Neurotransmitters are described in Table 24–1.

Functionally, neurons are classified based on their action. Motor (*efferent*) neurons are responsible for transmitting signals from the CNS to organs or skeletal muscles. Sensory (*afferent*) neurons transmit signals from the periphery to the CNS. Associational (*interneurons*) neurons transmit impulses between motor and sensory neurons (Ignatavicius, 2018a; Sugerman & Huether, 2012). *Myelin* is composed of lipid material that covers some axons and insulates impulse transmission. The term *white matter* refers to myelin-covered axons and glial cells, while *gray matter* is composed of neuronal cell bodies. Impulses are moved forward to their final destination by the connection of dendrites to other dendrites, cell bodies, or axons. Impulse conduction is enhanced by *nodes of Ranvier*, which are gaps in the myelin sheath. Impulse transmission is blocked when there is damage to the myelin sheath (Capriotti, 2020; Ignatavicius, 2018a).

The reticular formation, located in the brainstem, consists of specialized cells that are responsible for controlling cardiovascular and respiratory functions. Based on its role in regulating alertness and awareness, this group of cells is commonly known as the *reticular activating system* (RAS). The RAS transmits signals throughout the cerebellum and cerebral cortex (Capriotti, 2020; Sugerman & Huether, 2012).

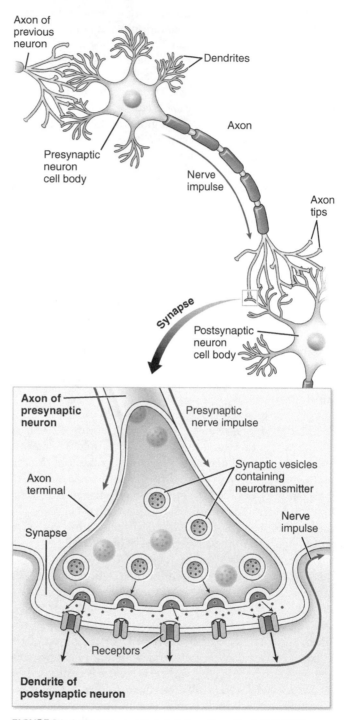

FIGURE 24–1 Neurons and their function *(From Capriotti, T. (2020).*
Pathophysiology: Introductory concepts and clinical perspectives (2nd ed.).
Philadelphia, PA: F.A. Davis.)

The brain tends to shrink as a part of normal aging, creating structural changes particularly to the frontal, parietal, and temporal lobes, while losing about 10% of its weight by the time a person reaches age 90. The ventricles enlarge, while *gyri* (ridges) of the cerebral cortex narrow and the surrounding *sulci* (indentations) become wider (Ignatavicius, 2018b). Changes in neurotransmitters are also attributed to some

TABLE 24–1 Neurotransmitters and Their Functions

Neurotransmitter	Location	Action	Disease
Acetylcholine (ACTH)	ANS, CNS, PNS	Excitatory Inhibitory	Alzheimer's ($\downarrow$ neurons that secrete ACTH) Myasthenia gravis ($\downarrow$ ACTH receptors).
Dopamine	Basal ganglia of midbrain and ANS synapses	Excitatory	Parkinson's disease, Tourette's, substance abuse, schizophrenia, ADHD
Gamma amino butyric acid (GABA)	CNS neurons	Inhibitory (primary inhibitory neurotransmitter) Anti-anxiety/ anticonvulsive effects in CNS	In epilepsy, give drugs to $\uparrow$ GABA function to inhibit excessive neuronal activity.
Glutamate	CNS	Excitatory	Accumulation causes cell death, implicated in altered cognition, memory and learning impairment (dementia); drugs that block glutamate can be used to treat ALS.
Norepinephrine	Brain, spinal cord, ANS	Excitatory Inhibitory	Stress ("fight or flight") Parkinson's dementia
Serotonin (5-hydroxytryptamine)	CNS	Excitatory	Mood and sleep disorders

(Capriotti, 2020; Sugerman & Huether, 2012)
   autonomic nervous system (ANS); central nervous system (CNS); peripheral nervous system (PNS); amyotrophic lateral sclerosis (ALS); attention deficit-hyperactivity disorder (ADHD)

age-related factors, including an altered response to stress (Sugerman & Huether, 2012; Townsend, 2020). These changes, along with cerebrovascular changes, contribute to altered cognition as the development of atherosclerosis, a precursor to infarcts, predisposes the older adult to additional impairments in cognition and functioning based on the area of the brain impacted by an infarct (Sugerman & Huether, 2012).

Pathophysiology

The components of cognitive function include awareness, attention, and memory. Components of awareness include self-awareness, awareness of surroundings, and mood, and are mediated by executive attention, attention, and memory pathways (Boss & Huether, 2012). While normal physiological aging of the neurological system causes some delays or slowing of cognitive processing, these changes do not result in the symptoms attributed to delirium or dementia. Components of attention and memory are most affected by normal aging, and while some components may remain relatively stable, others may require a longer period of time to accomplish (Emory University, 2017; Glisky, 2007). Table 24–2 describes the cognitive changes normal to the aging process.

Dementia is a slow, progressive disease that results from pathophysiological changes that lead to declines in orientation, decision making, judgment, language, and memory. Behavioral changes in dementia can be attributed to these cognitive declines.

HIGH YIELD FACT FOR TESTING

Normal cognitive functioning is affected by complex interactions of neurotransmitters to accurately transmit and process signals along neural pathways. While normal processing of information slows as one ages, decline in cognitive function is a sign of disease.

TABLE 24–2   Cognitive Changes of Normal Aging

Aspect of Thinking	Type	Normal Change
Attention	**Simple/focused** on one stimulus while disregarding other irrelevant stimuli **Divided** attention where focus is on more than one information source or task at a time	Stable May decline as ability to prioritize declines
Intelligence	**Crystalized** (based on education or experience; knowledge over time) **Fluid** (newer knowledge)	Stable Decline in ability to store new knowledge to memory
Language	**Verbal** (including vocabulary) **Word retrieval** or **name recall**	Stable Slows and is difficult to retrieve (not lost)
Memory	**Remote** recall **Recent** or new memories	Stable May decline
Reasoning and problem-solving	**Traditional** problems and situations **New** problems	Stable Takes longer to solve the problem
Speed of processing	**Cognitive** and **motor** processes	Stable but takes longer to perform

(Emory University, 2017; Glisky, 2007; Sugerman & Huether, 2012)

Presentation of dementia varies based on the type and location of underlying pathology in the brain (Boss & Huether, 2012; Ignatavicius, 2018b). It is common for individuals with one type of dementia to also exhibit pathological changes of another type of dementia, with the most common combinations being attributed to Alzheimer's and vascular dementias (Alzheimer's Association, 2018b).

Alzheimer's disease is the most common form of dementia (Alzheimer's Association, 2018b). The progressive cognitive impairments associated with Alzheimer's disease can be attributed to several changes within the brain. First, there is a decline in the production of *acetylcholine*, particularly noticeable in the cerebral amygdala, cortex, and hippocampus regions of the brain; this reduces neurotransmitters and disrupts cognitive processes. It is also thought that N-methyl-D-aspartate (NMDA) receptors are overstimulated as a result of excessive *glutamate* levels, which causes elevated intracellular calcium levels and eventual death of neurons. The role of other neurotransmitters in the development of Alzheimer's is not clear (Capriotti, 2020; Ignatavicius, 2018b; Townsend, 2020).

In the microtubules, chemical changes in tau proteins cause structural collapse, which leads to interruption of normal communication between neurons and a loss of cognitive abilities including a loss of recent memory and the ability to make new memories. Additionally, *neurofibrillary tangles* develop as tau proteins attach to each other and create fibrous masses. The resulting buildup of these tangles leads to neuron destruction (Capriotti, 2020; Ignatavicius, 2018b; Townsend, 2020). Within the hippocampus, as nerve terminals are destroyed, *beta amyloid plaques* form that further impair transmission of signals along neural pathways. Some degeneration of the brain's vasculature contributes to the pathological changes found in Alzheimer's disease. Together, these changes accelerate normal aging processes, including brain atrophy and neuron destruction, and progressive cognitive decline (Ignatavicius, 2018b).

Vascular (multi-infarct) dementia is the result of one significant *cerebrovascular accident* (CVA), multiple smaller CVAs, cerebral hemorrhage, or other conditions that damage blood vessels with the potential to impede cerebral blood flow, including atherosclerotic disease, diabetes, or hypertension. Inadequate flow of oxygen and nutrients to the neurons results in neuron destruction and cognitive impairment. Neuron damage is irreversible, and changes in thinking and perception may be sudden and significant in the event of a large CVA or may be mild and slowly progressive as the result of the cumulative neuron loss from multiple smaller vessel vascular events (Alzheimer's Association, 2018e; Capriotti, 2020; Ignatavicius, 2018b).

Lewy bodies are made up of alpha-synuclein protein, a neurotransmitter that aids in signal transmission across synapses. Neurons at particular risk for accumulation of Lewy bodies are those that produce acetylcholine and dopamine. *Lewy body dementia* is the result of excessive deposits of alpha-synuclein proteins in the brain's neurons, particularly in the brainstem and cerebral cortex (Perkins, 2017; Townsend, 2020). Lewy bodies are also found in patients with Alzheimer's and Parkinson's diseases. Symptoms of Parkinson's disease are frequently overlapped with those of *Lewy body dementia* (LBD), with the symptoms occurring in opposite order; movement symptoms occur first in Parkinson's disease, with dementia symptoms appearing later in the disease process, while the person with Lewy body dementia experiences dementia symptoms first and movement symptoms later as their disease progresses. These commonalities make it difficult to distinguish between the two conditions (Perkins, 2017).

In contrast to the progressive, nonreversible course of dementias, *delirium* is an acute, reversible condition of fluctuating cognitive function, confusion, and inability to focus attention (Guthrie & Rayborn, 2018; Mendes, 2017). While the metabolic changes that cause the symptoms of delirium have not been isolated, it is thought that an increase in dopamine and serotonin activity, a decrease in acetylcholine levels, and/or abnormal beta-endorphin and cortisol levels are responsible for delirium symptoms. Exogenous glucocorticoids have also been implicated as a cause of delirium. Finally, an increase in serotonin levels has been found in elderly patients with delirium, and inflammatory cytokines (interleukin-1 and interleukin-6) may contribute to delirium symptoms (Apold, 2018; Capriotti, 2020). Predisposing factors that result in pathological changes of delirium include metabolic conditions that impact brain function (hypercarbia, hypoxia, hypoglycemia), fever, brain abscess, CVA, electrolyte imbalances, hepatic encephalopathy, infections, and medications (Townsend, 2020).

Memory function may also be impaired as a result of TBI. These injuries occur in one of four ways: blunt trauma, acceleration–deceleration (also known as *coup-contrecoup*), penetrating events, or blast events. The Glasgow Coma Scale is used to guide classification of the severity of the initial injury (Capriotti, 2020). Research into the relationship between TBI and dementia suggests that the changes to the brain's chemistry that occur with sports-related, repetitive, mild TBI cause an increase in beta-amyloid and tau proteins (also elevated in Alzheimer's disease), which in turn cause a form of dementia called *chronic traumatic encephalopathy* (CTE). However, any TBI can result in these chemical changes and impair a person's cognitive abilities in the same manner as dementia, with symptoms often only appearing long after apparent recovery from the initial injury has occurred (Alzheimer's Association, 2019)

> **HIGH YIELD FACT FOR TESTING**
>
> The pathophysiological processes of dementia result in progressive and irreversible decline of cognitive function, while changes in cognitive function in delirium are acute and reversible.

Assessment

A general overview of the patient's health history (past and present), social history, and family history forms the foundation of a neurological assessment. Because neurological symptoms, particularly nonspecific symptoms of dizziness, fatigue, paresthesias, or syncope, may also be symptomatic of cardiovascular disease, endocrine disorders, or malignancy, it is important to rule out correctable reasons for the symptoms as a part of the neurological examination. Cranial nerves, motor strength and coordination, and deep tendon reflexes should be evaluated (Goolsby & Grubbs, 2019).

Identification of risk factors is an important component of neurological assessment. While the exact causes of dementia are not well established, risk factors for dementia include age, female gender, genetic abnormalities, family history of Alzheimer's disease, environmental factors, and a history of Down's syndrome (Alzheimer's Association, 2018b; Ignatavicius, 2018b). Research has also identified traumatic brain injury as a risk factor for Alzheimer's, and there have been links to the development of Alzheimer's, particularly early-onset disease, by individuals with some gene mutations (Townsend, 2020). Modifiable risk factors are related to conditions of cardiovascular health (including diabetes and hypertension), activity level, obesity, and smoking. Management of these conditions and increasing physical activity are shown to decrease dementia risks. Cardiovascular disease and history of CVA are known risk factors for vascular dementia (Alzheimer's Association, 2018b).

Alzheimer's Disease and Other Dementias

Often the earliest symptom of Alzheimer's disease is impairment of recent memory including events and name recall (Alzheimer's Association, 2018b; Ignatavicius, 2018b). Symptoms of the disease are typically divided into three overlapping stages: early, middle, and late. *Early (mild)* symptoms typically appear within the first 4 years of the disease. At this stage, patients remain independent in their *activities of daily living* (ADLs) and deny that they are having memory problems. Short-term memory difficulties are accompanied by minor changes in behavior and personality, and patients lose initiative and begin to withdraw from social situations. Judgment and executive decision-making abilities are impaired, and stressful situations cause symptoms to increase.

In contrast to Alzheimer's, initial symptoms of vascular dementia are often related to motor changes (muscle weakness, gait disturbances, or abnormal reflexes) rather than memory impairment (Townsend, 2020). With Lewy body dementia, as Lewy bodies accumulate in these cells, alterations occur in the individual's memory and ability to learn (acetylcholine influence) and in their mood, movement, motivation, and sleep patterns (dopamine influence). The patient with Lewy body dementia may also have changes in their sense of smell, because the olfactory pathways are sensitive to Lewy body accumulation, while an estimated 80% of patients experience vivid and realistic hallucinations.

The *middle (moderate)* stage of Alzheimer's generally lasts for 2 to 3 years and symptoms include progression of cognitive decline; increased difficulty with executive decision making; inability to successfully manage finances; disorientation to events, time, and place; getting lost easily; and increased difficulty driving and performing ADLs. In this stage, patients may wander and have difficulty sleeping. As the patient progresses through this stage, they have increasing difficulty with language and may become aphasic and incontinent. In the *late (severe)* stage, as decision-making ability declines, patients may begin to dress inappropriately for the weather and lose interest in their appearance. As this stage progresses, the patient is unable to ambulate and becomes bedridden, is unable to perform ADLs, and loses the ability to recognize faces (*agnosia*) (Alzheimer's Association, 2018d; Ignatavicius, 2018b).

Behavior and personality changes become more prevalent as cognitive decline progresses. Confusion usually increases later in the day (*sundowning*) when patients are very fatigued or when light is inadequate to recognize surroundings. Patients may become aggressive or have rapid mood swings, and they often hoard or hide items (Alzheimer's Association, 2018b; Ignatavicius, 2018b). Anxiety may cause agitation that leads to hitting or yelling. Patients may also develop delusions or hallucinations that are often anxiety producing (Ignatavicius, 2018b).

While vascular dementia may initially present with difficulty in executive decision making (planning, concentrating, and following steps), as the disease progresses, the symptoms become similar to those of Alzheimer's. While LBD progresses slowly and similarly to Alzheimer's dementia, there are some differences. The person with LBD will have wide variations (often within one 24-hour period) in their attention span and alertness along with vivid visual hallucinations and slow motor movements and tremors (Alzheimer's Society, 2020). For the individual who develops dementia following a TBI, the progress accelerates the symptoms of cognitive decline at an earlier age, but the progression of dementia is similar to other dementias (Alzheimer's Association, 2019).

Delirium

In contrast to dementias, *delirium* develops rapidly and in response to a variety of underlying causes. Predisposing factors that place patients at increased risk for delirium include advanced age; existing cognitive impairment or depression; medical conditions such as dehydration, hypoxia, hyperglycemia, or hypoglycemia; infection; poor nutrition; and functional or sensory impairment (Brooks, 2012; Brooks et al., 2014; Townsend, 2020). Modifiable factors that may precipitate the development of delirium in hospitalized patients include sedation, certain medications, postoperative pain, bedrest for extended periods of time, the use of physical restraints, or sleep deprivation. Managing these modifiable factors is key to preventing delirium (Brooks et al., 2014; Guthrie & Rayborn, 2018). Depression also places the patient at increased risk of developing postoperative delirium (Smith, 2012).

There is a relationship between dementia and delirium; dementia is a known risk factor for development of delirium, and risk increases as dementia progresses. When delirium is superimposed on underlying dementia, the delirium may go unrecognized, which leads to increased morbidity and mortality. In some cases, delirium may last for up to 6 months following the initial symptoms (Apold, 2018; Smith, 2012).

The hallmark symptoms of delirium are an inability to maintain attention or to shift attention and a loss of awareness of the environment (Guthrie & Rayborn, 2018). Delirium is classified and subtyped based on the level of motor activity exhibited by the patient. *Hyperactive* delirium is characterized by agitation, restlessness, and refusal to cooperate. The patient is disoriented to date, place, and/or time; may attempt to remove lines and tubes; and often has sleep disturbance characterized by a reversal of day and night. This type of delirium accounts for about 1.6% of all deliriums, typically occurs in younger individuals, and is often related to acute withdrawal or drug intoxication. In contrast, the patient with *hypoactive* delirium appears lethargic, is not completely aware of their surroundings, and exhibits little motor movement. They may also experience delusions, hallucinations, and sleep disturbances. Unfortunately, this type of delirium, which impacts 43.5% of those with delirium, often goes undiagnosed and has the poorest outcomes. *Mixed* delirium is defined by either normal motor activity or rapid fluctuation between hyperactive and hypoactive movement, while exhibiting attention impairment and confusion. About 55% of individuals with delirium exhibit mixed symptoms (Guthrie & Rayborn, 2018; Hickin, White, & Knopp-Sihota, 2017; Townsend, 2020). Characteristics of dementia and delirium are further summarized in Table 24–3.

TABLE 24–3   Characteristics of Dementia and Delirium

Presentation	Dementia	Delirium
Onset	Slow, progressive	Sudden; symptoms fluctuate during the day
Duration	Years	Hours or days dependent on correction of underlying cause
Etiology	May have some genetic basis, but generally unknown	Drugs, illness, post-surgical procedures among others
Orientation	Normal early, but impaired as disease progresses	Disoriented to date, place, time
Alertness	Normal	Impaired
Attention	Normal early, but impaired as disease progresses	Inattentive, easily distracted
Behaviors	Normal but impaired as disease progresses	Agitated, depressed, or combination of behaviors
Speech	Normal	Incoherent, may be rapid or slow
Hallucinations or delusions	None in early disease	Present
Treatment	Symptom management	Treat and eliminate the underlying cause

(Alzheimer's Association, 2018d; Boss & Huether, 2012; Hickin et al., 2017; Ignatavicius, 2018b)

Assessment Tools

Around 10% to 20% of alterations in mental status can be corrected, and not every affected patient presents with symptoms of mental status changes; however, a screening is an integral component of the neurological examination for patients who exhibit any change including confusion; difficulty with concentration, finding words, or reasoning; or exhibiting inappropriate behaviors (Goolsby & Grubbs, 2019). The *Mini-Cog* examination is often the first test used to evaluate cognitive impairment. It is often used during the preadmission assessment to predict delirium risk (Apold, 2018; Smith, 2012). The test is easy and takes less than 5 minutes to administer. In it, the patient is asked to repeat three unrelated words, follow directions to draw a clock, and finally to repeat the three unrelated words.

The *Mini-Mental State Examination* (MMSE) requires more time to administer and must be administered in an organized fashion, but is the most commonly used examination to evaluate other aspects of cognition beyond short- and long-term memory. Other components of the examination include orientation, attention, naming, recall, repetition, comprehension, drawing, reading, and writing. However, this examination does not distinguish between cognitive impairment due to dementia and that due to delirium (Alzheimer's Association, 2018c; Byrd & Pierson, 2019).

The *Confusion Assessment Method* (CAM) and the *CAM for the Intensive Care Unit* (CAM-ICU) examinations are commonly used to identify delirium in the postoperative patient. The CAM-ICU is used for patients who are mechanically ventilated and unable to communicate verbally. These tools are reliable and easy to administer in the clinical setting (Apold, 2018; Guthrie & Rayborn, 2018).

The *Delirium Index* (DI) measures delirium severity and is an adaptation of the CAM tool. It is designed as an observation tool to be used by non-psychiatrist practitioners

(Guthrie & Rayborn, 2018). The *4AT* tool uses four components—alertness, attention, abbreviated mental test (ability to correctly state age, date of birth, current location and year), and fluctuations or changes in mental status—to predict delirium in the elderly (4AT, n.d.; Guthrie & Rayborn, 2018). The *Delirium Elderly At Risk* (DEAR) scale has been successfully used to identify risk for development of dementia in the hospitalized patient and is used in conjunction with the MMSE. Five categories are used in determining risk for delirium (Freter, Dunbar, Koller, MacKnight, & Rockwood, 2015):

- MMSE score ≤23
- Presence of sensory impairment, either hearing (use of hearing aid) or visual
- Requiring assistance with ADLs (functional dependence)
- Substance use (consumes alcohol 3+ times a week or uses a benzodiazepine 3+ times a week)
- Age >80 years.

Delirium can be superimposed on *underlying dementia* (DSD); therefore, obtaining the patient's baseline cognitive level from either the medical record or from a family member or caregiver is essential to an accurate diagnosis of this medical emergency (Apold, 2018; Capriotti, 2020).

In addition to the assessment tools listed above, the *Richmond Agitation and Sedation Scale* (RASS) is used to determine whether the patient's sedation level will prevent accurate assessment using the CAM-ICU tool (Apold, 2018; Brooks et al., 2014). Finally, depression is a known risk factor for development of delirium. The *Geriatric Depression Scale* (GDS) is a simple 15-item tool that can be used to identify recent depression symptoms and takes only a few minutes to administer (Smith, 2012).

ASSESSMENT PEARLS
> Most cognitive assessment tools are simple to use, require minimal time to administer, and must be administered in a consistent manner to be useful in identifying signs of cognitive decline.

Nonpharmacological Management

While neither pharmacological nor nonpharmacological interventions can cure dementia, several interventions are known to help delay cognitive decline. The goals of nonpharmacological treatment of dementia are threefold: to improve or maintain (1) cognitive function, (2) the ability to perform ADLS, and (3) the patient's quality of life, for as long as possible (Alzheimer's Association, 2018b).

The nurse's role in dementia prevention is focused on patient education, including discussions on avoiding alcohol consumption, stopping smoking, consuming a healthy diet, engaging in consistent physical exercise, and managing blood sugar, blood pressure, and cholesterol levels and weight (Alzheimer's Association, 2018b, 2018d). While dietary supplements and herbal products are advertised as helpful to memory preservation, their effectiveness and safety have not been proved by the *U.S. Food and Drug Association* (FDA), and they may have potentially harmful interactions with a patient's prescribed medications (Alzheimer's Association, 2015, 2018a). Specifically, despite claims that essential fatty acids can be used to prevent or treat dementias, no evidence to support these claims has been established (Woo, 2020).

Care of the dementia patient requires an interdisciplinary team approach that includes the nurse, patient, and caregivers. It is important for caregivers (both paid and unpaid) to understand that, while dementia does not have a cure, interventions can be implemented to manage symptoms of dementia (Alzheimer's Association, 2018b). These interventions can enable the dementia patient to maintain a good quality of life by providing familiar routines so that they perceive they have some control of their lives (Mendes, 2017). The nurse should advise caregivers to use calendars and clocks to orient the patient to time; large signs can help the patient locate rooms (bathroom, bedroom, dining room, etc.). Photo albums and reminiscing can help with reality orientation. As cognitive decline progresses, patients with dementia benefit from structured environments, reorientation and validation strategies, cognitive stimulation, memory training, and encouraging communication (Ignatavicius, 2018b). Consistency in daily activities (i.e., meal and toileting schedules), caregivers, and presence of familiar personal items when the patient is moved to a care facility provide comfort and security and help prevent wandering. Finally, support resources for both the patient and family caregivers are important for successful management of dementia symptoms (Alzheimer's Association, 2018b; Townsend, 2020).

Symptom management for patients with Lewy body dementia include maintaining adequate lighting, particularly in the evening when hallucinations are most common. These patients also commonly exhibit Parkinson's-type movement difficulties, making safety and fall prevention priority care interventions. Paranoid delusions are common in the later stages of Lewy body disease, and the challenges of managing advanced symptoms of the disease often result in the need for institutional care (Perkins, 2017).

Delirium is best treated by identification and elimination of the underlying cause of the symptoms. Fluids and nutrition needs should be addressed. Reorientation to the environment using verbal cues, calendars, or clocks, along with family pictures, and providing the patient with their sensory devices (glasses or hearing aids) are key interventions. Physical restraints should be avoided when possible, as restraints are known to increase confusion; however, if they must be utilized to keep patients from self-harm, their need should be reassessed frequently (Capriotti, 2020).

Effective communication can be challenging when working with any patient with cognitive impairment. Simple language with short sentences, directions that have a minimal number of steps, written instructions that include pictures, and use of gestures can aid in understanding and decrease anxiety. Ask yes or no questions when possible, anticipate the patient's needs, and avoid assuming that confusion prevents the patient from understanding what is being said (Ignatavicius, 2018b).

Pharmacology

Pharmacological management of dementias varies with the disease process. Two classes of drugs are used to treat Alzheimer's disease. The first class of drugs, acetylcholinesterase inhibitors, increases the concentration of acetylcholine activity in the brain's cortex, improving memory as the increased levels help compensate for acetylcholine lost as neurons are destroyed (Alzheimer's Association, 2017; Karch, 2020; Knowlton, 2020). Three approved indirect-cholinergic agonists are included in this class: *donepezil*, *galantamine*, and *rivastigmine*. The second class slows plaque buildup by blocking glutamate stimulation in the brain. The only drug in this class is *memantine*, an *N*-methyl-D-aspartate (NMDA) receptor antagonist that may be prescribed for its action of controlling the amount of calcium allowed to enter nerve cells, thus improving storage of information. (Alzheimer's Association, 2017). There is also one combination drug on the market, *Namzaric*, which combines donepezil and memantine to affect both processes (Karch, 2020; Knowlton, 2020).

Treatment of vascular dementia focuses on the underlying disease process (e.g., diabetes and hypertension) with no FDA-approved drugs for treating symptoms (Alzheimer's Association, 2018e). Management of Lewy body dementia is aimed at symptom control rather than slowing disease progression. *Selective serotonin reuptake inhibitors*

(SSRIs) may be prescribed to treat symptoms of depression. The cholinesterase inhibitor rivastigmine has been approved to treat agitation, cognitive impairment, and psychotic symptoms. It should be noted that levodopa to control movement symptoms should be prescribed cautiously, as the drug has been known to increase confusion and hallucinations associated with LBD. Antipsychotic and neuroleptic drugs increase risk of severe adverse reactions, including neuroleptic malignant syndrome, and should be prescribed with caution (Perkins, 2017).

Drugs are not indicated as first line treatment options for delirium, and antipsychotics have a black box warning against use with elderly patients (Apold, 2018; Guthrie & Rayborn, 2018). However, drugs are often prescribed to manage the agitation of hyperactive delirium, and the drugs most commonly used to treat these symptoms are the antipsychotic drug haloperidol and the benzodiazepine lorazepam (Capriotti, 2020). Drugs commonly used to treat Alzheimer's and delirium are highlighted in Table 24–4.

Careful assessment of the patient's current medications is an important part of the medical history, because some drugs are known to precipitate or exacerbate other symptoms. Patients with known cardiovascular disease, peptic ulcers, asthma, epilepsy, or Parkinson's disease should avoid use of anticholinesterase inhibitors, because these drugs can exacerbate symptoms (Karch, 2020). Patients with chronic and

TABLE 24–4 Medications for Altered Cognition Disorders

Class	Example	Action	Dosage	SENC
Alzheimer's Disease				
Acetylcholinesterase inhibitors	Donepezil	Make more ACTH available by inhibiting acetylcholinesterase.	Oral: 5 mg daily at bedtime for 4–6 weeks, then may increase to 10 mg daily.	May slow cognitive decline, but does not cure. Use lower dose if patient is female, frail, and advanced age.
	Galantamine		Oral: 4–12 mg bid with meals.	Must ↓ dose with renal or hepatic disease; risk of Stevens-Johnson syndrome. Must wait 4 weeks before titrating dose upward.
	Rivastigmine		Oral: 1.5 mg bid *with food*; may increase to 3 mg bid if tolerated well. Transdermal: apply one 4.6 mg/24 patch daily.	Can be used to treat Alzheimer's and Parkinson's-related dementia.
***N*-methyl-D-aspartate (NMDA) antagonists**	Memantine	Binds to NMDA receptors; blocks glutamate binding.	Initial: 5 mg daily and increase each week to max dose of 10 mg bid (20 mg daily).	May slow cognitive decline, but does not cure. May take with or without food.
Namzaric	Combination of NMDA antagonist (memantine hydrochloride) and cholinesterase inhibitor (donepezil hydrochloride)	Combination effects to prevent acetylcholine breakdown.	Oral: 7 mg/10 mg daily in the evening OR 28 mg/10 mg daily.	May slow cognitive decline, but does not cure; take with or without food; must start at lower dose if patient not already on both drugs.

Continued

TABLE 24–4 Medications for Altered Cognition Disorders—cont'd

Class	Example	Action	Dosage	SENC
Delirium				
Antipsy-chotics	Haloperidol	Anticholin-ergic; alerts dopamine in CNS; decreases psychosis symptoms.	0.5 mg–2 mg bid; PO, IM, IV.	May cause extrapyramidal symptoms; blurred vision; neuroleptic malignant syndrome; dehydration. Many drug–drug interactions.
Benzodiaze-pines	Lorazepam	Inhibits GABA neurotransmit-ter; decreases anxiety and seizure activity.	1–3 mg bid–tid Elderly: 0.5–2 mg daily PO, IM, IV.	Caution: avoid confus-ing with alprazolam or clonazepam. For short-term use; avoid stopping the drug abruptly to avoid with-drawal symptoms.

(Capriotti, 2020; Drugs.com, 2021; Karch, 2020; Knowlton, 2020; Vallerand & Sanoski, 2017)

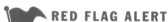 **RED FLAG ALERT**

Because acetylcholinesterase inhib-itors increase secretion of gastric acid, gastrointestinal upset is the most common side effect of these drugs (Knowlton, 2020). However, for unknown reasons, these drugs only work for some patients, and in those select patients, improvement in cog-nition is only temporary (Alzheimer's Association, 2018b).

advanced renal disease (creatinine clearance of 5–29 mL/min.) should have a dose reduction of memantine, because the drug is excreted renally (Knowlton, 2020). Classes to be avoided when the patient is at risk for or has symptoms of delirium include anticholinergics, antihistamines, antiemetics, anti-arrhythmics, beta blockers, digoxin, corticosteroids, histamine H-2 receptor antagonists, narcotics, and sedatives such as diazepam (Smith, 2012). The Beers Criteria Medication list of drugs can be used to help identify drugs that should be avoided in the care of older adults who are hospitalized (Guthrie & Rayborn, 2018).

Summary

While normal aging impacts the brain's ability to process information, alterations in cognition are not part of normal aging. As the number of older adults grows, the num-ber of adults with dementia is expected to grow exponentially, increasing the burden on society to provide adequate care for this vulnerable population. The nurse's role in helping caregivers understand how to best support these patients begins with under-standing the underlying causes and presentations; the risk factors such as age, fam-ily history, cardiovascular risk factors, and TBI; and effective treatment options of all types of dementia and delirium. Because each patient's disease may present differently, developing a therapeutic relationship with the patient and the caregiver is key to iden-tifying their needs and to providing care that supports an optimal quality of life for patients and their caregivers.

Key Points

- Delays in cognitive processing are a part of normal aging, while alterations in cog-nitive functioning attributed to dementias are the result of progressive pathological changes that impair memory, decision making, judgment, and language abilities.

- Delirium is a reversible state of confusion and agitation caused by metabolic imbalances and medical conditions. An individual with dementia is at increased risk of developing delirium.
- Nonpharmacological treatment options for dementia require an interdisciplinary team that addresses both patient and caregiver needs in the care plan.
- Drugs approved for dementia only temporarily slow cognitive decline and are not effective for all dementia patients.

Review Questions

1. The nurse is taking the health history of a 70-year-old patient who states, "My memory is not what it used to be. It is taking me longer to remember the names of people I don't see very often." The nurse understands that the patient is experiencing which of the following?
   a. Alzheimer's disease
   b. Delirium
   c. Lewy body dementia
   d. Normal aging

2. When conducting a Mini-Cog examination on a patient, which of the following is correct?
   a. Ask the patient to name the current and past two presidents of the United States.
   b. Ask the patient to repeat three unrelated words, draw a clock, and then repeat the words.
   c. Observe and record the patient's level of alertness and ability to recall names and events.
   d. Review the chart and record the number of drinks per day as a part of the screening score.

3. When asked to explain the difference between dementia and delirium, which of the following is the nurse's best response?
   a. "Both are progressive declines in memory and are treated with the same medications."
   b. "Dementia is a slow, progressive disease and delirium only occurs in patients with dementia."
   c. "Delirium is an acute, reversible condition that may also occur in patients with dementia."
   d. "Drugs to treat dementia can help reverse the cognitive changes and cure the disease."

4. Which of the following statements by a nurse best describes the difference between normal aging and dementia with regard to reasoning and problem-solving skills?
   a. "Dementia does not change our ability to solve problems we have solved in the past."
   b. "As we age, it takes longer to solve new problems, but we can still solve traditional problems."
   c. "New problems cannot be solved by older adults even if they don't have dementia."
   d. "Problem-solving is harder as we age because we can't do more than one thing at a time."

5. **The nurse is caring for a postoperative patient who has become agitated and unable to follow directions. Which of the following interventions would the nurse implement as a part of this patient's care? (Select all that apply.)**

   a. Make sure that the patient's hearing aids are in place.
   b. Obtain an order for haloperidol to calm the agitated patient.
   c. Place the patient in wrist restraints to prevent a fall.
   d. Reorient the patient using verbal cues and a clock.

See the appendix for answers to review questions.

References

Alzheimer's Association. (n.d.). *Aging, memory loss and dementia: What's the difference?* Retrieved from https://www.alz.org/mnnd/documents/aging_memory_loss_and_dementia_what_is_the_difference.pdf

Alzheimer's Association. (2015). *Medical foods*. Retrieved from https://www.alz.org/documents_custom/statements/Medical_Foods.pdf

Alzheimer's Association. (2017). *FDA-approved treatments for Alzheimer's*. Retrieved from https://www.alz.org/dementia/downloads/topicsheet_treatments.pdf

Alzheimer's Association. (2018a). *Alternative treatments*. Retrieved from https://www.alz.org/alzheimers_diasese_alternative_treatments.asp

Alzheimer's Association. (2018b). *2018 Alzheimer's disease facts and figures*. Retrieved from https://www.alz.org/facts/

Alzheimer's Association. (2018c). *Medical tests*. Retrieved from https://alz.org/alzheimers-dementia/diagnosis/medical_tests

Alzheimer's Association. (2018d). *Stages of Alzheimer's*. Retrieved from https://www.alz.org/alzheimers-dementia/stages

Alzheimer's Association. (2018e). *Vascular dementia*. Retrieved from https://www.alz.org/dementia/vascular-dementia-symptoms.asp

Alzheimer's Association. (2019). *Traumatic brain injury*. Retrieved from https://www.alz.org/alzheimers-dementia/what-is-dementia/related_conditions/traumatic-brain-injury

Alzheimer's Association. (2020). *Parkinson's disease dementia*. Retrieved from https://alz.org/alzheimers-dementia/what-is-dementia/types-of-dementia/parkinson-s-disease-dementia

Alzheimer's Society. (2020). *About dementia*. Retrieved from https://www.alzheimer.org.uk/about-dementia

American Delirium Society (2015). *What is delirium?* Retrieved from: https://americandeliriumsociety.org/what-delirium

Apold, S. (2018). Delirium superimposed on dementia. *The Journal for Nurse Practitioners, 14*(3), 183–189.

Boss, B. J., & Huether, S. E. (2012). Alterations in cognitive systems, cerebral hemodynamics, and motor function. In S. E. Huether & K. L. McCance (Eds.), *Understanding pathophysiology* (5th ed.). St. Louis, MO: Elsevier Mosby.

Brooke, J. (2018). Differentiation of delirium, dementia and delirium superimposed on dementia in the older person. *British Journal of Nursing, 27*(7), 363–367.

Brooks, P. B. (2012). Postoperative delirium in elderly patients. *American Journal of Nursing, 112*(9), 38–49.

Brooks, P., Spillane, J. J., Dick, K., & Stuart-Shor, E. (2014). Developing a strategy to identify and treat older patients with postoperative delirium. *AORN Journal, 99*(2), 256–276.

Byrd, L., & Pierson, C. (2019). Older patients. In M. J. Goolsby & L. Grubbs (Eds.), *Advanced assessment: Interpreting findings and formulating differential diagnoses* (4th ed.). Philadelphia, PA: F.A. Davis.

Capriotti, T. (2020). *Pathophysiology: Introductory concepts and clinical perspectives* (2nd ed.). Philadelphia, PA: F.A. Davis.

Centers for Disease Control and Prevention. (2019). *TBI: Get the Facts*. Retrieved from https://www.cdc.gov/traumaticbraininjury/get_the_facts.html

Drugs.com (2021). Namzaric. Retrieved from: https://www.drugs.com/namzaric.html

Emory University. (2017). *Fact sheet: Cognitive skills & normal aging*. Retrieved from www.http://alzheimers.emory.edu/healthy_aging/cognitive-skills-normal-aging.html

Freter, S., Dunbar, M., Koller, K., MacKnight, C., & Rockwoods, K. (2015). Risk of pre-and post-operative delirium and the delirium elderly at risk (DEAR) tool in hip fracture patients. *Canadian Geriatrics Journal, 18*(4). doi:http://dx.doi.org/10.577-/cgj.18.185

4AT. (n.d.). 4AT: Rapid clinical test for delirium. Retrieved from https://www.the4at.com/

Glisky, E. L. (2007). Changes in cognitive function in human aging. In D. R. Riddle (Ed.), *Models, methods and mechanisms*. Boca Raton, FL: CRC Press.

Goolsby, M. J., & Grubbs, L. (2019). Neurological system. In M. J. Goolsby & L. Grubbs (Eds.), *Advanced assessment: Interpreting findings and formulating differential diagnoses* (4th ed.). Philadelphia, PA: F.A. Davis.

Guthrie, P. F., & Rayborn, S. (2018). Evidence-based practice guideline: Delirium. *Journal of Gerontological Nursing, 44*(2), 14–25.

Hickin, S. L., White, S., & Knopp-Sihota, J. (2017). Delirium in the intensive care unit—A nursing refresher. *Canadian Journal of Critical Care Nursing, 28*(2), 19–23.

Ignatavicius, D. D. (2018a). Assessment of the nervous system. In D. D. Ignatavicius, L. Workman, & C. R. Rebar (Eds.), *Medical-surgical nursing: Concepts for interprofessional collaborative care* (9th ed.). St. Louis, MO: Elsevier.

Ignatavicius, D. D. (2018b). Care of patients with problems of the central nervous system: The brain. In D. D. Ignatavicius, L. Workman, & C. R. Rebar (Eds.), *Medical-surgical nursing: Concepts for interprofessional collaborative care* (9th ed.). St. Louis, MO: Elsevier.

Jarvis, C. (2020). *Physical examination & health assessment* (8th ed.). St. Louis, MO: Elsevier.

Karch, A. M. (2020). *Focus on nursing pharmacology* (8th ed.). Philadelphia, PA: Wolters Kluwer / Lippincott Williams & Wilkins.

Knowlton, R. (2020). Drugs affecting the autonomic nervous system. In T. M. Woo & M. V. Robinson. (Eds.), *Pharmacotherapeutics for advance practice nurse prescribers* (5th ed.). Philadelphia, PA: F.A. Davis.

Mendes, A. (2017). Recognising and assessing care needs in patients with dementia: The three Ds. *British Journal of Nursing, 26*(22), 1260–1261.

Perkins, A. (2017). Get to know Lewy body dementia. *Nursing Made Incredibly Easy! 15*(6), 32–39. doi:10.1097/01.NME.0000525548.83667.87

Smith, B. (2012). Special needs populations: Delirium issues in elderly surgical patients. *AORN Journal, 96*(1), 75–85.

Sugerman, R. A., & Huether, S. E. (2012). Structure and function of the neurologic system. In S. E. Huether & K. L. McCance (Eds.), *Understanding pathophysiology* (5th ed.). St. Louis, MO: Elsevier Mosby.

Townsend, M. C. (2020). *Psychiatric mental health nursing: Concepts of care in evidence-based practice* (9th ed.). Philadelphia, PA: F.A. Davis.

Vallerand, A. H., & Sanoski, C. A. (Eds.). (2021). *Davis's drug guide for nurses* (17th ed.). Philadelphia, PA: F.A. Davis.

Woo, T. M. (2020). Nutrition and nutraceuticals. In T. M. Woo & M. V. Robinson (Eds.), *Pharmacotherapeutics for advanced practice nurse prescribers* (5th ed., pp. 79–95). Philadelphia, PA: F.A. Davis.

Chapter 25

Anxiety and Depression

Introduction

Anxiety, a feeling of apprehension, worry, or vague dread that occurs when anticipating a situation, is a common emotion. However, when these feelings become irrational or when they interfere with daily routines, the condition is diagnosed as general-ized anxiety disorder, one of the most commonly diagnosed mental health disorders (Anxiety and Depression Association of American [ADAA], 2018b; Capriotti, 2020). In the United States alone, an estimated 40 million individuals are diagnosed with an anxiety disorder each year; however, more than 60% of these individuals do not seek treatment for their symptoms (ADAA, 2018a). Incidence of generalized anxiety disorder is most common in adults age 45 to 49 years and lowest in adults over age 60, and rates among women are twice that of men (Capriotti, 2020). Approximately 50% of individuals with *generalized anxiety disorder* (GAD) also exhibit symptoms of major depression (ADAA, 2018a).

Sadness or "the blues" is a common response to life's disappointments, losses, or failures and, if the adult can adapt and overcome the feelings in a short period of time, is considered normal. However, if the feelings persist over a longer time and the indi-vidual is unable to effectively adapt to the change, a pathological depression can ensue (Townsend, 2018). Major depression is defined as "presence of persistent (at least 2 weeks) depressed mood and/or loss of interest or pleasure" (Kverno & Velez, 2018, p.197), accompanied by three of the following symptoms: changes in appetite and/or weight, fatigue, sleep disturbance, difficulty thinking or concentrating, inappropriate feelings of guilt or worthlessness, or suicidal ideation or thoughts of death (Brodrick, 2020; Kverno & Velez, 2018).

In 2016, an estimated 16.2 million adults (6.7%) in the United States experienced a period of depression lasting at least 2 weeks. Rates were higher among women (8.5%) than among men (4.8%). Highest rates (10.9%) were in the 18-to-25-year-old age-group, and the highest prevalence (10.5%) occurred in individuals of mixed race (National Institute of Mental Health [NIMH], 2017). Between 2013 and 2016, older adults (age 60 years or older) reported high rates of depression, with women

(9.6%) and men (6.1%) reporting symptoms. Interestingly, statistical prevalence of depression between men and women remains consistent in different age-groups, except non-Hispanic black men where rates are higher (7.1%) than men in other racial/ethnic groups (Brody, Pratt, & Hughes, 2018). When the presence of poverty is factored in with race and Hispanic origin, there is not a significant difference in depression rates among the groups (Centers for Disease Control and Prevention [CDC], 2015).

Depressive episodes may be experienced across the life span. An estimated 1% to 2% of children (equal rates for girls and boys) are diagnosed with depression, and that rate increases to 4% to 5% of this vulnerable population by puberty, during which girls are twice as likely to experience depression symptoms as are boys (Charles & Fazeli, 2017). Approximately 12.8%, or 3.1 million adolescents (19.4% female and 6.4% male), exhibit major depressive symptoms each year (Brody et al., 2018; Mental Health America [MHA], 2018). Of the estimated 34 million older adults in the United States, an estimated 2 million have experienced a period of depression, particularly if they have recently lost their spouse or have any number of chronic illnesses common to older adults (MHA, 2018; NIMH, 2017). Finally, in individuals age 14 to 44, depression has been identified as the chief cause of disability (ADAA, 2018b), with home, work, and social activities being impacted to some extent by 80% of adults diagnosed with depression (Brody et al., 2018).

The purpose of this chapter is to provide nurses with information on brain physiology and the underlying pathophysiological changes of anxiety and depression and to provide information that will guide early assessment, diagnosis, and treatment of this common mental health condition.

Physiology

Anatomically, the *diencephalon*, or interbrain is located, within the cerebrum and is divided into four sections. The *epithalamus* is in the upper edge of the third ventricle and works in conjunction with the limbic system. The *thalamus* encloses the third ventricle and is responsible for afferent impulse transmission to the cerebral cortex. Forming the foundation of the diencephalon, the role of the *hypothalamus* includes body temperature and endocrine regulation and emotional response to stimuli (Sugerman & Huether, 2012). The anatomy and functions of the brain are shown in Figures 17–1 and 17–2 in Chapter 17.

Both the neural pathways and endocrine system play a role in hypothalamus function. The serotonin pathways originate in the brainstem's *raphe nuclei*, while norepinephrine pathways originate just below, in the *locus ceruleus*. Physiological response to stress begins in the locus coeruleus, which accounts for about one-half of all the central nervous system's adrenergic neurons. The pathways extend out across the brain into the cerebellum, forebrain, limbic system, and prefrontal cortex, and impaired transmission of impulses along these pathways triggers psychobiological imbalances that lead to depression (Townsend, 2018). The *limbic system* is a complex structure that includes portions of the *hippocampus*, *hypothalamus*, and *thalamus* and is responsible for transmission of impulses to the prefrontal cortex that initiate behavioral and visceral emotional responses, appetite, circadian rhythms, and olfactory sensations (Sugerman & Huether, 2012). The hypothalamus is also responsible for releasing corticotropin-releasing hormone, resulting in pituitary release of *adrenocorticotropin* (ACTH), which in turn causes the adrenal gland to secrete epinephrine, cortisol, and norepinephrine. Thus, the *hypothalamus-pituitary-adrenal* (HPA) feedback loop functions to begin and to stop the stress response (Capriotti, 2020; Wilson, 2009). One's emotional response to the environment (and to stress and fear) is the responsibility of the *amygdala*, also part of the limbic system, where neural pathways send signals throughout the brain to trigger a physiological response through the "fight-or-flight" sympathetic nervous system as well as to the prefrontal cortex, where emotions are integrated to behavioral responses (Capriotti, 2020).

Normal brain function is dependent on *neurotransmitters* (excitatory and inhibitory), which are essential in the transmission of impulses across synapses. The balance (or imbalance) of these neurotransmitters affects energy levels, the ability to focus and concentrate, moods, metabolism, and sleep patterns. Additionally, levels of *biogenic amines*, *peptides*, and *hormones* impact how well signals are transmitted. Biogenic amines include *epinephrine* and *norepinephrine*, excitatory neurotransmitters that help the body deal with stress; *dopamine*, which can be either an excitatory or inhibitory neurotransmitter and has a role in attention, behavior, cognition, mood, motivation, and reward responses in addiction; and *serotonin*, an inhibitory neurotransmitter whose precursor *tryptophan* is an antidepressant that improves antidepressant drug efficacy. Serotonin also has a role in aggression, anxiety, appetite, mood, cognition, and circadian rhythm. *Acetylcholine* is a cholinergic, can be either an excitatory or inhibitory transmitter, and has also been shown to have an impact on mood, neuroendocrine function, and sleep. Excessive transmission of acetylcholine is attributed to depression, while inadequate transmission is attributed to the development of mania (Capriotti, 2020; Townsend, 2018; Wilson, 2009).

Other neurotransmitters involved in behavioral and emotional responses include *gamma aminobutyric acid* (GABA), an inhibitory neurotransmitter involved in anticonvulsive and antianxiety responses in the brain. *Glutamate*, an excitatory neurotransmitter, is particularly involved in cognition, learning, and memory (Capriotti, 2020). Understanding normal brain physiology is helpful to nurses involved in the care of patients exhibiting symptoms of depression as pharmacological treatment is aimed at restoring the normal balance of neurotransmitters.

Pathways from the locus coeruleus extend to the amygdala, hippocampus, and limbic system and finally to the cerebral cortex.

 CLINICAL PEARLS

Normal transmission of impulses along pathways from the brainstem throughout the brain is required to maintain homeostasis in the balance of neurotransmitters.

Pathophysiology

Genetic tendency, inadequate dietary intake of amino acids (vitamin C, calcium, and zinc), environmental exposures (pesticides or heavy metals), some medications, and stress all can negatively impact message transmission between neurons. While it is well known that stress plays a role in many chronic diseases, including cardiovascular disease, cancer, and obesity, prolonged stress is also thought to lead to neurotransmitter imbalances that lead to depression, anxiety, and other mental health conditions (Wilson, 2009). *Eustress* is the term for stress that plays a positive role in behavior (motivation and feelings of success), while *distress* occurs when an individual has an abnormal or prolonged stress hormone response that results in negative feelings (Capriotti, 2020).

Seyle's stress response theory attempts to explain the impact of intermittent stress on homeostasis and body function. According to Seyle, the body's response to a stressful situation begins with *Alarm*. As the body is aroused to awareness of the stressful situation, the "fight-or-flight" response of the *sympathetic nervous system* (SNS) stimulates the hypothalamus, anterior pituitary gland, and the adrenal glands to secrete cortisol, epinephrine, and aldosterone; this causes increases in heart rate and blood pressure, bronchodilation, and vasoconstriction. In the kidney, potassium excretion is potentiated while sodium and water are reabsorbed, an effect that enhances blood pressure elevation. Initially, anti-inflammatory and white blood cell release increases, but the long-term effects of cortisol result in immunosuppression, a risk factor for infection in situations where the stress response is prolonged for more than 5 days. In the second stage, *Resistance*, a balance of hormones and catecholamines are secreted, and if stress is controlled or eliminated, the *parasympathetic nervous system* (PSNS) takes over to return to a relaxed state. Finally, *Exhaustion* results if the stressor is not removed and the body is overwhelmed by its attempts to continue catecholamine and hormone secretion. It is at this stage that the long-term effects of stress response result in feelings of anxiety, depression, inability to cope, fatigue, and physical illness (Capriotti, 2020).

In contrast, McEwen's theory attempts to explain the cumulative effects of prolonged stress on body functioning. According to McEwen, *homeostasis* is that constant physiological balance that is our "normal" physiological heart rate, blood pressure, and so on. *Allostasis* is the change in "normal" set points of physiological balance that occur with prolonged exposure to stress, and *allostatic load* is the long-term changes in body functioning that result from prolonged exposure to stress. For example, prolonged exposure to elevated cortisol causes immunosuppression and changes in sleep patterns, while chronic exposure to elevated epinephrine levels results in chronic vasoconstriction, which contributes to hypertension. Additionally, the allostatic load increases if the individual has repeated exposure to stressful experiences, is unable to successfully adapt to stress, has a prolonged or inappropriate reaction to stress, or simply does not secrete sufficient hormones to initiate the feedback mechanisms that respond to stress (Capriotti, 2020).

The HPA feedback loop links the endocrine system's release of stress hormones from the hypothalamus and pituitary gland with the nervous system. Released ACTH stimulates cortisol and norepinephrine release, causing the physiological changes of the stress response (elevated heart rate, blood pressure, and glucose levels). When the body is constantly responding to stress, the HPA feedback loop is unable to maintain proper functioning and cortisol levels fall, resulting in fatigue, hyperactive immune response that leads to autoimmune disease, and symptoms of depression. Chronic stress also impacts mood and motivation, feelings of fear, memory, and body response to appetite and pain because of HPA feedback loop interaction with the limbic system (Wilson, 2009). When tryptophan is depleted, serotonin levels fall, and depressive symptoms appear. In some patients, a genetic abnormality in serotonin transporter proteins can prevent the recycling of serotonin, lowering serotonin levels and increasing risk for clinical depression. Finally, endocrine changes when estrogen levels fluctuate (postpartum and menopause) or low testosterone levels in men have also been associated with the development of depression (Capriotti, 2020).

While the normal response to stress is a feeling of anxiousness, prolonged, intense feelings of anxiousness and the inability to cope with these feelings are defined as pathological anxiety (Hart, 2019). Cognitive theory suggests that thinking patterns become counterproductive and because thinking is distorted, the situation is inappropriately assessed. This leads to a behavioral response that is inappropriate for the situation (Townsend, 2018). Within the brain, levels of the neurotransmitters GABA and serotonin are below normal and there is an increase in norepinephrine activity in individuals with anxiety disorders (Capriotti, 2020).

Panic attacks have been connected to changes in the hippocampus and may have a genetic component with the overproduction of the protein cholecystokinin

(Capriotti, 2020; Townsend, 2018). The pathophysiology of *obsessive-compulsive disorder* (OCD), while not completely understood, is thought to be related to abnormal neurotransmission within the limbic system, frontal cortex, and thalamus. OCD also is thought to have a genetic component. The underlying pathophysiology of *post-traumatic stress disorder* (PTSD) is also not well understood but is thought to originate with a dysfunctional response to a repeated and prolonged response to stress. Sympathetic nervous system stimulation releases endogenous opioids; over time and with repeated exposure to stress, natural opioid levels decrease, resulting in hyperactivity. Neuroimaging of individuals with PTSD shows changes in blood flow (decreased to Broca's area and increased to amygdala), and a decrease in the size of the hippocampus (Capriotti, 2020).

CLINICAL PEARLS
While not well understood, vitamin B_{12} deficiency impacts synthesis of neurotransmitters and may contribute to the development of depression (Capriotti, 2020).

Assessment

Assessment of anxiety begins with a comprehensive history, including medications and medical and psychiatric conditions, plus neurological and physical examinations (Hart, 2019). Anxiety disorder can be subclassified into generalized anxiety, OCD, panic attacks, social anxiety, and PTSD. Because most anxiety disorders are missed or not treated effectively by primary care providers (Brodrick, 2020; Capriotti, 2020), it is important to distinguish between physical symptoms that are related to anxiety and those related to other medical conditions. Anxiety symptoms may mimic symptoms of cardiovascular disease, endocrine disorders, metabolic conditions, neurological conditions, anemias, excessive caffeine intake, vitamin B_{12} deficiency, respiratory disorders, and other psychiatric disorders; therefore, a physical examination to eliminate medical conditions should be conducted (Brodrick, 2020; Capriotti, 2020; Hart, 2019). The patient's feelings of fear, panic, and worry and the impact of these feelings on daily functioning must be explored (Hart, 2019). The *Hamilton Anxiety Rating Scale* (HAM-A) is administered by a provider and used to rate symptoms of anxiety (mood, tension, fear, insomnia, concentration and memory, and physiological symptoms) on a scale of not present to very severe. Self-report anxiety scales (Beck Anxiety Inventory, Zung Self-Rating Anxiety Scale) are also useful in describing the individual's anxiety symptom severity (Townsend, 2018). Signs and symptoms of the subclasses of anxiety are highlighted in Table 25–1.

Depression is classified based on symptoms and/or underlying cause of symptoms. *Major depressive disorder* (MDD), with symptoms lasting at least 2 weeks, can be a single episode or recurrent. *Persistent depressive disorder* (dysthymia) is a milder form of mood disturbance in which the individual feels sad for a prolonged period of at least 1 to 2 years but does not exhibit psychotic symptoms. *Substance or medication-induced depressive disorder* describes depression in which physiological symptoms are directly related to drug exposure or withdrawal from drugs. Individuals with *depressive disorder associated with medical conditions* exhibit depressive symptoms that can be attributed to an underlying medical condition (Townsend, 2018) such as cancer, cardiovascular disease, endocrine disorders (thyroid or adrenal gland disorders), neurological disease (Alzheimer's, multiple sclerosis, or Parkinson's disease), and certain nutritional deficiencies (iron, thiamine, or vitamin B_{12} deficiencies) (Capriotti, 2020).

Medications that are known to cause depressive symptoms include some antihypertensives, antiparkinsonian drugs, anti-anxiety drugs, Accutane, birth control pills,

TABLE 25–1 Symptoms of Anxiety

Type of Anxiety	Clinical Presentation
Generalized anxiety disorder (GAD)	Anxious, apprehensive feelings or worry that is not controlled Feelings are present most days over at least 6 months Symptoms are not related to a drug or medical condition Adults have at three or more of the following symptoms (adults) and children have one symptom: • Difficulty concentrating • Fatigue • Irritability • Muscle tension • Restlessness • Sleep disturbances
Panic attacks	Intense, sudden anxiety that peaks around 10 minutes from onset Fear of loss of control of the situation or impending death Physiological symptoms may mimic a myocardial infarction and include elevated heart rate, chest pain, choking sensation, dizziness, nausea, shortness of breath, sweating, trembling

Obsessive-compulsive disorder (OCD)	Recurring thoughts (obsessions) that is accompanied by an overwhelming need to perform rituals that once completed relieve the anxious feelings
	    The patient does not have control over the thoughts and actions
	    Obsessive-compulsive behaviors take up at least 1 a day and disrupt normal activities
	    Symptoms are not the result of drug or medical or mental health condition

Post-traumatic stress disorder (PTSD)	Flashbacks Hyperarousal Hypervigilance Insomnia Behavioral responses are similar to those the individual had in the initial stressful event
Social anxiety	Physical symptoms of dyspnea, elevated heart rate, panic, anxiety, sweating in response to a fear of being in a social situation (i.e., public speaking, dining in public, use of public restroom facilities)

(Capriotti, 2020; Hart, 2019; Townsend, 2018)

corticosteroids, and the hormones estrogen and progesterone (Hart, 2019). Prolonged bedrest, chronic pain, inactivity, and social isolation are also risk factors for depression (Capriotti, 2020). Additional risk factors for depression include a family or personal history of depression, and a major life change, stress, or trauma (NIMH, 2017).

A diagnosis of depression is made following a comprehensive medical and mental health evaluation and review of laboratory tests. Careful interviewing and active listening to the patient's symptoms are critical to a successful diagnosis because many medical conditions have similar signs and symptoms, patients may not be forthcoming with their behavioral symptoms, or symptoms may be related to certain medications or substance abuse. In fact, focusing on symptoms such as abnormal sleep patterns or anxiety can result in missing the underlying diagnosis of depression and initiating a treatment plan that worsens the depression (Hart, 2019).

While children, adolescents, and adults share some important symptoms, in children and adolescents the symptoms of depression may be more easily missed. Sudden changes in mood and behavior, drop in grades, and loss of self-confidence that lasts more than 2 weeks are often attributed to normal pubescent behavior but are red flags that the child or teen is experiencing depression (Townsend, 2018). The American Academy of Pediatrics recommends that all children age 12 and older be routinely screened for depression at their annual visit (Zuckerbrot et al., 2018). Late-life depression is common among older adults, particularly if they have experienced recent loss of a spouse or other loved one, have multiple health conditions, or have lost cognitive skills and are unable to perform independent activities of daily living (Beyer & Johnson, 2018). A significant distinction, however, is that individuals with late-life depression exhibit more cognitive impairments than is found in younger adults with depression. Cognitive decline may be misinterpreted as dementia rather than depression, delaying appropriate treatment (Kverno & Velez, 2018).

Diagnosis of depression is based on the number of symptoms (at least five) and the length of their presence (at least 2 weeks); these are highlighted in Table 25–2. Important to note is that symptoms negatively impact the individuals' participation in social activities and the ability to perform their jobs, which in turn increases their distress.

There are several assessment tools available to identify depression. Generally, these tools include questions about appetite, ability to concentrate, sleep patterns, and the

TABLE 25–2   Symptoms of Depression

Symptom	Adults	Older Adults	Adolescents	Children

Mood	Sadness that is present almost every day and lasts almost all day
	    Agitation or listlessness
	    Loss of interest in activities that cause pleasure (anhedonia)
	    Has recurrent thoughts of suicide and has devised a plan to commit suicide
		Sadness similar to adults
		    Bereavement overload may lead to depressive symptoms
			Anger
			Aggressiveness
			Delinquency
			Running away
			Social withdrawal
			Substance abuse
			Suicidal ideations
				Cranky
				Irritable
				    Loss of interest in activities and seeing friends
				Miserable
				Temper outburst
				Unhappy
				Suicidal ideations

Cognition	Feels worthless or has inappropriate guilt
	    Inability to concentrate and make decisions
		Apathy, confusion, memory loss may be misdiagnosed as cognitive decline	Apathy
			Restlessness
				Difficulty concentrating
				    Feels worthless or has inappropriate guilt
				    Thinks they are not loved

Physical	Fatigue
	    Weight changes (gain or loss)
	    Sleep disturbances (hypersomnia or insomnia) that are consistently present
		Early waking and reduced appetite may be misdiagnosed as depression, when actually part of normal aging	Eating disturbance
			Sleep disturbance
			Psychomotor complaints
				Appetite (overeating or not eating enough)
				    Weight does not increase per expectations
				    Sleep disturbances
				    Fatigue, headache, musculoskeletal pain, stomachaches

(Capriotti, 2020; Charles & Fazeli, 2017; Townsend, 2018)

inability to experience pleasure (*anhedonia*). The objective of these tools is to identify the presence and degree of depression with a goal of developing an effective treatment plan. Numeric scores for the individual items are tabulated to rank depression as mild, moderate, or severe. The health-care provider conducting the assessment should choose the tool that best fits the age and cognitive abilities of the patient. For example, some tools are specific to children, others to older adults and those with cognitive impairment. The Preschool Feelings Checklist, and the Cornell Scale for Depression in Dementia are completed by the caregiver. Each tool has specific directions included with the questions (Capriotti, 2020; Charles & Fazeli, 2017; Hart, 2019; Smith & Goad, 2019). Table 25–3 highlights basic information for each tool.

When assessing the patient for depressive symptoms, it is important to also assess for suicide risk. It is thought that one in seven people who experience symptoms of depression commit suicide and that more than 70% of these individuals have been seen by their health-care provider within 6 weeks of the event. Ask about the patient's past and present thoughts of hurting themselves, thoughts about suicide, and if they are having these thoughts, ask questions about any plans to carry out these thoughts. Presence of suicidal thoughts is a psychiatric emergency and requires immediate action to protect the patient from self-harm (Hart, 2019; Townsend, 2018).

TABLE 25–3 Depression Assessment Tools

Tool	Components
Beck Depression Inventory	A self-rating scale that gives points to score feelings related to depression.
Cornell Scale for Depression in Dementia	Used to screen individuals with moderate to severe dementia, contains 19 items; caregiver is interviewed to respond based on the prior week's observations of the person.
Geriatric Depression Scale	Yes or no answers to 15 questions related to feelings experienced over the past week. Points are given to each yes or no answer that is bolded on the questionnaire, with any score >5 suggesting depression. May also be used for older adults with dementia.
Hamilton Depression Rating Scale (HDRS)	Most widely used adult depression assessment tool. Gives point values for the patient's description of: Depressed mood, feelings of guilt, suicide ideations, Insomnia (early, middle of night and early morning), work and activities, psychomotor retardation, agitation, anxiety, somatic symptoms (GI and general), genital symptoms, hypochondriasis, weight loss, insight (acknowledgment of feelings of depression or illness).
Preschool Feelings Checklist	Used with preschool children. Has 16 yes or no answers that are answered by the parent/caregiver.
Mood and Feelings Questionnaire (MFQ)	Used with children ≥8 years of age. Has 13 questions that are answered "not true," "sometimes true," and "true" based on recent actions and feelings that occurred during the past 2 weeks.
Children's Depression Inventory 2 (CDI 2)	Used with children between 7 and 17 years of age and includes self-report questions for the child, parent, and teacher; children must be able to read at the second-grade level to take their portion of the questionnaire. Score is based on responses to questions in areas of Emotional (negative mood, physical, or self-esteem) and Functional (interpersonal problems or feelings of ineffectiveness) problems.

(Alexopoulos, Abrams, Young, & Shamoian,1998; Angold & Costello, 1987; Byrd & Pierson, 2019; Charles & Fazeli, 2017; Kovacs, n.d.; Ludy, Heffelfinger, Mrakotsky, & Hildebrand, 1999; Smith & Goad, 2019; Townsend, 2018)

ASSESSMENT PEARLS

Individuals who are experiencing depression may not self-report; therefore, careful assessment of presenting symptoms is critical to appropriate treatment interventions.

Pharmacology

Anxiolytics are the most commonly prescribed drugs used to treat anxiety. They work in the limbic system and in the reticular formation to potentiate GABA and cause the individual to become calmer. With the exception of buspirone, most anxiolytics typically cause CNS depression and should not be used in conjunction with other drugs known to cause CNS depression (Townsend, 2018). Benzodiazepines, *tricyclic antidepressants* (TCAs), *selective serotonin reuptake inhibitors* (SSRIs), and *serotonin-norepinephrine reuptake inhibitors* (SNRIs) are also used to treat anxiety as well as depression (Brodrick, 2020).

Antidepressants are the drugs of choice for treating depressive conditions to elevate mood and improve other symptoms of depression (Townsend, 2018). These drugs work to change neurotransmitter deficiencies by either increasing norepinephrine, blocking the reuptake of neurotransmitters, or by preventing neurotransmitter breakdown at the receptor sites. Drugs are classed based on how they act on various neurotransmitters and include

• TCAs,
• SSRIs, or
• *Monoamine oxidase inhibitors* (MAOIs)

SSRIs are also used to treat anger and irritability in PTSD patients, because these symptoms have been related to a serotonin deficiency (Capriotti, 2020).

Choice of drug is individualized and may be based on age and on how well the individual tolerates any adverse effects (Karch, 2020). Results of the physical and psychological examinations should be considered along with the patient's prior responses to treatment (if applicable) and the drug's risk/benefit and cost considerations (Brodrick, 2020).

Prescribing antidepressants for older adults requires lower dosage, and the Beers Criteria Medication list is suggested as a guide to identification of inappropriate drugs for older adults. Antidepressants often interact with other medications that the patient may be taking, so a careful review of current medication list is essential (Kverno & Velez, 2018; Townsend, 2018). Despite the challenges of prescribing antidepressants for older adults, these drugs have been shown to be effective in treating older adults with long-term, moderate to severe depression (Beyer & Johnson, 2018). Drug classes and prototypes used in treating anxiety and depression are highlighted in Table 25–4.

Serotonin syndrome may occur when SSRIs are combined with other drugs that increase levels of 5-hydroxytryptamine (5-HT), including other SSRIs. Therefore, when switching from one class of drug to another (i.e., between an SSRI and a MAOI or between an SSRI and a TCA), it is important to space out the transition, titrating therapy over at least 10 days or allowing 2 to 4 weeks' transition to avoid this life-threatening complication. Ingestion of St. John's wort and triptans when combined with an SSRI may also lead to serotonin syndrome (Karch, 2020; Woo, 2020). Serotonin syndrome is suspected when the following symptoms are observed in patients who have excessive serotonin levels: chills, hyperthermia, or perspiration along with *gastrointestinal* (GI) symptoms of diarrhea and nausea, hypertension, and neurological symptoms that encompass cognitive changes (disorientation, confusion, delirium), and motor symptoms of ataxia, tremor, and myoclonic jerking (Woo, 2020).

TABLE 25–4 Drugs Used to Treat Anxiety and Depression

Class	Example	Action	Dosage	SENC
Benzodiazepines used as anxiolytics	Alprazolam	Potentiate effectiveness of GABA to ↓ neuron activity.	0.25 mg tid with may dose 10 mg/day ↓ dose in older adults.	Used for anxiety. Must be tapered after long-term use.
Cyclopyrrolones	Eszopiclone	Interacts with GABA to improve sleep (not a benzodiazepine).	1 mg PO immediately prior to bedtime.	Caution: daytime drowsiness, coordination difficulties, and memory loss. May get out of bed after taking and perform activities that they are unaware of, especially if taken with alcohol or CNS depressants.
Tricyclic antidepressants (TCAs)	Amitriptyline	Potentiates action of norepinephrine and serotonin.	75 mg in divided doses with max of 150 mg/day. Lower dose for older patients.	Anticholinergic properties: dry eyes and mouth; suicidal ideations; cardiac arrhythmias; urinary retention. Class is on Beer's Criteria Medication list; avoid in older patients.
	Imipramine		25–50 mg tid to qid, max dose 300 mg/day. Geriatric dose: 25 mg at bedtime.	Avoid use with MAOIs. Safety not established in young children.
Monoamine oxidase inhibitors (MAOIs)	Phenelzine	Inhibits MAO; allows accumulation of dopamine, norepinephrine, and 5-HT at synapse.	Initial: 15 mg tid. Maintenance: 15 mg daily.	CNS symptoms (dizziness, vertigo), orthostatic hypotension, and anticholinergic effects.
Selective serotonin reuptake inhibitors (SSRIs)	Fluoxetine	Inhibits the reuptake of 5-HT.	20 mg PO every a.m. Max dose 60 mg/day.	Fluoxetine is approved for use in children 8 years and older.
	Escitalopram		Initial: 10 mg daily. Maintenance: 10–20 mg daily.	
Heterocyclic drugs	Bupropion	Inhibits dopamine, and to a lesser extent inhibits reuptake of serotonin and norepinephrine.	Initial: 100 mg bid and titrate after 3 days to max does of 450 mg/day. Once therapeutic level is achieved, may change to sustained or extended-release form.	In low doses, may be used as part of smoking cessation treatment. Avoid use with MAOIs; has anticholinergic effects; assess for suicical ideations and seizure activity.
Serotonin-norepinephrine reuptake inhibitors (SNRIs)	Duloxetine	Inhibits norepinephrine and serotonin reuptake.	40–60 mg/day in divided doses or one daily dose.	Avoid use with MAOIs; assess for symptoms of neuroleptic malignant and serotonin syndromes, suicidal ideations, and seizure activity.

(Brodrick, 2020; Karch, 2020; Kverno & Velez, 2018; Vallerand & Sanoski, 2017)

Patient education is crucial in pharmacological treatment of depression and is multifaceted. The nurse needs to:

- Stress the importance of taking medication as prescribed and reporting adverse symptoms.
- Teach patients that it may take about 2 to 4 weeks following initiation of drug therapy before symptoms improve, and to continue medication even if they do not see immediate symptom improvement (Townsend, 2018; Vallerand & Sanoski, 2017).
- Advise patients of interventions that can decrease side effects, including taking drugs with food to avoid GI upset; drinking water frequently or using sugarless candy for dry mouth; and voiding before taking the drug to avoid issues with urinary retention.
- Caution patients on becoming pregnant, as many antidepressants are harmful to the fetus (Karch, 2020; Townsend, 2018).
- Instruct patients to avoid alcohol consumption while on antidepressants to avoid potentiation of the effects of both.
- Educate patients not to abruptly stop taking anxiolytics and antidepressants to avoid withdrawal symptoms (NIMH, 2018; Vallerand & Sanoski, 2017).
- Caution patients not to take any other medications without checking with their provider.
- Warn patients not to "double up" if they miss a dose, because the primary reason for dividing the daily dose is to avoid adverse effects, including seizures (Townsend, 2018).

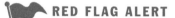

RED FLAG ALERT

Fluoxetine is the first line and only antidepressant (SSRI) approved for use in treating depression in children age 8 and older. Use requires careful monitoring for behavioral changes and suicidal thoughts.

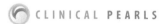

CLINICAL PEARLS

Treatment plans for individuals should be individualized and based on the underlying causes of depressive symptoms.

Complementary and Alternative Therapies

Drug therapy alone is often inadequate to treat anxiety or depressive symptoms. *Cognitive-behavioral therapy* (CBT) is an evidence-based intervention designed to help patients change their spontaneous and often distorted thoughts regarding feelings of failure, worthlessness, or inability to accept positive thoughts; it is frequently initiated to treat anxiety and depression. Interpersonal therapy and family therapy are also known CBTs that may be helpful in improving these conditions (Charles & Fazeli, 2017; NIMH, 2018; Townsend, 2018). Patients with OCD are introduced to CBT as a first line treatment option (Capriotti, 2020). Psychosocial interventions are key to treating depression, particularly in children too young to be treated with antidepressants and who may have been negatively impacted by bullying, abuse, neglect, or parents with a history of substance abuse or mental illness (Charles & Fazeli, 2017). Goals of psychotherapy include developing coping skills, understanding and changing behaviors that have contributed to depression symptoms, and improving relationships (CDC, 2018).

Other behavioral changes that are known to improve mental outlook on life are smoking cessation, avoiding alcohol and drug use, and improving health through diet and exercise (CDC, 2018). Participating in yoga, a practice that combines breathing exercises with meditation and physical postures, has been found effective in alleviating symptoms of depression and anxiety. Meditation and relaxation techniques are also helpful in reducing symptoms of anxiety and depression (ADAA, 2018a).

Transcranial magnetic stimulation (TMS) is a noninvasive procedure, typically used for short-term depression. During this procedure, a stimulating coil is placed on the skull and magnetic impulses are delivered to the areas of the brain responsible for mood regulation. It is thought that these impulses work to stimulate secretion of growth factors that are important to growth of nervous tissues and that have some antidepressant effects. *Vagus nerve stimulation* (VNS) was originally used to treat seizure disorders that did not respond to drug therapy; based on the resulting improvement in mood, the procedure is now approved as an alternative treatment for depression that has not been helped by other treatment options. The system is surgically implanted and delivers electrical stimulation to the vagus nerve, with the goal of improving mood (Capriotti, 2020; Townsend, 2018). In severe depression when antidepressants and other interventions have failed to resolve symptoms, *electroconvulsive therapy* (ECT) may be considered. The procedure is performed under anesthesia, and the seizure that is produced is thought to stimulate neurotransmitters. ECT sessions are typically scheduled for three times a week over a 2- to 4-week period and have been found to be an effective alternative treatment (Capriotti, 2020; NIMH, 2018).

CLINICAL PEARLS
Only very small amounts of amino acids found in protein-rich foods reach the brain to assist in conversion of amino acids to neurotransmitters, making the supplementation of vitamins and minerals such as calcium, zinc, and vitamin C an important part of amino acid therapy (Wilson, 2009).

Summary

Depression is a common mental health disorder that occurs across the life span, affecting over 16 million adults and over 3 million adolescents in the United States. While its etiology is not clearly understood, it is thought to stem from neurotransmitter imbalances caused by stress. Symptoms of anxiety and depression negatively impact the individual's quality of life, increase health-care costs, increase risk for substance abuse, and, if left untreated, may lead to suicidal ideation or even suicide itself (CDC, 2018; Kverno & Velez, 2018). Symptoms go beyond feelings of sadness or anxiety and often present differently in adults, adolescents, and children. Early recognition of symptoms of anxiety and depression and appropriate interventions are critical to developing and implementing an appropriate treatment plan that is aimed at improving the individual's health and quality of life. While antidepressant medication is the front line of pharmacological treatment of depression, alternative and complementary therapies exist that can support or replace drug treatment.

Key Points

- Anxiety and depression impact quality of life across the life span, and symptoms may be caused by a neurotransmitter imbalance in the brain that stems from environmental stressors, medical conditions, or drugs.
- While depression may be a one-time event, risk of recurrence is at least 50%, making early identification and treatment essential to decreasing this risk.
- Screening for depression is recommended for all children age 12 or older as well as for adults and older adults as a part of the annual examination.
- Antidepressants, the first line drugs used to treat depression, have adverse interactions with many other drugs.

- Psychotherapy is key to successful management of stress and anxiety or depressive symptoms.
- Patient education should include information about the role of stress, exercise, and healthy eating in anxiety and depression, as well as information about any prescribed drugs.

Review Questions

1. **The nurse is preparing a patient with short-term depression for electroconvulsive therapy (ECT). Which of the following statements is correct?**

   a. Ask the patient if they have a pacemaker, because the procedure uses magnets.
   b. Inquire whether the patient has prepared for the procedure by eating breakfast.
   c. Make a post-procedure assessment of the insertion site for signs of infection.
   d. Schedule sessions as ordered over the next 2 to 4 weeks.

2. **Which of the following screening tools is appropriate for use for an 8-year-old child?**

   a. Beck Depression Inventory
   b. Hamilton Depression Rating Scale
   c. Mood and Feelings Questionnaire
   d. No screening tool is available for children

3. **The nurse is taking a health history for an adult patient who reports fatigue, weight gain, and hypersomnia. When reviewing the patient's medication list, which of the following is suspected to contribute to the patient's symptoms?**

   a. The multivitamin taken to supplement their dietary intake
   b. The propranolol taken to control their blood pressure
   c. The statin taken to lower their cholesterol
   d. The thiazide diuretic they are taking for ankle swelling

4. **When assessing a patient with depression for suicide risk, which of the following questions should be including in screening? (Select all that apply.)**

   a. "Have you ever attempted suicide?"
   b. "Have you ever thought about harming yourself?"
   c. "Have you ever thought about harming others?"
   d. "If you have thought about harming yourself, do you have a plan?"

5. **When educating the patient who has been prescribed an antidepressant for depression, which of the following statements lets the nurse know that the patient understands instructions?**

   a. "I don't need a reminder, because I can double up on my dose if I forget to take it."
   b. "I can still have one glass of wine with dinner, because I take my dose in the morning."
   c. "I should void within 2 hours of taking my antidepressant to avoid feeling 'full.'"
   d. "I will continue taking my medication as ordered even though I may not feel better."

See the appendix for answers to review questions.

References

Alexopoulos, G. S., Abrams, R. C., Young, R. C., & Shamoian, C. A. (1998). Cornell Scale for Depression in Dementia. *Biological Psychiatry, 23,* 271–284.

Angold, A., & Costello, E. J. (1987). Mood and Feelings Questionnaire: Short version. Retrieved from http://devepi.duhs.duke.edu/instruments/MFQ%20Child%20Self-Report%20-%20Short.pdf

Anxiety and Depression Association of America. (2018a). Complementary and alternative treatments. Retrieved from https://adaa.org/finding-help/treatment/complementary-alternative-treatment

Anxiety and Depression Association of America. (2018b). *Types of depression.* Retrieved from https://adaa.org/understanding-anxiety/depression

Beyer, J. L., & Johnson, K. G. (2018). Advanced in pharmacotherapy of late-life depression. *Current Psychiatry Reports, 20*(34). Retrieved from https://doi.org/10.1007s11920-018-0899-6

Brodrick, N. (2020) Anxiety and depression. In T. M. Woo & M. V. Robinson (Eds.), *Pharmacotherapeutics for advanced practice nurse prescribers* (5th ed.). Philadelphia, PA: F.A. Davis.

Brody, D. J., Pratt, L. A., & Hughes, J. P. (2018) *Prevalence of depression among adults aged 20 and over: United States, 2013–2016* (NCHS Data Brief No. 303). Hyattsville, MD: National Center for Health Statistics. Retrieved from https://www.cdc.gov/nchs/products/databriefs/db303.htm

Byrd, L., & Pierson, C. (2019). Older adults. In M. J. Goolsby & L. Grubbs (Eds.), *Advanced assessment: Interpreting findings and formulating differential diagnoses* (4th ed.). Philadelphia, PA: F.A. Davis.

Capriotti, T. (2020). *Pathophysiology: Introductory concepts and clinical perspectives* (2nd ed.). Philadelphia, PA: F.A. Davis.

Centers for Disease Control and Prevention. (2015). *Depression in the U.S. Household population, 2009–2012.* Retrieved from https://www.cdc.gov/nchs/products/databriefs/db172.htm

Centers for Disease Control and Prevention. (2018). *Mental health conditions: Depression and anxiety.* Retrieved from https://www.cdc.gov/tobacco/campaign/tips/diseases/depression-anxiety.html

Charles, J., & Fazeli, M. (2017). Depression in children. *Australian Family Physician, 46*(12), 901–907.

Dillon, P. M. (2007). *Nursing health assessment: A critical thinking, case studies approach* (2nd ed.). Philadelphia, PA: F.A. Davis.

Hart, V. A. (2019). Psychiatric mental health. In M. J. Goolsby & L. Grubbs (Eds.), *Advanced assessment: Interpreting findings and formulating differential diagnoses* (4th ed.). Philadelphia, PA: F.A. Davis.

Karch, A. M. (2020). *Focus on nursing pharmacology* (8th ed.). Philadelphia, PA: Wolters Kluwer / Lippincott Williams & Wilkins.

Kovacs, M. (n.d.). Children's Depression Inventory 2. Retrieved from https://www.mhs.com/MHS-Assessment?prodname=cdi2

Kverno, K. S., & Velez, R. (2018). Comorbid dementia and depression: The case for integrated care. *The Journal for Nurse Practitioners, 14*(3), 196–201.

Luby, J., Heffelfinger, A., Mrakotsky, C., & Hildebrand T. (1999). Preschool Feelings Checklist. Retrieved from https://medicine.tulane.edu/sites/g/files/rdw761/f/pictures/Preschool%20feelings%20checklist.pdf

Mental Health America. (2018). *Depression in older adults: More facts.* Retrieved from http://www.mentalhealthamerica.net/conditions/depression-older-adults-more-facts

National Institute of Mental Health. (2017). *Major depression.* Retrieved from https://www.nimh.nih.gov/health/statistics/major-depression.shtml

National Institute of Mental Health. (2018). *Depression.* Retrieved from https://www.nimh.nih.gov/health/topics/depression/index.shtml

Smith, J. W., & Goad, B. J. (2019). *Geriatric notes.* Burlington, MA: Jones & Bartlett Learning.

Sugerman, R. A., & Huether, S. E. (2012). Structure and function of the neurologic system. In S. E. Huether & K. L. McCance (Eds.), *Understanding pathophysiology* (5th ed.). St. Louis, MO: Elsevier Mosby.

Townsend, M. C. (2018). *Psychiatric mental health nursing: Concepts of care in evidence-based practice* (9th ed.). Philadelphia, PA: F.A. Davis.

Vallerand, A. H., & Sanoski, C. A. (Eds.). (2021). *Davis's drug guide for nurses* (17th ed.). Philadelphia, PA: F.A. Davis.

Wilson, D. (2009). Anxiety and depression: It all starts with stress. *Integrative Medicine, 8*(3), 42–45.

Woo, T. M. (2020). Drugs affecting the central nervous system. In T. M. Woo & M. V. Robinson (Eds.), *Pharmacotherapeutics for advanced practice nurse prescribers* (5th ed.). Philadelphia, PA: F.A. Davis

Zuckerbrot, R. A., Cheung, A., Jenson, P.S., Stein, R.E.D., & Laraque, D. (2018). Guidelines for adolescent depression in Primary Care (GLAD-PC): Part 1. Practice preparation, identification, assessment and initial management. *Pediatrics, 141*(3) e20174081; DOI: https://doi.org/10.1542/peds.2017-4081

Psychotic Disorders

Introduction

Psychosis is defined as "a severe condition in which there is disorganization of the personality, deterioration of social functioning, and loss of contact with, or distortion, of reality" (Townsend, 2018, p. 420).

Psychosis may have a physiological, or organic, origin or may be completely psychological in nature. Hallucinations and delusions are the primary signs and symptoms of psychosis, but these are not necessarily present in all patients who are deemed psychotic. While psychosis may occur with various conditions, it is most frequently associated with schizophrenia, bipolar disorder, and depression (Capriotti, 2020; Townsend, 2018). Many external substances may result in psychosis, including street drugs, alcohol, prescriptions (e.g., antidepressants, antihypertensives, corticosteroids) and over-the-counter medications (e.g., NSAIDs, antihistamines) (Capriotti, 2020; Woo, 2020).

Rates of psychosis are variable because it often occurs with other psychiatric and medical conditions. Psychosis occurs in approximately 53% of individuals with bipolar disorder, which is noted as *bipolar-psychosis* (BP-P) (Burton et al., 2018). The overall rate of bipolar disorder is 2.8% of the U.S. population, with similar prevalence among men (2.9%) and women (2.8%). The rate of bipolar disorder is slightly higher for adolescents at 2.9%; among this group, girls have a higher rate of 3.3% as compared to boys at 2.6% (Burton et al., 2018; National Institute of Mental Health [NIMH], 2018). While bipolar disorder usually starts in late adolescence or early adulthood, children may be diagnosed with bipolar disorder. Prevalence of child-onset bipolar is not well established due to the frequency of concomitant disorders such as attention deficit-hyperactivity disorder, oppositional defiant disorder, conduct disorder, and anxiety disorders. Because there is a genetic predisposition to bipolar disorder, children who are at high risk for its development can be identified for early evaluation and/or intervention (NIMH, 2018).

While it is difficult to provide accurate incidence and prevalence rates for schizophrenia, because it is a complex diagnosis that often overlaps with other disorders (NIMH, 2018), the estimated prevalence of schizophrenia and/or a related psychotic disorder is less than 1% of the U.S. population, at about 0.24% to 0.64%. Globally, the prevalence of these same disorders has a wider range of 0.33% to 0.75%, but still remains less than 1%. While the prevalence of schizophrenia globally is relatively small, the economic burden associated with schizophrenia is significant because it is one of the top 15 reasons for claiming disability benefits. According to the World Health Organization, the cost of schizophrenia in Western countries ranges from 1.6% to 2.6% of total health-care expenditures (approximately 7% to 12% of the gross national product). Specifically, in the United States the economic burden of schizophrenia is more than $60 billion/year (Chong et al., 2016). The lost work productivity is an estimated $117 billion and is especially impactful as individuals are diagnosed early in life and lose many potential years as workers. The caregiver cost of schizophrenia is also significant and estimated at 1,040 hours per year ($52.3 billion), which is 34% of the cost of the disease. Additional costs of schizophrenia include the criminal justice system ($14.3 billion/9.2% total cost), suicide ($3.3 billion/2.1% total cost), emergency care ($2.6 billion/1.75 total cost), and homeless shelters ($1.9 billion/1.2% total cost) (NIMH, 2018).

Individuals with schizophrenia are also at risk for premature death and have a life expectancy that is 28.5 years shorter than the national average in the United States. This increased mortality is partially explained by medical comorbidities (e.g., diabetes, heart disease, and liver disease) and also by the high rate of suicide (up to 4.9%) (Capriotti, 2020; Hardy, 2013). Schizophrenia occurs across the life span but is most frequently diagnosed in the late teen years to thirties (NIMH, 2018). There is a sex-related difference in its emergence. In male individuals, it occurs in late adolescence to early twenties; in female individuals it usually occurs later, in their twenties and into thirties (Mental Health America [MHA], 2018).

Schizophrenia is rare in children and occurs at a prevalence rate of 1 in 40,000. Children experience similar symptoms to adults, including hallucinations and delusions, but they may be more difficult to diagnose because of developmental considerations. In a review of the literature that focused on the early identification of children at risk for psychosis, studies showed that those determined to be at *clinical high risk* (CHR) had mild positive symptoms, reported perceptual abnormalities, and measured lower in intelligence, without structural brain abnormalities. When identified as CHR, there was a definite diagnosis of psychosis at 1 year (17% to 20%) and 2 years (7% to 21%), supporting that there are early symptoms in children; however, further research is needed to clarify who will benefit from early intervention strategies (Tor et al., 2018). In a recent meta-analysis, the duration of untreated psychosis was associated with neurocognitive impairment (Allott et al., 2018), which emphasizes the importance of early recognition and treatment of psychosis. The nurse should be knowledgeable of the pathophysiology that is associated with psychosis along with a guide for assessment and treatment of psychosis based on current guidelines.

Physiology

Similar to other mental disorders such as depression, knowledge of normal brain physiology is necessary to understand pharmacological treatment of psychosis, which is aimed at restoring the normal balance of neurotransmitters (see Chapter 24 for normal brain physiology). Specifically, overactivity of dopamine has been suggested to be responsible for psychosis, through each of the four dopaminergic pathways: *mesolimbic, mesocortical, nigrostriatal,* and *tuberoinfundibular*. These pathways are shown in Figure 26–1. Any change in normal functioning along these pathways causes altered

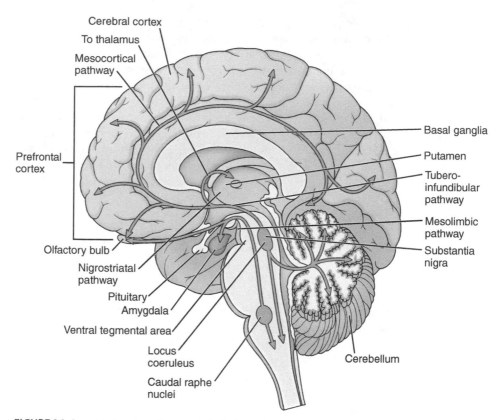

FIGURE 26–1 Dopaminergic pathways within the brain *(From Capriotti, T. (2020). Pathophysiology: Introductory concepts and clinical perspectives (2nd ed.). Philadelphia, PA: F.A. Davis.)*

mentation, sensations, and/or motor function. First, the mesolimbic pathway transmits dopamine from the *ventral tegmental area* (VTA) in the midbrain (*meso-* or *middle*), to the ventral striatum in the limbic system. Excess activity along this pathway is related to positive symptoms of schizophrenia (e.g., delusions and hallucinations) and also these symptoms when they occur in BP-P. Next, the mesocortical pathway transmits dopamine from the VTA to the prefrontal cortex; diminished dopamine activity along this pathway is associated with the negative symptoms of schizophrenia (e.g., flat affect, apathy, anhedonia). The nigrostriatal pathway transmits dopamine from the *substantia nigra pars compacta* (SNc) to the caudate nucleus and putamen; when dopamine does not move normally along this pathway alterations in movement, such as Parkinson's symptoms (tremors, lack of facial expression, difficulty moving/walking) occur. Finally, the tuberoinfundibular pathway transmits dopamine from the hypothalamus to the pituitary gland; alterations in this pathway affect functioning of the endocrine system. Abnormalities in any of these pathways for the transmission of dopamine may result in psychotic symptomatology (Capriotti, 2020; Townsend, 2018).

There are several neurotransmitters that are involved in the development and/or expression of psychosis. First, serotonin, found in the brain and *gastrointestinal tract* (GI), is a neurotransmitter that contributes to feelings of well-being and also regulates mood, memory, sleep, and appetite. Norepinephrine, associated with the alarm stage of *general adaptation syndrome* (GAS), is responsible for the fight-or-flight response, which includes both physiological (dilated pupils, dilated bronchioles, increased blood pressure) and psychological (increased alertness and elevated mood) components. Similarly, glutamate is a major mediator of excitatory signals in the *central nervous system* (CNS) and also increases cognition, memory, and learning. Once glutamate is released from the neuron, it must be removed from the extracellular space as its accumulation leads to brain cell injury and death. While these three transmitters have an excitatory effect on the nervous system, *gamma aminobutyric acid* (GABA) is the chief inhibitory neurotransmitter in the CNS and causes relaxation and decreased anxiety (Capriotti, 2020; NIMH, 2018; Woo, 2020).

CLINICAL PEARLS

An organic cause, or abnormality in the brain anatomy and physiology, must be ruled out before a patient is given a psychological diagnosis and cause of psychosis, such as schizophrenia.

Pathophysiology

Psychosis may occur with several mental disorders; the most common one is schizophrenia, but individuals with bipolar disorder may also have psychosis, especially in the manic phase. Pathophysiology for these two disorders is presented in this chapter, and the reader is directed to the pathophysiology for depression (see Chapter 25), as it may also be a cause of psychosis. The pathophysiology of schizophrenia is based on several theories and the exact cause has not been determined to date. Based on identical twin studies, there is a 50% rate of inheritance. Additionally, the vulnerability-liability theory proposes that the genetic component makes an individual *vulnerable* to developing schizophrenia, but the environment is also responsible for its ultimate development. It is theorized that the chance for inheriting schizophrenia increases if the father's age is over 60 at the time of conception, based on smaller numbers of healthy sperm available (Capriotti, 2020; NIMH, 2018).

While the dopamine theory of schizophrenia has existed for years and is the basis for pharmacological management with certain *antipsychotics* (APs), it has minimal supporting evidence. In this theory, an excess of dopamine is responsible for psychosis, but the specific mechanism is not well understood. It is thought that overactivity of *dopamine*$_2$ (D$_2$) receptors in the basal ganglia, hypothalamus, limbic system, brainstem, and medulla occurs along with underactivity of these same D$_2$ receptors in another area of the brain, the prefrontal cortex, and these are responsible for the symptoms of schizophrenia. Specifically, the overactivity of the D$_2$ receptors causes the positive symptoms, including psychosis (hallucinations and delusions), whereas the underactivity is responsible for the negative symptoms (social withdrawal, mutism, etc.) (Capriotti, 2020; NIMH, 2018; Woo, 2020).

It has also been proposed that an excess of serotonin and/or lack of GABAergic neurons may cause psychosis, along with an excess of norepinephrine and glutamate. With a decrease of GABA, which has a chiefly inhibitory action at the receptors, coupled with increased amounts of the stimulating neurotransmitters norepinephrine and glutamate, there is overstimulation of the receptors, which may precipitate abnormal thoughts (delusions) and sensations (hallucinations). Additionally, an excess of serotonin has been hypothesized to cause symptoms of schizophrenia. In addition, the loss of GABAergic neurons in the hippocampus leads to hyperactivity of serotonin (Capriotti, 2020).

The kindling theory is an emerging theory that proposes neurons that are stimulated too frequently become overly sensitive to further stimulation. The theory was originally used to explain how repeated seizures made the brain more sensitive to lower levels of stimulation, which lowered the seizure threshold. In bipolar disorder, rapid cycling between the manic and depressive stages stimulates neurons so that eventually less stimulation is needed to evoke a response. Rapid cycling occurs in approximately 20% to 30% of individuals diagnosed with bipolar disorder and places them at higher risk to repeated episodes of depression and/or mania (Capriotti, 2020).

Most of the support for these theories is based on patient responses to medications that block these neurotransmitters. Some theories point to alteration of brain circuits and processes rather than structural defects. Immune abnormalities, including cell antibodies that act against healthy brain cells, may also result in abnormal neurotransmitter activity that results in psychosis (Capriotti, 2020; Townsend, 2018). Additionally, the role of neuroinflammation is being studied as part of the relationship between systemic autoimmune diseases and psychiatric illness (Najjar, Pearlman, Alper, Najjar, & Devinsky, 2013).

There is support for physiological bases from neuroimaging studies that show the following changes in individuals with schizophrenia: loss of brain volume, lateral and third ventricle enlargement, and decreased cortical tissue, especially in the temporal, frontal, and occipital lobes. The loss of brain tissue is usually not symmetrical. Within the four dopaminergic pathways (described above) there are different dopamine receptors D_{1-6} that have concentrations in specific areas of the brain; pharmacological management may be aimed at certain receptors (usually D_1 and D_2) to control psychotic symptoms (Capriotti, 2020; Townsend, 2018; Woo, 2020).

In order to better understand pathophysiology of psychosis, van Dellen and colleagues (2016) conducted a study that compared individuals with subclinical psychotic symptoms with healthy individuals using diffusion tension imaging, and found the structural change of decreased centrality of parietal hubs in those with psychosis. These findings are preliminary but support the theory that brain network disturbances of white matter connections play a central role in the pathophysiology of psychosis.

In contrast, the pathophysiology for bipolar disorder has been supported with neuroimaging studies that revealed changes in the communication pathways between the prefrontal cortex and the amygdala. Also, *positron emission tomography* (PET) and *single photon emission computed tomography* (SPECT) scans showed increased activity in the temporal lobe with associated enlargement in the amygdala. Similar to schizophrenia, there is a strong genetic component to this condition, which is supported by the identification of a genome that encodes for an enzyme (*diacylglycerol kinase* [DGKH]) that is part of the lithium-sensitive pathway (Capriotti, 2020). According to Derosse and colleagues (2012), a review of molecular genetic studies revealed evidence for the relationship of genetic variation and symptom-based phenotypic variation within psychiatric illness, including psychotic disorders. Additionally, chromosomes 13 and 15 have been mapped for involvement with both bipolar illness and schizophrenia (Townsend, 2018).

Stressful events are also known to precipitate psychotic breaks and disorders, but the precise mechanism is not clear. The nurse can apply principles of Selye's stress response theory and McEwen's theory to care of individuals with psychosis (refer to Chapter 25). Specifically, Appiah-Kusi and colleagues (2016) synthesized current evidence related to alterations in the neuroendocrine stress response system and the endocannabinoid system in psychotic disorders. In studies that were included in the analysis, endocannabinoid levels were found to be higher in patients with psychosis as compared to healthy patients, and increased further in response to stress. The studies suggested these neurotransmitters may contribute to the development of psychosis; however, a link between stress and this system has not been supported by research. Furthermore, there are changes in the reactivity of the *hypothalamic–pituitary–adrenal* (HPA) axis and the endocannabinoid system in patients with psychosis, but the relationship of these two systems is not understood (Appiah-Kusi et al., 2016).

CLINICAL PEARLS
While not well understood, overactivity of several neurotransmitters, especially dopamine, may be responsible for the development of psychosis (Capriotti, 2020).

Assessment

Assessment of the individual who is experiencing active psychosis is a complex undertaking. When a patient is in the acute phase of an illness, they may not be able to contribute to the health history, and information must be obtained from other sources such as family members or prior health-care episodes, if available (Hart, 2015; Townsend, 2018). The nurse has the opportunity to establish rapport with the patient during the assessment while gathering valuable data about their mental status (Townsend, 2018). Because therapeutic communication techniques are vital to the effectiveness of this process, a brief overview of those that are especially helpful when interviewing patients experiencing psychosis are presented in Table 26–1. While there are many other manifestations of psychotic disorders, hallucinations and delusions are the primary symptoms of a psychosis and are the focus of this Assessment section.

An integral part of the mental status assessment is determining if the person is experiencing alterations in thought content, or delusions. Specifically, delusions are "false beliefs that are inconsistent with the person's intelligence or cultural background" (Townsend, 2018, p. 430), so understanding the patient's background and context (intellectual, social, environmental) is important in determining if there is a loss of reality. The most common delusions are presented in Table 26–2. The individual continues to

TABLE 26–1   Therapeutic Communication Techniques to Use With Patients With Psychotic Disorders

Technique	Description and Rationale for Use	Representative Quote
Accepting	Conveys positive regard for patient in the present	"I realize the voices are real to you."
Giving recognition	Acknowledges patient's progress	"I notice you have taken your medication regularly for the past month."
Offering self	Unconditional support and caring	"I'll sit with you even if you don't have anything to tell me."
Making observations	Presents reality and encourages patient to do so	"You seem anxious."
Encouraging description of perceptions	Promotes clarification of patient's experience	"Are you hearing voices? What are they saying?
Presenting reality	Gives accurate perceptions	"I do not hear voices, although I realize they are real to you."
Voicing doubt	Presents uncertainty without being confrontational; especially helpful with delusional thought content	"That is hard for me to believe."
Active listening	Listening to understand; imperative and effective across patient situations	"I am listening to you." Nurse's verbal and nonverbal communication must convey this. Eye contact, leaning forward, appropriate use of touch, relaxed and interested.

(Townsend, 2018)

TABLE 26–2   Common Types of Delusional Thought

Delusion	Description	Representative Quote
Persecution	Belief of being threatened and fears harm from others	"The FBI listens in on my phone conversations."
Grandeur	Beliefs of importance and power; may include thoughts of being a deity	"I am Jesus Christ."
Reference	Beliefs that all events have personal meaning for them	"This article in the newspaper has a message for me."
Control or Influence	Belief that one's behavior is controlled externally	"The doctor implanted a transmitter in my brain."
Somatic	Beliefs about body functioning	"I know I'm pregnant even though the test is negative."
Nihilistic	Beliefs that self or others do not exist	"I am not alive."

(Capriotti, 2020; Townsend, 2018)

have these false beliefs despite being presented with evidence that they are irrational (Capriotti, 2020; Dillon, 2015; Hart, 2015).

It is normal for a preschooler to have and talk to imaginary friends, but when this behavior persists into later childhood, there may be cause for concern. The onset of symptoms of psychosis before age 12 is rare, but valuable insight into the prodrome of schizophrenia can be obtained by understanding this phenomenon. Children may not be able to report and describe specific hallucinations but have a feeling that "something is wrong"; still, it is important to identify early warning signs and assess if treatment is needed, which often includes pharmacological intervention (Capriotti, 2020; MHA, 2018; Woo, 2020).

While delusions are false thoughts, hallucinations are false sensory perceptions that are not associated with stimuli from the patient's environment. Because they are a sensory experience, they may occur in any of the five senses, but auditory hallucinations are the most common. Patients may describe "hearing voices," but they may also hear other sounds, such as music, pounding, or clicks. *Command hallucinations* tell the person to do something, which has the potential to place them in dangerous situations. A person experiencing visual hallucinations may see entire people, faces, light flashes, or unintelligible forms. Tactile hallucinations result in sensations of being touched; a specific type, formication, is defined as "something crawling on or under the skin" and often causes agitation (Townsend, 2018, p. 431). Gustatory and olfactory hallucinations are usually unpleasant tastes and smells, respectively (Dillon, 2015; Hart, 2015; Townsend, 2018).

When a person is experiencing altered thoughts and perceptions, the nurse may ask them directly if they are having delusions and/or hallucinations, but must also rely on observation of the patient for cues that these psychotic symptoms are occurring, especially hallucinations (Dillon, 2015). The person may stop and act as if they are listening to someone and may actively speak back to the voices. They may appear to be talking to themselves but are actually responding to what they see and/or hear. While actively hallucinating, a person is hypersensitive to touch, so the nurse should avoid physical contact unless they tell the patient that they are planning to do so (Hart, 2015; Townsend, 2018). While the nurse does not support the patient's false beliefs and perceptions, asking questions about them to gain further understanding is useful; it is important to determine whether command hallucinations are present to maintain a safe environment.

During the assessment, the nurse communicates to the person that the voices or visions are not real. Using language such as "I realize the voices are real to you, but I do not hear them" presents reality-based thinking and affirms the person (Dillon, 2015; Hart, 2015). In a review of literature by Chadwick and Hemingway (2017), it was determined that it may be valuable to explore the content and meaning of the voices, rather than summarily dismissing them. It was noted that there are potential adverse reactions, and the nurse must be prepared to manage these, especially memories of past trauma. Because hallucinations often occur during episodes of increased anxiety, the nurse should also discuss ways to identify early stages of anxiety and coping strategies that can be implemented to prevent escalation (Dillon, 2015; Townsend, 2018).

Mason, Cardell, and Armstrong (2014) described the unique situation of patients with malingering psychosis and provided guidelines for advanced assessment of their hallucinations and delusions. In this small population, patients report that they are experiencing psychotic symptoms when they do not exist. Nurses navigate this complicated situation using the following approaches: accept the patient, while questioning inconsistencies, explore secondary gain, and present realistic options.

During the assessment of a patient with a psychotic disorder, the nurse has several priorities. First the potential for harm to self or others is determined so the safety of the patient is maintained; therefore, it is important to assess for suicide risk. There is a high rate of suicidal ideation and attempts in this patient population; specifically, 1 in 3 (30%) individuals with schizophrenia attempt suicide and 1 in 10 (10%) die. There is an even higher rate of suicide attempt (40%) among individuals with bipolar disorder, with an 11% death rate (Dome, Rihmer, & Gonda, 2019). The nurse should be well versed in how to address suicide ideation and intention with a thorough assessment of past and present thoughts of self-harm, including any specific plans. As stated in earlier chapters, suicidal thoughts are a psychiatric emergency and require action to protect the patient (Dillon, 2015; Hart, 2015; Townsend, 2018). Substance abuse is a frequent comorbidity for individuals with psychotic disorders and may impair the assessment and resulting diagnostic processes. Before individuals are properly diagnosed and treated for a psychotic disorder, they may self-medicate with various substances, often street drugs and alcohol (NIMH, 2018). Using a tool with established reliability and validity, such as CAGE [Cut down, Annoyed, Guilty, Eye-opener] or Drug Abuse Screening Test [DAST], is an accurate method for identifying substance abuse (see Chapter 27) (NIMH, 2018).

Neuroimaging studies may be part of the assessment of the individual with psychotic disorder. There are physiological changes that may are consistent with a diagnosis of schizophrenia, such as an overall loss of brain volume. *Computed tomography* (CT) scans may show enlargement of the lateral and third ventricles, along with a decrease in cortical tissue. The loss of symmetry in the temporal, frontal, and occipital lobes is another change in brain structure that has been noted on CT scan and is a possible cause for altered brain functioning (Capriotti, 2020).

Hardy (2013) describes the importance of physical health assessment for patients with long-term psychotic disorders who are at high risk for *cardiovascular disease* (CVD) due to medication side effects and unhealthy lifestyle (e.g., sedentary, tobacco abuse, stress). The prevalence of chronic illness comorbidities (e.g., diabetes, hypertension, CVD) in patients with psychotic disorders is estimated at 74%, so it is important to regularly assess the management of these conditions.

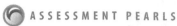 **ASSESSMENT PEARLS**

In addition to gathering information about the patient's current status during assessment, the nurse can present reality to the patient using therapeutic communication techniques.

Nonpharmacological Management

Similar to other mental health conditions, drug therapy alone is often inadequate to treat psychotic symptoms. While there is evidence that *cognitive-behavioral therapy* (CBT) is effective for the treatment of psychosis, there is disagreement about whether CBT should be modified and distinctive for psychotic patients. Experts agree that patients do not benefit from CBT while they are actively experiencing delusions and/or hallucinations; initiation of CBT must wait until medications take effect and the patient has rational thoughts and normal sensory perceptions. In an effort to better understand the role of CBT within this patient population, several tools have been developed to promote accurate psychometrics. Such scales include the following: the Cognitive Therapy Scale (CTS), Cognitive Therapy for At Risk of Psychosis Adherence Scale (CTARPAS), Revised Cognitive Therapy Scale (CTS-R), Cognitive Therapy for Psychosis Adherence Scale (CTPAS), and the Cognitive Therapy Scale for Psychosis (CTS-Psy) (Morrison & Barratt, 2010). Obviously, there is interest in accurately measuring the effect of CBT in promoting positive outcomes for patients with psychosis (NIMH, 2018; Townsend, 2018).

In addition to CBT, *social skills training* (SST) may be used to promote coping for individuals with psychosis. Turner and colleagues (2018) conducted a meta-analysis of studies that measured the effectiveness of SST and found that while it is often as effective as CBT for the positive and negative symptoms of schizophrenia, it is not routinely implemented. Based on these preliminary results, further research is recommended to assess SST as a treatment strategy for psychosis that occurs with schizophrenia and/or bipolar disorder. Using another approach to treating psychosis, Welfare-Wilson and Jones (2015) described a 1-day anxiety management workshop that was offered for individuals who had had their first episode of psychosis; this was part of an Early Intervention in Psychosis Service (EIPS) in the U.K. The 12 participants reported statistically significant reduction (p<0.0005) in anxiety post-intervention and intent to use skills they learned in the future to decrease anxiety. More long-term psychotherapy may help individuals develop coping skills to better manage anxiety and to learn new behaviors that will promote healthy interpersonal relationships (NIMH, 2018; Townsend, 2018). Frequently, patients with psychotic disorders are also diagnosed with substance abuse disorders; therefore, a 12-step treatment program, such as Alcoholics Anonymous, may be part or the treatment regimen (refer to Chapter 27 for information about substance abuse). The patient with psychosis may need both long- and short-term strategies to help them manage their symptoms and promote better quality of life.

Healthy lifestyles are encouraged for patients who are at risk for or experiencing psychotic disorders and include a balanced diet, regular exercise, smoking cessation, and avoidance of alcohol and drug use (MHA, 2018; Townsend, 2018). Because anxiety often precipitates altered thoughts (delusions) and perceptions (hallucinations), patients may benefit from practicing deep-breathing exercises with meditation. Yoga that incorporates focused deep breathing and slow movements/postures may also decrease anxiety. Overall, any activity that the person finds relaxing, such as walking, gardening, or crafting, may reduce anxiety and subsequent episodes of psychosis (MHA, 2018; NIMH, 2018; Townsend, 2018).

The caregiver burden on the families of individuals with psychotic disorders cannot be underestimated. It is important to identify the needs of the family and to connect them with resources to support their coping and problem-solving abilities. The effects on the caregiver can be significant and include psychological morbidity, impaired interactions with social support, financial strain, and lost time from work and leisure (Lin et al., 2018). The National Alliance on Mental Illness (NAMI) has been a leader in advocating for and providing these services. Specifically, NAMI offers a free, eight-session educational program that is designed to meet the needs of the family and friends of a person with mental illness. Mutual support and shared experiences are offered in a group setting that provides compassionate care along with evidence-based guidance focused on the family members (NAMI, 2020).

CLINICAL PEARLS

When the patient is actively psychotic, maintaining their safety is the priority in any treatment plan.

Pharmacology

Antipsychotics (APs) are the drugs of choice for treating psychotic symptoms regardless of their origin (Townsend, 2018). Similar to antidepressants, these drugs change the amounts of circulating neurotransmitters but are usually aimed at decreasing, rather than increasing, these substances and their uptake at the receptor sites. The APs are categorized into three main groups based on their development: the first generation (from 1950s) or typical, and the second generation (from 1970s) or atypical, and a third more recent generation, also atypical. The first and second generation APs work by blocking dopamine receptors in the various dopamine pathways, whereas the third generation atypical APs also block serotonin receptors and prevent overactivity of dopamine (Vallerand & Sanoski, 2020; Woo, 2020).

The typical APs are usually administered orally, although there are long-acting versions that are administered intramuscularly. Within this category, there are designations as high- and low potency medications. The high-potency APs have a higher incidence of *extrapyramidal side effects* (EPSs) (i.e., akathisia, dystonia, tremor) and tardive dyskinesia (involuntary mouth movements, difficulty speaking and swallowing). In contrast, lower potency versions have higher risk of the anticholinergic side effects (i.e., dry mouth, dry eyes, blurred vision, constipation, urinary retention) and anticholinergic adverse effects (orthostatic hypotension) (Vallerand & Sanoski, 2020).

The choice of an AP is based on several factors, including initial response to a dose, past responses to the AP, family history, and potential for side effects. Second generation APs are associated with greater risk of cardiovascular complications, so lower doses of first generation APs may be used for patients with either high risk or existing cardiovascular disease (Pringle, 2013; Woo, 2020). The third generation, atypical AP is thought to work by blocking serotonin, which has an inhibitory effect on dopamine (Woo, 2020). All types of APs are effective in the majority of patients, but it may be up to 4 weeks before a significant change is achieved. Overall, APs are indicated for suppressing psychotic symptoms, preventing relapse, improving quality of life, and promoting ability to participate in additional cognitive therapies (MHA, 2018; Vallerand & Sanoski, 2020; Woo, 2020). Notably, clozapine is the only medicine approved by the U.S. Food and Drug Administration (FDA) that is indicated when the patient has been tried on two APs without improvement; it is also recommended by the FDA to reduce the risk of suicide in people with schizophrenia (Duckworth, 2017).

Compliance with taking medications as prescribed is a significant barrier to effective management of psychotic disorders. Pringle (2013) reported a 64% rate of noncompliance among patients with schizophrenia in the U.K. Promoting patient compliance with long-term maintenance use of APs is difficult for many reasons. The patient's altered thought processes and content due to the disease affect decision making, and there are often multiple psychosocial factors such as homelessness and substance abuse that affect their ability to obtain and take medications as prescribed (Townsend, 2018; Woo, 2020).

Nurses need to be competent in using a variety of strategies to support these individuals and their ability to achieve wellness despite the diagnosis of a significant mental illness; medication compliance is key to their achieving this goal. First, the nurse should assess the external factors that support the patient's ability to be compliant with their medication regimen. These may include supportive family/friends, stable living situation, and supervised medication administration program. Then the nurse can guide the patient to identify their positive internal factors, such as commitment, determination, and resilience (Dillon, 2015; MHA, 2018; Woo, 2020). Helping the patient use effective coping skills will also support their self-efficacy in medication management (Townsend, 2018). Stringfellow and Young (2017) studied the impact of including family in the interventions for patients with psychosis and determined that contextual factors have a significant impact on the successful outcomes of complex plans of care for this patient population. They found that families often lacked knowledge, skills, and confidence, but when they were supported by training they were able to assume a reasonable level of responsibility for the care of their family member with psychosis. Lithium has been used as the primary pharmacological treatment for bipolar disorder for years, although its mechanism of action is not well understood. It works to stabilize mood with common side effects of increased urination, hand tremors, increased thirst, weight gain, and emotional numbing; the side effect of weight gain is a significant issue for individuals with a concurrent eating disorder. Administration may also result in life-threatening side effects such as hypothyroidism, diabetes insipidus, and lithium toxicity. Maintaining adequate fluid intake is vital to preventing lithium toxicity. Patients with altered mood combined with impaired thought processes may have difficulty complying with this requirement. Nurses should monitor blood levels for maintenance of therapeutic levels and identification of potential toxicity in its early stages (Townsend, 2018; Woo, 2020). While lithium is the primary treatment for bipolar disorder, it is not always effective or tolerated well. Antipsychotics may also be used to treat bipolar disorder; these medications are aimed at controlling mania and decreasing psychotic symptoms that can be present during the manic phase of the illness. Anti-anxiety and antiseizure medications are also used during the manic phase, whereas antidepressants are necessary during the depressed cycle of the disorder. The pharmacological management of BP-P is complicated and requires clinical expertise and patient compliance for optimal results (Vallerand & Sanoski, 2020). More information about APS and other medications that are used in the treatment of psychotic disorders is presented in Table 26–3.

Leahy (2017) described the use of evidence-driven and medically recommended pharmacogenetic testing to determine pharmacological options for patients. Using these data, patients may respond more quickly to medication and have resolution of their psychotic symptoms, thus improving quality of life. Barriers to this approach include limited access to testing and cost that is not covered by private or government

TABLE 26-3 Drugs Used to Treat Psychotic Disorders

Class	Example	Action	Dosage	SENC
First generation of typical antipsychotics	Haloperidol	Blocks postsynaptic dopamine (D_2) receptors in the limbic system, so dopamine is unable to be activated.	Psychosis: 0.2–5 mg 2 or 2 × daily. Severe psychosis: 3–5 mg 2 or 3 × daily up to 100 mg/day. Decanoate: long-acting IM injection q 4 weeks 50–100 mg.	Give with full glass (8 oz) of water or with food or milk. Anticholinergic side effects: dry eyes and mouth; suicidal ideations; cardiac arrhythmias; urinary retention. Monitor for extra-pyramidal side effects (EPS) and irreversible tardive dyskinesia and Parkinson's.
Second generation of atypical antipsychotics	Clozapine	Interferes with binding of dopamine to D_1 and D_2 postsynaptic receptors in limbic system.	Initiate at 12.5 mg/day in 1 or 2 doses. Increase to a target dose of 350–450 mg/day in 3 doses.	Life-threatening side effect: agranulocytosis. Requires regular laboratory findings to monitor for it. Report flu-like symptoms: fever, sore throat, lethargy, infection.
Third generation of atypical antipsychotics	Aripiprazole	Mechanism of action is not clear but is thought to block serotonin receptors in the cortex, which inhibits serotonin's ability to block dopamine.	Adults: 10–15 mg/day. Children: 2 mg/day.	Weight gain and sedation are most problematic side effects. Risk of EPS is much less than with other APs.
Anticholinergics	Benztropine	Centrally acting anticholinergic acts by decreasing excess cholinergic effect associated with decreased dopamine. It is used to prevent anticholinergic (tremors and rigidity) side effects of medications.	0.5–1 mg/day. Increase to 6 mg/day. 1–2 mg IV for acute dystonic reaction.	Give with food. Gradually increase and/or decrease dosage, as effects are cumulative.
Mood stabilizers	Lithium	Its mechanism is unclear, but it competes with cations and affects cell membranes, neurotransmitters, and body water composition. It is used to control and prevent mania in bipolar disorder.	Adults: Loading: 600 mg 3 × a day or 900 mg sustained release twice daily. Maintenance: 300 mg 2 or 3 × daily. Children: 15–60 mg/kg/day in 2 to 3 divided doses.	Monitor for seizures. Report loose stools or diarrhea, as dehydration may occur quickly. Use sunscreen for photosensitivity.

Continued

TABLE 26-3   Drugs Used to Treat Psychotic Disorders—cont'd

Class	Example	Action	Dosage	SENC
Anticonvulsants	Valproic acid	Action is thought to be related to increased availability of GABA. It may also suppress neuronal firing by inhibiting sodium channels. Used for mania in bipolar disorder.	Adults: 750 mg/day in divided doses.	Monitor for therapeutic levels of 50–100 mcg/mL. Monitor carefully during dose adjustments for oversedation.

(Karch, 2017; Vallerand & Sanoski, 2020; Woo, 2020)

insurance plans, although some progress is being made. Currently, Medicare does not have a national coverage determination for pharmacogenetic testing for psychotropics, but exceptions are made for individual cases (Dangor, 2019).

Patient education should include the importance of taking any antipsychotic drug as prescribed, reporting adverse symptoms early, and implementing interventions to decrease side effects. As with many medications, patients should be educated that antipsychotics should not be stopped abruptly (NIMH, 2018). Finally, there are many potential interactions with other medications, so patients should check with their provider or pharmacist for confirmation that they can safely take additional medications or supplements (Townsend, 2018; Vallerand & Sanoski, 2020).

 RED FLAG ALERT

Antipsychotics should not be used with older patients who have dementia-related psychosis (Townsend, 2018; Woo, 2020).

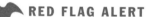 CLINICAL PEARLS

While psychotic symptoms due to different underlying causes may be managed similarly with medications, treatment plans for individuals should be individualized and based on their response to pharmacological and other treatment modalities.

Summary

Psychosis may occur due to various causes, and its early identification may prevent long-term complications that include direct and indirect health-care costs; risk for substance abuse; loss of quality of life and social connections; impulsive behavior that can lead to financial ruin; violent behavior that can lead to incarceration and/or harm to others; and potential for suicidal ideation (MHA, 2018; NIMH, 2018). While the pathophysiology is based primarily on theories, patients experience significant improvement on antipsychotic medications. Successful pharmacological management of psychotic disorders often requires a combination of medications with continuous monitoring and frequent adjustments to obtain optimal benefits and minimal side effects. Medication compliance is complex and multifactorial; focusing on factors that the patient can change and/or control is a realistic starting point and affords the patient opportunities for success. In addition, nonpharmacological approaches are often effective in supporting the patient and family in their ability to cope with this condition and may decrease the need for multiple medications. A psychotic disorder does not prevent a person from achieving a high level of wellness and enjoying quality of life with appropriate assessment and ongoing intervention.

Key Points

- The cause of psychosis is not well understood but is thought to be caused by neurotransmitter imbalances in the brain, medical conditions, or by medications and/or other drugs.
- Hallucinations and delusions are the primary symptoms of psychosis.
- Schizophrenia is the mental disorder that is most frequently responsible for hallucination and delusions, but these symptoms may also occur in bipolar disorder, depression, and substance abuse disorder.
- Antipsychotics, first line drugs used to treat psychosis, have adverse side effects and potential interactions with many other drugs.
- Psychotic symptoms must be resolved or well-controlled before CBT or any form of psychotherapy can be a successful adjuvant in disease management.
- Patient education should include information about the role of stress, exercise, and healthy eating in promoting mental health as well as information about any prescribed drugs.

Review Questions

1. **The nurse is educating the patient about the pathophysiology of psychotic disorders. Which of the following statements is correct?**
   a. "Psychotic disorders are caused by underactivity of the same neurotransmitters as depression."
   b. "There are no genetic components of these disorders."
   c. "There are structural differences in the brain that cause psychosis."
   d. "The dopamine theory along with environmental and genetic factors are probably responsible."

2. **Which of the assessment findings would you expect with a 14-year-old child with a psychotic disorder?**
   a. Decreased appetite with associated weight loss
   b. General feeling that something is not right in thinking
   c. Vivid nightmares
   d. Temper tantrums

3. **When reviewing the patient's medication list, the patient reports that he has side effects of restlessness and involuntary tongue movements. Which medication is probably responsible for these symptoms?**
   a. Multivitamin taken to supplement their dietary intake.
   b. Propranolol taken to control their blood pressure.
   c. Statin taken to lower their LDL cholesterol.
   d. First generation antipsychotic

4. **When assessing a patient experiencing auditory hallucinations, which of the following questions should be including in screening? (Select all that apply.)**
   a. "Are you hearing the voices now?"
   b. "Are the voices telling you to harm yourself?"
   c. "Do you think other people hear these voices?"
   d. "What do you think these voices mean?"

5. When educating the patient who has been prescribed lithium to manage psychotic symptoms of bipolar disorder, which of the following statements lets the nurse know that the patient understands instructions?

   a. "I'll take the medication as soon as my hallucinations return."
   b. "I will follow up for laboratory findings that determine a therapeutic dose."
   c. "I will limit fluid intake, so I won't feel bloated."
   d. "I will discontinue taking this medication if I don't feel better."

See the appendix for answers to review questions.

References

Allott, K., Fraguas, D., Bartholomeusz, C. F., Díaz-Caneja, C. M., Wannan, C., Parrish, E. M., . . . Rapado-Castro, M. (2018). Duration of untreated psychosis and neurocognitive functioning in first-episode psychosis: A systematic review and meta-analysis. *Psychological Medicine, 48*(10), 1592–1607. doi:10.1017/S0033291717003002

Appiah-Kusi, E., Leyden, E., Parmar, S., Mondelli, V., McGuire, P., & Bhattacharyya, S. (2016). Abnormalities in neuroendocrine stress response in psychosis: The role of endocannabinoids. *Psychological Medicine, 46*(1), 27–45. doi:10.1017/S0033291715001786

Burton, C. Z., Ryan, K. A., Kamali, M., Marshall, D. F., Harrington, G., McInnis, M. G., & Tso, I. F. (2018). Psychosis in bipolar disorder: Does it represent a more "severe" illness? *Bipolar Disorders, 20*(1), 18–26. Retrieved from https://doi.org/10.1111/bdi.12527

Capriotti, T. (2020). *Pathophysiology: Introductory concepts and clinical perspectives* (2nd ed.). Philadelphia, PA: F.A. Davis.

Chadwick, C., & Hemingway, S. (2017). A review of the effectiveness of interventions aimed at understanding the content and meaning of the experience of voice hearing. *Mental Health Nursing, 37*(6), 8–14.

Chong, H. Y., Teoh, S. L., Wu, D. B., Kotirum, S., Chiou, C. F., & Chaiyakunapruk, N. (2016). Global economic burden of schizophrenia: a systematic review. *Neuropsychiatric Disease and Treatment, 12*, 357–373. https://doi.org/10.2147/NDT.S96649

Dangor, G. (2019). Pharmacogenetic test makes cheer UnitedHealth coverage. Others payers aren't there yet. *MedTech Dive.* Retrieved from https://www.medtechdive.com/news

Derosse, P., Malhotra, A., Lencz, T., DeRosse, P., Malhotra, A. K., & Lencz, T. (2012). Molecular genetics of the psychosis phenotype. *Canadian Journal of Psychiatry, 57*(7), 446–453.

Dillon, P. M. (2015). *Nursing health assessment: A critical thinking, case studies approach* (3rd ed.). Philadelphia, PA: F.A. Davis.

Dome, P., Rihmer, Z., & Gonda, X. (2019). Suicide risk in bipolar disorder: A brief review. *Medicina (Kaunas, Lithuania), 55*(8), 403. Retrieved from https://doi.org/10.3390/medicina55080403

Duckworth, K. (2017). Taking another look a too-often-forgotten treatment for schizophrenia. Proceedings from National Alliance for the Mentally Ill (NAMI) Convention. Retrieved from https://www.nami.org/Blogs/NAMI-Blog/March-2017/Taking-Another-Look-a-Too-Often-Forgotten-Treatment

Hardy, S. (2013). Physical health checks for people with severe mental illness. *Primary Health Care, 23*(10), 24–26.

Hart, V. A. (2015). Psychiatric mental health. In M. J. Goolsby & L. Grubbs (Eds.), *Advanced assessment: Interpreting findings and formulating differential diagnoses.* Philadelphia, PA: F.A. Davis.

Karch, A. M. (2017). *Focus on nursing pharmacology* (7th ed.). Philadelphia, PA: Wolters Kluwer / Lippincott Williams & Wilkins.

Leahy, L. G. (2017). Genetic testing for psychopharmacology. *Journal of Psychosocial Nursing & Mental Health Services, 55*(3), 19–23. doi:10.3928/02793695-20170301-02

Lin, E., Durbin, J., Guerriere, D., Volpe, T., Selick, A., Kennedy, J., . . . Lero, D. S. (2018). Assessing caregiving demands, resources and costs of family/friend caregivers for persons with mental health disorders: A scoping review. *Health & Social Care in the Community, 26*(5), 613–634. Retrieved from https://ezproxy.queens.edu:6464/10.1111/hsc.12546

Mason, A. M., Cardell, R., & Armstrong, M. (2014). Malingering psychosis: Guidelines for assessment and management. *Perspectives in Psychiatric Care, 50*(1), 51–57. doi:10.1111/ppc.12025

Mental Health America. (2018). *Psychosis.* Retrieved from http://www.mentalhealthamerica.net/conditions/psychosis

Morrison, A., & Barratt, S. (2010). What are the components of CBT for psychosis? A Delphi study. *Schizophrenia Bulletin, 36*, 136–142. Retrieved from https://doi.org/10.1093/schbul/sbp118

Najjar, S., Pearlman, D. M., Alper, K., Najjar, A., & Devinsky, O. (2013). Neuroinflammation and psychiatric illness. *Journal of Neuroinflammation, 10*(1), 43. doi:10.1186/1742-2094-10-43

National Alliance for the Mentally Ill (NAMI). (2020). *Peer to peer.* Retrieved from: https://www.nami.org/Support-Education/Mental-Health-Education/NAMI-Peer-to-Peer

National Institute of Mental Health. (2018). *What is psychosis?* Retrieved from https://www.nimh.nih.gov /health/topics/schizophrenia/raise/what-is-psychosis.shtml

Pringle, R. (2013). Psychosis and schizophrenia: A mental health nurse's perspective. *Nurse Prescribing, 11*(10), 505–509.

Stringfellow, A., & Young, N. (2017). Developing the integrated delivery of family intervention within community mental health teams for people with psychosis: A pilot project. *Foundation of Nursing Studies: Improvement Insights, 12*(1–10), 1.

Tor, J., Dolz, M., Sintes, A., Muñoz, D., Pardo, M., de la Serna, E., . . . Baeza, I. (2018). Clinical high risk for psychosis in children and adolescents: A systematic review. *European Child & Adolescent Psychiatry, 27*(6), 683–700. doi:10.1007/s00787-017-1046-3

Townsend, M. C. (2018). *Psychiatric mental health nursing: Concepts of care in evidence-based practice* (9th ed.). Philadelphia, PA: F.A. Davis.

Turner, D. T., McGlanaghy, E., Cuijpers, P., van der Gaag, M., Karyotaki, E., & MacBeth, A. (2018). A meta-analysis of social skills training and related interventions for psychosis. *Schizophrenia Bulletin, 44*(3), 475-491. doi:10.1093/schbul/sbx146

Vallerand, A. H., & Sanoski, C. A. (Eds.). (2020). *Davis's drug guide for nurses* (17th ed.). Philadelphia, PA: F.A. Davis.

Van Dellen, E., Bohlken, M. M., Draaisma, L., Tewarie, P. K., van Lutterveld, R., Mandl, R., . . . Sommer, I. E. (2016). Structural brain network disturbances in the psychosis spectrum. *Schizophrenia Bulletin, 42*(3), 782–789. doi:10.1093/schbul/sbv178

Welfare-Wilson, A., & Jones, A. (2015). A CBT-based anxiety management workshop in first-episode psychosis. *British Journal of Nursing, 24*(7), 378–382. doi:10.12968/bjon.2015.24.7.378

Woo, T. M. (2020). Drugs affecting the central nervous system. In T. M. Woo & M. V. Robinson (Eds.), *Pharmacotherapeutics for advanced practice nurse prescribers* (5th ed.). Philadelphia: F.A. Davis.

Chapter 27

Substance Abuse Disorders

LEARNING OBJECTIVES

Upon completion of this chapter the student will be able to:

- Integrate knowledge of the physiology, pathophysiology, assessment, and nonpharmacological and pharmacological management for care of children, adolescents, and adults with substance abuse disorders.
- Appraise current standards of care for individuals with substance abuse disorders.

Introduction

Substance abuse has had various definitions through the years as knowledge of its etiology and treatment has evolved; current definitions of key terms, including *substance abuse*, are provided as a foundation for this chapter. First, *substance use disorder* is also known as *addiction*, which is defined as "chronic, relapsing brain disease that is characterized by compulsive drug seeking and use, despite harmful consequences" (National Institute on Drug Abuse [NIDA], 2018). *Intoxication* and *withdrawal* are considered substance-induced disorders (Townsend, 2018). Intoxication may be due to many different substances and/or combinations and is defined by the World Health Organization (WHO, 2018) as "a condition that follows the administration of a psychoactive substance and results in disturbances in the level of consciousness, cognition, perception, judgement, affect, or behavior, or other psychophysiological functions and responses." Withdrawal is defined by WHO (2018) as "a group of symptoms of variable clustering and degree of severity which occur on cessation or reduction of use of a psychoactive substance that has been taken repeatedly, usually for a prolonged period and/ or in high doses."

Drugs most often associated with substance abuse are alcohol, cannabis, barbiturates, benzodiazepines, cocaine, methaqualone, opioids, and amphetamines; however, some authorities also include caffeine and tobacco (NIDA, 2018). There are commonalities among substance abuse concepts across the various drugs, but this chapter will focus on the two substances that have the highest mortality rates and that nurses are most likely to encounter: alcohol and opiates. While alcoholism is a long-standing illness that has steadily increased in prevalence and affects approximately 15.1 million (6.2% of the U.S. population) individuals and their families, 2.5 million individuals abuse prescription opiates and/or heroin. The use and resulting abuse of opiates has increased exponentially in the past two decades and has been identified as a national emergency by politicians and health care providers (Murthy, 2017; NIDA, 2018). In the late 1990s, pharmaceutical companies falsely reassured providers that opioid pain relievers were not addictive; in fact, 20% to 30% of patients misuse opioids that are prescribed for chronic pain. Approximately 80% of people who use heroin have a history of prescription opioid misuse (NIDA, 2018).

Accurate statistics are difficult to determine as much of the data are self-reported and there are criminal implications for some substances. Mortality associated with substance abuse is significant. According to WHO (2018), alcohol is responsible for 3.3 million deaths annually, and over 31 million individuals have alcohol and/or drug use disorders globally. Likewise, the cost of substance abuse is difficult to capture in statistics because the costs extend to incarceration and lost wages for decades. The estimated cost of drug abuse (defined as illegal drugs, alcohol, and tobacco) is over $740 billion annually in the United States and growing (NIDA, 2018).

An emerging problem is accidental drug overdose, which is the leading cause of death in the United States for all individuals less than 50 years of age (Drug Policy, 2020). This growing problem includes the following trends:

• Accidental overdose is increasing at 20% per year.
• Heroin overdose rates have quadrupled in the past decade.
• Death rates are highest for individuals ages 25 to 44.
• The highest increase is in the Northeast and Midwest regions of the United States (Drug Policy, 2020).

According to the Centers for Disease Control and Prevention (CDC), the cost of alcohol abuse in the United States is $249 billion annually, but these costs are largely underestimated because many alcohol-related health problems are underreported or misdiagnosed (CDC, 2018). The overwhelming majority of these costs (72%) were attributed to absenteeism from work, worker's compensation injuries, Social Security disability, and unemployment benefits. The cost burden varies greatly by U.S. geographic region with a low of $488 million in North Dakota to a high of $35 billion in California. Washington, D.C., had the highest per capita (which accounts for differences in population among areas) annual cost at $1,526, nearly twice the national average. (CDC, 2018; NIDA, 2018).

Physiology

Review normal brain physiology in Chapters 17 and 25 to understand alterations that occur with substance abuse and mechanisms for pharmacological treatment. Normal physiology of the liver will be presented here, because many substances, especially alcohol, affect liver function and often cause damage. The functioning cells in the liver are hepatocytes. While the liver is responsible for many functions when considered how it works with other organs, the primary ones will be discussed.

First, the liver is involved in the metabolism of carbohydrates, proteins, amino acids, and lipids. By synthesizing and storing glycogen via glycogenesis, it releases glucose into the bloodstream via glycogenolysis when it is needed to maintain homeostasis. Through another mechanism, gluconeogenesis, the liver synthesizes glucose from other substances, such as amino acids, lactate, or glycerol; the liver also uses fat for this process.

Next, the liver is the primary organ responsible for protein metabolism, both synthesizing and destroying proteins. Amino acids are also synthesized by the liver. Another important function is the production of red blood cells and clotting factors (e.g., I [fibrinogen]), II [prothrombin], V, VII, VIII, IX, X, XI, XIII, protein C, protein S, and antithrombin). In a related function, the liver manufactures thrombopoietin, which stimulates platelet production in bone marrow. In its role in lipid metabolism, the liver synthesizes cholesterol, triglycerides, and multiple lipo-proteins (Capriotti, 2020).

The liver is a *gastrointestinal* (GI) organ, and so its function is necessary for diges-tion, as it produces and excretes bile that emulsifies ingested fats and promotes vitamin K absorption. Bile is emptied directly into the duodenum via the biliary duct and is also stored in the gallbladder. The liver produces growth factor 1, which pro-motes normal growth in children and has anabolic effects in adults (Capriotti, 2020).

In addition to digestion, the liver is involved in the metabolism of substances, including insulin and bilirubin. As the liver metabolizes bilirubin via glucuronidation, it is excreted via the biliary system. Many other by-products of metabolism are further broken down by the liver so they can be excreted. The liver also metabolizes many medications and toxic substances. Urea, the metabolite of ammonia, is metabolized by the liver and then excreted in urine (Capriotti, 2020).

Finally, the liver provides storage for many life-sustaining substances; it stores vita-mins (A, D, K, B_{12}) and the elements iron and copper (Capriotti, 2020). It also manu-factures and stores albumin, which comprises the most protein in blood and therefore maintains oncotic pressure. Through its mononuclear phagocyte system, the liver fil-ters antigens as they enter the portal system. The liver's production of angiotensino-gen, a hormone that causes blood pressure to increase in response to renin, helps to maintain normal blood pressure (Capriotti, 2020).

CLINICAL PEARLS

Normal liver function is necessary for many basic body functions, including metabolism of internal and external substances.

Pathophysiology

The exact cause of substance abuse is not clear, with the two predominant theories being either a genetic disposition that is triggered or reinforced by others, or a habit that, if addiction develops, manifests itself as a chronic debilitating disease. Current research supports that an individual's genetics are responsible for 50% of risk for sub-stance abuse, and the remainder of risk is dependent on environmental factors and their interactions with the individual's genetics (Capriotti, 2020; CDC, 2018). The pathophysiology for substance abuse is presented below, and the environmental risk factors are presented in Table 27–1.

TABLE 27–1   Environmental Factors for Substance Abuse

Cultural	Social	Behavioral

Historically high incidence of alcohol addiction in certain populations (e.g., Native Americans, Alaska Natives, Northern Europeans)
    Emphasis on alcohol in daily life
    Alcohol included in celebrations
	Emphasis on alcohol in setting (e.g., college, homeless)
	    Availability of drugs in neighborhood (predomi-nantly but not exclusively low socioeconomic)
	    Social isolation
	    Ineffective coping with stress
		Head trauma
		    Mental illness (anx-iety, depression, psy-chotic disorders)
		    Risk-taking personality
		    Personality disorders

(NIDA, 2018; Townsend, 2018)

Multiple genes play a role in the risk for developing *alcohol use disorder* (AUD) and/or *opioid use disorder* (OUD); there are genes that increase risk, as well as those that may decrease risk, either directly or indirectly. There is testing for DRD2 TaqI polymorphism, an allele that is correlated to alcoholism and opiate addiction. When this human dopamine receptor gene variation (DRD2 TaqI polymorphism) is identified, the person has a significantly increased chance of developing addiction to opiates and/or alcohol. An example of a gene mutation that may decrease the risk of alcohol abuse is the gene variant ADH1 B*3 found primarily in people of Asian race/ethnicity that affects alcohol metabolism and results in unpleasant symptoms, including flushing, nausea, and tachycardia. People who experience these effects from drinking alcohol are likely to avoid it (Capriotti, 2020; NIDA, 2018).

Epigenetics, the study of inherited phenotype changes without alterations in DNA sequencing, provides information about AUD and factors that affect genetic expression. A change in a gene transcription factor in the nucleus accumbens has a role in addiction by increasing drug reward and drug-seeking behaviors. Physiologically, alcohol causes increased stimulation of *gamma aminobutyric acid* (GABA) receptors, resulting in *central nervous system* (CNS) depression. Physical dependence and associated tolerance develop with regular ingestion of alcohol as the numbers of GABA receptors diminish and those remaining are desensitized. Because GABA inhibits neuron transmission, especially in the dopamine pathways, blocking GABA results in a surplus of dopamine CNS overstimulation. Abrupt cessation of regular alcohol consumption causes uncontrolled synapse firing because the inhibitory effect of GABA is inactivated, resulting in an overactive CNS with the following signs/symptoms: anxiety, seizures, delirium tremens, and hallucinations (Capriotti, 2020; CDC, 2018; NIDA, 2018).

Other neurotransmitters that are affected by alcohol use disorder include dopamine, *N*-methyl-D-aspartate (NMDA), and glutamate. First, alcohol stimulates the release of dopamine, which activates reward pathways and euphoria. Next NMDA, an amino acid that is an excitotoxin, kills nerve cells by overexciting them. Similarly, glutamate, another amino acid and a stimulant, acts as an opposing and balancing neurotransmitter to GABA. Excessive glutamate leads to CNS hyperactivity and increases the risk of seizures (Capriotti, 2020; Townsend, 2018).

There are also physiological changes that result in psychological and physical dependence on opioids and resulting withdrawal. Specifically, when there are increased signals of *brain-derived neurotrophic factor* (BDNF) from the *ventral tegmental area* (VTA), there is a resulting decrease in withdrawal symptoms via several proteins; however, opiates cause increased excitability in VTA neurons and associated shrinkage. In an opiate-naïve person, initial use of opiates causes euphoria due to decreased BDNF signals. Psychological dependence is due to increased activity of the *cyclic adenosine monophosphate* (cAMP) pathway mediated by *cAMP response element binding protein* (CREB), a gene transcription factor, in the nucleus accumbens. Similarly, physiological dependence is due to increased activity in the same pathway in the locus coeruleus (Capriotti, 2020).

Alcohol abuse has both short-term and long-term psychological and physiological effects. The short-term sequelae are due mostly to the associated risky behaviors and include unintentional injury (e.g., motor vehicle crashes, falls, drownings), violence (against self and others), and sexual promiscuity (unintended pregnancy, sexually transmitted infections, fetal alcohol spectrum disorder) (Capriotti, 2020). Physiologically, blood alcohol levels can reach lethal levels quickly, especially in children and adolescents, resulting in a potentially fatal condition, alcohol poisoning, which is a medical emergency (Capriotti, 2020). Many chronic diseases may develop as a result of long-term alcohol use, including hypertension, cardiovascular heart disease, stroke, and liver disease. Alcohol abuse is also associated with increased risk for development of the following cancers: breast, mouth, throat, esophageal, liver, pancreatic, and colon. Mental health problems, such as dementia, depression, and anxiety, along with alcohol dependence or alcoholism, may result from alcohol abuse (CDC, 2018; Murthy, 2017; Townsend, 2018).

Explicitly, alcohol abuse often leads to liver disease in the form of fatty liver disease, alcoholic hepatitis, cirrhosis, and hepatic encephalopathy. First, alcohol abuse may lead to fatty liver because toxic metabolites of alcohol, including aldehydes, are produced as alcohol is metabolized by the liver. There are several stages to the development of this condition. Initially, hepatocytes present liposomes which is a microvascular fatty change, and the resulting fat droplets eventually push the nucleus to the cell periphery, also known as *signet ring*. The cellular fats dissolve causing large vacuoles that form irreversible fatty cysts. Severe fatty liver disease may have associated liver inflammation, known as *alcoholic steatohepatitis* (ASH); there is also a form of this condition not related to alcohol use, known as *non-alcoholic steatohepatitis* (NASH) (Capriotti, 2020).

In alcoholic hepatitis, there are several key physiological changes in the hepatocytes. First, characteristic filaments (Mallory's hyaline bodies) accumulate in hepatocytes. The hepatocytes swell (i.e., ballooning degeneration) with fluids, lipids, and proteins that should normally be in the circulating bloodstream. Necrotic changes and associated inflammation of the hepatocytes results in blocked biliary ducts, which may lead to cholestasis. This inflammation affects hepatic function and triggers neutrophils to enter the system. These changes lead to multiple symptoms, including general malaise, hepatomegaly, ascites, and liver enzyme elevation; with more severe disease, there may be jaundice and organ failure (Capriotti, 2020).

A related condition, cirrhosis, is also common in individuals who have consumed alcohol for a long period of time; it is often preceded by alcohol hepatitis and/or fatty liver disease. The physiological changes cause scar tissue to replace normal parenchyma and block portal circulation. Specifically, the stellate cell that normally stores vitamin A is responsible for increased production of myofibroblasts and resulting fibrotic tissue. Stellate cells cause proliferation of connective tissue and block enzymes that break down the matrix of these tissues, allowing further proliferation. This fibrous tissue does not function normally, so blood flow is diminished through the hepatic parenchyma, leading to splenic congestion and enlargement; this condition, portal hypertension, is a life-threatening complication of cirrhosis (Capriotti, 2020; Townsend, 2018).

Hepatic encephalopathy is a life-threatening liver disease that occurs with long-term alcohol abuse. The underlying pathophysiological process is related to the inability of hepatocytes to metabolize waste products and the development of collateral circulation that bypasses liver filtration, causing waste (especially nitrogen) to accumulate in the bloodstream. In particular, ammonia crosses the blood–brain barrier and is absorbed and metabolized by the astrocytes, which respond with increased osmotic pressure and swelling. In addition, the increased ammonia levels cause increased activity of the GABA neurotransmitter system, which decreases normal brain activity (Capriotti, 2020; Townsend, 2018).

◠ CLINICAL PEARLS

Substance abuse results in alterations to many body systems but is especially detrimental to the GI system (Capriotti, 2020).

Assessment

The assessment of the patient will depend on many factors, including current intoxication and/or overdose, potential for withdrawal, physical comorbidities, presence of family members, and patient's readiness to acknowledge their condition and accept treatment. Depending on the substance, the signs and symptoms may be varied; also, people react differently to various substances, so there will also be variation based on individual response. In order to obtain valid data from patients, nurses must first examine their own thoughts and potential biases about substance abuse, so a nonjudgmental approach is evident when interviewing patients (Anandan, Cross, & Munro, 2016; Dillon, 2017; Hart, 2015).

The nurse must be able to speak directly with patients about their substance abuse and its impact on their life without being confrontational. The physical assessment should be first, as intoxication, overdose, and/or withdrawal are potentially life-threatening situations. In addition to assessing the person's current psychological state, the nurse performs a focused head-to-toe examination with an emphasis on early identification of an abuse disorder before irreversible organ damage has occurred (Dillon, 2017; Townsend, 2018).

Assessment for Alcohol Use Disorder

One of the salient signs of AUD is the patient's denial that a problem exists. The nurse needs to obtain data about how much the person drinks and the effect their drinking has on the patient's life and others in their lives. An experienced interviewer may weave these questions into the overall interview or may use a tool that is targeted to determine likelihood the person has AUD. There are many assessment tools (examples are given in Table 27–2) that may be used with various age ranges in

TABLE 27–2 Substance Abuse Assessment Tools

Tool	Components
Clinical Institute Withdrawal Assessment for Alcohol, Revised (CIWA-Ar) scale	Vital signs, nausea/vomiting, tremor, tactile/auditory disturbances, orientation, anxiety/agitation, headache
Michigan Alcohol Screening Test (MAST)	Points for how often a person drinks and the effect of drinking: interpersonal, health, occupation, arrests
CAGE Assessment	Consists of four questions: Have you felt you should Cut down on your drinking? Have people Annoyed by criticizing your drinking? Have you ever felt bad or Guilty about your drinking? Have you ever had a drink first thing in the morning to steady your nerves or to get rid of a hangover (Eye opener)?
NIDA Drug Use Screening Tool	Used with both alcohol and drugs. Has an adapted version for adolescents. May be self-administered or by clinician.
Opioid Risk Tool (ORT)	Self-administered tool for adults.
CRAFFT	Recommended by American Academy of Pediatrics Committee on Substance Abuse and Prevention for use with adolescents. Six-question tool to determine whether a longer conversation is needed about alcohol and drug use.

(NIDA, 2018; Townsend, 2018)

different settings to facilitate an evidence-based assessment of the impact of alcohol use on the patient's life (NIDA, 2018; Townsend, 2018). And while these tools are supported by evidence, a systematic review of substance misuse by Voon, Karamouzian, and Kerr (2017) determined that current systematic reviews have found a lack of high-quality evidence on the prevalence, risk factors, and optimal clinical assessment and treatment for substance misuse, particularly opioid misuse for chronic pain, and recommend more primary research to determine the clinical utility of these standardized assessment instruments.

Alcohol is absorbed from the GI tract and travels through the bloodstream to have its effect eventually on all body systems; however, it acts most predominantly in the neurological system and more specifically the CNS. First, peripheral neuropathy occurs due to vitamin B deficiency and results in nerve damage with associated pain and burning/tingling sensations. Wernicke's encephalopathy is due to another vitamin deficiency, thiamine, and if not reversed may be fatal. The signs and symptoms of this condition include paralyzed ocular muscles, ataxia, and stupor. Korsakoff's psychosis is a related neurological disorder, and the two conditions are often referred to as Wernicke-Korsakoff syndrome. The person experiences altered mental function with confusion, memory loss, and confabulation to fill in any the missing information due to memory loss and/or blackouts. A full neurological assessment may be needed to identify problems in the CNS and peripheral nervous system (Dillon, 2017; Townsend, 2018).

There are certain neurological findings that may occur with hepatic encephalopathy. Level of consciousness often worsens and may progress quickly from alertness to lethargy, somnolence, and eventually coma. Asterixis is jerking movement of the limbs that resolves as the level of consciousness worsens. Reflexes are also affected by hepatic encephalopathy; clonus and a positive Babinski sign may be present in the late stages. Cerebral edema may result in seizures and/or coma in its late stages (Dillon, 2017; Hart, 2015).

A potentially life-threatening condition that develops as a result of long-term alcohol abuse is alcoholic cardiomyopathy. With altered lipid metabolism, there are lipid deposits in the myocardial cells that both enlarge and weaken the heart muscle. Congestive heart failure and arrhythmias are the primary result of these changes and lead to decreased activity tolerance, tachycardia, dyspnea, dry cough, palpitations, and peripheral edema (Dillon, 2017; Townsend, 2018).

The GI system may also be affected both directly and indirectly by alcohol ingestion. First, alcohol is a local irritant to the esophagus, so esophagitis may result. An additional cause of esophagitis is irritation by the acidic gastric contents that occurs with frequent vomiting due to alcohol. Next, alcohol is also a local irritant to the gastric mucosal lining, causing gastritis, with the following signs/symptoms: nausea, vomiting, and epigastric pain/distension. Similar symptoms may occur with alcohol-induced acute pancreatitis (nausea, vomiting, abdominal pain/distension). If this condition progresses to a chronic state, the signs/symptoms are steatorrhea, malnutrition, weight loss, and diabetes mellitus (Hart, 2015; Townsend, 2018).

The liver is the gastrointestinal organ most affected by alcohol abuse, and the manifestations are alcoholic hepatitis and cirrhosis. With hepatitis, the person may have vague symptoms of lethargy, nausea, and abdominal fullness; however, the physical findings of jaundice, ascites, and an enlarged, tender liver are often quite specific to this condition. When assessing jaundice, the nurse should assess for changes in the sclera, as jaundice is often first evident as a yellowish discoloration there and is not affected by skin pigmentation and exposure to sun. Jaundice is also manifested in dark-colored urine. When assessing the skin for jaundice, the nurse should focus on areas that are not regularly exposed to the sun, such as the abdomen (Dillon, 2017; Hart, 2015).

When assessing the patient, the nurse observes the abdomen for swelling, which may be ascites (an accumulation of protein-containing fluid in the peritoneal cavity). The symptoms of ascites vary based on the amount of fluid and the patient's size. Small amounts of fluid may not cause symptoms and may be minimal on physical examination; radiological examination may be needed to confirm presence of ascites. With larger amounts of fluid, the patient may experience the following symptoms: early satiety, abdominal fullness and/or pain, or shortness of breath. Physical examination of the abdomen and ascites is more difficult in an obese patient. The abdominal girth should be measured at the umbilicus and tracked over time. As the nurse initially observes the abdomen, the presence of bulging flanks is a sign of ascites. If the patient's flanks are noticeably bulging when viewed from the patient's feet, it is a sign of excess fluid in the abdominal cavity. When the patient is supine, the fluid shifts to the flanks, causing them to bulge due to gravity. Ascites is graded on a scale of 1 to 4 or 1 to 3, with a higher score indicating more fluid and also a tenser abdomen when palpated (Dillon, 2017; Hart, 2015).

The *fluid wave/thrill* and *puddle* tests are considered somewhat definitive for the presence of ascites. First, the *fluid wave* test is performed by having the patient (or a colleague) push their hands down on the midline of the abdomen. The nurse taps one flank, while feeling on the other flank for the tap; if fluid is present, the tap will be felt on the other side and considered a positive fluid wave test. When one side of the abdomen is palpated, the other side may also be painful due to the transfer of the fluid across the abdominal cavity. The *puddle* sign can detect small amounts of fluid (as little as 120 mL). The *puddle test* is performed after the patient lies prone for 5 minutes. The patient then rises onto elbows and knees and the nurse places the diaphragm of the stethoscope on the most dependent part of the abdomen while repeatedly flicking their finger on the near flank and on the abdomen. As the nurse moves the stethoscope across abdomen and away from the examiner, the loudness of the flicking increases at the farthest edge of fluid or *puddle*. The transmission of sound does not change when patient sits up. Obviously, the patient must have mobility and the flexibility to change positions for this test to be performed accurately. Both the fluid wave and puddle test are noninvasive and cost-effective methods of assessing ascites. If physical assessment is not definitive, abdominal ultrasonography may be necessary to confirm the presence of ascites (Dillon, 2017; Hart, 2015).

Percussion and palpation of the liver are valuable techniques in determining if the liver is enlarged and/or tender. First, the nurse percusses down from the third intercostal space along the right *midclavicular line* (MCL). If the liver is normal size, the sound changes from tympany to dullness at fifth intercostal space in the MCL. Then the nurse percusses upward from below the umbilicus in the same line to assess the lower border and measure the distance in centimeters (using a ruler or fingerbreadth). Using the *5-7-9 rule*, the upper border of a healthy liver is defined by dullness at the following anatomical areas:

- 5th intercostal space in the midclavicular line,
- 7th intercostal space in the midaxillary line, and
- 9th intercostal space in the scapular line.

Clinically, liver span is commonly underestimated but normal size is as follows: 6 to 12 cm MCL and 4 to 8 cm in the midsternal line (Dillon, 2017; Hart, 2015).

Next after percussion, the nurse progresses to palpation of the liver. With patient supine, the nurse places the right hand on patient's abdomen, just lateral to the rectus abdominis, and below lower border of liver that was identified by percussing dullness. As the patient inhales, the nurse feels the liver edge as it descends. It is normal for the edge of the liver to be palpable as a smooth, non-tender surface against the examiner's hand.

With liver enlargement due to disease more of the liver may be palpable, and its palpation may also be associated with pain that is relieved once palpation is complete. Laboratory values are also assessed to determine liver function and/or injury. Elevated liver enzymes, especially *aspartate aminotransferase* (AST or SGOT) and *alanine aminotransferase* (ALT or SGPT), are released when there is liver injury (Dillon, 2017; Hart, 2015).

Assessment for Opioid Use Disorder

The nurse alters and individualizes the assessment of a person with suspected OUD based on their presenting symptoms. When the patient is under the influence of opioids, the nurse should assess for the following signs/symptoms: decreased pain perception, euphoria, confusion, excessive sleepiness, nausea, constipation, and miosis. These manifestations of opioid(s) can be assessed using basic observational skills during the interview process. There can be rapid progression from intoxication to overdose in which the patient displays the following: severe miosis, bradycardia, hypothermia, bradypnea, unresponsiveness, pulmonary edema, shock, and possible death. Pupils may also be dilated in an opioid overdose (Dillon, 2017; Hart, 2015).

When the potential for a life-threatening situation has resolved, the nurse must provide ongoing assessment during the withdrawal phase, as this may include very uncomfortable sensations as the body adjusts to not having the substance in the circulating bloodstream and tissues. Onset of withdrawal depends on which opioid was used; heroin has a very short time to withdrawal, which occurs at about 5 hours after use, while methadone withdrawal may not ensue for 2 days. Duration of withdrawal symptoms also varies with the specific opioid and is usually 2 to 4 days, but may extend for 2 weeks. The most common symptoms of opioid withdrawal by system are neurological (agitation, anxiety, insomnia), yawning, sweating, tremors, piloerection (*goose bumps*), eye/ear/nose/throat (dilated pupils, excessive tearing, rhinorrhea, sneezing), gastrointestinal (cramps, cravings, diarrhea), and cardiovascular (hypertension, tachycardia) (Dillon, 2017; Hart, 2015).

 ASSESSMENT PEARLS
There are many evidence-based assessment tools that may be used for substance abuse and/or alcohol abuse that are age specific (NIDA, 2018).

Nonpharmacological Management

Unlike many other mental health conditions, the nonpharmacological treatments are the primary foundation for many substance abuse disorders. The following approaches have been supported by evidence to be effective in decreasing anxiety, cravings, withdrawal symptoms, and potential for relapse while improving coping skills. *Marital therapy* involves the spouse in the therapeutic process and educates the couple on how to develop a home environment that supports sobriety. *Motivational interviewing* uses focused questions to help the individual optimize adaptive coping skills and to learn new behavioral skills. *Community reinforcement approach training* (CRAFT) helps families and friends to support change in the individual and decreases the effects of abuse on the individual and those in their community. *Exposure therapy* has been used to decrease anxiety in individuals by having individuals confront anxiety-producing situations to decrease their effect. *Contingency management* uses rewards (or removal of privileges) contingent on the individual's compliance with their treatment plan (CDC, 2018; Murthy, 2017). Because alcohol causes damage to the prefrontal cortex and results in difficulty with executive functions including social behavior, *social skills training* may be a useful adjuvant.

Self-help organizations (Alcoholics Anonymous [AA] and Narcotics Anonymous [NA]) provide support for sobriety and also support the family members through related groups (e.g., Al-Anon). Briefly, AA is based on abstaining from alcohol through spiritual (not necessarily religious) awakening by following the *Twelve Steps*. Sobriety is supported by volunteerism within the AA organization, regular meeting attendance, and supporting other members. The organization uses a sponsor system in which an experienced fellow alcoholic mentors and supports a newer member through the program steps (Townsend, 2018). While the "higher power" referred to in AA and NA is not necessarily a religious entity and may refer to the support group itself, some individuals are not comfortable with this aspect of these treatments. Alternative approaches include LifeRing (secular group that provides peer network focused on abstinence), Women for Sobriety (abstinence-based program comprised of women only), and Moderation Management (program based on moderating and controlling problem drinking behaviors) (Substance Abuse and Mental Health Services Administration [SAMHSA], 2020).

According to a recent National Survey of Drug Use and Health, nearly one-third of people with a substance abuse disorder also have a diagnosed mental illness, which complicates the treatment plan for the patient and family (National Alliance for the Mentally Ill [NAMI], 2017). This co-occurrence of a mental illness and substance use is often referred to as *dual diagnosis*. Individuals often self-medicate with alcohol and other substances to deal with the symptoms of mental illness, (e.g., anxiety, depression, bipolar disorder) before a correct diagnosis is made and a treatment plan is initiated. Once properly treated for a diagnosed mental illness, they may no longer need or use the additional substances. However, often the person has developed both a physical and psychological addiction to the substance(s) and now requires treatment for substance abuse as well. While evidence supports the relationship between these conditions, further research is needed to develop interventions that effectively address this complex situation (NAMI, 2017).

In a meta-analysis of Web-based behavioral interventions for various mental health conditions, including substance abuse, Rogers, Lemmen, Kramer, Mann, and Chopra (2017) concluded that such programs had major drawbacks of being difficult to locate and access and being time intensive, requiring weeks to months of engagement by the user. Positives aspects of these interventions included availability in various languages, opportunities for self-pacing and self-monitoring, and interaction with and personalized feedback from providers. While the Web-based programs evaluated had generally positive outcomes, the authors cautioned that more research is needed to support their use, and access needs to be improved in order for them any substantial impact.

The *Healthy People 2020* campaign addressed substance abuse and supported the use of educational and community-based programs that included settings outside of health care, such as schools, worksites, and community centers. In these settings, there are more opportunities to work with people within their existing social structures and cultures (HealthyPeople.gov, 2018). By tailoring the interventions to the specific population and taking it to their community, time and resources necessary for program development are appropriately focused and allocated (HealthyPeople.gov, 2020; Patchell, Robbins, Lowe, & Hoke, 2015). The CDC has launched the Rx Awareness campaign with the goal to increase awareness that prescription opioids can be addictive and dangerous. Also, the campaign is aimed at decreasing the number of individuals who use opioids recreationally or misuse/overuse them (CDC, 2020). The most effective programs use multiple settings to reach the most people (HealthyPeople.gov, 2020; Murthy, 2017).

In addition to helping the individual with substance use disorder, it is important to support the families who must cope with the disorder. Options include support groups or family therapy and counseling, which can improve individual treatment effectiveness by supporting the whole family. Supporting a loved one with substance use disorder can lead to caregiver role strain, so nurses should encourage caregivers to take steps to prioritize their own health. Family members may be more likely to notice early mood and/or behavioral changes in the individual with substance use disorder and can activate services to begin and/or maintain recovery (SAMHSA, 2020). There are also various community coalitions that partner with schools, faith-based organizations, and public health agencies to educate both youth and adults to reduce excessive use of alcohol and abuse of substances, particularly opioids (CDC, 2018).

Healthy lifestyles are also encouraged for patients who have substance use disorders or are in recovery and include a balanced diet, regular exercise, and smoking cessation (NAMI, 2017; Townsend, 2018). Because patients with substance use disorders often have underlying anxiety and depression, they may benefit from practices that promote relaxation, such as deep breathing exercises with meditation, yoga, and tai chi. These strategies may also be effective for patients while in withdrawal and during ongoing recovery. Social support may also be important for promoting coping skills and improving quality of life during various phases of recovery (NAMI, 2017; Townsend, 2018). The nurse focuses care on the individual and their family; these nonpharmacological approaches have much higher success rates when families are included in the education about them and participate with the individual as appropriate. Al-Anon and Alateen are support groups for family members; meetings are often held concurrent to AA meetings to facilitate family involvement. Nurses need to be knowledgeable about the various resources that are available in their community to meet the needs of these individuals and their families. These services often vary greatly and while the Affordable Care Act mandated that insurance companies offer coverage for substance abuse treatment and mental health, there are differences among policies (CDC, 2018).

◐ CLINICAL PEARLS

When the patient is actively under the influence of alcohol or an opiate, maintaining their safety is the priority in the treatment plan.

Pharmacology

Patients with substance use disorders may be treated in a variety of methods and settings that may include observed detoxification and rehabilitation in an inpatient and/or outpatient setting. The treatment plan may include pharmacological intervention during this time. The most commonly used pharmacological management of alcohol withdrawal is the use of long-acting benzodiazepines, usually chlordiazepoxide or diazepam, to prevent and control symptoms (Vallerand & Sanoski, 2020). Vitamins, specifically thiamine, folic acid, and pyridoxine, are necessary to replace missing nutrients and prevent withdrawal symptoms, especially Wernicke syndrome. These are administered intravenously before food or fluids are given via mouth. Once the person is out of the withdrawal period, one of the following medications may be used to prevent resumption of alcohol use: disulfiram, naltrexone, and/or acamprosate (Karch, 2017; Townsend, 2018; Vallerand & Sanoski, 2020). These medications should not be administered if the person has ingested alcohol in the past 12 hours; they work by blocking the enzyme acetaldehyde dehydrogenase, which metabolizes alcohol. As a result, acetaldehyde blood levels rise, and the person experiences the unpleasant symptoms of acute alcohol withdrawal (i.e., a *hangover*), such as flushed skin, tachycardia, shortness of breath, nausea/vomiting, headache, and mental confusion. It is important that patients understand the premise of treatment with disulfiram and are aware of its use in their treatment plan (Townsend, 2018). If ammonia levels are elevated, the patient is usually placed on lactulose to prevent hepatic encephalopathy. Lactulose binds ammonia in the gut by using normal intestinal bacteria to acidify the colon, changing ammonia into ammonium so it can be excreted safely and does not diffuse into the bloodstream (Karch, 2017; Townsend, 2018; Woo, 2020).

In contrast, individuals with opioid use disorders are often treated with *opioid replacement therapy* (ORT) during withdrawal because the symptoms are so difficult to endure, and abrupt cessation of use may be life threatening. Additionally, it is believed that ORT promotes gradual resumption of a sober lifestyle because strong euphoric effects of opioids are not experienced on the low-dose replacement medications while drug cravings and withdrawal are mitigated. Risk of mortality due to overdose is decreased with ORT. Both methadone and buprenorphine may be used during the withdrawal phase of opioid use and as part of ORT. Naloxone, an antidote and reversal agent for opioids, is used for opioid overdose and is available without prescription for use by family members in addition to first responders and heath care providers (Karch, 2017; Townsend, 2018). Medications used in the treatment of alcohol and/or opioid use disorders are presented in Table 27–3.

It is important for nurses to know and follow their respective state's practice guidelines regarding opioids. Specifically, there are state-run databases, *prescription drug monitoring programs* (PDMPs), that provide information regarding a patient's prescription history. However, there are no standards related to the drugs that are monitored, data collected, or if it is shared between/among states (American Nurses Association [ANA], 2020).

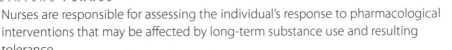 **RED FLAG ALERT**

There are many potential drug–drug interactions with medications that are used for substance use withdrawal.

CLINICAL PEARLS
Nurses are responsible for assessing the individual's response to pharmacological interventions that may be affected by long-term substance use and resulting tolerance.

Summary

Substance abuse is a long-standing but growing problem both in the United States and globally. The opioid crisis has brought renewed attention to this significant health problem that affects millions of individuals and their families. The pathophysiology that results from abuse of substances, particularly alcohol and opioids, confirms the life-threatening nature of these conditions. Individuals with suspected substance abuse disorder must be assessed with an objective, nonjudgmental approach in order to initiate early identification and treatment (Anandan et al., 2016). There are multiple tools that bring objective measurement to what can often be a subjective and complicated diagnosis. While nonpharmacological management is the foundational treatment approach, pharmacological interventions may be useful in treating these disorders and supporting psychological strategies that promote and support sobriety. It is important to involve families in the plan of care to support and maintain the patient's recovery.

TABLE 27-3 Drugs Used to Treat Substance Abuse

Class	Example	Action	Dosage	SENC
Benzodiazepines	Chlordiazepoxide	Increases GABA in the limbic, thalamic, and hypothalamic areas.	50–100 mg/day, up to 300 mg/day.	Monitor for orthostatic hypotension and tachycardia, especially with parenteral administration. Agranulocytosis is a potential side effect. Potentiates effects of alcohol.
Vitamin	Thiamine (B_1)	Essential coenzyme in carbohydrate metabolism. Prevents Wernicke-Korsakoff syndrome.	100 mg over 5 min IV.	Monitor for anaphylaxis and cardiovascular collapse.
Vitamin	Folic acid (B_2)	Essential for nucleoprotein synthesis and normal erythropoiesis.	Up to 1 mg/day PO or IV.	Flushing with IV administration.
Vitamin	Pyridoxine (B_6)	Essential for carbohydrate and protein metabolism including amino acid metabolism. Aids in energy transformation and normal function of nervous system.	10–20 mg/day × 2–3 weeks.	Monitor platelets for hemolytic abnormalities. Administer concurrently with folic acid.
Anti-alcoholic agents	Disulfiram	Inhibits aldehyde dehydrogenase that is needed for normal alcohol metabolism. Causes unpleasant symptoms similar to hangover. Works 30 min after ingestion of alcohol and lasts 30 min to several hr.	Initially 500 mg/day × 1–2 weeks and then 125–500 mg/day maintenance.	Use as an adjuvant for patients who commit to maintaining sobriety. Side effects: hepatotoxicity, hypotension, acute congestive heart failure.
Ammonia-binding agents/hyperosmotic agents	Lactulose	Acidifies colon contents, which slows diffusion of ammonia from GI tract into bloodstream.	30–40 mL 3 × a day to produce 2–3 loose stools/day.	Promote adequate fluid intake to prevent dehydration.
Opiate agonist-antagonists	Buprenorphine	Synthetic opiate agonist 30 × that of morphine and antagonist 3 × naloxone.	16 mg/day sublingual. Daily dose adjusted based on patient response and lack of withdrawal symptoms.	Side effects: hypotension, respiratory depression, sedation, miosis.
Opioid replacements	Methadone	Synthetic opioid that causes CNS depression. Low dose is used in ORT to decrease withdrawal.	15–40 mg/day.	Side effects: sedation, constipation. Most resolve in several weeks.
Opioid receptor antagonists	Naloxone	Thought to compete for CNS opiate receptor sites, blocking effect of opioids.	0.4–2 mg IV. May repeat q 2–3 min.	Preferred treatment of overdose regardless of drug. Give prescription for IM auto-injector and educate family.

(Karch, 2017; Vallerand & Sanoski, 2020; Woo, 2020)

Key Points

- Substance use disorder is caused by the interaction of genetic predisposition with environmental factors.
- Abuse of alcohol and/or opioids can be life threatening, ranging from acute intoxication to long-term complications.
- The primary systems affected by alcohol use disorder are the neurological and gastrointestinal systems.
- The primary system affected by opioid use disorder is the neurological system.
- Opiate replacement therapy may be used to prevent withdrawal symptoms and overdose.
- Alcohol withdrawal can precipitate a medical emergency and may require pharmacological intervention.
- Families should be educated on how to support the patient's recovery and sustained sobriety.

Review Questions

1. **The nurse is assessing the patient's knowledge of the development of substance use disorders. Which of the following statements is correct?**

    a. "I didn't have a chance; I have alcoholism because my father had it."
    b. "There are no genetic components to these disorders."
    c. "There are structural differences in my brain that cause substance use disorder."
    d. "Its's probably a combination of environmental and genetic factors that caused this."

2. **Which of the assessment findings would the nurse expect to observe in an adult who is in opiate withdrawal? (Select all that apply.)**

    a. Mydriasis
    b. Agitation
    c. Miosis
    d. Nightmares
    e. Tachycardia

3. **What does the nurse include in the teaching for a patient on lactulose to prevent hepatic encephalopathy?**

    a. "Take a multivitamin to prevent malnutrition."
    b. "Maintain adequate fluid intake to prevent dehydration."
    c. "Discontinue use if you experience loose stools."
    d. "Take an anti-diarrheal as needed."

4. **When assessing a patient with alcohol use disorder, what does the nurse include in the interview? (Select all that apply.)**

    a. Ask the patient directly how much they drink each day.
    b. Use a reliable tool to assess the presence of alcohol use disorder.
    c. Ask family members if they also have problems with alcohol.
    d. Assess for concomitant physical conditions due to alcohol use.

5. **When educating the patient who has been prescribed disulfiram to maintain sobriety, which of the following statements lets the nurse know that the patient understands instructions?**
   a. "I'll take the medication if I have a craving for alcohol, as it will decrease it."
   b. "I will take the medication regularly and know that I will get sick if I drink alcohol."
   c. "I will limit fluid intake, so I won't feel bloated."
   d. "I don't need AA if I take this medication as prescribed."

See the appendix for answers to review questions.

References

American Nurses Association. (2020). *Opioid epidemic.* Retrieved from https://www.nursingworld.org/practice-policy/work-environment/health-safety/opioid-epidemic/

Anandan, R., Cross, W., & Munro, I. (2016). Nursing attitudes towards people with comorbid substance abuse: A brief review of literature. *Australian Nursing & Midwifery Journal, 24*(6), 39.

Capriotti, T. (2020). *Pathophysiology: Introductory concepts and clinical perspectives* (2nd ed.). Philadelphia, PA: F.A. Davis.

Centers for Disease Control and Prevention. (2018). *Excessive alcohol use.* Retrieved from https://www.cdc.gov/chronicdisease/resources/publications/factsheets/alcohol.htm

Centers for Disease Control and Prevention. (2020). *Rx awareness.* Retrieved from https://www.cdc.gov/rxawareness/about/index.html

Dillon, P. (2015). *Nursing health assessment: A critical thinking, case studies approach* (3rd ed.). Philadelphia, PA: F.A. Davis.

Drug Policy. (2020). *Drug overdose.* Retrieved from https://www.drugpolicy.org/issues/drug-overdose

Hart, V. A. (2015). Psychiatric mental health. In M. J. Goolsby & L. Grubbs (Eds.), *Advanced assessment: Interpreting findings and formulating differential diagnoses.* Philadelphia, PA: F.A. Davis.

HealthyPeople.gov. (2018). Substance abuse. Retrieved from https://www.healthypeople.gov/2020/topics-objectives/topic/substance-abuse

Karch, A. M. (2017). *Focus on nursing pharmacology* (7th ed.). Philadelphia, PA: Wolters Kluwer / Lippincott Williams & Wilkins.

Murthy, V. H. (2017). Surgeon General's Report on Alcohol, Drugs, and Health. *JAMA: Journal of the American Medical Association, 317*(2), 133–134. doi:10.1001/jama.2016.18215

National Alliance for the Mentally Ill. (2017). Integrated treatment for mental illness and substance use. Retrieved from https://www.nami.org/Blogs/NAMI-Blog/October-2017/Integrated-Treatment-for-Mental-Illness-and-Substa

National Institute on Drug Abuse. (2018). Understanding drug use and addition. Retrieved from https://www.drugabuse.gov/publications/drugfacts/understanding-drug-use-addiction

Patchell, B. A., Robbins, L. K., Lowe, J. A., & Hoke, M. M. (2015). The effect of a culturally tailored substance abuse prevention intervention with Plains Indian adolescents. *Journal of Cultural Diversity, 22*(2), 3–8.

Rogers, M. A., Lemmen, K., Kramer, R., Mann, J., & Chopra, V. (2017). Internet-delivered health interventions that work: Systematic review of meta-analyses and evaluation of website availability. *Journal of Medical Internet Research, 19*(3), 1. doi:10.2196/jmir.7111

Substance Abuse and Mental Health Services Administration. (2020). *Resources for families coping with mental and substance use disorders.* Retrieved from https://www.samhsa.gov/families

Townsend, M. C. (2019). *Psychiatric mental health nursing: Concepts of care in evidence-based practice* (9th ed.). Philadelphia, PA: F.A. Davis.

Vallerand, A. H., & Sanoski, C. A. (Eds.). (2020). *Davis's drug guide for nurses* (17th ed.). Philadelphia, PA: F.A. Davis.

Voon, P., Karamouzian, M., & Kerr, T. (2017). Chronic pain and opioid misuse: A review of reviews. *Substance Abuse Treatment, Prevention & Policy, 12*(1), 36. doi:10.1186/s13011-017-0120-7

Woo, T. M. (2020). Drugs affecting the central nervous system. In T. M. Woo & M. V. Robinson (Eds.), *Pharmacotherapeutics for advanced practice nurse prescribers* (5th ed.). Philadelphia, PA: F.A. Davis.

World Health Organization. (2018). Acute intoxication. Retrieved from http://www.who.int/substance_abuse/terminology/acute_intox/en/

Case Study 6 (Mental Health): Attention Deficit-Hyperactivity Disorder (ADHD)

LEARNING OBJECTIVES

Upon completion of this case study the student will be able to integrate knowledge of the pathophysiology, assessment, and pharmacological and nonpharmacological care options for a patient with *attention deficit-hyperactivity disorder* (ADHD) and their family.

Introduction to ADHD

ADHD is a neurological condition that affects the *central nervous system* (CNS) and causes behaviors that are developmentally inappropriate, so the age of the child must be considered when evaluating for a potential diagnosis. ADHD may continue into adulthood and/or be initially diagnosed in adults (Capriotti, 2020; National Institute of Mental Health (NIMH), 2018; Ramos-Olazagasti et al., 2018). Regardless of the age of the patient, there are three major components to ADHD: *inattention*, *hyperactivity*, and *impulsivity*. Some patients display only one of these behaviors, while others have a combination of the three; most children with ADHD have the combined type. A brief explanation of each of these behaviors will help the nurse to understand the presenting signs/symptoms and subsequent treatment plan. *Inattention* is displayed in the following behaviors: difficulty focusing and staying on task, lack of persistence, and disorganization. *Hyperactivity* is exhibited in excessive movement, fidgeting, restlessness, and/or talking. *Impulsivity* is manifested in rash decision making, lack of delayed gratification, and risk-taking behaviors (American Academy of Pediatrics [AAP], 2018; Capriotti, 2020; NIMH, 2018; Townsend, 2018). Each of these behaviors in isolation or in combinations may lead to both short-term and long-term problems for a child or adult with ADHD and their families (Ramos-Olazagasti et al., 2018; Townsend, 2018).

The prevalence rates of ADHD vary based on the diagnostic criteria used. According to the *Diagnostic and Statistical Manual of Mental Disorders* (DSM-V) criteria, it affects about 5% to 7% of children, as compared to 1% to 2% when using the International Classification of Diseases 10 (ICD-10) criteria. Globally, according to the World Health Organization and using the ICD-10 criteria, there are 51.1 million people with ADHD; in the United States, 6.1 million children have been diagnosed with ADHD (Centers for Disease Control and Prevention [CDC], 2019). There is gender disparity in diagnosis, with boys (12.9%) diagnosed with ADHD three times more often than girls (5.9%). While predominantly a pediatric disease, the initial diagnosis may also occur after the age of 18 (Capriotti, 2020; NIMH, 2018; Townsend, 2018).

Because the expectations for executive functions increase with age, symptoms of ADHD may not manifest until adolescence or early adulthood. Of those diagnosed in childhood, 30% to 50% continue to have symptoms into adulthood, resulting in an adult prevalence rate of 2% to 5% (AAP, 2018; Capriotti, 2020; Ramos-Olazagasti et al., 2018). Generally, inattentiveness is the prominent manifestation in adults with ADHD, as hyperactivity and impulsivity decrease with overall developmental maturity (AAP, 2018; Townsend, 2018).

The AAP has given an explanation for the increased prevalence of ADHD diagnoses and treatment that is based on several factors, including increased knowledge of the disease and its treatment and an interdisciplinary approach with input from family, teachers, and caregivers. There is controversy, however, around the question of whether more children actually have ADHD or the higher rate of diagnosis and treatment is based on unrealistic expectations for behavior at home and school. Davidovitch, Koren, Fund, Shrem, and Porath (2017) studied the ADHD prevalence rates and reached several conclusions. First, the global prevalence of ADHD diagnoses has increased, while the U.S. prevalence has decreased slightly. Although there is concern regarding overuse of pediatric ADHD medication (from 3.57% to 8.51%), currently in the United States children with ADHD are treated with medication only (30%), behavioral treatment only (15%), or a combination of medication and behavioral treatment (32%) (CDC, 2019). The authors concluded that both providers and parents were more open to diagnosing and treating ADHD with the goal of improving school performance, often requiring medications. Increased diagnosis and treatment of ADHD in females may also be a result of these changed attitudes. Because ADHD is the most studied condition in children, there is ample research to develop evidence-based standards of care (AAP, 2018; NIMH, 2018).

Meet CE

CE is a 14-year-old Caucasian boy who was diagnosed with ADHD when he was 7 years old. He has been on medication for most of the past 7 years during the school year; drug holidays were implemented during the summer months. His school performance is good, both grades and behavior. CE takes methylphenidate 10 mg upon awakening and at lunch on school days. He does not take any other medication or have any chronic illnesses. CE's mom accompanies him to the pediatrician today for a well-child checkup, but CE wants to go to the examination room alone.

Physiology and Pathophysiology

Review normal brain physiology, especially as related to neurotransmitters, in other chapters (see Chapter 24) to understand the alterations of ADHD. The physiology/pathophysiology specific to ADHD focuses on dopamine and norepinephrine pathways, which originate in the ventral tegmental area and locus coeruleus and are responsible for numerous functions in various areas of the brain, including cognition, motor function, and behavioral control (Capriotti, 2020; NIMH, 2018). The impaired functioning seen in children with ADHD is due to altered anatomy such as decreased size of brain structures, especially the left-sided prefrontal cortex, which is responsible for executive functions including behavior control (Capriotti, 2020; Townsend, 2018).

The pathophysiological processes of ADHD stem from abnormalities in the neurotransmitter pathways, in particular depletion of dopamine and norepinephrine, and possibly serotonin, too. There is a genetic predisposition to the development of ADHD, although a specific gene has not been identified; similar to many disorders, it is thought to be a result of the interaction of genetics and environment. The manifestations of

ADHD symptoms are dependent on the child's environment; for example, a disorganized and chaotic family household may precipitate and/or magnify the child's symptoms. Environmental lead, such as paint from older homes, is a risk for its development. Traumatic brain injuries and/or prematurity are also risk factors for ADHD, as are prenatal exposure to alcohol or nicotine (AAP, 2018). In a study by Ask and colleagues (2018), it was determined that prematurity was associated with a higher level of ADHD symptoms in preschool children; however, in school-age children, prematurity was associated with inattention but not hyperactivity. This study demonstrates the variability of symptom presentation across ages due to an identified risk factor.

ADHD symptoms are a result of abnormal brain activity primarily in the prefrontal cortex and with executive functions that control behaviors such as attention, organization, emotions, inhibitions, and short-term working memory. Using *single-photon computed emission tomography* (SPECT), decreased activity of the neurotransmitter in the prefrontal cortex has been documented. Children with ADHD have smaller brains by 3% to 5%; more severe disease is associated with smaller frontal lobes. The decreased size and abnormal functioning of this area of the brain is the rationale for medications that increase dopaminergic and noradrenergic activity in this area (Capriotti, 2020; NIMH, 2018).

Gathering Information

Nurse AB decides to gather recent health history from CE first and then talk to his mother while the health-care provider assesses him. CE says, "I'm tired of having to take medicine; I don't like having to go to the nurse every day for my midday dose. Haven't I outgrown this ADHD stuff? My grades are good." Otherwise, he has no complaints about his health and reports he has a friend group from school. CE's mom is concerned that he still needs medication because he is a teenager and is more likely to be impulsive. CE was in cognitive-behavioral therapy (CBT) until last year when he decided he didn't want to participate.

Assessment and Diagnosis

Diagnosis of ADHD often occurs when the child enters school and the symptoms are manifested and/or amplified in a setting where they are required to follow instructions, control behaviors, and interact with others. Within ADHD, there are three subtypes: predominantly inattentive (more common in females), predominantly hyperactive, and combination (both more common in males) (Goolsby & Grubbs, 2019). Assessment includes asking the child, family, and teachers about the child's behavior. Physical reasons for the child's behavior should be evaluated, such as hyperthyroidism, neurological disease, medication, and environment influences. After ruling out other disorders (e.g., anxiety disorder, depression, learning disabilities), the diagnosis of ADHD is made based on presence of symptoms for at least 6 months and in two settings (e.g., home, school, sports teams). Nurses are advocates for coordinated care for the child and family before, during, and after the diagnosis, so the appropriate supportive resources/therapies are utilized, and the family is involved in care decisions (NIMH, 2018; Townsend, 2018). Notably, there are implications whenever a mental health diagnosis is established, and nurses are in key positions to educate the family, prevent stigmatization of the child/family, and promote positive outcomes (Capriotti, 2020).

Diagnosis

CE's diagnosis of ADHD has been established using the appropriate criteria. At this visit, the provider's goal is to assess whether CE needs to continue pharmacological treatment.

CE, at age 14, is involved in the decision making. The Conners' Parent Rating Scale *and* Conners' Teacher Rating Scale *(27-item, 0 to 3 behavioral rating) have been used for current symptom evaluation and do not indicate current manifestations of ADHD. CE's teacher has provided documentation that he is attentive in class and has not had any behavioral difficulties this academic year.*

Treatment Options

Treatment is aimed at supporting the child's normal growth and development by allowing them to participate in age-appropriate activities, with an emphasis on safety, school performance, and social interaction. When the child's symptoms are managed, they are able to meet developmental milestones, and quality of life is improved for the patient and family (AAP, 2018). The short-term goals are focused on safety, school performance, and social interactions; the long-term goals address normal growth and development and maintenance of self-esteem (Townsend, 2018).

Medication management is recommended for symptoms that are moderate to severe and after nonpharmacological interventions have not been effective. The diagnosis of ADHD and evaluation of need for medication most frequently occurs when the child is school age; however, when the symptoms present in children of preschool age, parents may be faced with the decision to start medication (AAP, 2018). In a study by Hart, Ros, Gonzalez, and Graziano (2018), 45% of parents of preschool-age children were open to the initiation of medication for treating their child's ADHD. These parents had reported higher levels of aggressive behavior in their children as compared to parents who were not receptive to their children taking medication for ADHD. There are implications for early interventions that may include pharmacological management in preschool children.

Stimulants (see Table CS6–1) are often first-line choices and are made based on the patient's response to the medication and also side effect profile. In general, amphetamines cause the release of norepinephrine from central noradrenergic neurons; in higher doses, amphetamines also cause dopamine to be released in the mesolimbic system (Capriotti, 2020; NIMH, 2018; Woo & Robinson, 2020). In a German study that compared the health-care resource utilization and costs of two stimulants, *atomoxetine* (ATX) and *long-acting methylphenidate* (LA-MPH), the results were conclusive that patients on ATX required more prescriptions and physician visits, with resulting higher health-care costs as compared to LA-MPH patients (Greven et al., 2017). The most common side effects of amphetamines are restlessness, insomnia, headache, palpitations, hypertension, abdominal pain, anxiety, tolerance, and dependence. With long-term use, there may be physical growth delays (AAP, 2018; Capriotti, 2020; Woo & Robinson, 2020).

While stimulants are by far the most commonly prescribed medications for ADHD, nurses may encounter patients who are on another medication either due to the side effects of stimulants or their ineffectiveness. For example, nonstimulants are also used to manage ADHD (AAP, 2018; Woo & Robinson, 2020). In a recent study, evidence showed that guanfacine reduced symptoms more than ATX in treating ADHD (Shafrin, Shrestha, Chandra, Erder, & Sikirica, 2017). Omega-3 and omega-6 fatty acids are recommended for children with ADHD because they are necessary for normal neurocognitive development and it is theorized that a deficiency would exacerbate symptoms (AAP, 2018; Woo & Robinson, 2020). While these nutritional supplements may be helpful, a balanced, healthy diet that is low in simple sugars is one of the basic recommendations for promoting normal growth and development.

TABLE CS6–1 Drugs Commonly Used to Treat ADHD

Class	Example	Action	Dosage	SENC
Amphetamine	Methylphenidate	CNS stimulant, especially in cerebral cortex.	Adults: 20–30 mg/day PO in divided doses. Children: 5–10 mg PO before breakfast and lunch. Transdermal: 10 mg patch worn × 9 hr/day.	Apply transdermal 2 hr before needed effect. Weigh child 2–3 times weekly initially. Monitor for desired effect. Wean to prevent withdrawal.
Amphetamine	Dexmethylphenidate	CNS stimulant. Blocks reuptake of norepinephrine and dopamine.	Child and adult dose: 2.5 mg twice daily; may increase to 20 mg/day.	Extended release available; administer whole. Monitor complete blood count and liver function with prolonged treatment.
Alpha-adrenergic agonists	Guanfacine	Activates receptors in prefrontal cortex to increase executive functioning.	Immediate-release tablet: 1–2 mg twice daily. Extended-release tablet: 1–4 mg twice daily.	May be used with a stimulant. Side effects: sleepiness, tiredness, headache, and stomachache may be undesirable for school-age child.
Psychotherapeutic agents	Atomoxetine	Inhibits norepinephrine reuptake.	Adults: start with 40 mg/day to build to 80 mg/day. Children: 0.5 mg/kg/day increased to 1.2 mg/kg/day.	Administer dose in morning. Monitor for hypertension, especially with dosage increase.
Essential fatty acids	Omega-3	Normal neurocognitive development.	550 mg to 1 g/day.	May also be obtained from diet rich in fish (e.g., salmon, mackerel, sardines, albacore tuna).

(AAP, 2018; Townsend, 2018; Woo & Robinson, 2020)

Because a pharmacological treatment period may span years, ongoing compliance with daily medication is a common problem. In a longitudinal study, Brinkman, Sucharew, Hartl Majcher, and Epstein (2018) studied compliance with the initiation and continuation of ADHD medication and determined that compliance was 81% at 0 to 90 days and then decreased to 54% after day 91. Initially, compliance was positively affected by child's age, adequacy of medicine education, decreased symptoms, parental confidence in medication efficacy, and parental/provider collaboration. Conversely, long-term (over 91 days) compliance was related to the child's acceptance of treatment with medication and symptom improvement. In a systematic review of 31 articles related to ADHD medication regimens, Rashid, Lovick, and Llanwarne (2018) concluded that as the child enters adulthood, decision making evolves so that the child is supported toward autonomy and self-management while continuing to weigh the risk/benefit ratio of any treatment plan. If the locus of decision making about the treatment plan shifts gradually as the child matures, the patient is able to collaborate with the provider to develop the best treatment plan.

In addition to understanding the importance of medication, the parents of a child with ADHD and the child, depending on age, should make safety a priority. Because a child with ADHD may not always be aware of dangers and may take risks, extra precautions should be implemented (AAP, 2018; Townsend, 2018). While these situations pose a potential risk to any child, a child with ADHD should be supervised when near busy streets, power tools, swimming pools, and chemicals/cleaning supplies. Child-proofing the home for firearms (or their removal, as recommended by the AAP) and medications is vital for a safe home environment even when a child is older, as the child with ADHD does not have age-appropriate impulse control. Driving safety may be a particular concern for the family of a teen with ADHD; the age at which the child gets their license may need to be delayed or based on developmental rather than chronological age (Townsend, 2018).

According to Turvey and Fortney (2017), research supports the effectiveness of telemedicine using a population health approach to promote collaborative care, self-monitoring, and chronic disease management in pediatric ADHD populations. Using secure patient portals, information about the child's condition is shared between providers and patients/families to optimize care. Researchers recommend further evidence to support clinical protocols for using these technologies to decrease the population burden of mental health.

A family-centered approach to caring for the child with ADHD is supported by a meta-analysis (Theule, Cheung, & Aberdeen, 2018) of studies with families who have a child with ADHD. Based on their evaluation, these families had higher stress levels based on higher scores on the *Parenting Stress Index* (PSI), as compared to the control group. Therefore, the treatment plan should include collaboration with and care for the parents, so their needs are also addressed as they care for their child.

A common parental concern is how ADHD will affect their child once they reach adult age. Based on evidence by Roy and colleagues (2017), there are no consistent predictors of adult functioning based on a child's diagnosis and treatment for ADHD, except a lower *intelligence quotient* (IQ) in childhood. For children with ADHD and a lower IQ, there was an association with poorer outcomes as an adult. There are many approaches to ADHD treatment for adults, including both psychosocial and pharmacological interventions. As adults with ADHD are a relatively new patient demographic, further studies are needed and under way to determine the best treatment options. An adaptive treatment approach has been used successfully with adults with ADHD, which individualizes and adapts both pharmacological and nonpharmacological interventions based on patient response (Zinnow et al., 2018). There is evidence of gender differences with transition into adulthood with ADHD; females with childhood ADHD reported increased ADHD symptoms upon reaching adulthood, as compared to males (Millenet et al., 2018).

Treatment and Follow-Up

CE's mom asks about the long-term effect of medication and what will happen as he enters adulthood. Because she is also interested in the use of complementary therapies,

Nurse AB shares that there is evidence that any of the following may be helpful: chiropractic manipulation, biofeedback, yoga, massage, and visual and/or auditory therapies. Dietary modifications have not been successful with CE in the past, but they may try herbal supplements such as pine bark, melatonin, echinacea, St. John's wort, and ginkgo biloba; however, they should alert all providers if they add any of these to CE's treatment.

The treatment plan for CE is developed collaboratively by a team composed of CE, his provider, and CE's family and teacher. The team decides that CE is meeting both short-term goals (safety and school performance) and long-term goals (normal growth and development and social interactions) and that a trial medication discontinuation is warranted. Education is given about signs/symptoms to report to the provider (e.g., agitation, difficulty focusing, and risk-taking behaviors). CE plans to start yoga aimed at stress management.

Summary

While pediatric nurses are probably most familiar with ADHD and its treatment, this condition can extend into adulthood and/or be first diagnosed when the patient is an adult, so all nurses should be knowledgeable about this condition and its treatment (Ramos-Olazagasti et al., 2018). For mild symptoms that do not significantly affect the child's family or school performance, the child may be treated with behavior interventions and age-appropriate rewards for positive changes (AAP, 2018; Townsend, 2018). If symptoms are problematic, especially in the school setting, pharmacological intervention is necessary to provide symptoms control. As with most pharmacological interventions, the lowest effective dose for the shortest period of time should be used, and the child should be reassessed frequently, as the diagnostic parameters are related to age and change as the child grows and develops (AAP, 2018; Woo & Robinson, 2020).

Key Points

- The three age-specific behavioral components of ADHD are inattention, hyperactivity, and impulsivity.
- ADHD develops as a result of genetic and environmental factors.
- Pharmacological treatment is used for to moderate to severe ADHD and is usually a stimulant medication.
- Assessment of the child with ADHD includes input from multiple sources, including the child, parents, teacher(s), and other caregivers.

Review Questions

1. **The nurse is reviewing the health history of CE and his request to stop medication for ADHD. The nurse understands that which of the following will be weighed in the decision. (Select all that apply.)**
   a. CE's desire not to take medication
   b. CE's school performance
   c. Medication cannot be continued into adulthood
   d. Unable to get a driver's license if on a stimulant
   e. Risk of developing medication tolerance

2. **When explaining transition to adulthood with ADHD to CE's family, which of the following statements made by the nurse is correct?**

    a. "The diagnosis of ADHD is age dependent, so the criteria change as he ages."
    b. "Your child may need hospitalization for medication management as an adult."
    c. "Medications will be discontinued at age 18 as he transitions from pediatric care."
    d. "We'll have to wait until the insurance company designates him as an adult."

3. **Which of the following statements made by CE's mother indicates accurate understanding of his treatment plan as an adolescent?**

    a. "I will expect his medication to change as he becomes an adult."
    b. "I will plan for his ADHD to become worse after puberty and as he enters adulthood."
    c. "I will continue to bring him for assessments of growth and development independent of his ADHD."
    d. "I will seek a referral to a mental health specialist for medication management."

4. **The nurse is providing education about the decision to stop medication management for CE. Which of the following statements made by CE's mother indicates a need for further education?**

    a. "If his school performance declines, I'll call the office."
    b. "I'll start his medication back at half dose if he seems anxious."
    c. "CE will be weaned off the medication because he has been on it for so long."
    d. "I can expect that CE may have increased appetite when the medication is discontinued."

5. **The nurse understands that CE and his family should expect which of the following to be included in his treatment plan for ADHD as an adolescent? (Select all that apply.)**

    a. Parental education about assessing for risky behaviors
    b. Caution regarding obtaining driver's license
    c. Need to eat a healthy diet and limit simple sugars
    d. Potential for constipation when medication is discontinued
    e. Continuing nonpharmacological strategies if effective

See the appendix for answers to review questions.

References

American Association of Pediatrics. (2018). *Diagnosing and treating ADHD*. Retrieved from https://www .healthychildren.org/English/health-issues/conditions/adhd/Pages/Diagnosing-ADHD-in-Children -Guidelines-Information-for-Parents.aspx

Ask, H., Gustavson, K., Ystrom, E., Havdahl, K. A., Tesli, M., Askeland, R. B., & Reichborn-Kjennerud, T. (2018). Association of gestational age at birth with symptoms of attention-deficit/hyperactivity disorder in children. *JAMA Pediatrics, 172*(8), 749–756. doi:10.1001/jamapediatrics.2018.1315

Brinkman, W. B., Sucharew, H., Hartl Majcher, J., & Epstein, J. N. (2018). Predictors of medication continuity in children with ADHD. *Pediatrics, 141*(6), 1–10. doi:10.1542/peds.2017-2580

Capriotti, T. (2020). *Pathophysiology: Introductory concepts and clinical perspectives* (2nd ed.). Philadelphia, PA: F.A. Davis.

Centers for Disease Control and Prevention. (2019). *Data and statistics about ADHD*. Retrieved from https:// www.cdc.gov/ncbddd/adhd/data.html

Davidovitch, M., Koren, G., Fund, N., Shrem, M., & Porath, A. (2017). Challenges in defining the rates of ADHD diagnosis and treatment: Trends over the last decade. *BMC Pediatrics, 171*–179. doi:10.1186 /s12887-017-0971-0

Goolsby, M., & Grubbs, L. (2019). *Advanced assessment: Interpreting findings and formulating differential diagnoses (4th ed.).* Philadelphia, PA: F.A. Davis.

Greven, P., Sikirica, V., Chen, Y., Curtice, T., Makin, C., Chen, Y. J., & Curtice, T. G. (2017). Comparative treatment patterns, healthcare resource utilization and costs of atomoxetine and long-acting methylphenidate among children and adolescents with attention-deficit/hyperactivity disorder in Germany. *European Journal of Health Economics, 18*(7), 893–904. doi:10.1007/s10198-016-0836-8

Hart, K. C., Ros, R., Gonzalez, V., & Graziano, P. A. (2018). Parent perceptions of medication treatment for preschool children with ADHD. *Child Psychiatry & Human Development, 49*(1), 155–162. doi:10.1007/s10578-017-0737-9

Millenet, S., Laucht, M., Hohm, E., Jennen-Steinmetz, C., Hohmann, S., Schmidt, M. H., . . . Zohsel, K. (2018). Sex-specific trajectories of ADHD symptoms from adolescence to young adulthood. *European Child & Adolescent Psychiatry, 27*(8), 1067–1075. doi:10.1007/s00787-018-1129-9

National Institute of Mental Health. (2018). Attention deficit hyperactivity disorder. Retrieved from https://www.nimh.nih.gov/health/topics/attention-deficit-hyperactivity-disorder-adhd/index.shtml

Ramos-Olazagasti, M. A., Klein, R. G., Castellanos, F. X., & Mannuzza, S. (2018). Predicting the adult functional outcomes of boys with ADHD 33 years later. *Journal of the American Academy of Child & Adolescent Psychiatry, 57*(8), 571–582.e1. doi:10.1016/j.jaac.2018.04.015

Rashid, M. A., Lovick, S., & Llanwarne, N. R. (2018). Medication-taking experiences in attention deficit hyperactivity disorder: A systematic review. *Family Practice, 35*(2), 142–150. doi:10.1093/fampra/cmx088

Roy, A., Hechtman, L., Arnold, L. E., Swanson, J. M., Molina, B. S., Sibley, M. H., & Howard, A. L. (2017). Childhood predictors of adult functional outcomes in the multimodal treatment study of attention-deficit/hyperactivity disorder (MTA). *Journal of the American Academy of Child & Adolescent Psychiatry, 56*(8), 687–695.e7. doi:10.1016/j.jaac.2017.05.020

Shafrin, J., Shrestha, A., Chandra, A., Erder, M. H., & Sikirica, V. (2017). Evaluating matching-adjusted indirect comparisons in practice: A case study of patients with attention-deficit/hyperactivity disorder. *Health Economics, 26*(11), 1459–1466. doi:10.1002/hec.3408

Theule, J., Cheung, K., & Aberdeen, K. (2018). Children's ADHD interventions and parenting stress: A meta-analysis. *Journal of Child & Family Studies, 27*(9), 2744–2756. doi:10.1007/s10826-018-1137-x

Townsend, M. C. (2018). *Psychiatric mental health nursing: Concepts of care in evidence-based practice* (9th ed.). Philadelphia, PA: F.A. Davis.

Turvey, C., & Fortney, J. (2017). The use of telemedicine and mobile technology to promote population health and population management for psychiatric disorders. *Current Psychiatry Reports, 19*(11), 1–8. doi:10.1007/s11920-017-0844-0

Woo, T., & Robinson, M. (2020). *Pharmacotherapeutics for the advanced practice nurse prescribers* (5th ed.). Philadelphia, PA: FA Davis.

Zinnow, T., Philipp-Wiegmann, F., Rösler, M., Thome, J., Banaschewski, T., Fallgatter, A. J., . . . Sobanski, E. (2018). ESCAlate—Adaptive treatment approach for adolescents and adults with ADHD: Study protocol for a randomized controlled trial. *Trials, 19*(1). doi:10.1186/s13063-018-2665-9

Appendix: Answers to Review Questions

Chapter 1
1. C, D, E
2. C
3. A, C, E
4. D
5. B, C, D, E

Chapter 2
1. D
2. B
3. C
4. A, B, C
5. B

Chapter 3
1. A
2. B
3. C
4. A
5. A, B, C

Chapter 4
1. B
2. B
3. D
4. A, B, C, D
5. B

Chapter 5
1. A, B, E
2. D
3. B, C, E
4. A, E
5. B

Case Study 1 (Adult): Glaucoma
1. A, B, D
2. A
3. C
4. C
5. B, C

Chapter 6
1. B
2. A, C
3. B
4. A
5. A

Chapter 7
1. B
2. A, B, C, D
3. A, B, C, D
4. A
5. A

Chapter 8
1. A, C
2. A, B, C, D
3. A
4. A, B, C, D
5. A, B, C, D

Chapter 9
1. B
2. A, B, C, D
3. A, B, C, D
4. A
5. A

Case Study 2 (Maternity): Vaginal Bleeding

1. C
2. A, B, C, D
3. A, B, C, D
4. A
5. B, C, D

Chapter 10

1. D
2. D
3. B
4. A
5. A

Chapter 11

1. B
2. C
3. B
4. A
5. A

Chapter 12

1. B
2. B
3. B
4. A
5. A

Chapter 13

1. A, B, C, D
2. C
3. B
4. A, B, C, D
5. A

Case Study 3 (Newborn): Nutrition

1. B, C
2. A
3. A, B
4. A
5. D

Chapter 14

1. B, C, D
2. A
3. C, E
4. B
5. A, C, D, E

Chapter 15

1. B, D
2. C
3. A, E
4. B
5. A, D, E

Chapter 16

1. A, E
2. D
3. A
4. A
5. B
6. A, B, C, D, E

Chapter 17

1. A, C, E
2. A, C, D
3. C
4. A, B
5. B
6. A, B, C, D, E

Chapter 18

1. B
2. A, D, E
3. B
4. D
5. B

Case Study 4 (Pediatrics): Acute Lymphoblastic Leukemia

1. A, B, D, E
2. A
3. C
4. C
5. A, B, C, E

Chapter 19

1. A, B
2. C
3. D
4. B
5. B

Chapter 20

1. A, C, E
2. C
3. A, B, C, D, E
4. A
5. A, B

Chapter 21

1. D
2. B
3. C
4. A, B, D
5. D

Chapter 22

1. C
2. B
3. C
4. B
5. A, B

Chapter 23

1. B
2. A, D, E
3. B
4. D
5. B

Case Study 5 (Geriatrics): Osteoporosis

1. A, B, D
2. B
3. C
4. B
5. D

Chapter 24

1. D
2. B
3. C
4. B
5. A, D

Chapter 25

1. D
2. C
3. B
4. A, B, D
5. D

Chapter 26

1. D
2. B
3. D
4. A, B, D
5. B

Chapter 27

1. D
2. A, B, E
3. B
4. A, B, D
5. B

Case Study 6 (Mental Health): Attention Deficit-Hyperactivity Disorder (ADHD)

1. A, B, E
2. A
3. C
4. B
5. A, B, C, E

Index

Note: Page numbers followed by *f* refer to figures; page numbers followed by *t* refer to tables; page numbers followed by *b* refer to boxes.